ONCOLOGY NURSING SECRETS

Second Edition

ONCOLOGY NURSING SECRETS

Second Edition

ROSE A. GATES, RN, MSN, CNS/NP

Oncology Clinical Nurse Specialist/Nurse Practitioner
The Oncology Clinic, P.C.
Colorado Springs, Colorado

REGINA M. FINK, RN, PhD, AOCN

Research Nurse Scientist
University of Colorado Hospital
Denver, Colorado

HANLEY & BELFUS, INC./Philadelphia

Publisher: HANLEY & BELFUS, INC.
                    Medical Publishers
                    210 South 13th Street
                    Philadelphia, PA 19107
                    (215) 546-7293; 800-962-1892
                    FAX (215) 790-9330
                    Web site: http://www.hanleyandbelfus.com

Note *to the reader*: Although the information in this book has been carefully reviewed for correctness of dosage and indications, neither the authors nor the editors nor the publisher can accept any legal responsibility for any errors or omissions that may be made. Neither the publisher nor the editors make any warranty, expressed or implied, with respect to the material contained herein. Experimental compounds and off-label uses of approved products are discussed. Before prescribing any drug, the reader must review the manufacturer's current product information (package inserts) for accepted indications, absolute dosage recommendations, and other information pertinent to the safe and effective use of the product described. This is especially important when drugs are given in combination or as an adjunct to other forms of therapy.

Library of Congress Cataloging-in-Publication Data

Oncology nursing secrets / edited by Rose A. Gates, Regina M. Fink.—2nd ed.
      p. ; cm.—(The Secrets Series®)
    Includes bibliographical references and index.
    ISBN 1-56053-477-X (alk. paper)
      1. Cancer—Nursing—Miscellanea. I. Gates, Rose A., 1952– II. Fink, Regina M., 1955–
    [DNLM: 1. Neoplasms—nursing—Examination Questions. 2. Oncologic
  Nursing—methods—Examination Questions. WY 18.2 O58 2001]
    RC266.O57 2001
    610.73'698—dc21
                                                                          2001024146

ONCOLOGY NURSING SECRETS, 2nd edition   ISBN 1-56053-477-X

Last digit is the print number: 9   8   7   6   5   4   3   2   1

CONTENTS

VII. CARING FOR THE PERSON WITH CANCER

CONTRIBUTORS

Susan Adnan-Koch, RN, MSN, OCN
Clinical Nurse Specialist, Case Management/Nursing, University of Colorado Hospital, Denver, Colorado

Debra Adornetto, RN, MS
Nursing Director, Bone Marrow Transplant, and Resource Office, University of Colorado Hospital, Denver, Colorado

Tauseef Ahmed, MD
Professor of Medicine, Department of Oncology/Hematology, New York Medical College, Valhalla, New York

Lowell Anderson-Reitz, RN, MS, ANP, AOCN
Bone Marrow Transplant Nurse Practitioner, Rocky Mountain Cancer Center, Denver, Colorado

Robert A. Avery, MD, FACP
Chief, Hematology/Oncology Service, Landstuhl Regional Medical Center, Landstuhl, Germany

Carolyn Becker, RN, OCN
Clinical Nurse Educator, Bone Marrow Transplant, University of Colorado Hospital, Denver, Colorado

Maude Becker, RN, BSN, OCN
Cutaneous Oncology, Oncology Clinical Nurse, University of Colorado Cancer Center, University of Colorado Hospital, Denver Colorado

Jeffrey L. Berenberg, MD, COL, MC
Clinical Associate Professor, and Chief, Division of Medical Oncology, John A. Burns School of Medicine, University of Hawaii; Associate Researcher, Cancer Research Center of Hawaii; Chief, Hematology-Oncology Service, Tripler Army Medical Center, Honolulu, Hawaii

Mona Bernaiche Bedell, RN, BSN, MSPH
Nurse Epidemiologist, Denver Public Health Department, Denver, Colorado

Rocky Billups, RN
Patient Care Director, Blood and Marrow Transplant/Critical Care, Presbyterian/St. Luke's Medical Center, Denver; Clinical Nurse Coordinator, Rocky Mountain Blood and Marrow Transplant Program, Denver, Colorado

Carol Blendowski, RN, BS, OCN
Nurse Clinician, Department of Oncology, Rush Cancer Institute, Rush Presbyterian St. Luke's Medical Center, Chicago, Illinois

Deborah A. Boyle, RN, MSN, AOCN, FAAN
Oncology Clinical Nurse Specialist, Inova Fairfax Cancer Center, Falls Church, Virginia

Jane Braaten, RN, MS, CNS
Cardiovascular Clinical Nurse Specialist, Centura Porter Adventist Hospital, Denver, Colorado

Harri Brackett, RN, BSN, OCN
Clinical Nurse Educator–Oncology, University of Colorado Hospital, Denver, Colorado

Carol Brueggen, MS, RN, AOCN, CNS-BC
Oncology Clinical Nurse Specialist, Department of Nursing, Mayo Clinic–St. Marys Hospital, Rochester, Minnesota

Mark W. Brunvand, MD
Director of Unrelated Transplants, Rocky Mountain Blood and Marrow Transplant Program, Denver, Colorado

Dawn Camp-Sorrell, MSN, FNP, AOCN
Oncology Nurse Practitioner, Central Alabama Hematology-Oncology Association, Alabaster, Alabama

Muhammad S. Choudhry, MD
Professor, Department of Urology, New York Medical College, Valhalla, New York

Mary Jo Cleaveland, RN, MS
Private Practice, Littleton, Colorado

Allen Cohn, MD
Rocky Mountain Cancer Center, Denver, Colorado

Susanne K. Cook, RN, BSN, OCN
Oncology Clinical Nurse, University of Colorado Cancer Center, University of Colorado Hospital, Denver, Colorado

Tonya P. Cox, RN, BSN, OCN
Clinical Nurse Coordinator/Staff Educator, Rocky Mountain Blood and Marrow Transplant Program, Denver, Colorado

Frances Crighton, RN, PhDc
Coordinator, Genitourinary Oncology, University of Colorado Cancer Center, University of Colorado Hospital, Denver, Colorado

Barbara I. Damron, PhD, RN
Educational Psychologist, St. Vincent's Hospital, Santa Fe, New Mexico

Susan A. Davidson, MD
Associate Professor and Director, Gynecologic Oncology, Department of Obstetrics/Gynecology, University of Colorado Health Sciences Center, Denver, Colorado

Georgia M. Decker, MS, RN, CS-ANP, AOCN
Advanced Practice Nurse, Integrative Care, NP, PC, Albany, New York

Deborah A. DeVine, RN, MS, AOCN, CRNI
Practice Administrator, Rocky Mountain Cancer Center, Littleton, Colorado

Ann Marie Dose, MS, RN, AOCN, CNS-BC
Clinical Nurse Specialist, Department of Nursing, Mayo Clinic–Rochester Methodist Hospital, Rochester, Minnesota

Barbara Eldridge, RD, LD
Clinical Research Associate, Department of Radiation Oncology, University of Colorado Cancer Center, Denver, Colorado

Lynn Ellis, RN, MEd, OCN
Virginia Oncology Associates, Newport News, Virginia

Constance Engelking, RN, MS, OCN
Adjunct Instructor of Medicine, Department of Medicine/Division Oncology and Hematology, New York Medical College, Valhalla, New York

Lynn Erdman, RN, MN, OCN
Consulting Associate, Duke University Medical Center School of Nursing, Durham; Executive Director, George Batte Cancer Center, NorthEast Medical Center, Concord, North Carolina

David Faragher, MD
Rocky Mountain Cancer Center, Denver, Colorado

Kyle Fink, MD
Rocky Mountain Cancer Center, Denver, Colorado

Regina M. Fink, RN, PhD, AOCN
Research Nurse Scientist, University of Colorado Hospital, Denver, Colorado

Mary T. Garcia, RN, MPH, CCRA
Head Clinical Research Associate, Southwest Oncology Group, Clinical Investigations Core, Cancer Center, University of Colorado Health Sciences Center, Denver, Colorado

Robert H. Gates, MD, FACP
Chief, Department of Medicine, Brooke Army Medical Center, San Antonio, Texas

Rose A. Gates, RN, MSN, CNS/NP
Oncology Clinical Nurse Specialist/Nurse Practitioner, The Oncology Clinic, P.C., Colorado Springs, Colorado

Colleen Gill, MS, RD
Clinical Dietitian, Oncology and Bone Marrow Transplant, University of Colorado Hospital, University of Colorado Health Sciences Center, Denver, Colorado

Rene Gonzalez, MD
Associate Professor of Medicine, Division of Medical Oncology, University of Colorado Health Sciences Center, Denver, Colorado

Michelle Goodman, RN, MS
Assistant Professor, Section of Medical Oncology, Rush Cancer Institute, Rush Presbyterian St. Luke's Medical Center, Chicago, Illinois

Elder Granger, MD, COL
Commander, Landstuhl Regional Medical Center, Hematology-Oncology Service, Landstuhl Regional Medical Center, Landstuhl, Germany

Julie Griffie, RN, MSN, CS, AOCN, CHPN
Clinical Nurse Specialist, Palliative Care, Medical College of Wisconsin, Milwaukee, Wisconsin

Irene Stewart Haapoja, RN, MS
Oncology Clinical Nurse Specialist, Section of Medical Oncology, Rush Cancer Institute, Rush Presbyterian St. Luke's Medical Center, Chicago, Illinois

Lenore L. Harris, RN, MSN, AOCN
Head and Neck Advanced Practice Nurse, Oak Park, Illinois

Pamela J. Haylock, RN, MA
Oncology Consultant, Medina, Texas

Laura J. Hilderley, RN, MS
Clinical Nurse Specialist, Radiation Oncology (Retired)

Ioana Hinshaw, MD
Rocky Mountain Cancer Center, Denver, Colorado

Brenda M. Hiromoto, RN, MS, CETN, OCN
Oncology Coordinator, Oncology Clinic, Kaiser Permanente Hawaii, Honolulu, Hawaii

Andrea Iannucci, PharmD, BCOP
Oncology Clinical Pharmacy Specialist/Adjunct Assistant Professor, School of Pharmacy, University of Colorado Health Sciences Center, Denver, Colorado

Joanne Itano, RN, PhD, OCN
Associate Professor, Department of Nursing, University of Hawaii at Manoa, Honolulu, Hawaii

R. Lee Jennings, MD
Assistant Clinical Professor of Surgery, University of Colorado Health Sciences Center, Denver, Colorado

Gari Jensen, RN, BSN, OCN
Charge Nurse, Oncology Unit, University of Colorado Hospital, Denver, Colorado

Patrick H. Judson, MD
Great Plains Regional Medical Center, North Platte, Nebraska

Leigh K. Kaszyk, RN, MS
Nurse Consultant, Littleton, Colorado

Matthew Kemper, PharmD
Clinical Pharmacy Specialist, Rush University, Rush Presbyterian St. Luke's Medical Center, Chicago, Illinois

Linda U. Krebs, RN, PhD, AOCN
Assistant Professor, School of Nursing, University of Colorado Health Sciences Center, Denver, Colorado

Scott Kruger, MD
Virginia Oncology Associates, Newport News, Virginia

Susan A. Leigh, BSN, RN
Cancer Survivorship Consultant, Tucson, Arizona

Kevin O. Lillehei, MD
Professor, Department of Neurosurgery, University of Colorado Health Sciences Center, Denver, Colorado

Kelly Mack, RN, MSN, AOCN, NP-C
Nurse Practitioner, Rocky Mountain Cancer Center, Denver, Colorado

Heidi Ann Mahay, PharmD
Oncology Pharmacist, Good Samaritan Hospital, Phoenix, Arizona

Jeffrey V. Matous, MD
Rocky Mountain Blood and Marrow Transplant Program, Assistant Clinical Professor of Medicine, Division of Medical Oncology, University of Colorado Health Sciences Center, Denver, Colorado

Marcia L. Maxwell, RN, BSN, CCRN
Critical Care Educator, ACLS Course Director, Presbyterian St. Luke's Medical Center, Denver Colorado

Janelle G. McCallum-Orozco, RN, BSN, MSM
Vice President, Home and Nursing Home Services, Hospice of Metro Denver, Denver, Colorado

Michael T. McDermott, MD
Professor of Medicine, Division of Endocrinology, Diabetes and Metabolism, University of Colorado Health Sciences Center, Denver, Colorado

Beth E. Mechling, RN, MS, AOCN, APN
Advance Practice Nurse III and Nursing Manager for Bone Marrow Transplant, Rocky Mountain Blood and Marrow Transplant Program, Denver, Colorado

Susan Kay Morgan, MD
Hematology/Oncology Service, Tripler Army Medical Center, Honolulu, Hawaii

Sandra Muchka, RN, MS, CS, CHPN
Clinical Nurse Specialist, Palliative Care, Medical College of Wisconsin, Milwaukee, Wisconsin

Jamie S. Myers, RN, MN, AOCN
Oncology Clinical Nurse Specialist and Head Nurse, Research Medical Center, Kansas City, Missouri

Lillian M. Nail, PhD, RN, FAAN
Dr. May E. Rawlinson Endowed Professor and Senior Scientist, School of Nursing, Oregon Health Sciences University, Portland, Oregon

Diane K. Nakagaki, RN, BSN, ET, OCN
Registered Nurse Level III, Oncology Clinic, Kaiser Permanente Medical Center, Honolulu, Hawaii

Patrice Y. Neese, MSN, RN, CS, ANP
Nurse Practitioner, Breast and Melanoma Teams, Department of Surgery, University of Virginia, Charlottesville, Virginia

Paula Nelson-Marten, RN, PhD, AOCN
Associate Professor, Oncology Nursing, School of Nursing, University of Colorado Health Sciences Center, Denver, Colorado

Patricia Winck Nishimoto, RN, BSN, MPH, DNS
Oncology Clinical Nurse Specialist, Department of Hematology/Oncology, Tripler Army Medical Center, Honolulu, Hawaii

Patricia Novak-Smith, RN, MS, AOCN
Clinical Nurse Manager, Trauma, Oncology, and Post-Surgery, Centura St. Anthony Central Hospital, Denver, Colorado

Cindy L. O'Bryant, PharmD
Assistant Professor, Department of Pharmacy Practice, School of Pharmacy, University of Colorado Health Sciences Center, Denver, Colorado

Dev Paul, DO, PhD
Rocky Mountain Cancer Center, Denver, Colorado

Kelly Pendergrass, MD
Clinical Professor of Medicine, and Chief, Section of Oncology, University of Missouri at Kansas City, Kansas City, Missouri

Jennifer Petersen, RN, MS
Clinical Nurse Specialist, Department of Oncology, Rush Cancer Institute, Rush Presbyterian St. Luke's Medical Center, Chicago, Illinois

Cathy E. Pickett, RN, BSN
Oncology Clinical Nurse, Conway, Arkansas

Kim Pollmiller, RN, MS, CNRN
Clinical Nurse Specialist, Department of Neurosurgery, University of Colorado Health Sciences Center, Denver, Colorado

Brenda K. Ronk, RN, MS
Oncology Clinical Nurse Specialist, Grasso, Cowall, and Martin, MD, PA, Salisbury, Maryland

Pamela A. Rossé, RN, MS, CRA
Project Manager, Clinical Investigations Core, Cancer Center, University of Colorado Health Sciences Center, Denver, Colorado

Tina Russell, RN, OCN
Oncology Clinical Nurse, University of Colorado Cancer Center, University of Colorado Hospital, Denver, Colorado

Deborah M. Rust, RN, MSN, CRNP, AOCN
Nurse Consultant, Schering Corporation, and Instructor, School of Nursing, University of Pittsburgh, Pittsburgh, Pennsylvania

Diana Ruzicka, RN, MSN, AOCN, CNS
Assistant Chief Nurse, McDonald Army Community Hospital, Fort Eustis, Virginia

Carmel Sauerland, RN, MSN, AOCN
Oncology Clinical Nurse Specialist, Zalmen A. Arlin Cancer Institute, Westchester Medical Center, Hawthorne, New York

Lisa Schulmeister, RN, MN, CS, OCN
Oncology Nursing Consultant, New Orleans, Louisiana

Paul Seligman, MD
Professor of Medicine, Division of Hematology/Oncology, University of Colorado Health Sciences Center, Denver, Colorado

Jeffrey Gordon Shaw, MS
Genetic Counselor, Penrose Hospital and St. Mary Corwin Hospital, Colorado Springs, Colorado

Jean K. Smith, RN, MS, OCN
Lymphedema Case Manager, Penrose Cancer Center of Centura Health, Colorado Springs, Colorado

Karen J. Stanley, RN, MSN, AOCN
Nursing Consultant, Oncology Issues, Claremont, California

Julie R. Swaney, MDiv
Coordinator, Department of Pastoral Care, University of Colorado Hospital, Denver, Colorado

Daniel T. Tell, DO, FACP
Oncology Clinic, P.C., Colorado Springs, Colorado

Debra K. Thaler-DeMers, BSN, RN, OCN, PHN
President, Cancer ACCESS: Advocacy, Counseling, Clinical Education and Survivorship Skills, San Jose, California

Marion Tolch, RN, BSN, CWOCN
Ostomy, Skin, and Wound Care Specialist/Case Manager, University of Colorado Hospital, Denver, Colorado

Charlene A. Trouillot, RN, MS, ANP, OCN
Adult Nurse Practitioner, University of Colorado Cancer Center, University of Colorado Hospital, Denver, Colorado

Leslie Tuchmann, RN, MS, HNC
Oncology Clinical Nurse Specialist, Healing Arts Practitioner and Educator, Honolulu, Hawaii

Carol S. Viele, RN, MS
Assistant Clinical Professor, Department of Physiological Nursing, University of California–San Francisco, San Francisco, California

Michael R. Watters, MD, FAAN
Professor of Medicine, Division of Neurology, University of Hawaii, John A. Burns School of Medicine, Honolulu, Hawaii

Rita Wickham, PhD, RN, AOCN
Associate Professor, College of Nursing, Rush University, Chicago, Illinois

Anne Zobec, MS, RN, CS, ANP, AOCN
Oncology Clinical Nurse Specialist, Penrose Cancer Center, Penrose Hospital, Colorado Springs, Colorado

PREFACE

With over 45 years of combined oncology nursing experience, we were motivated to create this book in order to share knowledge that we wished had been at our fingertips when we began our careers. We have often heard new oncology staff nurses say: "I don't know enough to even ask a question"; "I don't know where to begin looking for the answers"; "I don't have time to look up something in a book that weighs 50 pounds"; or "I'm embarrassed to ask a question." The Secrets Series® is an ideal format for presenting questions and answers in a convenient, readable, and concise manner. This new second edition of *Oncology Nursing Secrets* includes questions and answers appropriate for novices as well as advanced practitioners. As Socrates exemplified, the best way to teach is to ask questions.

Because oncology nursing derives "secrets" from many disciplines, we made full use of our collaborative ties with physicians and other care providers. The authors range from staff nurses to oncologists to nurse academicians, all of whom are actively contributing to the care of oncology patients. This book is not meant to be a complete reference or comprehensive textbook. Rather it is intended to focus on commonly asked questions and to stimulate further discussion and research. The reader is encouraged to make full use of the excellent oncology textbooks and references cited throughout the book. With so many facts to present, it is impossible to express the complex human dimensions and love that permeate every aspect of oncology nursing care. We hope that you will discover those secrets for yourself. We invite you to share your secrets and to always ask questions. May you find wisdom and compassion in the answers.

We are grateful to all our patients and their families, who have been our best teachers. They have taught us to make the most of each day and to live even as we are dying. We would like to express our appreciation to all the contributors for their time and work. We also acknowledge the oncologists, nurses, pharmacists, and other health care providers who have been our partners, as well as our teachers. As before, we would like to thank Linda Belfus and her staff for their editorial assistance, support, and willingness to believe in *Oncology Nursing Secrets*.

We hope that this book will continue to provide information and secrets to enhance nursing care and symptom management for patients with cancer.

Rose A. Gates, RN, MSN, CNS/NP
Regina M. Fink, RN, PhD, AOCN

DEDICATION

To our husbands, Rob and Kyle, who participate in the ultimate collaboration by staying married to us, and to our children, Brandon, Melissa, and Brian, for their gifts of love and understanding.

I. General Overview of Cancer

1. BIOLOGY OF CANCER

Jeffrey Shaw, MS

My father always told me a smart person is not afraid to say "I don't know" but then actively seeks the answer.

1. What are the chances of getting cancer?

Approximately one of three Americans will develop a malignancy at some time in their lives, and one in four deaths in the U.S. is due to cancer. Cancer is second to heart disease as the most common cause of death in the U.S. In 2001, there were an estimated 1,268,000 new cases of invasive cancer in the U.S. and 553,400 deaths due to cancer (1,516 people/day).

2. How are cancer cells different from normal cells?

Normal cells (1) reproduce in an organized, controlled, and orderly manner, (2) do not divide when space or nutrients are inadequate, (3) do not spread into parts of the body where they do not belong, (4) become fully differentiated to perform a specific task, and (5) have limited potential and lose their ability to replicate, eventually dying.

The first rule for cancer cells is that they follow no rules; cancer is complete anarchy. The basic features of malignant cancer cells are summarized below:

1. **Unregulated cell growth.** Cancer cells have uncontrolled continual growth and continue to multiply even when space and nutrients are lacking.

2. **Ability to invade other tissues.** Cancer cells lack contact inhibition; they are not inhibited in either growth or movement by contact with other cells. Many metastatic cancer cells have altered surface enzymes and can secrete enzymes that dissolve their way through other cells.

3. **Poor cellular differentiation.** Well-differentiated cancer cells are more like the normal cells of the tissues in which they originate. Many cancer cells resemble normal undifferentiated cells, retaining the ability to divide. Undifferentiated (anaplastic) cancer cells are disorganized and exhibit few features of the normal tissue, sometimes to the point that their site of origin cannot be determined. They also may express antigens (e.g., alpha-fetoprotein, CA-125) not normally expressed by the parent cell.

4. **Ability to initiate new growth at distant sites.** Lack of contact inhibition and lack of adhesiveness allow cancer cells to grow and spread without the restraint exhibited by normal cells.

5. **Ability to escape detection and destruction by the immune system.** Carcinogenesis and the metastatic potential of tumor cells may be a balance between the effectiveness of an individual's immunosurveillance and the ability of the tumor cells to evade destruction.

3. How can the concepts that underlie cancer cells be explained to patients?

Patients can be told that cancer cells have lost the ability to control their own growth and behavior. They do not recognize the "personal space" of neighboring cells in their tissue of origin and see no problem in spreading to other tissues of the body. They are selfish and continue to divide and multiply even when there is a lack of adequate food or space to support them.

4. Explain carcinogenesis. In other words, how do cancers get started?

Cancer is caused by mutations in a variety of genes responsible for controlling the growth of cells either directly (gatekeeper genes) or indirectly (caretaker genes). People with a strong

1

family history of cancer often say that cancer is "genetic" in their family when probably they mean that the family has an inherited predisposition for cancer. All cancer is "genetic" because cancer is the uncontrolled division of a cell, and genes control cell division. Therefore, at the molecular level, all cancer is due to mutations (a change in the genetic code) in genes. Carcinogens cause these mutations.

5. What is a carcinogen?

A carcinogen is any substance, situation, or exposure that can damage genetic material (DNA). The hundreds of known carcinogens include internal factors created in the body by metabolic processes (e.g., free radicals, hormones), viruses (e.g., hepatitis B, human papillomavirus), chemicals (e.g., tobacco, alcohol, industrial asbestos), and radiation (e.g., diagnostic radiation, ultraviolet light).

6. What genes are involved in cancer?

Hundreds of identified genes either directly or indirectly participate in a cell's ability to control growth. With the current success of the human genome project (the mapping of the complete human genetic code), the list of genes involved in the control of a cell's growth will increase. Currently these genes are divided into the following four major categories: oncogenes, tumor suppressor genes, mismatch repair genes, and "housekeeping" genes. Probably they will undergo substantial reclassification over the next several years.

7. Define oncogene.

Oncogenes originate from a mutation in normal genes called **proto-oncogenes**. Proto-oncogenes fall into four main classes with different functions, but all of them are involved with signaling the cell that it is time to divide. This process of normal cell replication is used to replace damaged or dying cells. **Activation** is the term used to describe a mutation in a proto-oncogene that transforms it to an oncogene. These mutations cause a gain of function, pushing the cell to divide uncontrollably. Therefore, the mutation of one proto-oncogene of a particular pair (most genes occur in identical pairs, one from the mother and one from the father) can lead to the initiation of cancer. Examples of oncogenes include *abl, myc, ras*, and *ret*.

8. What are tumor suppressor genes?

Currently tumor suppressor genes are lumped into one category. They probably have a significant number of different functions and can be considered the opposite of oncogenes. Tumor suppressor genes are growth-suppressing and play an important role in the regulation of cell growth, either directly or indirectly. One functional copy of a particular tumor suppressor gene (either paternal or maternal) appears to be sufficient to control cell growth. Loss of function of both genes can lead to unregulated cell growth. Examples of tumor suppressor genes include *BRCA1, BRCA2, APC*, and *WT1*.

9. Explain the function of mismatch repair genes.

Every time a cell replicates itself into two daughter cells, all 3 billion letters of genetic code need to be duplicated exactly—a daunting task. Needless to say, errors are made. Mismatch repair genes function as "spell-checkers" after DNA replication is complete. If both pairs of a mismatch repair gene have mutated, resulting in loss of function, the cell can build up mutations, eventually affecting proto-oncogenes, tumor suppressor genes, and others involved with cell growth regulation. Examples of mismatch repair genes include *MLH1* and *MSH2*.

10. What are housekeeping genes?

This category is difficult to define because there are probably hundreds of different housekeeping genes, and researchers are just beginning to identify their existence and function. In general, housekeeping genes work to keep the cell clean and functional. For example, housekeeping genes (1) break down the carcinogens in tobacco products, (2) regulate estrogen in the cell, and

(3) protect against viral activation of cancer in the cervix. Probably they do not participate directly in cell growth regulation. Instead, their function seems to be directed toward protection of the cell from carcinogenic invaders or processes.

11. List the four stages of cancer cell growth.

Initiation, promotion, progression, and metastasis.

12. Describe the initiation stage.

The initiation stage is the irreversible mutation of a gene that leads to malignant transformation. Although the cell appears somewhat abnormal, it is still able to carry out its original functions. The mutation must not impair the cell's ability to replicate, or the cell will die.

13. What is the promotion stage?

To become malignant, the cell must enter the promotion stage. Usually there is a latency period between initiation and promotion, the length of which depends on many factors. The promoting agent does not act on the DNA but instead stimulates the growth and division of a cell. Promoting elements have a threshold effect, a minimal dose that is required before they stimulate the growth of the cancer cell. Promoting agents may be a chemical carcinogen, endogenous hormones, ultraviolet light, or other factors.

14. What is the progression stage?

Progression refers to a series of changes that lead to the characteristics of an undifferentiated cell. The normal cell is transformed into a cell with malignant potential and has the characteristics and abilities listed in question 2. Continued mutations in the cell lead to altered appearance, function, and growth rate.

15. How does metastasis occur?

Usually a subpopulation of cells within the heterogeneous tumor has the properties needed to spread to other organs in the body.

16. Explain the concept of tumor doubling times.

Tumor doubling time is the time required for the tumor to double in size. It varies from hours to months, according to the type of cancer (primary and metastatic). It may take years for a tumor to double 20 times.

17. Why is it so difficult to detect cancer?

Once the cancer goes through about 30 doublings, it has reached roughly the size of a marble (about 1 cm in diameter). A tumor of this size contains approximately one billion cancer cells. This is about the earliest point at which screening x-ray studies can detect developing cancers. At this stage the cancer needs to go through only about ten more doublings to reach one trillion cells, which is usually the number that leads to death. Thus, much of the lifespan of the cancer is "silent" and takes place before the cancer is large enough to be detected. (See figure at top of following page.)

18. Explain tumor heterogeneity. Why is it important?

Tumor heterogeneity refers to the subpopulations of biologically diverse cancer cells in tumors. A key point is that not all of the cells that make up a malignant tumor are the same. A tumor mass may contain multiple clones with different chromosomal numbers and different characteristics. In addition, the genetic make-up of these cells can be quite different. Therefore, some cells within a malignant tumor may be sensitive to one chemotherapy drug, whereas other cells are resistant (hence the rationale for combination chemotherapy). Some cells are growing, whereas others are dormant and emerge years later. This lack of uniformity makes it difficult to eradicate every cell in treating cancers.

Growth Curve for Cancers (either Primary or Metastatic Tumor Masses)
and the Effect of Surgery, Radiation, or Chemotherapy

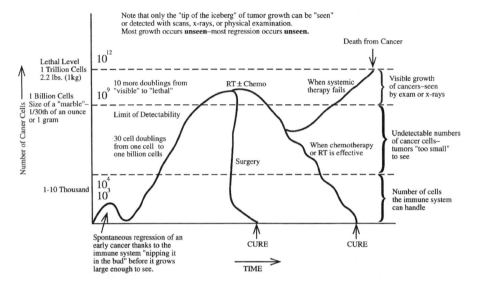

Growth curve for cancers. (Adapted from DeVita VT, et al: Principles of chemotherapy. In DeVita VT, et al (eds): Cancer: Principles and Practice of Oncology. Philadelphia, Lippincott Williams & Williams, 1982, p 149.)

19. How do cancer cells invade tissues and metastasize to different sites?

The most unique characteristic of malignant cells that results in morbidity and mortality is their capability to invade tissues and to metastasize to other sites. The ability to metastasize requires multiple steps: (1) invasion of adjacent tissues through basement membranes, (2) entrance into nearby vessels (lymph or blood), (3) invasion of the immune system, (4) reentrance into distant tissues, and (5) implantation of malignant cell in new tissue.

Invasive tumor cells secrete enzymes that degrade basement membranes, which normally bar access to adjacent tissues. After access to adjacent tissue, malignant cells erode vessel walls and circulate as individual cells or small clumps of tumor cells (tumor embolus). These tumor cells may be coated by fibrin or circulate in clumps of platelets, thereby escaping the immune cells in the blood. This process is relatively inefficient, because only about 0.1% of tumor cells that enter the blood system survive more than 24 hours.

20. What is homing?

It is not known why tumor cells of different malignancies prefer to metastasize to specific organs in a process called homing. In some cases, this process is simply a result of anatomic blood circulation—as in the spread of colon cancer to the liver via the portal venous circulation. In other cases, tumor cells home to specific target organs as a result of specific chemical signals released by certain cells. Specific receptors have been identified on the surface of certain circulating tumor cells that recognize sites on endothelial cells of specific organs.

21. Define angiogenesis.

For tumor cells ultimately to develop into organ metastasis, they must develop their own blood supply—in a process called angiogenesis. The tumor cells and neighboring normal cells synthesize and secrete angiogenic molecules that produce capillary networks for tumors at least 1–2 mm in size.

22. How do you explain to a patient that cancer has spread to another site?

Patients and families frequently misunderstand the concept of cancer spreading to another site. For example, if breast cancer spreads to the bone, the patient may believe that she has a new bone cancer. It is important to explain to the patient that the bone cancer is still breast cancer that has spread to the bone (metastasized). Bone metastases from breast cancer are breast cancer cells that have spread through the body to another site. This process can occur long before the original tumor mass in the breast is large enough to be palpated on physical examination or detected on screening mammograms. When a surgeon tells the patient he/she "got it all" and that the "margins were clear," the surgeon means that all cancer visible to the eye and microscope has been removed. Currently there are no good tests to detect micrometastases, which are very small groups of cancer cells growing in a location away from the primary site.

23. What terms are used to describe the three patterns of cancer occurrence?

Sporadic, inherited, and familial cancer.

24. Describe the sporadic pattern of occurrence.

Most cancer occurs in a sporadic pattern. The patient has no unusual family history of cancer, which appears to come from nowhere. The tumor suppressor, mismatch repair, and other important genes inherited from the parents are fully functional. Cancer is caused primarily from exposure to carcinogens. Sporadic cancers tend to occur later in life (after the age of 50), when many mutations are likely to have accumulated and the immune system is not as proficient in protecting against cancer cells. However, many sporadic cancers occur in childhood or at a much younger age (e.g., testicular cancer).

25. What is meant by familial predisposition?

The patient has inherited several housekeeping genes that are functional but not doing a good job of protecting the patient from carcinogens. Affected families usually have an excess of cancer cases but not necessarily at a young age. The cancer in the family does not have to be genetically related (e.g., the tumor suppressor genes that control the growth of cervical cells are different from those that control breast cells). Familial predispositions are multifactorial conditions. In other words, the patient must inherit several suboptimal housekeeping genes *and* be exposed to specific carcinogens. As a result, familial predispositions tend to dilute over each generation because it is difficult to pass down several specific genes, and families do not tend to share the same environmental exposures from generation to generation. Therefore, familial predispositions tend to confer a small-to-moderate increase in risk for cancer.

26. Define inherited cancer predisposition.

The patient has inherited a faulty tumor suppressor, oncogene, or mismatch repair gene from either parent. Because the mutated (nonfunctional) gene was present in the egg or sperm, it is present in every cell of the body. An environmental insult is still necessary to mutate the other gene of the pair and initiate cancer. Because of the inherited mutation, there is a significant increase in risk for malignancy, usually in specific organs. The cancer often has an early onset, and the risk for second primary tumors is increased significantly. Inherited cancer predispositions do not dilute. Either a child inherits the gene from a parent and has a significantly increased risk for cancer, or the child does not inherit the gene and is not at increased risk (based on the family history of cancer).

27. How common is inherited cancer predisposition?

There are hundreds of known inherited cancer syndromes, but luckily most are quite rare. For example, approximately 5–10% of all breast cancer is due to an inherited predisposition, 10–15% is due to familial predisposition, and the remaining 75–80% is sporadic. If a patient, family, or medical provider is concerned about a particular family history of cancer, a referral should be made to a health care professional specifically trained to evaluate family histories of cancer (e.g., genetic counselors).

28. What does the future hold in terms of understanding the biology of cancer?

Over the next decade, the explosion of information about the basic processes of cancer derived from genetic research will continue to increase. It is an exciting time as we see this new wealth of genetic information applied to cancer screening, diagnosis, and treatment.

ACKNOWLEDGMENT

The author wishes to acknowledge the contributions of Richard Callahan, MD, and David Faragher, MD, to the Biology of Cancer chapter in the first edition.

REFERENCES

 1. Appelbaum JW: The role of the immune system in the pathogenesis of cancer. Semin Oncol Nurs 8:51–62, 1992.
 2. Devita VT, et al: Principles of chemotherapy. In DeVita VT, et al (eds): Cancer: Principles and Practice of Oncology. Philadelphia, Lippincott Williams & Williams, 1982.
 3. Ellerhorst-Ryan JM: The nature of cancer. In Varricchio C (ed): A Cancer Source Book for Nurses, 7th ed. London, Jones & Bartlett, 1997, pp 27–34.
 4. Greenlee RT, Hill-Harmon MB, Murray T, Thun M: Cancer statistics 2001. CA Cancer J Clin 50:15–36, 2001.
 5. Kelly PT. Assess Your True Risk of Breast Cancer. New York, Owl Books, 2000.
 6. Lind J: Tumor cell growth and cell kinetics. Semin Oncol Nurs 8:3–9, 1992.
 7. Lydon J: Metastasis. Part I: Biology and prevention. In Hubbard SM, Goodman M, Knobf MT (eds): Oncology Nursing. Philadelphia, Lippincott-Raven Publishers, 1995, pp 1–13.
 8. Offit K: Clinical Cancer Genetics: Risk Counseling and Management. New York, Wiley-Liss, 1998.
 9. Reilly JA: The biology of metastasis: Basic science of oncology. Contemp Oncol 11:32–46, 1993.
10. Schneider KA: Counseling About Cancer: Strategies for Genetic Counselors. Dennisport, MA, NSGC, Inc., 1995.

2. CANCER PREVENTION AND DETECTION

Mona Bernaiche Bedell, RN, BSN, MSPH

1. Which risk factors for cancer can be modified?

Over 70% of all cancers are associated with lifestyle choices. Adopting a healthy lifestyle and changing risky personal habits and behaviors can reduce the risk for cancer. Examples include elimination of both smoking and chewing tobacco, modification of alcohol intake, limiting exposure to ultraviolet light, adoption of sexual practices that limit exposure to sexually transmitted viruses (e.g., abstinence, limited number of sexual partners, use of condoms), stress reduction, eating foods high in fiber and low in fat, and regular exercise.

2. Elimination of which lifestyle factor would have the greatest impact on reducing the incidence of cancer?

Cigarette smoking is the most preventable cause of cancer-related death in the United States. Smoking not only contributes to 90% of lung cancer in men and 79% in women but is also the leading cause of head and neck cancers and is associated with cancers of the stomach, bladder, kidney, pancreas, liver, and cervix. Smoking also contributes to deaths from cardiovascular disease, pneumonia, stroke, emphysema, and bronchitis.

3. Are vaccines available to prevent cancer?

Vaccines are not yet available to prevent cancer directly. A highly effective vaccine is currently available to prevent hepatitis B virus (HBV) infection. Approximately 30–90% of young children and 2–10% of adults who are infected with HBV develop chronic infection. Persons with chronic HBV infection are at significant risk for the development of hepatocellular carcinoma. At present there are over one million chronic carriers of HBV in the U.S., or about 1 in every 250 Americans.

4. How useful is the Papanicolaou (Pap) test?

The Pap test is highly effective in detecting precancerous cells of the cervix. This simple, painless, and inexpensive test has reduced deaths from cervical cancer by 90% in the past 40 years, primarily through preventing invasive cancer. Screening efforts must be made to reach high-risk women in lower socioeconomic groups and elderly women. In both groups the incidence of advanced disease at diagnosis remains high. Over one-half of all American women with newly diagnosed cervical cancer have never had a Pap test.

5. Describe primary and secondary levels of cancer prevention.

Primary prevention refers to simple measures taken early to avoid the development of cancer. Primary cancer prevention can be achieved by making changes in lifestyles that eliminate risky behavior before cancers occur. Examples of primary prevention activities include smoking cessation, dietary changes to reduce fat and increase fiber, and limiting exposure to ultraviolet light and sexually transmitted viruses. **Secondary prevention** targets specific populations and refers to activities such as testing or screening to identify high-risk groups with cancer or precursors to cancer. Mammography, Papanicolaou testing, sigmoidoscopy, and prostate-specific antigen (PSA) testing are examples of secondary prevention activities.

6. How successful is screening for lung cancer in high-risk populations?

Extensive clinical trials have failed to show a significant decrease in lung cancer mortality even when patients at high risk for lung cancer were screened with chest radiography and sputum cytology. Primary prevention through the elimination of cigarette smoking offers the only hope for reducing the incidence of lung cancer. Currently routine screening to detect early lung cancer is not recommended.

7. When is cancer screening most beneficial?

Screening produces the greatest benefit when a certain cancer is highly prevalent in the population and early diagnosis and treatment result in a reduced mortality rate. Screening tests must be simple, inexpensive, and safe as well as clinically acceptable to the patient. Tests must be sensitive (able to identify cancer when it is present) and specific (able to determine when cancer is not present).

8. Does exposure to environmental tobacco smoke increase a nonsmoker's risk for lung cancer?

Passive cigarette smoke, involuntary smoke, and sidestream smoke refer to environmental exposure to tobacco smoke, which is responsible for about 30% of lung cancers. Risk of lung cancer is higher for nonsmokers who have lived or worked for years among heavy smokers. Second-hand smoke has significantly higher concentrations of carcinogenic compounds than mainstream smoke. A burning cigarette gives off at least 43 known carcinogens.

9. What is the most common cancer?

Skin cancer is the most common cancer. Most patients develop nonmelanoma skin cancers, basal cell carcinoma, or squamous cell carcinoma. Basal cell is the most common skin neoplasm worldwide, followed by squamous cell carcinomas. Malignant melanoma accounts for < 10% of skin cancers but is associated with higher mortality rates. Three-quarters of all deaths associated with skin cancer are caused by malignant melanoma. An estimated 51,400 cases of invasive malignant melanoma will be diagnosed in 2001. The incidence of this deadly cancer is rising more rapidly than the incidence of any other cancer in the United States. One in 75 Americans will develop malignant melanoma during his or her lifetime if current rates continue. However, skin cancers are highly curable when diagnosed early and surgically excised.

10. Are tanning booths a safer way to obtain a tan?

Avoid tanning booths or salons! There is no such thing as a safe tan. Damage from sunlight or artificial sources of sunlight is cumulative over a lifetime and increases the risk for developing skin cancer. Tanning is the skin's response to injury. Excessive exposure also contributes to skin changes that cause wrinkles, premature aging, and rough, leathery skin.

11. Are sunscreens effective in protecting against skin cancer?

Skin cancer is mostly preventable when sun protection measures are used consistently. The lifetime incidence of basal cell carcinoma and squamous cell carcinoma can be reduced by as much as 78% with regular use of sunscreen with sun protection factor (SPF) of at least 15 during the first 18 years of life. Sunscreen use should begin in infancy but it is never too late to start. Sunscreen preparations of at least SPF 15 should be applied liberally and frequently. Another simple precaution to protect against ultraviolet light damage is wearing protective clothing (e.g., closely woven long-sleeve shirts and pants, brimmed hats, sunglasses). Avoid or minimize outdoor activities between 10 AM and 4 PM, when ultraviolet light is most intense. Sun effects are also more intense at higher altitudes and when the sun reflects off snow, sand, and water.

12. Explain the sharp increase in prostate cancer incidence, followed by a decline, in recent years.

The rising incidence probably reflects extensive use of prostate specific antigen (PSA) screening in previously unscreened men and an increase in men diagnosed at an earlier age. Shortly after testing became available in 1986, the number of men diagnosed with prostate cancer doubled. The incidence peaked in 1992 and began to decline after that time. The increase in incidence also may reflect the start of mass screening programs, improved detection techniques, and increased public awareness.

13. What is the significance of PSA screening for early detection of prostate cancer?

Widespread PSA testing in asymptomatic men has led to the identification of earlier-stage prostate cancer (smaller and more localized lesions). PSA cannot distinguish latent from aggressive prostate cancers that require treatment. In addition, PSA is not specific for cancer of the prostate; elevated levels are also found in men with benign hypertrophy, prostatitis, and prostatic trauma. Scientific evidence is insufficient to establish that PSA, alone or in combination with digital rectal examination (DRE) or transrectal ultrasonography, has had any impact on reducing the mortality rates of prostate cancer. However, because appropriate use of PSA alone provides approximately 90% specificity for prostate cancer and offers a 5–10-year lead-time in diagnosis, the American Cancer Society and the American Urological Association recommend that men 50 years and older, with a life expectancy > 10 years, should be screened annually with PSA and DRE.

14. Which tests are recommended to screen for colorectal cancer in asymptomatic people?
The American Cancer Society recommends DRE and annual fecal occult blood testing (FOBT), along with periodic flexible sigmoidoscopy (once every 3–5 years), double-contrast barium enema (every 5–10 years), or colonoscopy, for persons 50 years and older at average risk for colorectal cancer. A recent study suggests that screening colonoscopy is better than flexible sigmoidoscopy in detecting early and potentially curable colorectal cancers. Despite the widespread endorsement of screening by medical organizations and the availability of effective screening tools, less than one-third of eligible persons actually undergo screening. More effort is needed to raise awareness and promote colorectal screening at regular intervals.

15. What are serum tumor markers?
Tumor markers are biochemical indicators, found in the blood, of neoplastic activity; they are produced by a tumor or by other cells in response to a tumor. Some tumor markers are not sufficiently sensitive or specific to be used as screening tools in the general population, but they are helpful in monitoring response to therapy. Commonly used serum tumor markers are listed below.

TUMOR MARKER	MALIGNANCIES ASSOCIATED WITH ELEVATION
Alpha-fetoprotein (AFP)	Hepatocellular carcinoma
	Choriocarcinoma, teratoma
	Embryonal cell tumors of ovary or testis
Carcinoembryonic antigen (CEA)	Colon, rectum, pancreas, gastric, lung, breast, ovary
CA-125	Epithelial ovarian neoplasms, breast, colorectal, gastric
CA-15-3	Breast
CA-19-9	Colorectal, pancreas, gastric, liver
CA-27-29	Breast
Human chorionic gonadotropin (HCG)	Choriocarcinoma, germ cell, testicular teratoma, hydatidiform mole
Prostate-specific antigen (PSA)	Prostate

16. What is carcinoembryonic antigen (CEA)? How is it used?
CEA is a protein normally found in small quantities in the blood of healthy people. It is elevated in over one-half of patients who have cancer of the colon, pancreas, stomach, lung, or breast. Elevations also have been associated with noncancerous conditions such as ulcerative colitis, liver disease, lung infections, and smoking (20% of smokers); therefore, elevated CEA is not specific enough to be used for screening or diagnosis. CEA testing is most useful for monitoring response to therapy and detecting disease recurrence.

17. List foods and drugs that may give false-positive reactions to guaiac-based tests for fecal occult blood.
Rare red meat, broccoli, turnips, cauliflower, parsnips, cabbage, horseradish, potatoes, and melons should be avoided for 3 days before and during testing. Aspirin, vitamin C, iron tablets, nonsteroidal anti-inflammatory drugs, and cimetidine also should be avoided.

18. What chemoprevention strategies are useful for decreasing the risk of developing colorectal cancer?

The most widely studied agents in the prevention of colorectal cancer are aspirin and the nonsteroidal anti-inflammatory drugs (NSAIDs). Cyclooxygenase-1 and cyclooxygenase-2 (enzymes necessary for the synthesis of prostaglandins) are found in many tissues, and levels have been elevated in persons with colon cancer and adenomas. NSAIDs that have inhibitory effects on COX-1 and COX-2 also have been shown to decrease the number of intestinal adenomas and colon tumors. The mechanism by which this process occurs is not well understood but may involve an increase in apoptosis and/or regulation of angiogenesis. In addition, folate and calcium supplementation and hormone-replacement therapy (estrogen) in women have shown a chemopreventive benefit.

19. What factors help to identify families at increased risk for hereditary forms of cancer?

Hereditary cancer accounts for 5–10% of all cancers diagnosed. Families at high risk have some of the following features in their history and should be referred for genetic or cancer-risk counseling:

1. Two or more generations diagnosed with the same or related forms of cancer
2. Early age of onset
3. Occurrence of rare tumors
4. Bilateral, multifocal, or multiple primary tumors in one or more family members.

20. At what age should screening for breast cancer be started?

There is nearly universal agreement about the benefit of breast cancer screening in women aged 50–69 years. Randomized controlled trials have evaluated the effectiveness of annual mammography and clinical breast examination and found a reduction in mortality among women aged 50–69. However, routine screening outside this age group is controversial. Evidence of benefit for women aged 40–49 years is less clear, and recommendations from scientific organizations are varied. There is a lack of agreement about the effectiveness of screening and the optimal interval for screening in this age group. Potential risks and benefits should be discussed with women under age 50 when screening is considered.

21. Name three methods used in screening for breast cancer in asymptomatic women.

Screening modalities include mammography, clinical breast examination (CBE), and breast self-examination (BSE). CBE remains an integral part of breast cancer screening and in combination with mammography has shown to improve cancer detection and reduce overall mortality. Most cancers are detected with mammogram alone, yet an estimated 3–24% of cancerous lesions are undetectable by mammogram, especially in women < 50 years of age. Mammography can detect small lesions when cancers are in an early, more curable stage. BSE has been encouraged in the United States for over 35 years and has been recommended as a screening modality beginning at age 20. Although women currently discover 90% of all breast lumps, it is estimated that only one-third of all women perform BSE. Studies of BSE have failed to confirm a reduction in breast cancer mortality.

22. When should BSE be performed?

Ideally, BSE should be done monthly. The best time for premenopausal women is 5–7 days after menses stop when breasts are least lumpy and tender. Postmenopausal women, women who menstruate irregularly, and pregnant women can select a date each month for BSE.

23. What are the components of BSE?

The three essential components of BSE are (1) visual examination using a mirror, (2) palpation in the shower, and (3) palpation in the supine position on the bed. Changes in breast appearance (including shape, size, or symmetry); skin discoloration or dimpling; sores or skin scaling in and around the areola; and nipple retraction, discharge, or puckering should be assessed.

24. Who is at risk for breast cancer?

The major risk factors for 75% of people diagnosed with breast cancer are female gender and increasing age. The risk of breast cancer increases as women age; the risk is highest after age 50. Other factors placing women at highest risk include a personal history of breast cancer or a mother or sister with premenopausal or bilateral breast cancer; identification of a *BRCA1* or *BRCA2* gene mutation; history of proliferative disease, such as atypical hyperplasia; menarche before age 12; menopause after age 55; first birth of a child after age 30; and nulliparity.

25. List the general dietary recommendations of the American Cancer Society to reduce cancer risk.

1. Avoid overeating and maintain an ideal body weight.
2. Reduce total fat intake to < 30% of caloric intake. Excessive fat intake and obesity increase the risk of developing cancers of the breast, colon, and prostate.
3. Include a variety of fruits and vegetables that provide fiber, vitamins, minerals, and other chemicals known to have a protective effect. Lower cancer rates have been associated with higher intake of fruits and vegetables.
4. Increase fiber intake by eating whole grain cereals, legumes, fresh fruits, and vegetables. Fiber decreases transit time of fecal material through the bowel and reduces contact between carcinogens and intestinal mucosa.
5. Minimize the intake of foods that are salt-cured, smoked, and nitrite-cured, such as luncheon meats, bacon, and hot dogs. Stomach and esophageal cancers are associated with consumption of smoked and pickled foods. Nitrates and nitrites, used as food preservatives, are believed to enhance carcinogenic nitrosamine formation.
6. Limit consumption of alcoholic beverages. Heavy drinkers are at increased risk for cancers of the oral cavity, larynx, esophagus, breast, and liver.

REFERENCES

1. Burack RC, Wood DP: Screening for prostate cancer. Med Clin North Am 83:1423–1442, 1999.
2. Frank-Stromborg M, Cohen RF: Assessment and interventions for cancer detection. In Yarbro CH, Frogge MH, Goodman M, Groenwald SL (eds): Cancer Nursing: Principles and Practice, 5th ed. Boston, Jones & Bartlett, 2000, pp 150–188.
3. Greenlee RT, Hill-Harmon MB, Murray T, Thun M: Cancer Statistics, 2001. CA Cancer J Clin 50:15–37, 2001.
4. Helm JF, Sandler RS: Colorectal cancer screening. Med Clin North Am 83:1403–1420, 1999.
5. Janne PA, Mayer RJ: Chemoprevention of colorectal cancer. N Engl J Med 342:1960–1968, 2000.
6. Jerant AF, Johnson JT, Sheridan CD, Caffrey TJ: Early detection and treatment of skin cancer. Am Fam Physician 62:357–358, 2000.
7. Mahon SM: Principles of cancer prevention and early detection. Clin J Oncol Nurs 4:169–176, 2000.
8. Lieberman DA, Weiss DG, Bond JH, et al: Use of colonoscopy to screen asymptomatic adults for colorectal cancer. N Engl J Med 343:162–168, 2000.
9. Patz EF, Goodman PC, Bepler G: Screening for lung cancer. N Engl J Med 343:1627–1633, 2000.
10. Potter SR, Partin A: National Comprehensive Cancer Network (NCCN) practice guidelines for early detection of prostate cancer. Oncology 13(11A):88–115, 1999.
11. Schafer DF, Sorrell MF: Hepatocellular carcinoma. Lancet 353:1253–1257, 1999.
12. Sirovich BE, Sox HC: Breast cancer screening. Surg Clin North Am 79:961–990, 1999.
13. Smith RA, Mettlin CJ, Davis KJ, Eyre H: American Cancer Society guidelines for the early detection of cancer. CA Cancer J Clin 50:34–49, 2000.

3. DIAGNOSIS AND STAGING

Daniel T. Tell, DO, FACP

1. How is cancer diagnosed?

Cancer may be diagnosed clinically or by looking at a sample of tissue suspected of being cancerous under a microscope. A clinical diagnosis is the physician's best educated guess at the most likely diagnosis. A patient may be asymptomatic or present with a group of signs and symptoms that suggest a diagnosis of cancer. Most signs and symptoms, however, are nonspecific and can be seen in a wide variety of illnesses. A diagnosis of cancer requires a diagnostic test—and that test is the biopsy.

2. Define biopsy.

A biopsy is a surgical procedure that involves removing all or part of the tissue suspected of being cancerous.

3. What are the three major types of biopsy?

A **needle biopsy** involves inserting a needle into a suspicious lesion and removing individual cells (aspiration biopsy) or a core of tissue (core biopsy). If a lesion is large or accessible only by endoscopy, a surgeon may remove only a small portion of the lesion with a scalpel or forceps (**incisional biopsy**). Lastly, the surgeon may remove the entire lesion (**excisional biopsy**).

4. What other sampling method may be used?

Cytology specimens. Malignant cells can be found in body fluids (e.g., ascites, spinal fluid, pleural effusions) or exfoliated from organs (e.g., cervical Papanicolaou smears, sputum).

5. Why is it important to establish a pathologic tissue diagnosis?

Cytology or biopsy specimens establish with certainty the diagnosis of cancer. A tissue diagnosis (tissue procurement and identification) eliminates all of the other diseases in the differential diagnoses originally considered by the clinician when the patient's signs and symptoms were first evaluated. With a firm diagnosis, accurate and specific treatment can be administered, and the patient can be given a prognosis.

6. What information does the pathologist report after doing the biopsy?

Specimens are sent to the laboratory to identify the histopathology (tumor type, classification, and grade) of the malignancy. Examples of **tumor types** are carcinoma, sarcoma, germ cell tumor, lymphoma, and glioma. **Classification** is the subtype of the malignancy, such as squamous or adenocarcinoma. **Grade** refers to the degree to which a malignant tumor is similar to normal tissue. For example, poorly differentiated or high-grade tumors contain few features of normal tissue.

7. How is biopsied tissue processed?

Biopsied tissue may be processed in many different ways, depending on the suspected diagnosis. Initially, all tissue is fixed in a preservative solution and embedded in wax (tissue block). This method of processing the tissue allows thin slices to be cut from the block for staining and subsequent viewing under a microscope. Standard stains allow the pathologist to identify features specific to the biopsied organ as well as individual cells, nuclei, and nucleoli. Results from a biopsy should be available in 24 hours.

8. What does the pathologist do if standard stains do not help?

If the pathologist cannot make a diagnosis with standard tissue stains, a wide variety of stains and techniques is available to define the cancer further. In general, a pathologist is able to diagnose cancer from the standard fixation and tissue stains. It is not unusual for the pathologist to have some difficulty in giving a final diagnosis without further testing. Additional testing often includes special stains as well as specialized studies (e.g., flow cytometry, monoclonal antibody testing, cytogenetics, and electronmicroscopy).

9. What are special stains?

Like the clinician, the pathologist generates a differential diagnosis when looking at the biopsy. The pathologist may not be sure of what he or she is looking at but usually has a good idea. Probabilities are ranked, and various tests are ordered to rule in (or out) the most likely diagnosis. The tests that the pathologist orders in this situation are collectively known as "special stains." The test may be as simple as a stain for mucin to differentiate squamous carcinoma from adenocarcinoma. Alternatively, immunoperoxidase techniques may be used to identify prostate-specific antigen in an otherwise nonspecific adenocarcinoma. Special stains generally take another 24–48 hours to complete. Considering the differential diagnosis obtained by looking at the biopsy, a pathologist generally orders several special stains at once.

10. What is flow cytometry?

Flow cytometry allows analysis of individual cells based on specific characteristics or characteristics identified by specific stains. The cells are placed in suspension and analyzed as they flow through a port or laser source that separates the cells on the basis of the selected characteristic.

11. How is flow cytometry used in diagnosis?

As a diagnostic technique, flow cytometry generally is used to characterize the various types of lymphoma and leukemia. Cells can be labeled with antibodies directed at various antigens specific for certain types of lymphoma. The cells then are sorted by this characteristic. An example is the selection and sorting of the CD5 antigen, which is present in most cases of chronic lymphatic leukemia. A suspension of lymphoma cells is exposed to an antibody directed at the CD5 antigen. The antibody is labeled to allow detection as the cells pass through the port. The CD5 cells are detected and counted separately, as is the total number of cells. The results are generally reported as a percentage of the number of CD5 cells relative to the total number of cells counted. It is, therefore, most useful in refining rather than establishing a diagnosis. Occasionally, an otherwise undiagnosable lymphoma may exhibit a characteristic flow cytometric pattern, thereby yielding a specific diagnosis.

12. How is flow cytometery used for solid tumors?

Flow cytometry is used to determine the chromosomal content and growth fraction of various tumors, most commonly breast cancer. Although neither a diagnostic nor a staging procedure, this ancillary test often is used to assess prognosis and guide treatment. Flow cytometry provides the clinician with the percentage of tumor cells in "S" phase (dividing cells) and an indicator for the presence of tumor cells with abnormal DNA content. High percentages of cells in S phase and with abnormal DNA content are generally believed to confer a worse prognosis in breast cancer, and often more aggressive treatment is prescribed.

13. What are monoclonal antibodies?

All cells possess surface antigens that may be detected by antibodies directed against them. The antibodies are labeled to facilitate detection. The label may be radioactive or designed to fluoresce or change color so that it can be seen. Cancer cells often possess antigens unique to that particular type of cancer. The pathologist may request a wide variety of monoclonal antibody tests to evaluate a biopsy, depending on the suspected diagnosis. Examples of commonly used monoclonal antibodies are antileukocyte common antigen (anti-LCA) and anticytokeratin. Both tests are often used in the evaluation of a poorly differentiated malignancy.

During routine staining, a pathologist may be able to say that a tissue specimen is malignant but unable to determine whether the cancer is lymphoma or carcinoma. This distinction is important for both treatment and prognosis. Such a biopsy probably would be tested for both LCA and cytokeratin. An LCA-positive biopsy is consistent with lymphoma, whereas a cytokeratin-positive biopsy is consistent with carcinoma.

14. What are cytogenetic studies?

Some tumors are associated with specific genetic abnormalities, which often can be detected by cytogenetic studies. The chromosomes from individual cells are cultured and isolated during cell division. They are fixed, stained, and magnified so that rearrangements (translocations) and deletions can be seen. Probably the best known translocation is the Philadelphia chromosome, which is associated with and usually is diagnostic of chronic myelogenous leukemia. Further refinements of cytogenetic techniques have allowed the identification of individual mutations.

15. What is electronmicroscopy?

Just as light is used to view microscopic structures, electrons can be used to visualize the extremely small cell components. Because the wavelength of electrons is much shorter than visible light, resolution and magnification are much greater. Electronmicroscopy (EM) can be used to visualize cellular organelles, cellular inclusions, and intercellular bridges, which are often characteristic of various malignancies. The limit of magnification with light microscopy is about 1000 ×. EM can enlarge into the tens of thousands and even higher with specialized techniques.

16. What happens after the pathologist decides that the diagnosis is cancer?

Usually the pathologist calls the patient's physician, who has to tell the patient. In most cases, the patient has been advised that a malignant diagnosis is likely and is mentally prepared to deal with the news. Preparing a patient to receive the news and actually delivering the news are an art that requires compassion, awareness of the patient's personality, and, to a certain extent, experience. The physician most qualified to inform the patient is the primary care physician; it is most important that he or she be involved. However, many physicians are uncomfortable in this role—which is why God made oncologists. Effective collaboration and communication between physicians and nurses are essential in assisting the patient through this initial crisis.

17. Describe the role of the nurse when the patient is told about a diagnosis of cancer.

The nurse's role in this setting is critical; it is not only supportive but also informative. The nurse should be able to address issues that invariably arise after the patient has been told the diagnosis. Because most patients are anxious, they hear little of the physician's discussion after they hear the diagnosis or are confused about what they did hear. Patients may not be comfortable questioning the physician or may believe they are taking up too much of the physician's time. The nurse should be prepared to address the patient's questions and have general information about the disease process, prognosis, further testing, potential complications, and available treatments. If a specific question cannot be answered, the nurse should say so and obtain the answer or refer the patient to an oncology clinical nurse specialist or other appropriate provider. It is always better to admit that the answer is not known than to provide incorrect information. The patient may not be interested in specific answers at this point. Listening, support, guidance, and reassurance may be more important than statistics and technical information.

18. After the diagnosis of cancer has been made, what is the next step?

Once a patient has been given the diagnosis of cancer, a series of tests is performed to determine the extent of the disease. This process is known as staging. Patients need to be told why the tests are done and instructed about preparation procedures and possible complications. Other instructions include description of physical sensations or discomfort that may be anticipated, when results are available, and identification of who will report the results. Patients should be assessed for contraindications or hypersensitivities to iodine or other radioactive agents.

19. What is staging?

Staging is used to determine the extent of disease in an individual patient. The tumor-node-metastasis (TNM) system of the American Joint Committee on Cancer (AJCC) is preferred for solid tumors (e.g., breast, lung, colon):

    T = characteristics of a given tumor (size, depth of invasion, involvement of surrounding structures)

N = presence or absence of involved nodes and size or number of involved nodes
M = presence or absence of metastases.
A typical TNM classification for a 3-cm breast cancer with one involved lymph node and bone metastases would be as follows: T2N1M1 (bone).

20. How are TNM results grouped?

TNM results can be incorporated into larger groupings, called stages, in which various Ts, Ns, and Ms with similar prognoses are collected. Most tumors proceed from stage I through stage IV. Prognosis worsens with stage progression for any given disease. Stage IV disease is generally metastatic, whereas stage I disease is generally confined to the organ of origin. A T2N1M1 breast cancer is stage IV, whereas a T2N1M0 breast cancer is stage II. Such a system allows the clinician to assign a prognosis and usually guides treatment. It also allows health professionals to discuss individual clinical situations and to exchange information about prognosis and management. The detail provided by such a system allows retrospective (or prospective) investigations, which may reveal differences in prognosis for certain situations. These differences may justify moving a particular TNM combination to a different stage or provide new information about its management.

The system is specific for all of the different anatomic sites with respect to T and many Ns; as a result, it is complicated. Fortunately, *Cancer Staging Handbook*, published by the AJCC, lists all of the anatomic sites and the accepted staging schema for each. If a staging manual is not available, most oncology texts explain TNM staging in the chapter for each tumor.

21. Why is staging important?

1. The extent to which a disease has spread is prognostic.
2. Extent of disease often dictates treatment.
3. Accurate staging allows collection of data that eventually provides information about treatment outcomes for each type of cancer and each stage of disease. Staging information is collected by a tumor registry.

22. How are tumor registries maintained?

Hospitals with an accredited cancer program are required by the American College of Surgeons to have a registry that collects data about all malignant diagnoses made at the institution. When a patient is entered into the registry, the cancer diagnosis, stage, and treatment are recorded. The registry follows the patient for life. Follow-up information is collected from the patient, the patient's medical records, and the treating physician. If the patient is no longer under treatment or has not seen the physician in the preceding year, a letter is sent to the patient requesting information about the status of the disease.

23. Why are tumor registries important?

The American College of Surgeons periodically collects data about an individual disease from all of the tumor registries in the country. This information is then analyzed and published. The data allow a hospital to determine whether treatment provided for its patients is comparable to that provided by other hospitals around the country.

24. Is there a different staging system for lymphomas?

Yes. Sometimes the term liquid tumor is used to distinguish lymphomas and leukemias from solid tumors. For most lymphomas, the Ann Arbor classification is used. It has a number of advantages over the TNM system: (1) clinicians are comfortable with it; (2) it is easy to remember; and (3) it provides generally accurate information for prognosis and treatment.

25. Summarize the Ann Arbor system.

Stage I disease is confined to one nodal group. **Stage II** disease involves more than one nodal group on the same side of the diaphragm. **Stage III** disease is present on both sides of the diaphragm, and **stage IV** disease is disseminated (i.e., present in nonlymphoid organs). This system also includes modifiers to denote the presence or absence of constitutional or "B" symptoms (e.g., fevers, sweats, weight loss). The system also denotes whether the disease involves a nonlymphoid organ by contiguity. Such involvement is referred to as "E" disease (extralymphatic) and is distinguished from disseminated disease. A patient with a non-Hodgkin's lymphoma involving the liver is classified as stage IV. A patient with mediastinal adenopathy and direct extension to the surrounding lung is classified as stage IE (lung). If the same patient also had a greater than 10% loss in body weight or unexplained fever or sweats, he or she is classified as stage IBE (lung). This system is in common usage among oncology health professionals and is worth knowing.

26. Is there a separate staging system for leukemias?

Chronic lymphatic leukemia (CLL) is the only leukemia to which a staging system is applied on a regular basis. The rationale is simple: staging of CLL has prognostic implications. CLL is a chronic disease that lends itself well to a staging system. A patient with only an absolute lymphocytosis may live 7–10 years or more, whereas a patient with thrombocytopenia may live only 2 years. The most commonly used classification is the Rai system:

Stage 0   > 10,000 lymphocytes
Stage I   Enlarged lymph nodes
Stage II   Enlarged liver and/or spleen
Stage III   Anemia
Stage IV   Thrombocytopenia

27. What are the prognostic indicators for unstaged leukemias?

Lack of staging systems for other leukemias does not mean that prognostic indicators do not exist or that extent of disease (tumor burden) is not important. Other leukemias are disseminated at diagnosis and have a short clinical course if not treated promptly and effectively. This fact somewhat lessens the value of a staging system. Staging systems with widespread acceptance eventually may be formulated for the acute leukemias as more information becomes available. The presence or absence of certain genes or immunophenotypes, certain ages, and certain locations are of known prognostic importance for various forms of leukemia. This information is often used to formulate a treatment plan. Eventually, these variables may be organized into a clinically useful staging system.

28. What factors are used in the staging of cancer?

All staging begins with a history and physical examination. Usually both have been done by the time a patient is diagnosed with cancer. More specific questions and more thorough physical testing may be performed after diagnosis to assess signs or symptoms peculiar to the diagnosed cancer. This information may make a physician suspect the presence of disease at another site, and other tests may be ordered to confirm such suspicions.

The physician generally orders a complete blood count, chemistry tests of liver and kidney function, and urinalysis when a patient is first suspected of having cancer. These tests help to detect the presence of metastatic disease and to assess organ function in preparation for treatment. Tumor markers may be ordered to serve as a point of reference for subsequent treatment. In some diseases, elevated tumor markers may suggest the extent of disease and tumor burden as well as have prognostic implications.

Besides the history, physical examination, and screening laboratory studies, a wide variety of tests is available to evaluate the extent of a particular disease. The most commonly used tests are radiographs (plain film, computed tomography [CT] scans, magnetic resonance imaging [MRI], and nuclear medicine scans). Biopsies are sometimes used to confirm a suspicious radiograph or scan abnormalities and to evaluate tissue that cannot be evaluated in any other way (e.g., bone marrow).

29. Define tumor marker.

Tumor markers are substances secreted by tumors that can be found in the blood. In general, they are used to evaluate response to therapy and to monitor recurrence. These tests are somewhat organ-specific, although overlap with other diseases is common. Many tumor markers also can be elevated in benign conditions.

30. What are the most commonly used tumor markers?

Many tumor markers are available to monitor various tumors. The most commonly used markers include carcinoembryonic antigen (colon), prostate-specific antigen (prostate cancer), CA-125 (ovarian cancer), CA-15-3 and CA-27-29 (breast cancer), and CA-19-9 (pancreatic cancer). All of these tests may be abnormal in benign conditions and may be useful to monitor other malignancies. CA-19-9 may be used to follow gastric or biliary tract cancers; CEA may be abnormal in breast and lung cancer. Tumor markers are more likely to be elevated in patients with metastatic disease and tend to rise progressively with worsening disease. No test is perfect, however, and some patients with metastatic disease may have normal tumor markers.

31. Discuss the role of carcinoembryonic antigen (CEA) testing.

Carcinoembryonic antigen (CEA) was the first tumor marker to be described and remains a useful test. CEA is elevated in many tumors of epithelial origin but is used most commonly to evaluate colon malignancies. It is often elevated in breast and lung cancer but may be abnormal in benign conditions such as bronchitis, hepatitis, and ulcerative colitis. It is mildly elevated in patients who smoke cigarettes. CEA is ordered preoperatively in patients with colon cancer. In this setting, an elevated CEA implies a worse prognosis. The test is repeated postoperatively, and levels should return to normal if all disease is resected. The test is repeated at periodic intervals to detect recurrence.

32. Are tumor markers useful for cancer screening?

This is as much an economic as a scientific question. Screening asymptomatic patients for various cancers with tests that lack sensitivity and, of greater importance, specificity may be a waste of valuable health care dollars. Screening for prostate cancer with an annual prostate-specific antigen (PSA) test is considered useful, although PSA is elevated in patients with benign prostatic hypertrophy. How much is society willing to spend for PSA tests that yield normal results and for evaluations in patients with abnormal results to detect cancer? Put another way, how much does it cost to diagnose one cancer in a population of asymptomatic adult men? As a corollary, what is the benefit to the patient diagnosed with cancer? Is the patient curable, or does a patient diagnosed in this manner require treatment at all? Should the test be restricted to a high-risk population or a certain age range? Such questions apply to all available tumor markers; they will assume increasing importance as economic pressures on medicine become more intense.

33. What are the current recommendations for screening for prostate and ovarian cancer?

A screening PSA test is performed annually for all men over the age of 50. Screening CA-125 for ovarian cancer is used on a more selective basis for women at higher-than-average risk for disease.

34. What are CT scans?

CT is a radiographic procedure in which a patient is exposed to x-rays and an image is generated based on the differential absorption of x-rays by different tissues in the body. In this respect the technique is similar to plain radiographs. In CT scanning, however, the images are manipulated by a computer to provide cross-sectional images (or images in any plane, for that matter). The result is multiple cross-sectional images, usually several centimeters apart, depicted from head to toe.

35. How are CT scans used in patients with cancer?

CT usually is ordered for a general anatomic area, such as head, chest, abdomen, or pelvis. It allows visualization of most internal organs in great detail and may spare the patient a surgical procedure. It is useful in the staging of a wide variety of cancers. In lung cancer, CT visualizes the mediastinum, which may show enlarged lymph nodes not apparent on plain chest radiograph. Such patients do not undergo surgical treatment; instead, they are treated with radiation and chemotherapy. In pancreatic cancer, a CT scan of the abdomen may show liver metastases. Again, surgery is not an option; the patient receives chemotherapy. In either case, a biopsy probably would be performed to confirm the presence of disease in the lymph nodes or liver; the presence of disease in either location radically affects treatment and prognosis.

36. What is an MRI scan?

In MRI, the area of the patient to be visualized is exposed to a strong magnetic field, which aligns all of the atoms of the organ in question in one direction. When the magnet is deactivated, the atoms return to their normal alignment and in so doing release energy. Different tissues with varying water content release energy at different times. This energy is monitored and can be imaged. The result is a scan that at first glance appears similar to a CT scan but provides different information.

37. How are MRI scans used in patients with cancer?

MRI may be used to image a suspicious area on a CT scan, such as an area of fibrosis or an enlarged lymph node. Tumor within a scar or enlarged lymph node emits a different signal, allowing the radiologist to detect its presence. MRI also may be used to detect lesions that are isodense. Such lesions have the same density as the tissue in which they grow and may not be seen on CT scanning. Brain and liver metastases are occasionally isodense; when an MRI scan is performed, the lesions become obvious as bright white masses. Because isodense lesions are relatively uncommon, MRI scanning is not a routine part of staging. Generally a negative CT scan is accepted as normal unless the patient displays symptoms suggesting the presence of disease. In this situation an MRI may be ordered to exclude isodense metastases.

MRI also has proved useful in the diagnosis of carcinomatous meningitis. Before the availability of MRI, patients often required myelography, which is invasive, uncomfortable, and potentially dangerous.

38. What are nuclear medicine scans?

Nuclear medicine scans are radiographic studies in which a radioactive label is administered to the patient intravenously. The radioactive isotope concentrates within the target organ, where it is temporarily trapped. The label emits radiation that can be imaged. Before the advent of CT scanning, brain and liver scans were commonly used for staging. However, CT scans have far better resolution and have largely replaced nuclear medicine scanning of the brain and liver.

39. How are nuclear medicine scans used in patients with cancer?

A **bone scan** is often used to stage patients with lymphoma and various solid tumors (e.g, lung and breast cancer). Gallium scans are often used to assess the extent of lymphoma, because gallium is often taken up by lymphomatous tissue. Gallium scans are considered part of the staging evaluation of Hodgkin's disease, and some oncologists find them useful in the evaluation of lymphoma. Like all staging studies, these studies are often repeated after treatment to assess response.

A **multiple-gated acquisition (MUGA)** or heart scan is often ordered during staging to assess cardiac function in patients who may need cardiotoxic chemotherapy. This scan provides information about cardiac wall motion, contractility, and ejection fraction; it is used to determine whether the patient's heart is functioning well enough to tolerate specific drugs (e.g., doxorubicin). It is not part of staging per se.

40. What is positron emission tomography (PET)?

PET is a special kind of nuclear medicine imaging tomography made possible by the unique fate of positrons. It cannot be performed with conventional gamma cameras; a specially designed PET scanner is required. Malignant cells have an enhanced rate of glycolysis. Fluorine-18 fluorodeoxyglucose (FDG) is a positron emitter that mimics this increased rate of glycolysis in tumor cells.

41. How is PET used in patients with cancer?

PET imaging is a reliable method for evaluating and staging recurrent lung and colon cancers, lymphoma, and malignant melanoma.

42. What is a bone marrow biopsy?

Bone marrow biopsy is a commonly used minor surgical procedure that determines the presence or absence of marrow involvement by tumor. The posterior iliac crest is the site most commonly chosen; when viewed from the back, it may be seen in most patients as two dimples on either side of the lower lumbar spine at the belt line. In most patients, the iliac bone is close to the surface at this point and separated from the surface of the skin only by fat.

43. How is a bone marrow biopsy performed?

The patient may be sedated for the procedure. After local anesthetic infiltration, a small stab incision is made. A needle is inserted through the bone cortex into the marrow cavity, and a small amount of liquid marrow is aspirated into a syringe. A biopsy needle then is inserted into the bone to remove a core or cylinder of bone marrow, usually about 2 cm long and a few millimeters wide. In patients in whom sedation is not possible, the procedure is moderately uncomfortable. The dominant sensation is an intense pressure punctuated by brief periods of toothache-like pain. In the bone marrow involved by tumor, collections of tumor cells may be seen in scattered areas throughout the marrow cavity, or tumor may completely fill the space.

44. What are the complications of bone marrow biopsy?

The only major complication of a correctly performed bone marrow biopsy is the remote possibility of infection in the bone. Postprocedural pain is generally mild and resolves within a few days. An occasional patient develops a subperiostial hematoma, which may cause point tenderness for several weeks.

45. How is bone marrow biopsy used in staging?

A bone marrow biopsy is a diagnostic procedure for leukemia, whereas it is generally a part of the staging evaluation of lymphomas. It also is used in small cell lung cancer when the likelihood of marrow involvement is substantial and when marrow involvement changes treatment. In most other diseases, marrow biopsy is used selectively. In solid tumors and lymphomas, marrow involvement often changes treatment and always changes prognosis. As a result, bone marrow biopsy may be used to stage a patient in whom bone marrow involvement is suspected. For example, the complete blood count (CBC) of a patient with breast cancer may show mild anemia and thrombocytopenia. The differential may show a small number of immature white cells and an occasional nucleated red blood cell. This constellation of CBC findings is highly suspicious for marrow involvement by tumor. In the absence of another good explanation, bone marrow biopsy is recommended. Treatment is affected dramatically if the bone marrow is involved. Local measures such as mastectomy become secondary to systemic treatment, and bone marrow transplantation may even be considered. Prognosis, of course, also is changed.

46. When does it all end?

Staging is complete when the doctor and patient know the diagnosis, prognosis, and correct treatment. Every attempt is made to make the process safe, comfortable, informative, efficient, and cost-effective.

47. Are there times when the type of cancer cannot be determined?

In occasional patients who present with metastatic cancer, a careful search reveals no obvious primary tumor. This situation, known as adenocarcinoma–unknown primary (ACUP) or simply unknown primary, accounts for about 5–10% of all patients with cancer. Most commonly such tumors are poorly differentiated carcinomas or adenocarcinomas. (See Chapter 36.)

48. What is scintigraphy?

In scintigraphy, a radioactive isotope is injected around a primary tumor and then imaged after it has traveled to the lymph node group that serves as primary drainage for the tumor site. This technique is useful in evaluating tumors with ambiguous lymph node drainage, such as melanomas on the trunk. A melanoma on the back, for instance, may drain to either the axilla or groin or even the cervical region. Demonstrating lymph node involvement in melanoma has become highly important, because effective adjuvant treatment has been discovered for patients with metastatic lymph nodes.

Scintigraphy or sentinel lymph node mapping has gained popularity in the evaluation of breast cancer. The first lymph node draining the breast cancer, known as the sentinel node, is biopsied rather than performing an axillary node dissection. The assumption is that a negative sentinel lymph node is predictive of a negative axillary lymphadenectomy (see Chapter 25).

49. Are there any controversies in the diagnosis of cancer?

No. A tissue diagnosis must always be made. Physicians may argue about the best way to obtain a diagnosis, but none would argue against making the diagnosis. The implications of a diagnosis of cancer and the potential for harm during the treatment of cancer are too great to assume the diagnosis. A clinical diagnosis, if incorrect, exposes the patient to great emotional, physical, and financial stress. The cardinal rule of oncology is simple: no DX (diagnosis), no RX (treatment).

50. Are there any controversies in the staging of cancer?

Yes. For most diseases, staging procedures and tests are standard. Controversy arises when technologic advances and new or ancillary tests become available. Patient risk, inconvenience, and cost enter the equation, and there is a period of uncertainty until the new technology is perceived or proved to be indispensable or ancillary. In the future, advancing technology will clash with increasing cost consciousness, and the manner in which cancer is diagnosed and staged will change—hopefully for the better.

REFERENCES

1. Fleming ID, Cooper JS, Henson DE et al: AJCC Cancer Staging Handbook, 5th ed. Philadelphia, Lippincott-Raven, 1998.
2. Griffin-Brown J: Diagnostic evaluation, classification, and staging. In Yarbro CH, Frogge MH, Goodman M, Groenwald SL (eds): Cancer Nursing: Principles and Practice, 5th ed. Boston, Jones & Bartlett, 2000, pp 214–239.
3. Madeya ML, Pfab-Tokarsky JM: Flow cytometry: An overview. Oncol Nurs Forum 19:459–463, 1992.

II. Treatment of Cancer

4. PRINCIPLES OF THERAPY

Kyle M. Fink, MD, and Ioana Hinshaw, MD

1. How is cancer treated? What therapies are currently under study?

The major treatment modalities for cancer are surgery, radiation therapy, chemotherapy, hormonal therapy, and biologic therapy; each may be used alone or in combination with other modalities. Studies are ongoing to evaluate the effectiveness of other modalities, such as gene therapy, novel drugs, cryotherapy, immunotherapy, photodynamic therapy, bone marrow and stem cell transplantations, and differentiation therapy as well as to improve strategies and reduce toxicities of standard therapies.

2. List strategies that help to establish rapport and trust in interacting with patients presenting with a new diagnosis of cancer or for follow-up care.

1. **Listen to patients** and maintain open communication to understand their concerns about cancer and treatments and their fears about the future. Two of the most worrisome problems for patients are fear of the unknown and probable survival time. You need to understand their perspective and level of knowledge, making sure that you talk with them, not at them. In a busy setting, the health care provider should be centered and focused on the patient. Try to ensure that outside interruptions, such as phone calls and paging, are kept to a minimum.

2. **Try to connect** with all of your patients, even in the smallest manner. Find out something personal—what kind of work they do, their support system, their interests, their children. Try to find something in common in a nonmedical area. For instance, you may be from the same town or state or have gone to the same school; both of you may play tennis, have an interest in movies or books, or like cats.

3. **Compassionate disclosure** of information requires that you communicate a new diagnosis of cancer or bad test results as directly and as soon as possible. Do not "beat around the bush" for the first half of the visit. Patients are unable to focus on your discussion until they know specifically with what they are dealing and until anxiety and fear of the unknown have been relieved.

4. **Honesty** about the diagnosis or test results increases the patient's level of trust. Whenever possible, the physician should enlist the collaborative assistance of a nurse or oncology clinical nurse specialist. By being present in the room, the nurse knows what has been said and can offer support, compassion, and follow-up information to clarify what the physician has said.

5. **Make sure that the patient initially understands the treatment objective**, whether it is curative, adjuvant, or palliative. Some patients, especially if they are to receive palliative care, may not wish to acknowledge the fact after the initial discussion. Sometimes they cope better by using denial—and this strategy is all right. However, the oncologist, nurse, patient, and family can be reassured that the subject has been broached openly and honestly.

6. **Incorporate patients into the treatment plan** by giving them options from which to choose. By helping to determine their treatment program, patients are better able to accept and comply with therapy. For example, patients can be given options about timing of chemotherapy and choice of antiemetic.

7. **Leave the room with a positive note**, no matter how dismal the information. The only positive element may be reassuring a terminal patient that medications are available to control pain or that the health care team will do everything possible to sustain quality of life.

3. What are the most important steps before initiating therapy for cancer?

All decisions in oncology are based on understanding the natural history of the disease, treated or untreated. Before initiating any therapy, important points need to be considered:

1. The diagnosis must be confirmed, almost always by tissue biopsy. Do not diagnose unconfirmed cancer.

2. The disease must be staged by appropriate diagnostic means (e.g., physical examination, computed tomography [CT] scans, bone scan). Extent or stage of disease critically determines prognosis and treatment.

3. The goal of therapy must be defined: curative, adjuvant, or palliative.

4. A treatment plan must be chosen from many therapeutic options, depending on the stage of the disease and patient characteristics such as age, performance status, and comorbid disease as well as the patient's wishes.

4. What is the difference between curative and palliative treatment?

Curative treatment is given with the intent of eradicating measurable, discernible malignant disease. Some cancers, such as lymphomas and testicular cancers, can be cured despite extensive disease at diagnosis. In the curative setting, therapy should be aggressive, and some treatment-related morbidity and even risk of death may be justified. To increase the chance for cure, the dose intensity of any chemotherapy regimen should be maintained and dose reductions avoided.

Palliative treatment is given when the disease is not curable and survival time is limited. The goals of palliative treatment are to alleviate symptoms and to improve quality of life while also extending survival. In this setting, care must be taken to keep toxicity at a minimum, and drug dose reductions are often necessary.

5. What is adjuvant therapy? When is it given?

Adjuvant therapy refers to the use of therapy, usually chemotherapy, along with another treatment modality. Adjuvant therapy is given with curative intent. The primary treatment (surgery) may have already cured the patient; the adjuvant therapy is added to increase the cure rate. Adjuvant treatments are given to patients who may or may not have cancer. It can cure only a microscopic tumor load. If the tumor becomes discernible or macroscopic, the treatment strategy must be adjusted, because adjuvant therapy is not strong enough to cure a larger tumor burden.

6. Give a common example of adjuvant therapy.

The best example is adjuvant chemotherapy for breast cancer given after mastectomy to a patient with positive nodes. The patient with breast cancer may be "cured" by the mastectomy, but the positive lymph nodes are an indication of possible microscopic disease somewhere in the body that may later develop into recurrent cancer; thus, adjuvant therapy is indicated. In contrast, adjuvant chemotherapy is not used in non-small cell lung cancer because, even if microscopic disease is present after surgical removal, chemotherapy is not effective in killing microscopic tumor cells.

7. What cancers are responsive to chemotherapy?

Responsiveness of Various Cancer Types to Chemotherapy

Cancers with macroscopic disease that can be cured with chemotherapy	
Testicular cancer	Acute leukemias
Hodgkin's disease	Small cell lung cancer (nonmetastatic)
High-grade non-Hodgkin's lymphoma	Ovarian cancer

Cancers with microscopic disease that can be cured with adjuvant chemotherapy	
Breast cancer	Osteosarcoma
Colorectal cancer	Bladder cancer
	Ewing's sarcoma

Table continued on following page

Responsiveness of Various Cancer Types to Chemotherapy (Continued)

Cancers with metastatic disease that can be controlled but not cured with chemotherapy

Breast cancer	Endometrial cancer
Colorectal cancer	Cervical cancer
Prostate cancer	Head and neck cancer
Lung cancer (non-small cell and small cell)	Bladder cancer
Low-grade non-Hodgkin's lymphoma	Stomach cancer
Multiple myeloma	Esophageal cancer
Chronic leukemias	Soft tissue sarcoma
Ovarian cancer	Osteosarcoma

Cancers that have low response rates or are unresponsive to chemotherapy

Brain tumors	Thyroid cancer
Renal cell cancer	Cholangiocarcinoma
Malignant melanoma	Mesothelioma
Hepatoma	Carcinoid tumors
Pancreatic cancer	

8. How can the concept of adjuvant therapy be explained to patients?

Explain to patients that the detectable limit of cancer with currently available tests is 1 cubic centimeter of tumor, which equals one billion cancer cells (10^9). Patients may be told that if they have cancer, they have anywhere from 1 to 1 billion cancer cells; the objective of adjuvant chemotherapy is to destroy the microscopic cancer cells. Always emphasize the positive: the patient may have zero cancer cells and may already be cured.

9. What is the difference between adjuvant therapy and neoadjuvant therapy?

Neoadjuvant chemotherapy is adjuvant therapy given before primary treatment (surgery or radiation) in patients with localized tumor. Neoadjuvant therapy reduces the extensiveness of surgery. For example, patients with breast cancer who initially are not surgical candidates because of tumor size may be able to undergo surgery after tumor size is reduced by neoadjuvant chemotherapy. Response to neoadjuvant therapy is also useful in establishing tumor chemosensitivity and prognosis. After removal of the residual tumor, the viability of the remaining tumor cells is examined to classify patients into complete responders, partial responders, or nonresponders; all have different prognoses.

10. In addition to the oral and parenteral routes, how else can chemotherapy be given?

- Instillation into the cerebrospinal fluid (CSF) for control of meningeal carcinomatosis
- Intrapleural or intrapericardial administration for control of malignant effusions
- Intraperitoneal administration as postsurgical therapy for ovarian carcinoma
- Intraarterial administration for isolated liver metastases due to colon carcinoma; also selected arterial infusion for sarcomas of the extremities

11. Why is performance status important in making treatment decisions?

In general, performance status predicts how the patient will tolerate therapy. Patients with poor performance status have an increased risk of chemotherapy-related toxicity.

Karnofsky and American Joint Committee on Cancer (AJCC) Performance Status Scales

DESCRIPTION	KARNOFSKY SCALE (%)	AJCC SCALE	DESCRIPTION
Normal; no complaints; no evidence of disease	100	H0	Normal activity
Able to carry on normal activity; minor signs or symptoms of disease	90		

Table continued on following page

Karnofsky and American Joint Committee on Cancer (AJCC) Performance Status Scales (Continued)

DESCRIPTION	KARNOFSKY SCALE (%)	AJCC SCALE	DESCRIPTION
Normal activity with effort; some signs or symptoms of disease	80	H1	Symptomatic and ambulatory; cares for self
Cares for self; unable to carry on normal activity or do active work	70		
Requires occasional assistance but is able to care for most of own needs	60	H2	Ambulatory > 50% of time; occasionally needs assistance
Requires considerable assistance and frequent medical care	50		
Disabled; requires special care and assistance	40	H3	Ambulatory ≤ 50% of time; nursing care needed
Severely disabled; hospitalizaiton indicated, although death not imminent	30		
Very sick; hospitalization with active supportive treatment necessary	20	H4	Bedridden; may need hospitalization
Moribund, fatal processes progressing rapidly	10		
Dead	0		

12. What are the most useful prognostic factors in cancer?

Prognostic factors are both tumor-related and patient-related. Important tumor-related prognostic factors are histologic type, grade, and stage of disease. Other factors include expression of hormone receptors, cytogenetic abnormalities, and tumor-associated markers. Important patient-related prognostic factors are performance status, age, and associated systemic symptoms (weight loss, fevers, night sweats). Certain cancers have defined prognostic groups associated with specific survival rates.

13. How is response to therapy defined?

The response is usually quantified into complete response, partial response, progressive disease, and stable disease. Complete response means the disappearance of all measurable disease for at least 1 month. This response is clinically the most important indicator of effectiveness of chemotherapy and is the prerequisite for cure. Partial response is defined as at least 50% reduction in measurable tumor mass without appearance of new lesions for at least 2 months. Progressive disease means an increase of tumor mass by more than 25% or appearance of new tumor lesions. Stable disease is characterized as either a decrease or increase of tumor not meeting criteria for partial response or progressive disease.

14. What are mixed responses to therapy?

If chemotherapy is effective in shrinking disease at one site, it usually has the same effect on all disease-involved sites; thus, the response is uniform. In rare cases, however, there may be tumor shrinkage at one site with tumor growth at another site. This is called a mixed response.

15. Why are multiple cycles of chemotherapy necessary?

Based on observations in experimental systems of animal tumors, it is believed that tumor cell killing is fractional in humans. According to the log cell kill hypothesis, at any given exposure chemotherapy drugs kill only a fraction of the cells. Because visible tumors are usually larger than 10^9 cells and one chemotherapy cycle is of the order of 2–5 log cell kill, it is apparent that treatment must be repeated many times to achieve control and/or cure.

16. Summarize the major advantages of combination chemotherapy.

Most successful chemotherapy programs involve the use of multiple drugs, sometimes following complex schedules of administration. This approach is commonly referred to as combination chemotherapy. By using combinations of drugs, one can get maximal cell kill for each drug within a tolerated range of toxicity, broader range of activity against different subgroups or a heterogeneous tumor population, and prevent or retard the development of new resistant cell lines.

17. What principles govern the use of combination chemotherapy?

1. Only drugs that are active against the tumor to be treated are included in the combination.

2. The drugs should have a different mechanism of action to minimize the possibility of drug resistance.

3. The drugs should have different toxic side effects, thus allowing administration of full or nearly full doses of each active agent.

4. Each drug should be given at an optimal dose and schedule and at consistent intervals.

18. How is a patient's progress with chemotherapy assessed?

Because chemotherapy agents are potentially toxic, one should strive to follow objective markers of response in patients with metastatic disease. Objective markers may include decrease in size of a tumor, disappearance of hypercalcemia or other paraneoplastic syndrome, or decrease or disappearance of a tumor marker such as prostate-specific antigen (PSA) or carcinoembryonic antigen (CEA). Subjective responses such as tumor-related pain or weight gain are less reliable indicators of drug action. An objective determination of performance status gives an accurate estimation of the patient's overall condition and quality of life.

19. What does 5-year survival mean? When is a cancer considered cured?

National statistics about cancer are based on 5-year survival rates. For the most part, patients who are still alive 5 years after initial diagnosis are considered cured. With common tumors such as breast, lung, and colon cancer, recurrences usually follow a bell-curve; the incidence of recurrence peaks at 18–24 months after diagnosis, with few recurrences after 5 years.

20. Define chemoprevention.

Chemoprevention refers to the use of specific chemical agents to prevent the development of a premalignant or malignant lesion or to cause regression of a premalignant lesion. Tamoxifen recently was approved for chemoprevention of high-risk breast cancer. Many large chemoprevention trials are in progress. Examples include breast cancer prevention with raloxifene, prevention of lung and head and neck cancers with the retinoid Accutane, and prevention of prostate cancer with the testosterone inhibitor finasteride (Proscar).

21. Explain biochemical modulation.

The activity of some drugs may be increased or decreased by the presence of other drugs or normal metabolites. This process is called biochemical modulation and is best illustrated by studies of 5-fluorouracil (5-FU). Several chemicals potentiate the activity of 5FU, including methotrexate, thymidine, PALA, allopurinol, uridine, and leucovorin. Leucovorin best modulates 5-FU with beneficial effect for the patient. This combination is commonly used in the adjuvant or palliative treatment of colon cancer. 5-FU works by binding to the enzyme thymidilate synthetase, which leads to depletion of thymidine, a necessary ingredient for DNA synthesis. Reduced folate is a cofactor for 5-FU binding to the enzyme; leucovorin enhances this binding, thus potentiating 5-FU activity. The combination of the two drugs is more potent but also more toxic with increased incidence of mucositis and diarrhea.

22. How is chemotherapy dosed?

Information about dosage is derived from prior empirical dose-escalating trials in patients. Drug dosage is determined as a function of body surface area (BSA) rather than body weight. This convention was adopted because of research relating the maximal tolerated dose of chemotherapy in multiple species to body weight and BSA; it became apparent that interspecies comparison of dose were far more accurate using BSA than weight. Patients who are grossly obese require higher doses of chemotherapy, and their dosing is not calculated on ideal body weight. The chemotherapy dose must be adjusted according to renal and liver function.

23. Does BSA need to be recalculated with weight changes?

Because chemotherapy dosing is based on body surface area, recent weight loss or gain (> 10 pounds) requires recalculation of doses.

24. Explain the concept of dose intensity.

The concept of dose intensity is significant because a major factor limiting the ability to cure cancer is adequate dosing. Dose intensity is defined as the amount of drug given per unit of time ($mg/m^2/week$), regardless of the schedule used. Generally, to cure cancer, it is best to give chemotherapy drugs at the highest dose at the shortest intervals; however, this approach is often difficult because of the low therapeutic index (toxicity to normal tissues) of many chemotherapy agents. There has been increasing concern that patients with cancer may receive inadequate doses of chemotherapy because of inappropriate dose reductions by physicians concerned about drug toxicity. Procedures using high-dose chemotherapy and autologous bone marrow transplant are an example of trying to take advantage of dose intensity treatment.

25. How does gene therapy affect cancer treatment?

Gene therapy can be defined as the introduction of new genetic material into cells for therapeutic intent. Gene therapy has huge potential for cancer treatment. Clinical trials are now in progress, but this approach is still highly investigational.

REFERENCES

1. DeVita VT Jr: Principles of cancer management: Chemotherapy. In DeVita VT, Hellman S, Rosenberg SA (eds): Cancer: Principles and Practice of Oncology, 6th ed. Philadelphia, Lippincott-Raven, 2001, pp 289–306
2. Fisher B, Costantino JP, Wicherham L, et al: Tamoxifen for prevention of breast cancer: Report of the national surgical adjuvant breast and bowel project P-1 study. J Natl Cancer Instit 90:1371–1388, 1998.
3. Fleming ID, Cooper JS, Henson DE, et al (eds): AJCC Cancer Staging Handbook, 5th ed. Philadelphia, Lippincott-Raven, 1998.
4. Lenhard RE, Lawrence W, McKenna RJ: General approach to patients. In Murphy GP, Lawrence W Jr, Lenhard RE Jr (eds): American Cancer Society Textbook of Clinical Oncology, 2nd ed. Atlanta, American Cancer Society, 1995, pp 64–74.
5. Stagno SJ, Zhukovsky DS, Walsh D: Bioethics: Communication and decision-making in advanced disease. Semin Oncol 27:94–100, 2000.
6. Weiss RB: Introduction: Dose-intensive therapy for adult malignancies. Semin Oncol 26:1–5, 1999.

5. SURGICAL ONCOLOGY

Ann Marie Dose, MS, RN, AOCN, CNS-BC, and
Carol Brueggen, MS, RN, AOCN, CNS-BC

1. What is the role of surgery in the prevention of cancer?
Certain people may be at higher risk for development of cancer because of underlying health conditions or congenital or genetic traits. If an organ with potential for development of cancer is not crucial for survival, surgery may be necessary or desirable to prevent malignancy. Surgery may be performed to prevent colon cancer (in cases of familial polyposis), breast cancer, or testicular cancer. Other cancers, such as cervical cancer, develop from a premalignant phase and, even in early stages of malignancy, remain locally confined. Limited surgical excision, laser, or cryotherapy techniques may effectively obliterate or reduce spread of disease.

2. What are the goals of surgery in the treatment of cancer?
1. **Prophylaxis** (see question 1).
2. **Diagnosis.** Tissue biopsy is necessary to validate the diagnosis and to identify the histology or specific type of cancer (see questions 4 and 5).
3. **Staging.** The extent of disease can be determined by surgical staging, which identifies tumor type, extent of growth, size, nodal involvement, and regional and distant spread. Exploratory surgery may be required to stage Hodgkin's disease or ovarian cancer. Sentinel node biopsy can be done for breast cancer or malignant melanoma.
4. **Definitive or curative treatment.** The primary goal of cancer surgery is cure. Definitive or curative surgery involves removing the entire tumor, associated lymph nodes, and a 2–5-cm margin of surrounding tissue. Early diagnosis is essential when the goal is cure. Surgery for early-stage cervical, breast, skin, renal cell, prostate, and colon cancer may be curative. Surgical placement of brachytherapy for cervical and prostate cancers has curative intent.
5. **Palliation.** Surgical intervention for palliation is most commonly done to minimize symptoms of advanced disease and relieve distress. For example, palliative surgeries include cytoreductive surgery; ablative procedures; surgery to relieve gastrointestinal, respiratory, and urinary obstructions or fistulas; and neurosurgical procedures for pain control. Decompressive laminectomy may be done to relieve spinal cord compression secondary to malignancy.
6. **Adjuvant or supportive therapy.** Surgical procedures performed in addition to other treatment modalities are called adjuvant or supportive. Examples include surgery to implant a vascular access device, feeding tube, or tracheostomy.
7. **Reconstructive or rehabilitative therapy.** Advances in plastic and reconstructive surgery have made it possible to repair anatomic defects and to improve function and cosmetic appearance after radical surgery (e.g., breast and head and neck cancer). The goal is to minimize deformity and improve quality of life.
8. **Salvage treatment.** Further surgery is done to treat local disease recurrence after use of a less extensive primary treatment. Examples include salvage radical cystectomy after primary radiation therapy for bladder cancer or salvage mastectomy after primary lumpectomy and radiation therapy for breast cancer.

3. What patient and tumor factors need to be assessed before surgery?
Tumor factors include growth rate, invasiveness, metastatic potential, and location. In general, tumors that are slow-growing and have cells with prolonged cell cycles lend themselves best to local control by surgery. Surgeons need to know the pattern of local invasion for a specific tumor to remove it as an entire mass with adequate normal surrounding tissue to minimize seeding or local recurrence. Some tumor invasions may necessitate more radical surgery; other

tumors may not need total resection if additional chemotherapy and radiation therapy have been demonstrated to improve survival. Metastatic potential of a tumor determines the amount and appropriate combination of multimodal therapies. Location of the tumor and spread into adjacent tissue and vital organs or structures also need to be considered in weighing the risks and benefits of surgical intervention and effect on functional status and overall quality of life.

Patient factors include overall health status and comorbidities, such as diabetes and cardiac, pulmonary, or kidney disease. General health habits, nutritional status, rehabilitation potential, and use of prior oncologic treatment modalities are other issues to explore. Age may be a factor, but it is relevant only in the face of overall general health status and quality of life.

4. Why are biopsies important in cancer care?

A biopsy is performed to confirm or diagnose cancer correctly. A biopsy consists of removing a tissue sample from an organ or other part of the body for histologic examination by a pathologist. A positive biopsy indicates the presence of cancer, whereas a negative biopsy may indicate that no cancer is present or that the biopsy specimen was not adequate. When a biopsy is negative but cancer is still suspected, further investigation is required.

5. What different types of biopsies and surgical procedures are performed?

The ideal biopsy method should be relatively inexpensive and noninvasive, convenient for patients, and easy to perform while providing enough information to deliver a preliminary cancer diagnosis. The type of surgical procedure is determined by preoperative evaluation of tumor involvement and individual health considerations and preferences. Numerous types of biopsies and surgical procedures are available, each with different uses and advantages and disadvantages.

Surgical Procedures in Patients with Cancer

TYPE	USE	ADVANTAGES	DISADVANTAGES
Incisional biopsy	Obtain tissue for pathology exam	Simple method to obtain diagnosis	Additional, more extensive surgical procedure generally done to remove tumor
Excisional biopsy	Establish tissue diagnosis and tumor removal	Quick, simple removal of tumor at biopsy; may not require hospitalization; decreased cost; minimal cosmetic effects	Tumor cells may be implanted along surgical path and incision, resulting in local recurrence
Needle biopsy	Obtain tissue for pathology exam	Simple to perform, reliable, inexpensive, performed under local anesthesia on outpatient basis	Risk of injury to adjacent structures; risk of tumor cell implantation along needle track and recurrence
Diagnostic laparotomy	Determine stage and extent of disease	Provides more accurate information for treatment planning	Major surgical procedure with risk for postoperative complications; requires hospital stay, costly, multiple lifestyle disruptions
Local excision	Primary treatment Cytoreductive surgery Removal of solitary metastasis Palliation	Minimal tissue removal with little effect on functional status and appearance; may require no or short hospital stay	Risk of microscopic residual disease in tissue, resulting in local recurrence
Wide excision	Primary treatment Cytoreductive surgery Prophylactic surgery	Eliminates visible and microscopic disease locally and in adjacent tissue at increased risk for disease spread	Longer, more involved rehabilitation required; may cause major changs in functional ability and appearance; may require reconstructive surgery

Table continued on following page

Surgical Procedures in Patients with Cancer (Continued)

TYPE	USE	ADVANTAGES	DISADVANTAGES
Laser surgery	Primary treatment Cytoreductive surgery Palliation	Can be used in all body systems; decreased blood loss and need for blood products; decreased local recurrence rates; minimal side effects, including minimal pain during and after surgery; decreased wound drainage; earlier return of functional ability; reduced incidence of functional disabilities; minimal preparation time and easy to deliver; decreased procedure time; decreased or no hospital stay; may be repeated on recurrent tumor; immediate graft possible; may be done when traditional surgery is contraindicated (e.g., by tumor location, poor health status of patient)	None noted
Photodynamic therapy	Primary treatment	More precise in locating cancer cells, particularly when all sites of disease are unknown; decreased risks and variety of side effects compared with traditional surgery	Photosensitivity for 4–6 weeks, causing possible lifestyle disruptions
Stereotaxis	Obtain biopsy Primary treatment Cytoreductive surgery Implantation of radioactive sources, hyperthermia, or chemotherapeutic agents Perform thalamotomy for intractable pain or tremor	Minimizes exposed and affected tissue; less trauma to brain tissue than traditional approaches with decreased neurologic deficits; shorter hospital stay and reduced hospitalization costs; lower mortality and morbidity rates	Use depends on size and location of tumor and current expertise and technology in imaging modalities and computer technology Neurologic side effects depend on size and location of tumor
Laparoscopic surgery	Primary treatment	Decreased postoperative pain and procedure-related complications; earlier recovery and return to activities of daily living Shorter hospital stay and lower treatment costs	Use depends on size and location of primary tumor and presence of regional disease; anatomic defects may limit access and use; inconclusive data about long-term effect on prognosis

From Itano JK, Taoka KN (eds): Core Curriculum for Oncology Nursing, 3rd ed Philadelphia, W.B. Saunders, 1998, with permission.

6. Why is surgery sometimes done when metastasis is present?

In certain situations, when the primary tumor has been resected or is in remission, resecting solitary metastatic tumors may be appropriate. In patients with evidence of multiple metastatic lesions or aggressive tumors, resection is not indicated. The following factors must be considered before surgical intervention is attempted: (1) histology of the tumor, (2) disease-free interval, (3)

tumor doubling time, (4) tumor size and location, (5) rate of metastasis, and (6) patient's performance status. Studies have reported successful resection of solitary metastatic tumors of the lung,
liver, brain, and bone.

7. How does surgical staging differ from clinical staging?

Clinical staging includes findings acquired before definitive treatment: physical examinations, imaging, endoscopy, biopsy, and some surgical exploration. Surgical evaluative and pathologic staging is done after surgery, including lymph node studies.

Staging of Cancer

TYPE	METHOD	DATABASE	COMMENT
Clinical diagnosis	Physical exam X-rays and scans Biopsy	All information available before definitive treat- ment	Almost all cancers are clinically staged Accuracy limited
Surgical evaluation	Biopsy Exploratory surgery with intraoperative palpation ± biopsies Sentinel node biopsy	All clinical information Histology from biopsies	More information needed for definitive treatment decision (e.g., laparotomy for Hodgkin's disease, mediastinoscopy for lung primary)
Postsurgical pathology	Resection of tumor, often including nodes	Histologic information about all resected tissues	Comprehensive histologic in- formation about tumor ± regional nodes or organs

Adapted form Knobf MKT: Cancer treatment—Surgery. In Johnson BL, Gross J: Handbook of Oncology
Nursing, 3rd ed. Boston, Jones & Bartlett, 1998, pp 22–36.

8. What nursing issues should be considered preoperatively?

The nurse provides education and psychosocial support to patient and family. Preoperative
teaching should include discussion of the extent of the planned surgery and any expected functional
limitations. Issues of concern should be clarified, and sources of support should be identified and discussed. Instructions about the use of any equipment, pulmonary exercises, coughing techniques, and
pain management options should be provided. Because of shortened postoperative hospital stays, it is
also beneficial to do an initial discharge assessment preoperatively. Factors that may influence discharge planning include home environment, financial status, self-care abilities, anticipated postoperative self-care abilities, available family and agency support, employment status, and type of work. It
is common for patients and families to experience anxiety. As the nurse interacts with patients and
families preoperatively, their concerns related to the uncertainty of long-term survival and the possible need for further treatment should be assessed and addressed. Because anxiety reduces a patient's
ability to understand and retain information, teaching should be reinforced as appropriate.

9. What nursing issues should be considered postoperatively?

Because of decreased hospital stays and the potential for fragmentation of care as patients are
seen by the primary care provider, surgeon, and other specialists, it is even more imperative for
nurses to communicate and collaborate with one another. Generic components of postoperative nursing care include assessment, patient education, emotional support, physical care, and rehabilitation.

10. What topics should be included in postoperative patient education?

The challenges of teaching patients and family members what they need to know to provide
care after hospital discharge are increased by shortened hospital stays and increased complexities
of surgical interventions. Patients and families need to know about prescribed medications, ongoing wound care, signs and symptoms of infection, appropriate nutrition, proper balance of rest
and exercise, care of catheters or ostomies, and where and when to return for postoperative examinations. Communication with agencies providing care after hospitalization, such as home
care agencies or nursing homes, is key to ensuring continuity of care. If additional chemotherapy

or radiation therapy is scheduled, baseline teaching can be done if the patient and family are ready and receptive. Use of anatomic models enhances patient learning.

11. Discuss the important aspects of physical care in the postoperative period.

Physical care centers on general surgical nursing principles, with specific focus on pain management, wound care, nutrition, hemostasis, and prevention of complications (see table below). Good pain control can improve patient satisfaction, promote healing, reduce recovery time, and decrease postoperative complications. Postoperative pain can be managed in many ways, including administration of opioids by patient-controlled analgesia (PCA) and continuous epidural analgesia; addition of injectable nonsteroidal anti-inflammatory drugs (NSAIDs), such as ketorolac (Toradol), to traditional intravenous opioids; and various nondrug methods to decrease anxiety and pain (see Chapter 46).

Complications after Surgery for Cancer

COMPLICATION	CONTRIBUTING FACTORS	
Acute respiratory distress syndrome	Hemorrhage Aspiration Prolonged atelectasis Infection Pulmonary edema	Deposition of platelets Trauma to lung parenchyma Cardiopulmonary bypass Pulmonary emboli
Aspiration pneumonia	Difficulty in swallowing Mechanical obstruction from cancer	Excessive sedation
Bleeding	Prolonged cardiopulmonary bypass Medications	Coagulopathy
Cardiovascular dysfunction	Congestive heart failure Myocardial infarction	Arrhythmias
Infection	Neutropenia Cell-mediated deficiencies Humoral-mediated deficiencies	Splenectomy Transfusion-transmitted infections Disruptions of mechanical barriers
Mucositis	Antimetabolite chemotherapeutic agents	Head and neck radiation Dehydration
Obstruction/ileus	Immobility Opioids	Other medications
Poor wound healing	Malnutrition Neutropenia Chemotherapy Previous radiation therapy	Steroid therapy Local tumor invasion Immune dysfunction Pressure ulcer formation

Adapted from Polomano R, Weintraub FN, Wurster A: Surgical critical care for cancer patients: Semin Oncol Nurs 10:165–176, 1994; and Burke C: Surgery: In Liebman MC, Camp-Sorrell D (eds): Multimodal Therapy in Oncology Nursing. St. Louis, Mosby, 1996, pp 34–43.

12. Does ketorolac increase the risk of bleeding?

Ketorolac tromethamine (Toradol) is a parenteral NSAID that is useful for acute postoperative pain. It is especially helpful for bone pain, chest tube pain, or inflammation. Depending on the type of surgical procedure, ketorolac is associated with a small increased risk for overall operative-site bleeding and gastrointestinal (GI) bleeding. To prevent adverse effects, ketorolac should be given in low doses of 105 mg/day or less for 5 or fewer days. The usual adult dose is 30 mg intravenously (IV) or intramuscularly (IM) every 6–8 hours as needed. Patients who are older than 65 years, frail, or renally impaired may not be candidates for ketorolac or should receive a smaller dose (15 mg IV or IM). Contraindications include an active GI ulcer, bleeding, renal impairment, volume depletion, aspirin or NSAID allergy, coagulopathy, pregnancy, or lactation.

13. What factors should be considered in the assessment and care of surgical wounds?

Wound assessment should include length, width, depth, location, and direction of the wound as well as descriptions of the base, edges, and any exudate. Factors that can delay wound healing include age, obesity, prior chemotherapy or radiation therapy, malnutrition, and diabetes. If the surrounding tissue is compromised or a deep pocket of infection exists, wounds may be left to heal on their own (from the inside out). Dressings may be used to protect the wound, to promote comfort, to immobilize wound edges, and to maintain a moist environment.

14. Does nutritional status affect surgical outcome?

Nutritional status before surgery can significantly affect outcome. Protein/calorie malnutrition, a common problem in patients with prior treatment and compromised immune status, may lead to wound dehiscence, ileus, sepsis, and increased hospital stay. Perioperative and postoperative support in the form of high protein/calorie oral diets, enteral tube feedings, and total parenteral nutrition (TPN) can significantly decrease morbidity and mortality.

15. Are patients with cancer at increased risk for hemostatic or bleeding problems?

Altered hemostasis in the form of hypercoagulability and thrombosis can put the patient with cancer at higher risk for postoperative complications. Some patients have been reported to have elevated clotting factors, shortened partial thromboplastin time, or hemorrhage. Common cancer types include adenocarcinoma of the lung, pancreas, and colon. Early postoperative ambulation is imperative to prevent thrombophlebitis.

16. What factors should be considered in postoperative rehabilitation?

Rehabilitation centers on meeting physical, psychosocial, sexual, spiritual, educational, vocational, and financial needs. It begins preoperatively and continues postoperatively. Nursing interventions should be individualized according to patients' needs and priorities. Common nursing diagnoses include body image disturbance related to disfigurement, impaired tissue integrity, and decreased self-esteem. For example, some patients may have no desire to address workplace issues and concerns in the first few days after surgery; others may have increased pain and/or lack of sleep related to anxieties and worries about how they will continue to provide for their families. Thorough and ongoing assessment is imperative to discover the "real" issues.

17. How soon after surgery can adjuvant chemotherapy and radiation therapy begin?

Certain antineoplastic agents and radiation doses interfere with wound healing; thus, special consideration must be given to the timing of adjuvant therapy. Adjuvant therapy can be started as early as a few days after surgery, but in many instances a recovery time of 3–6 weeks is standard. Some patients with cancer are at greater risk for postoperative complications such as bleeding and infection.

18. What has changed in cancer surgery over the past 25–30 years?

Surgeries that originated as radical procedures to remove tumors with adequate tissue margins have become more conservative, enhancing overall quality of life and promoting rehabilitation. In addition, as more is understood about how cancers originate and metastasize, the proper combination of surgery, chemotherapy, radiation and biological therapy has emerged. Multimodal therapy has improved cure and control rates for many cancers. Surgery has played a major role in the cure of breast, colorectal, and thyroid cancers and melanoma. Technologic advances in surgery, such as the use of lasers, stapling devices, and microsurgery, have further contributed to the array of surgical options.

19. If a tumor is exposed to air during surgery, will the cancer spread?

A common myth is that surgery may cause cancer to spread by exposing cancerous cells to air. This myth is not true. Cancer does not spread because it has been exposed to the air. Patients sometimes feel worse after surgery than before surgery because of incisional discomfort and organ manipulation. This feeling is normal. Surgery also can lower immune response, and if the cancer is found to be more advanced at the time of surgery than originally thought, the patient may be more susceptible to postoperative complications. Because early removal of all cancer cells provides the best chance of cure, people should not allow this myth to prevent them from seeking surgery.

20. What is "seeding"?

Seeding means that the cancer has spread, with the occurrence of small nodules in the peritoneum or wound. Seeding may occur in an area where surgery has been performed previously.

21. What types of surgeries are indicated for rehabilitation?

After radical surgery, many wounds do not close adequately, or enough skin, muscle, or subcutaneous tissue may not be available for satisfactory results. Reconstructive surgery may be indicated to promote self-esteem and body image, to enhance quality of life, and to improve certain physical functions. Examples include breast reconstruction, facial reconstruction for head and neck cancers, and skin grafting after melanoma removal.

22. Should a surgeon say, "I got it all"?

In general, when a surgeon says, "I got it all," he or she means that the tumor was removed in its entirety, the margins were clean or free of cancer cells, and there was no evidence of lymph node or metastatic spread. This statement should be made with caution because approximately 70% of patients have evidence of micrometastases at the time of diagnosis. Surgery alone can be curative in patients with localized disease, but often it is necessary to combine surgery with other treatment modalities to achieve higher response rates.

It may be less misleading to the patient if the surgeon says, "Apparently there is no evidence of cancer left behind. In one to two days, we'll have a pathology report that will give us more information. If the pathology is clear at the margins, there is a good chance that it's all been removed. There is a chance, however, that microscopic disease has already spread. That is why it is important to see a medical oncologist to talk about chemotherapy."

23. What is a second-look procedure?

Second-look surgery is an exploratory laparotomy performed to stage cancer more accurately after completion of initial treatment, to determine treatment response, and to plan for possible further therapy. Its use may be less common with advances in diagnostic imaging. It may be used in ovarian cancer and other solid tumors in the face of rising tumor markers and negative clinical work-ups for metastasis, but not all surgeons agree that it is the best practice.

24. What does it mean when a surgeon says, "We got adequate margins"?

The surgeon needs to remove not only the tumor but also enough surrounding tissue to prevent local spread of disease. The amount of surrounding tissue that needs to be removed varies with the type of cancer and site of involvement. Margins range from 2–5 cm of "normal" tissue in solid tumors to wide excision for primary melanomas in the skin. How to define "adequate margins" is still under question.

25. What is conscious sedation?

Conscious sedation is a medically controlled state of depressed consciousness that (1) allows protective reflexes to be maintained; (2) retains the patient's ability to maintain a patent airway independently and continuously; and (3) permits appropriate response by the patient to physical stimulation or verbal command. Indications for conscious sedation include complex wound care and bone marrow biopsy.

REFERENCES

1. Alavassevich M, McKibbon A, Thomas S: Information and needs of patients who undergo surgery for head and neck cancer. Can Oncol Nurs 5:9–11, 1995.
2. Burke C: Surgery. In Liebman MC, Camp-Sorrell D (eds): Multimodal Therapy in Oncology Nursing. St. Louis, Mosby, 1996, pp 34–43.
3. Fleming ID, Cooper JS, Henson DE, et al (eds): AJCC Cancer Staging Handbook, 5th ed. Philadelphia, Lippincott-Raven, 1998.
4. Frogge MH, Cunning SM: Surgical therapy. In Yarbro CH, Frogge MH, Goodman M, Groenwald SL (eds): Cancer Nursing: Principles and Practice, 5th ed. Boston, Jones & Bartlett, 2000, pp 272–285.
5. Itano JK, Taoka KN: Core Curriculum for Oncology Nursing, 3rd ed. Philadelphia, W.B. Saunders, 1998, pp 606–607.
6. Knobf MT: Cancer treatment–Surgery. In Johnson BL, Gross J (eds): Handbook of Oncology Nursing, 3rd ed. Boston, Jones & Bartlett, 1998, pp 22–36.
7. McCorkle R, Grant M, Frank-Stromberg M, Baird SB: Cancer Nursing: A Comprehensive Textbook, 2nd ed. Philadelphia, W.B. Saunders, 1996.
8. Polomano R, Weintraub FN, Wurster A: Surgical critical care for cancer patients. Semin Oncol Nurs 10:165–176, 1994.
9. Rosenberg SA: Principles of surgical oncology. In DeVita VT, Hellman S, Rosenberg SA (eds): Cancer: Principles and Practice of Oncology, 6th ed. Philadelphia, Lippincott Williams & Wilkins, 2001, pp 253–264.
10. Srom BL, Berlin JA, Kinman JA, et al: Parenteral ketorolac and risk of gastrointestinal and operative-site bleeding: A postmarketing surveillance study. JAMA 275:376–382, 1996.
11. U.S. Department of Health and Human Services, Agency for Health Care Policy and Research: Clinical Practice Guideline for Acute Pain Management: Operative or Medical Procedures and Trauma. AHCPR Pub. No. 92-0032. Rockville, MD, Agency for Health Care Policy and Research, Public Health Service, U.S. Dept. of Health and Human Services, 1992.

6. RADIATION THERAPY

Laura J. Hilderley, RN, MS

1. When was radiation first used to treat cancer?

The therapeutic use of ionizing radiation began in the early 20th century after the discoveries of Roentgen and the Curies, who observed its effect on human tissues. For many years, little was known about controlling the total radiation dose or protecting healthy tissue from radiation damage. Although therapeutic results were sometimes quite remarkable, severe side effects contributed to misunderstanding and fear of radiation. During the second half of the 20th century research efforts resulted in detailed understanding of the physical and biologic effects of ionizing radiation and its application in the treatment of cancer. Radiation therapy is now one of the primary modalities used in cancer treatment. It is used either alone or, more commonly, in combination with surgery, chemotherapy, or immunotherapy.

2. How does radiation work?

Ionizing radiation targets tissue at the cellular level, either directly by damaging DNA or indirectly by affecting the medium (primarily water) surrounding the cells. When DNA is damaged or destroyed, cell division is delayed or prevented, thus stopping the growth of targeted tissue. The challenge for the radiation oncologist is to achieve maximal therapeutic benefit (tumor destruction) while protecting and preserving healthy tissue. Cancer cells undergo frequent division and growth. These highly mitotic cells are more vulnerable to radiation damage than cells that do not divide or do so infrequently. Thus, most cancers are susceptible to radiation effect and are described as radiosensitive or radioresponsive. Some types of cancer are radioresistant and do not respond to the usual doses of radiation. Radioresistance may be overcome by combined chemoradiotherapy, higher-than-usual doses, or altered fractionation schedules (e.g., > 1 treatment/day).

3. What produces the side effects of radiation therapy?

Normal, healthy tissue is also radiosensitive. Healthy cells are inevitably present in any treatment site or field, and are therefore subject to radiation effect. The response of healthy tissue in the treatment site produces the familiar side effects of skin reaction, hair loss, and gastrointestinal disturbances. However, healthy cells can recover from radiation injury that occurs during controlled therapeutic exposure, and side effects are rarely permanent.

4. List and explain the three roles of radiation in cancer treatment.

1. **Curative intent.** Several cancers (e.g., early-stage cancer of the larynx, Hodgkin's disease, prostate and skin cancers) are curable with radiation alone.

2. **Adjuvant intent.** When used after definitive surgery (e.g., orchiectomy for seminoma, lumpectomy for breast cancer), radiation is an adjuvant treatment.

3. **Palliative intent.** Palliation of symptoms (see questions 41–43) with radiation therapy has long been a primary and highly effective application. Bleeding, ulceration, neurologic symptoms, and obstruction due to tumor mass can be effectively controlled, often with a short course of treatment. Relief of pain, especially from bone metastases, can be quite dramatic. When cure is not possible, symptom control with radiation therapy can substantially improve quality of life for many patients.

5. What is the goal of radiation treatment? Who makes up the treatment team?

The goal of radiation therapy is to eradicate the cancer while sparing healthy tissue. Achieving this therapeutic ratio requires skill and input from all members of the radiation oncology team. Radiation oncologists, radiation therapists (formerly called technologists), dosimetrists, radiation physicists, computer scientists, radiobiologists, nurses, and, from time to time, other professionals (e.g., dietitian, social worker, clergy) may be involved. The patient and family are key team members.

6. How is the specific course of treatment determined?

Each patient's treatment plan is determined through a combination of personal and other factors, including the following:
- Histology and characteristics of the cancer (stage, grade, location, usual route of spread)
- Prior, concomitant, or future treatment with other modalities
- Patient's general condition, prognosis, and personal choices
- Availability of and eligibility for clinical trials
- Access to specific types of radiation delivery systems

7. What takes place during simulation and treatment planning?

Before any treatment is given, certain physical parameters must be determined, treatment volume calculated, and appropriate equipment selected. In addition, the patient must be fully informed and carefully guided through the process.

The radiation oncologist, physicist, dosimetrist, and radiation therapist are largely responsible for the precise determination of the treatment field and volume. Target volume is defined with the aid of the simulator, physical measurements, computed tomography (CT) scans and other diagnostic images, sophisticated three-dimensional(3-D) computer programs, and virtual imaging techniques. During the simulation process temporary ink marks are drawn on the patient's skin to help identify the treatment field. These lines later are replaced with a few tiny permanent tattoos that mark several coordinate points used to ensure accurate reproduction of the field at each treatment.

Some patients may require assistive devices to help with positioning or immobilization during treatment. Children particularly may need to be restrained to ensure accuracy. Assistive devices, including armboards, head and neck masks, and various casts, are designed during the simulation process.

8. What is the nurse's primary role during simulation?

Simulation may take up to 1 hour, depending on the complexity of the treatment plan. The process can be tiring and stressful for the patient. The nurse's role in simulation is to provide information before the process begins and supportive care throughout. The well-informed patient is better able to tolerate the sometimes lengthy process.

9. How is damage to healthy tissue minimized during radiation treatment?

During the simulation and treatment planning process, careful attention is focused on targeting the tumor precisely to avoid as much healthy tissue as possible. Lead alloy blocks can be shaped to conform to specific areas in need of shielding from the treatment beam. These blocks are secured to a tray fitted to the head of the treatment machine and positioned between the beam and the patient so that the blocked area is protected from radiation. Simulators and teletherapy equipment often are linked with sophisticated computer systems, which enable the therapy team to produce 3-D images of the patient's anatomy. Treatment volume and actual shape and dimensions of the target site can be adjusted, excluding or at least minimizing the dose to healthy tissues.

10. What factors complicate delivery of focused treatment? How are they managed?

Various factors continue to challenge the radiation oncologist and other team members in defining target volume and delivering focused treatment, including tumors with highly irregular shapes, tumors adjacent to highly radiosensitive structures, and tumors surrounded by complex anatomy. The introduction and refinement of 3-D computer planning and treatment delivery has markedly increased the ability to deliver larger doses to more clearly delineated targets. Three-dimensional conformal radiation therapy has resulted in greater tumor control, with reduced complications. This technique is used primarily for treatment of nonmetastatic prostate cancer but also has been used to treat lung, esophageal, head and neck, and hepatobiliary sites.

11. Summarize the requirements of 3-D radiation treatment.

Three-dimensional treatment requires immobilization of the patient by means of a body cast, followed by reconstruction of the target using the 3-D computer planning program and CT scans obtained with the patient in the cast. Finally, multiple angled beams are selected to focus on the target volume in contrast to the usual four-field technique. Adding to the precision of 3-D treatment, the newer linear accelerators may be equipped with a multileaf collimator consisting of 20–40 matched pairs of lead leaves fitted to the jaws or opening in the accelerator head. The leaves are controlled individually by the computer to move in and out of the path of the beam, adjusting the treatment field to the desired shape.

12. Explain the two basic methods of delivering radiation therapy.

The most commonly used method is **teletherapy** or treatment delivered from a machine or source at a distance from the body. Teletherapy also is called external-beam therapy. **Brachytherapy** involves the use of radioactive sources placed in direct contact with the treatment target via implanted needles, wires, or seeds or intracavitary placement of applicators containing the source. Except for implanted radioactive seeds, brachytherapy applicators are removed when treatment is completed.

13. What type of equipment is used for teletherapy?

Linear accelerators (sometimes called linacs) have a range of energies (photon and electron) that allows treatment at varying depths within the body. Photons are used for lesions deeper within the body; electrons are suited for treatment close to the surface.

Cobalt teletherapy machines contain a radioactive cobalt source that emits gamma energy equivalent to the deeply penetrating photons. Because cobalt is a radioactive element, it is constantly emitting (losing) energy; therefore, the source must be replaced every few years.

14. How is brachytherapy delivered?

Brachytherapy can be delivered using low-dose rate (LDR) or high-dose rate (HDR) sources.

15. Compare LDR and HDR.

LDR treatment generally requires hospitalization for several days, during which the patient is isolated to protect others from exposure to radioactivity. The patient also may be confined to bed to prevent dislodgment of the applicator. Disadvantages include potential complications of prolonged bedrest, discomfort, hospitalization costs, and radiation exposure to staff delivering bedside care.

HDR treatment has the distinct advantages of outpatient delivery and completion in several treatments, each lasting only a few minutes. Hospitalization and bedrest with its concomitant risks can be avoided. The staff is not exposed to radiation because treatments are given with the patient inside a shielded room, using a remote delivery system.

16. Discuss the role of brachytherapy in the treatment of cancer.

Brachytherapy may be used as the only method of treatment delivery. More commonly, however, it is combined with teletherapy and given as a boost dose either before or after a larger field has been treated with external-beam teletherapy. The teletherapy field encompasses the tumor site and may extend to cover regional lymph nodes or local extension of disease. Brachytherapy delivers a full dose directly to the tumor or tumor bed.

17. Which radioactive sources are used to deliver brachytherapy?

Radioactive sources used to deliver brachytherapy include iridium-192, cesium-137, iodine-131 and iodine-125, gold-198, phosphorus-32, radium-226, and strontium-90.

18. How do nurses caring for patients undergoing brachytherapy protect themselves from radiation exposure?

Federal and state regulatory agencies govern the use of radioactive sources and have established maximum permissible dose (MPD) for radiation workers. Each institution using radioactive materials must be licensed to do so and must have a radiation safety officer, who is

responsible for ensuring that federal and state regulations are followed. Radiation safety principles are based on the **ALARA** concept: exposure should be **as low as** reasonably achievable. All
who are involved in the care of radioactive patients must receive continuing education and wear a
film badge that records exposure. Badges are checked regularly to ensure that the worker is practicing within safe parameters. Key components of radiation safety include understanding and following institutional guidelines and the three cardinal principles of radiation safety:

Time: minimize time spent near the source.

Distance: maximize distance from the source.

Shielding: use protective barriers between source and worker whenever possible.

19. How is radiation dose expressed?

Before 1985 the unit of radiation dose was called a rad (radiation absorbed dose), and this
term is still found in the literature. However, the accepted unit of radiation dose is the gray or Gy.
One Gy equals 100 centigray (cGy). One cGy equals 1 rad.

20. Describe the usual regimen of radiation treatment.

The average total dose for external-beam therapy is 4500 cGy (45 Gy) given in 25 treatments
over 5 weeks (5 days/week) at 180 cGy/day. Both shorter and longer courses of treatment may be
used, ranging from 2–8 weeks with varying total doses. In general, a shorter course of treatment
is given with palliative intent, whereas average or longer courses are given when cure or long-
term disease control is the goal.

21. What are the acute side effects of radiation therapy?

Side effects that occur during a course of treatment and subside within 1 or 2 weeks after
completion are considered acute. Acute side effects occur in tissues with rapid renewal characteristics. Skin, mucous membranes, salivary glands, and bone marrow are among the tissues most
susceptible to radiation effect and are likely to exhibit acute reactions. Side effects are site-specific and are seen in the irradiated tissues. For example, prostate treatment can cause diarrhea but
not scalp alopecia. Dysphagia is a common side effect with radiation for lung cancer, but oral
mucositis is not expected. Fatigue, anorexia, and possible bone marrow depression are the only
generalized side effects of local radiation. Examples of other site-specific side effects include
alopecia, xerostomia, mucositis, taste alterations, pharyngitis, esophagitis, gastritis, cystitis,
sexual dysfunction, edema, lymphedema, and cerebral edema.

22. What factors determine the severity of acute side effects?

Side effects usually can be predicted from the volume of normal tissue exposed to the beam,
the total dose delivered, and the sensitivity of the normal tissue to radiation. Age, nutritional status,
and prior or concomitant chemotherapy also contribute to the severity of acute side effects. The
larger the treated volume of normal tissue, the more likely the patient is to develop side effects.

23. How are the acute side effects of radiation therapy treated?

Most acute side effects are transient and can be managed symptomatically with appropriate
medications and supportive care. Acute side effects usually abate after completion of therapy. If side
effects such as nausea or diarrhea persist after 1 or 2 weeks, other causes should be investigated.

24. Discuss the late or chronic side effects of radiation therapy.

Late or chronic side effects of radiation are local, usually permanent reactions that may develop several months to years after radiation is completed. The severity of acute side effects does
not predict the development of late effects. Similarly, late effects can develop in tissues that exhibited no acute response. The daily dose fraction tends to predict the severity of chronic side effects.
As the daily dose increases, the normal tissue loses its ability to maintain adequate repair and
long-term damage tends to be worse. Late-reacting tissues include skin, spinal cord, bone, and
organs such as lung, liver, and gonads. Although the risk for developing most of these late effects
is small, patients must be fully informed about risks as well as benefits before therapy begins.

25. List examples of possible site-specific late effects.

- Cataracts
- Xerostomia
- Dental caries
- Taste changes
- Head and neck flap necrosis
- Esophageal stricture or fistula
- Hypothyroidism
- Pneumonitis and pulmonary fibrosis
- Pericarditis
- Bowel adhesions
- Proctitis or enteritis
- Cystitis
- Vaginal fibrosis
- Infertility
- Osteoradionecrosis
- Myelopathies
- Permanent depilation
- Skin pigmentation changes
- Second malignancies

26. How can the nurse help to prepare a patient for radiation treatment?

The most powerful tool that nurses can offer to patients and their families is information. Radiation is poorly understood and surrounded by tales from the past about severe skin reactions and acute nausea and vomiting. This concern can produce unwarranted worry and anxiety, interfering with timely initiation and completion of therapy. The nurse as educator must first understand radiation treatment and appreciate its role in relation to other modalities. A visit to the radiation department or freestanding facility can be helpful for both nurse and patient. Nurses also can ask colleagues working in radiation to provide information and clarification for a patient before the initial consultation.

27. What psychological issues should the nurse keep in mind?

When preparing patients for radiation, the nurse should acknowledge each patient as an individual. The diagnosis of cancer can be overwhelming, interfering with the ability to make sound decisions. Because patients often feel out of control of their lives, they should be given reasonable time and full information to help in their decision making. The nurse's open and caring attitude allows patients to feel safe in expressing concerns that they may feel reluctant to present to the doctor. Nurses can empower patients to reach good decisions about their care and treatments by:

- Educating patients about the disease, treatment, anticipated side effects, and expected outcome
- Acknowledging patients' feelings
- Including patients as primary participants in their health care
- Providing nonjudgmental support

28. Why do patients receiving combined chemotherapy and radiation seem to have worse side effects?

Certain chemotherapeutic agents (e.g., 5-fluorouracil, cisplatin, mitomycin-C) enhance the cell-killing effect of radiation. Precisely for this reason such drugs often are combined with radiation in an attempt to produce optimal therapeutic results. Ideally, the combined effect on the tumor will be greater than the sum of the two types of treatment used alone. However, the intensity of side effects in the targeted tissues also is increased. Patients must be fully informed about these anticipated effects and prepared to deal with them. An example of the combined approach with potential for severe local reaction is treatment of high-grade squamous cell cancers of the head and neck.

29. How can acute oropharyngeal reactions be managed?

Radiation reactions in the highly sensitive mucous membranes of the oral cavity, oropharynx, and esophagus are among the most challenging for patients and caregivers alike. Whenever possible, several steps should be taken in anticipation of the reaction:

- Fully inform patients and families, ensuring them of support.
- Maximize nutritional status before starting treatment.
- Refer patients to a dentist for dental prophylaxis and fluoride treatment.

• Consider insertion of a gastrostomy feeding tube before treatment if intake is likely to be severely compromised.
• Emphasize the importance of cessation from smoking and alcohol.

30. Describe the appropriate nursing assessment and management of mucosal reactions.

1. Daily assessment for potential reaction, including observation of erythema, xerostomia, mucositis, bleeding, ulceration, or moniliasis. Assess symptoms of discomfort, pain, taste changes, dysphagia, anorexia.
2. Begin daily mouth care regimen according to institutional guidelines.
3. Weigh patients weekly or more often, as indicated.
4. Assess intake, offering supplements and suggestions for well-tolerated foods.
5. Arrange to talk with the cook in the family, not just the patient.
6. Use written resources for patient information about oral care and nutrition.
7. Refer to dietitian as appropriate.
8. Reconsider use of gastrostomy feeding tube if indicated.
9. Obtain orders for medications such as analgesics, antifungals, antibiotics, oral solutions for topical application, as appropriate.
10. Monitor blood counts.
11. Offer continued psychosocial support, reinforcing the fact that acute symptoms will subside.

31. Is skin reaction inevitable? Describe the range of reactions.

Skin in the treatment field can be expected to show some response to most courses of radiation. There may be more than a single site or portal of entry, and the exit portal also should receive monitoring and care. Skin reactions vary from slight erythema to severe moist desquamation; occasionally the patient has nothing more than dry skin at the treatment site. Reaction varies with anatomic site, concomitant therapies, characteristics of treatment equipment, and total radiation dose. Skin folds, moist areas, and opposing skin surfaces subject to friction are likely to develop more intense reactions. Prepare the patient with information about what to expect as well as assurance that acute reactions will heal within a few weeks after treatment with minimal visible skin change. Patients also need to know that a skin reaction does not always start to subside when treatment ends. In fact, the reaction may peak during the week after treatment, then subside gradually.

32. What is the focus of skin care?

Skin care focuses on patient comfort, promotion of healing, and prevention of infection. Nurses should inspect skin in the treatment area for preexisting cutaneous conditions, including dryness, thinning, and infection (particularly fungal). Treat infections with antifungal/antibiotic creams as indicated.

33. Which skin care products are appropriate for patients undergoing radiation therapy?

Numerous skin care products are available both by prescription and over the counter. Erythematous skin or skin that has developed dry desquamation can be soothed with lotions and creams containing aloe, lanolin, petrolatum, vitamins A and D, and other moisturizing components. A 1% hydrocortisone cream eases pruritus. Avoid preparations containing alcohol, witch hazel, or menthol ingredients because they are drying and astringent. A light dusting of cornstarch may soothe erythematous skin. However, do not use both cornstarch and an ointment or cream because the resulting paste is irritating, especially in skin folds and creases. When moist desquamation occurs, apply antibiotic creams such as silver sulfadiazine. A solution of hydrogen peroxide and saline (1:2) is sometimes used to cleanse an area of moist desquamation before applying an antibiotic cream. Moisture- and vapor-permeable and gel-type dressings are soothing and aid in healing larger areas of moist desquamation.

34. How can patients and family help to minimize skin reactions?

• Cleanse the skin gently with mild soap.
• Avoid friction from clothing (e.g., belts, collars, shoulder straps, bras).

• Avoid exposure of treated areas to the sun and extremes of heat or cold.
• On the treated area use only skin care products recommended by the treating facility.
• Do not apply skin care products to the treatment site for several hours prior to daily treatment.
• Apply skin care products gently. Do not rub in; friction contributes to loss of skin integrity.

35. Why is radiation so tiring?

Fatigue during and after a course of radiation is well documented, but the cause is largely unknown. Some authoritites theorize that the increased energy expenditure needed to rid the body of toxins produced by tumor breakdown may be an important factor. In addition, the necessity for daily travel to the radiation facility may be a significant source of fatigue for some patients. Fatigue tends to increase as the course of treatment continues and generally is more pronounced in the late afternoon, regardless of the time of day when treatment is given. Some patients have described radiation fatigue as a constant that never diminishes even after a long nap or good night's sleep. The following factors are likely to contribute to radiation fatigue and should be addressed:

• Pain
• Insufficient intake/dehydration
• Anemia
• Decreased activity
• Fever
• Anxiety/depression

36. What suggestions may help patients to deal with fatigue?

1. Restful sleep is best achieved in bed. Avoid dozing in front of the television or taking cat-naps on the couch during the daytime. Neither approach is conducive to restful sleep. Instead, plan time for a 1- or 2-hour nap, in bed with curtains drawn, door closed, and an alarm set. The television set should not be playing. By setting an alarm for 1 to 2 hours, the patient can avoid worrying about oversleeping and being awake at night. A solid 2-hour nap during the day can actually enhance nighttime sleep.

2. Try to achieve a balance between rest and activity. Moderate exercise (such as walking), socializing, and diversions (television or reading) can help to counteract fatigue.

3. Avoid spurts of vigorous energy expenditure (e.g., raking leaves, heavy cleaning, tennis or other running sports). Instead, try walking, gardening, playing a few holes of golf (using a cart), or attending a sporting event.

4. Remind the patient that radiation fatigue, like most other side effects, usually resolves after treatment is completed. However, resolution is gradual and may take several months.

37. Are nausea and vomiting inevitable in patients undergoing radiation therapy?

No. Although treatment to some anatomic sites (e.g., abdomen, pelvis, lumbosacral spine) with large fields has the potential for inducing nausea, nausea is not an inevitable side effect of all radiation treatment. Several highly effective antiemetic medications are available and should be used before treatment as a preventive whenever nausea is anticipated.

38. What other factors may contribute to nutritional compromise during treatment?

Anorexia, oral and esophageal mucositis, moniliasis, diarrhea, and anxiety.

39. How can nurses encourage proper nutritional intake?

Patients undergoing radiation must be able to take in adequate calories and protein to maintain weight and promote healing. Pretreatment assessment of the patient's intake history and present diet is essential. Dietary supplements that offer high caloric and high protein content may help the patient to achieve a sense of well-being by maintaining weight, immune status, and positive nitrogen balance. Patients also can prepare their own supplements with a blender or food processor. Consultation with the dietitian can offer invaluable help.

40. What strategies are useful when oral intake is inadequate or physically impossible because of disease or treatment effects?

A gastrostomy feeding tube may be the best alternative. When symptoms subside, oral feedings can gradually be resumed. Some patients who have experienced severe oropharyngeal mucosal reactions requiring a feeding tube also have had surgery that interferes with oral intake and may need referral to a speech therapist for retraining of swallowing mechanisms.

41. Describe the role of radiation therapy in pain control.

The many sources of cancer pain include pressure of the tumor on an adjacent structure, invasion of an organ, tumor growth within an enclosed area, encroachment on a nerve plexus, tissue necrosis that exposes nerves, and muscle spasms, particularly in relation to bone metastasis. Radiation is effective in controlling pain by stopping further extension of the cancer, relieving pressure by shrinking the tumor, and, in the case of bone metastases, allowing bone to regrow after the tumor is destroyed. Radiation therapy can provide long-term complete or partial relief of pain, thereby improving quality of life. Some patients experience remarkable pain relief, which allows them to return to a near-normal lifestyle and activity level. Others experience partial pain relief, which allows reduction in pain medications with concomitant improvement in sense of well-being and control, even at the end of life. Pain management in cancer care is a major challenge in which radiation therapy plays a significant role. Relief of pain can occur quite quickly (a few days) in some situations, or it may take 2 weeks or longer to achieve. Improvement may continue even after treatment is completed. Adequate and aggressive use of opioids and other means of pain relief must be maintained until radiation takes effect.

42. Explain the rationale and technique of palliative radiation.

The goal of palliative radiation is to provide comfort or improve quality of life even when cure is not possible. The potential for relief of symptoms must be weighed against side effects and the time required for treatment. The goal is to achieve relief of symptoms as quickly as possible. Therefore, daily dose fractions are usually larger, with fewer total treatments and a smaller total dose. Although the risk of late or chronic side effects is greater with large fractions, this risk is offset by the patient's terminal status and need for palliation.

43. List common indications for palliative radiation.
- To control pain
- To reduce tumor volume and open an airway or the esophagus
- To control primary or metastatic brain tumors and relieve incapacitating headache, seizures, or loss of motor control
- To treat vertebral metastases and thereby relieve spinal cord compression, prevent paralysis, and relieve pain
- To relieve bleeding or obstruction from advanced bowel, bladder, prostate, or cervical cancers

44. Discuss the risk of developing a second malignancy after treatment with radiation.

Exposure to therapeutic radiation carries an increased risk of developing a second malignancy compared with the unexposed population. Estimates of risk vary somewhat, but most authorities agree that approximately 5% of all patients treated with radiation may develop second malignancies.

45. How is a radiation-induced second cancer defined? Give examples.

The tumor must be different from the primary, must arise within the previously irradiated tissue, and must occur from 10–15 years after the original tumor was treated. Examples of radiation-induced second malignancies are high-grade sarcomas, meningiomas, and thyroid cancers.

46. What factors may increase the likelihood of a radiation-induced second cancer?

Genetic factors, immune status, and treatment with other modalities must be considered in predicting an individual patient's risk of second malignancy. Cancer secondary to radiation also has been reported in people treated with radiation for nonmalignant processes (e.g., ankylosing spondylitis, tuberculosis, tinea capitis). Children and young adults who receive radiation therapy show a higher rate of second malignancies than unexposed controls of the same age, although it is not clear whether radiation therapy is the only inciting factor.

When considering any cancer therapy including radiation, the benefits of treatment should outweigh the potential risks. Special consideration should be given to irreversible or long-term risks (such as some malignancies) when children or young adults are to be treated. The risks of second malignancies should be carefully explained to patients and parents of young children.

47. What new delivery techniques are under investigation?

1. Heavy charged-particle (proton, helium, nitrogen) beam therapy is being used in a few research settings, primarily for small tumors in an attempt to exploit the different physical properties of different beams. The goal continues to be decreased effect on normal tissue with adequate tumor control. Treatment machines such as the proton beam are too costly for use in any but the research setting.

2. Radioimmunotherapy involves attaching a radioactive isotope (iodine-131, ytrium-90) to a tumor-specific antibody, which is then injected into the patient, delivering its lethal radiation dose directly to the tumor.

3. Photodynamic therapy involves laser technology delivered to the body surface. The laser seeks out light-sensitizing compounds selectively retained by tumor cells. This technique may prove especially useful for tumor seeding within body cavities (e.g., gastrointestinal or ovarian cancer).

48. Summarize the status of hyperthermia and intraoperative radiation therapy.

Once considered promising new approaches, hyperthermia and intraoperative radiation therapy are no longer in the forefront of investigational therapies. Hyperthermia, the use of heat to enhance tumor cell kill, has not shown any significant therapeutic advantage over radiation alone. In addition, poor quality control in clinical trials led to the cessation of cooperative group hyperthermia research in the United States. Intraoperative radiation therapy is a technique for delivering a single large fraction of radiation directly to the surgically exposed tumor or tumor bed. This technique has been explored since the 1940s in phase I and II clinical trials, and even more commonly outside a protocol setting. Despite some evidence of benefit, lack of patient accrual has prevented the introduction of phase III clinical trials. Intraoperative radiation treatment continues in approximately 250 centers in the United States and abroad.

49. What new applications of radiation therapy are under investigation?

In addition to treatment of cancer, interest has focused on the use of ionizing radiation for several nonmalignant conditions, including macular degeneration, prevention of heart and lung allograft rejection, and prevention of recurrence of vascular stenosis after angioplasty.

ACKNOWLEDGMENT

The author gratefully acknowledges the contributions of Joan Foley, RN, BSN, and Merle Sprague, MD, to the Radiation Therapy chapter in the first edition.

REFERENCES

1. Abel LJ, Blatt HJ, Stipetich RL, et al: Nursing management of patients receiving brachytherapy for early stage prostate cancer. Clin J Oncol Nursing 3:7–15, 1999.
2. Behrend SW (ed): Radiation oncology. Semin Oncol Nurs 15(4), 1999 [entire issue].
3. Bruner DW, Bucholtz JD, Iwamoto R et al (eds): Manual for Radiation Oncology Nursing Practice and Education. Pittsburgh, Oncology Nursing Press, 1998.
4. Dibble SL, Shiba G, MacPhail L, et al: MacDibbs mouth assessment: A new tool to evaluate mucositis in the radiation therapy patient. Cancer Pract 4:135–140, 1996.
5. Hassey-Dow K, Bucholtz JD, Iwamoto R, et al (eds): Nursing Care in Radiation Oncology, 2nd ed. Philadelphia, W.B. Saunders, 1997.
6. Hilderley LJ: Principles of radiation therapy. In Yarbro CH, Frogge, MH, Goodman, M, et al (eds): Cancer Nursing Principles and Practice, 5th ed. Boston, Jones & Bartlett, 2000, pp 286–351.
7. Huang HY, Wilkie D, Schubert MM, et al: Symptom profile of nasopharyngeal cancer patients during radiation therapy. Cancer Pract 8:274–281, 2000.
8. Kolcaba K, Fox C: The effects of guided imagery on comfort of women with early stage breast cancer undergoing radiation therapy. Oncol Nurs Forum 26:67–72, 1999.
9. Rose MA, Schrader-Bogen CL, Korlath G, et al: Identifying patient symptoms after radiotherapy using a nurse-managed telephone interview. Oncol Nurs Forum 23:99–102, 1996.

7. PRINCIPLES OF CHEMOTHERAPY

Matthew Kemper, PharmD, Irene Stewart Haapoja, RN, MS,
and Michelle Goodman, RN, MS

1. How has the role of chemotherapy changed in the treatment of cancer?

Chemotherapy was not successful in treating cancer until nitrogen mustard was used in the treatment of lymphomas in the 1940s. Currently, chemotherapy is responsible for increasing the survival time of many patients with cancer (see Chapter 4). In recent years, there has been a shift toward giving chemotherapy in earlier stages of cancer to prevent recurrences. Adjuvant chemotherapy for women with early breast cancer has produced substantial reductions in recurrence (35%) and mortality (27%). At the other end of the treatment spectrum, chemotherapy for women with metastatic breast cancer can provide palliation and symptom improvement. In addition, improvements in cancer treatment continue to focus on reducing toxicities associated with chemotherapy.

2. How does chemotherapy work?

Chemotherapy drugs interfere with steps of the cell cycle specifically involved in synthesis of DNA and replication of tumor cells. The cell cycle, the process whereby both normal and cancerous cells replicate, involves five basic phases:

G0   Resting stage in which cells are out of cycle temporarily
G1   RNA and protein synthesis; the gap between resting and DNA synthesis
S   DNA synthesis
G2   Second gap, during which the cell constructs the mitotic apparatus
M   Mitosis

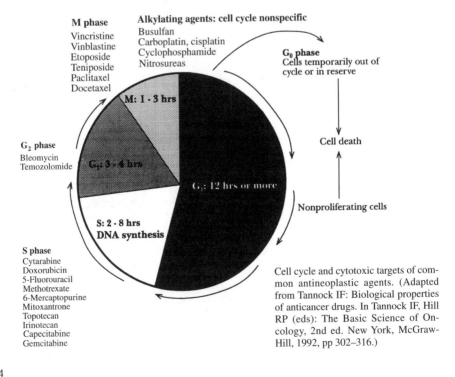

Cell cycle and cytotoxic targets of common antineoplastic agents. (Adapted from Tannock IF: Biological properties of anticancer drugs. In Tannock IF, Hill RP (eds): The Basic Science of Oncology, 2nd ed. New York, McGraw-Hill, 1992, pp 302–316.)

3. How are chemotherapeutic agents classified and by what mechanisms do they cause tumor cell death or prevent tumor growth?

Most antineoplastic agents are categorized based on their biochemical activity or origins. Many drugs are derived from natural products.

The **alkylating agents** exert their lethal activity by interacting with DNA bases, causing breakage of the DNA helix and preventing DNA replication. These agents are predominantly cell cycle nonspecific but are also effective against cells in the resting phase. Examples include cyclophosphamide, ifosfamide, cisplatin, carboplatin, nitrogen mustard, the nitrosoureas, and busulfan.

The **antimetabolites** inhibit enzyme production needed for DNA and RNA synthesis. These agents are cell cycle phase-specific, because they act during a specific phase of the cell cycle—usually the S-phase—and are therefore most effective against highly proliferative cancers. Examples include methotrexate, 5-fluorouracil (5-FU), cytarabine, fludarabine, capecitabine (Xeloda), and gemcitabine (Gemzar).

The **vinca alkaloids** are also cell cycle phase-specific agents that act primarily in the M-phase by binding to protein tubulin. This process leads to disruption of mitotic spindle formation so that the cell dies as it attempts division. Examples include vincristine, vinblastine, and vinorelbine (Navelbine).

The **antitumor antibiotics** are cell cycle phase-specific drugs that act in the S-phase of the cell cycle by binding to DNA and causing partial unwinding of the DNA helix, thereby inhibiting DNA and RNA synthesis. Examples include doxorubicin, idarubicin, and mitomycin.

The **camptothecins** are a newer class of agents that also exert their activity in the S-phase of the cell cycle. These agents inhibit the formation of topoisomerase I, an enzyme responsible for the prevention of DNA strand breakage during synthesis. The DNA strands break and are unable to effect repairs. The two drugs in this category are topotecan (Hycamtin) and irinotecan (Camptosar).

The **taxanes** are natural products derived from the yew tree. They are M-phase–specific and act by causing stabilization of the microtubule, which inhibits cell division. The two drugs in this category are paclitaxel (Taxol) and docetaxel (Taxotere).

The **podophyllotoxins** are plant alkaloids. They are M-phase–specific and cause double-stranded breaks in DNA by inhibition of topoisomerase II. The two drugs in this category are etoposide (VP-16, VePesid) and teniposide (VM-26, Vumon).

Miscellaneous agents do not fit into a particular class but are primarily phase-specific agents that may inhibit protein, RNA, or DNA synthesis. Examples include L-asparaginase, hydroxyurea, and procarbazine.

4. Discuss the role of monoclonal antibodies in the treatment of cancer.

Most monoclonal antibodies are still undergoing clinical trials, but two have been approved by the Food and Drug Administration (FDA):

1. Trastuzumab (rhuMAb HER-2), more commonly known as Herceptin, is the first monoclonal antibody indicated for the treatment of metastatic breast carcinoma. Herceptin is effective only in patients who overexpress the HER-2 protein on the tumor cell surface (approximately 25–30% of breast cancers). Herceptin binds to the HER-2 protein, inhibiting tumor cell proliferation. It may be used as a single agent or in combination with chemotherapy.

2. Rituximab (Rituxan) is a monoclonal antibody indicated for the treatment of relapsed or refractory B-cell non-Hodgkin's lymphoma (NHL). It is the first monoclonal antibody to be used as a chemotherapeutic agent. Rituxan binds to the CD20 antigen, a protein found on the cell surface of > 90% of B-cell non-Hodgkin's lymphomas, preventing cell growth and resulting in cell lysis.

5. What are antiangiogenesis factors? How do they work?

Antiangiogenesis factors are a group of agents that prevent new blood vessel formation in solid tumors. Tumors form new blood vessels by stimulating the production of angiogenic factors. The most potent angiogenic factor identified is vascular endothelial growth factor (VEGF), which is expressed in most solid tumors. Bevacizumab (rhuMAb VEGF) is a monoclonal antibody that blocks the effect of VEGF, thereby preventing tumor blood vessel formation and eventually preventing tumor cell growth and metastasis. It is currently under investigation as a single agent and in combination with chemotherapy, specifically in advanced breast carcinoma and non-small cell lung carcinoma. Other antiangiogenesis factors under investigation include matrix metalloproteinase inhibitors. These agents block the activity of enzymes that dissolve the extracellular matrix. Breakdown of the matrix is associated with tumor cell growth, invasion, metastasis, and angiogenesis. Most of these agents are taken orally and are being tested as single agents or in combination with chemotherapy.

6. Describe the effect of tumor growth on responsiveness to chemotherapy.

The growth and size of a tumor is a product of the proportion of cells actively dividing (growth fraction), the length of the cell cycle (doubling time), and the rate of cell loss. The higher the growth fraction and the higher the doubling time, the greater the cell kill. The higher the proliferative rate of a tumor, the more effective the chemotherapy. Tumors are most likely to be responsive to chemotherapy when they are small and vascular rather than later, when cell proliferation slows because of crowding, poor vascularization, and limited nutrients.

7. Why are certain cancers resistant to chemotherapy?

Drug resistance is one of the major barriers to cure. Drug resistance may be intrinsic or acquired over time, because each cancer cell has the ability to mutate spontaneously. Many cancers (e.g., melanoma, renal cell, pancreatic cancer) are intrinsically resistant to most if not all chemotherapeutic agents. Cancers that are intrinsically resistant to chemotherapy contain the multidrug resistance gene, known as the MDR pump, which contains P-glycoprotein. The MDR pump resides within the cellular membrane and actively pumps out certain drugs as they are given, thus preventing accumulation of the drug within the cell. In the presence of overexpression of P-glycoprotein, drugs such as doxorubicin, mitoxantrone, daunorubicin, vincristine, vinblastine, paclitaxel, etoposide, and dactinomycin are readily extruded from the cell.

Cancer cells may be resistant to drugs by other mechanisms, such as decreased drug uptake, reduced drug activation, impaired drug transport into cells, increased catabolism of the drug, alterations in target enzymes to reduce drug binding, and increased DNA repair, all of which reduce therapeutic efficacy.

8. Describe the mechanism of increased DNA repair.

In the past decade, resistance to apoptosis (programmed cell death) and presence of telomerase have been described as significant properties that permit cancer cells not to die or age despite appropriate signals. Apoptosis refers to the cell death that normally follows cellular damage. When cancer cells lack apoptosis, they survive despite damage from chemotherapy drugs or other mechanisms that initiate programmed cell death, thus contributing to malignant transformation and chemotherapy resistance. Normally, cell senescence (process of aging) results when telomeres shorten with each division and chromosomes are not able to replicate their DNA. Unlike normal somatic cells, most cancer cells possess telomerase, an enzyme that lengthens telomeres to sustain DNA replication. Telomerase permits cells to ignore the biologic clock, thereby promoting tumor cell growth and possible chemotherapy resistance.

9. How can drug resistance be overcome?

Research suggests that tamoxifen, cyclosporine, verapamil, and quinidine may be effective in reversing the MDR pump mechanism. Other important strategies in overcoming resistance are combination chemotherapy and dose-intensive chemotherapy, which kill the cells before they have the chance to become resistant. Future chemotherapy may be developed to target cancer cell resistance to apoptosis and the presence of telomerase.

10. What test is used to assess tumor response to chemotherapy?

Flow cytometry is used to estimate the growth fraction, cell cycle phase distribution, and kinetic properties of cell populations. Tumors that contain a higher percentage of proliferating cells

(cells in S phase) are more sensitive to cycle-dependent chemotherapy and have a better prognosis than tumors with a low S-phase fraction.

11. Define ploidy.

Ploidy refers to the ratio of DNA content of tumor cells in G1 phase. Patients with diploid tumors (DNA index < 1 or normal DNA content) tend to have a better prognosis than those with aneuploid tumors (DNA index > 1 or abnormal DNA content). The incidence of subclinical dissemination and tumor recurrence is greater in patients with an aneuploid tumor having a high S-phase fraction.

12. What patient factors affect response to chemotherapy?

Optimal performance status, stable weight, absence of significant concomitant illnesses, and optimal symptom management. A depressed immune system and weight loss decrease tolerance to the side effects of chemotherapy. In addition, dose reductions and treatment delays due to toxicity and patient adherence promote tumor resistance. Finally, women with breast cancer who are HER-2 positive are more likely to respond to chemotherapy. Women who are HER-2 positive, receiving trastuzumab are optimal candidates for simultaneous administration of paclitaxel. Trastuzumab enhances response to paclitaxel.

13. Can circadian rhythm affect the patient's response to chemotherapy?

Administering chemotherapy according to circadian rhythm may enhance response and minimize toxicity. 5-FU, which targets the gut and bone marrow, may be best tolerated if given in the evening because the cells of the gut and the bone marrow divide most actively during the first half of the working day.

14. What other factors affect response to chemotherapy?
- Tumor burden: the larger the primary tumor, the greater the risk for metastatic disease.
- Tumor cell heterogeneity increases risk for primary and secondary resistance to chemotherapy.

15. What is the advantage of combination chemotherapy?

Combining drugs that are synergistic and act at different phases of the cell cycle maximizes tumor cell kill. Examples include paclitaxel/trastuzumab and methotrexate/5-FU. These drugs work synergistically and result in higher response rates than when they are used as single agents. Combination drug therapy also minimizes the proliferation of resistant tumor stem cells, thereby reducing the potential for drug resistance. Another advantage of combination chemotherapy is that the drugs produce differing toxicities and maximal doses of each drug can be given.

16. How does the combination of chemotherapy and radiotherapy increase responsiveness?

Certain drugs act as radiosensitizers (paclitaxel, 5-FU, carboplatin), allowing the radiation therapy to be more effective. Unfortunately, they also increase the potential for toxicity. An advantage of combined chemotherapy and radiotherapy is that the patient can receive local (primary tumor) and systemic (micrometastatic disease) treatment simultaneously.

17. Does the sequence of administering certain drugs affect response to chemotherapy?

The sequence in which drugs are given may enhance efficacy and/or minimize toxicity:
- When paclitaxel is given in combination with carboplatin or cisplatin, it is always given first. Administration of paclitaxel after carboplatin or cisplatin not only decreases its efficacy but also may enhance its myelosuppressive effects.
- When paclitaxel is combined with doxorubicin, doxorubicin is given first. If paclitaxel is given first, its clearance may be reduced, resulting in dose limiting (grade 3) mucositis without increased efficacy.
- Administration of lower doses of paclitaxel on a weekly basis may permit optimal dosing and increase efficacy compared with administration of larger doses every 3 weeks. Patients

appear to tolerate weekly dosing with less toxicity, including myelosuppression, peripheral neuropathies, and hair loss.
- When methotrexate is combined with 5-FU for treatment of early breast cancer, it is given intravenously 1 hour before 5-FU. The dose of methotrexate is escalated to promote synergism between the two drugs. The methotrexate sensitizes the cell membrane to enhance the transport of 5-FU into the cell, thereby promoting intracellular concentration and presumably cell kill.

18. What agents can be given to minimize the toxicity of chemotherapy?

The following protective agents have the potential to minimize toxicity and maximize treatment options:

- Leucovorin (with high-dose methotrexate)
- Dexrazoxane (with doxorubicin)
- Amifostine (with cisplatin)
- Mesna (with ifosfamide)

19. Explain the protective effect of leucovorin.

High-dose methotrexate may be given only with leucovorin rescue. Leucovorin, which blocks the action of methotrexate and rescues normal cells from toxicity, is started 24 hours after methotrexate and continued according to blood levels of methotrexate.

20. How does dexrazoxane work?

Doxorubicin damages the myocytes of the heart, causing it to function less efficiently once the maximal dose is reached. Administering doxorubicin with a cardioprotective agent such as dexrazoxane (Zinecard) may permit longer courses of treatment beyond the traditional recommendation of 550 mg/m^2. Dexrazoxane is dosed at a 10:1 ratio (i.e., 1,000 mg of dexrazoxane per 100 mg of doxorubicin) and given by intravenous push or intravenous piggy-back (IVPB) within 30 minutes before doxorubicin. Dexrazoxane is an important agent for many patients who continue to respond to doxorubicin and have few other effective options for treatment but risk the long-term effects of congestive heart failure as a consequence of continued therapy.

21. Describe the protective role of amifostine in combination with cisplatin.

Amifostine (Ethyol) is used to prevent nephrotoxicity associated with cisplatin therapy. It also minimizes other side effects of cisplatin, such as neurotoxicity, ototoxicity, and myelosuppression. Amifostine is a prodrug that is metabolized to its active free thiol metabolite, preferentially in normal tissues, by alkaline phosphatase. The free thiol binds to and detoxifies reactive metabolites of cisplatin and acts as a free radical scavenger. The potential protective role of amifostine with paclitaxel, carboplatin, and doxorubicin is under investigation. The dose used to prevent nephrotoxicity is 910 mg/m^2 by IVPB over 15 minutes immediately before administration of chemotherapy. If the full dose cannot be administered because of increased nausea and vomiting, subsequent doses should be reduced to 740 mg/m^2.

22. What is the role of amifostine in patients receiving radiotherapy?

Amifostine reduces xerostomia in patients receiving radiation therapy. It is dosed at 200 mg/m^2/day and given by IVPB over 3 minutes 15–30 minutes before radiation therapy. Patients need to be monitored for side effects of nausea and hypotension.

23. Describe the protective effects of mesna.

Ifosfamide has a toxic metabolite, acrolein, which binds to and damages the urinary tract epithelium. Mesna is given with ifosfamide to prevent urotoxicity. Mesna does not have antitumor activity, but it binds directly to acrolein and blocks its ability to damage cells in the urinary tract.

24. How and when is mesna administered with ifosfamide?

Because mesna has a shorter plasma half-life than ifosfamide, the two drugs are usually given concomitantly. Mesna is continued for 12–24 hours after the ifosfamide is administered. Typically mesna is given at 0 (before), 4, and 8 hours after ifosfamide:

Route	Dose	Schedule
Oral	40% of ifosfamide dose	Give at 0, 4, and 8 hours
Intravenous push	20% of ifosfamide dose	Give at 0, 4, and 8 hours
Continuous IV infusion	Same as ifosfamide dose	Give continuously

Oral mesna tastes and smells of sulfur and may not be well tolerated by patients prone to nausea and vomiting. Administration in 7-Up or Coca-Cola helps to mask the taste. Patients should be advised to push fluids, empty the bladder frequently, and report symptoms of irritation or pain during voiding. Patients unable to tolerate oral mesna may be taught to administer the drug intravenously at home, provided that they have a central line.

25. Why is the dose of carboplatin calculated with the Calvert formula instead of in mg/m²?

Use of the Calvert formula ensures optimal dosing of carboplatin based on physiologic parameters, which vary from patient to patient. Severe myelosuppression may result if the carboplatin dosage is not adjusted for patients with impaired renal function. The Calvert formula adjusts carboplatin dosages based on glomerular filtration rate (GFR) and a desired serum concentration/area under the curve (AUC). The target AUC is based on whether the patient has been previously treated. The dose calculated using the Calvert formula is the actual dose in mg, not the mg/m² dose.

26. What are the most common side effects of chemotherapy?

In general, adverse effects from chemotherapy result from damage to the rapidly dividing stem cells or drug toxicity to cells or tissues of specific organs unrelated to cell growth rate. The degree or severity of effects varies according to dosage, timing or duration, route of administration, prior chemotherapy or radiation therapy, coadministration of other agents, condition of patient, and individual sensitivities. Acute, late, and chronic effects, ranging from mild to dose-limiting or fatal toxicities, may or may not be predictable. See table below for common side effects and toxicities; refer to Chapter 45 for specific organ toxicities and late effects.

Cancer Chemotherapy Side Effects

AGENT (TRADE NAME)	N/V	MUCO-SITIS	D/C	ALO-PECIA	BMS	HSR	V/I	ORGAN AND OTHER TOXICITIES
L-Asparaginase (Elspar)	±	0	0	0	0	++	0	Hepatic, neurologic, hyperglycemia, pancreatitis
Bleomycin (Blenoxane)	±	+	0	±	0	+	I	Skin, fever, pulmonary, Raynaud's phenomenon
Busulfan (Myleran)	±	0	D±	±	++	0	0	Skin, gonadal, hepatic, ocular, pulmonary
Capecitabine (Xeloda)	+	+	D++	±	+	0	0	Hand and foot syndrome (may be severe); grade 3 and 4 hyperbilirubinemia (17% of patients)
Carboplatin (Paraplatin)	±	0	0	0	+	=	I	Hepatic, neurologic, hypomagnesemia
Carmustine, BCNU (BiCNU)	+	+	D±	0	++	0	I	Gonadal, hepatic, neurologic*, pulmonary*, renal
Chlorambucil (Leukearn)	±	0	0	0	±	0	0	Gonadal, pulmonary*
Cisplatin, CDDP (Platinol)	++	0	D±	0	±	+	I	Gonadal, neurologic, ototoxic, renal, hypomagnesemia
Cladribine, 2-CdA (Leustatin)	±	0	0	0	+	0	0	Skin, neurologic, renal*

Table continued on following page

Cancer Chemotherapy Side Effects (Continued)

AGENT (TRADE NAME)	N/V	MUCO-SITIS	D/C	ALO-PECIA	BMS	HSR	V/I	ORGAN AND OTHER TOXICITIES
Cyclophosphamide, Cytoxan (Neosar)	+	0	0	++	++	0	0	Cardiac*, gonadal, SIADH, hemorrhagic cystitis
Cytarabine, Ara-C (Cytosar-U)	+	++	D+	±	++	0	0	Skin, flu-like syndrome, neurologic*, ocular*, pulmonary
Dacarbazine (DTIC)	++	0	0	±	+	0	I	Skin, hepatic, flu-like illness
Dactinomycin, actino-mycin D (Cosmegen)	+	++	D±	+	++	0	V	Skin, fever, hepatic
Daunorubicin, dauno-mycin (Cerubidine)	+	+	0	++	++	+	V	Cardiac, red urine, skin
Docetaxel (Taxotere)	±	+	D±	+	++	++	I	Skin, neurologic, fluid re-tention syndrome, fatigue
Doxorubicin, ADR (Adriamycin, Rubex)	+	+	0	++	++	+	V	Cardiac, skin, red urine
Epirubicin (Epidoxorubicin)	+	+	D±	+	++	+	V	Cardiac, red-orange urine
Estramustine (Emcyt)	+	0	D±	±	±	0	0	Cardiac, gynecomastia
Etoposide, VP-16-213 (Vepesid)	±	0	C±	+	+	+	I	Hypotension (rapid infu-sion), neurologic
Floxuridine (FUDR)	±	+	D+	±	±	0	0	Skin, hepatic
Fludarabine (Fludara)	±	0	D±	±	±	0	0	Neurologic*, decreased T cells
5-Fluorouracil, 5-FU (Adrucil)	±	++	D++	±	+	0	I	Cardiac, skin, neurologic, ocular
Gemcitabine (Gemzar)	+	0	0	±	++	0	0	Skin, fever, flu-like syn-drome, ARDS; BMS may lead to cumulative thrombocytopenia
Hydroxyurea (Hydrea)	±	±	D±/C±	±	+	0	0	Skin, megalobastosis
Idarubicin HCl (Idamycin)	+	+	D±	+	++	0	V	Cardiac, skin
Ifosfamide (Ifex)	+	±	D/C±	+	++	0	I	Neurologic*, hemorrhagic cystitis, renal*
Irinotecan HCl (Camptosar)	++	±	D+	+	+	0	I	Pulmonary
Lomustine, CCNU (CeeNu)	+	±	D±	±	++	0	0	Gonadal, hepatic, pulmo-nary, renal
Mechlorethamine, nitrogen mustard, HN2 (Mustargen)	++	0	0	+	++	0	V	Skin, fever, gonadal
Melphalen, L-PAM (Alkeran)	±	0	0	±	+	+ (IV)	0	Skin, hepatic*, gonadal
Mercaptopurine, 6MP (Purinethol)	±	+	D±	0	+	0	0	Hepatic, skin
Methotrexate, MTX (Folex, Rheumatrex)	±	++	D±	±	+	0	0	Skin, hepatic*, neurologic*, ocular, pulmonary*, renal*

Table continued on following page

Cancer Chemotherapy Side Effects (Continued)

AGENT (TRADE NAME)	N/V	MUCO-SITIS	D/C	ALO-PECIA	BMS	HSR	V/I	ORGAN AND OTHER TOXICITIES
Mitomycin C (Mutamycin)	+	+	0	+	++	0	V	Skin, hemolytic uremic syndrome, hepatic*, pulmonary
Mitoxantrone HCl (Novantrone)	±	+	D±	+	++	0	I	Cardiac, blue-green discoloration (nails, sclera, urine
Paclitaxel (Taxol)	±	±	D±	+	+	++	I	Bradycardia, skin, neurologic
Procarbazine (Matulane)	+	±	D±	±	+	+	0	Gonadal*, neurologic, monoamine oxidase inhibitory effect
Temozolomide (Temodar)	+	0	0	0	++	0	0	Headache, fatigue (common)
Thiotepa (Thioplex)	±	±	0	0	+	0	0	Skin*, gonadal, neurologic*
Topotecan (Hycamtin)	+	+	D±	+	+	0	0	Skin, fever, flu-like illness, neurologic*
Vinblastine, VLB (Velban)	±	+	C+	±	+	0	V	Neurologic, jaw pain
Vincristine, VCR (Oncovin)	±	±	C+	±	±	0	V	Neurologic, SIADH
Vinorelbine tartrate (Navelbine)	±	±	C+	±	+	0	V	Neurologic

Disclaimer: This table illustrates principal or unique toxicities but is not all-inclusive. It may not list rare, occasional, or late effects. Side-effect profiles change with dosage, route and duration of administration, prior chemotherapy or radiotherapy, coadministration of other therapies, and patient condition and sensitivities.
N/V = nausea/vomiting, D/C = diarrhea/constipation, BMS = bone marrow suppression, HSR = hypersensitivity reaction, V/I = vesicant/irritant, SIADH = syndrome of inappropriate antidiuretic hormone, 0 = none or rare, ± = mild, + = moderate to moderately high, ++ = severe.
* High doses.
Developed and updated by Fink R, Gates R, Goodman M, Petersen J, 1997, 2000.

27. What is the future of chemotherapy?

Chemotherapy is an effective but nonspecific treatment. The major risks associated with chemotherapy are a result of the drug's effect on normal tissue. Recent advances in biotherapy and gene therapy have enabled the development of targeted therapies that are directed specifically at the tumor cell and spare normal tissue. Treatment with Herceptin and Rituxan has proved to be effective with virtually no toxicities compared with chemotherapy. New biologic therapies focus on three major areas: antiangiogenesis, inhibition of growth factors, and enhanced apoptosis (programmed cell death). Combining chemotherapy with various biologic agents that affect different aspects of tumor growth will allow individualized, more effective, and more tolerable treatments.

REFERENCES

1. Berg DT: New chemotherapy treatment options and implications for nursing care. Oncol Nurs Forum 24(Suppl):5–12, 1997.
2. Bonomi PD: Novel treatment approaches for non-small cell lung cancer. Lung Cancer 29 (Suppl 2):129, 2000.
3. Brizel DM, Wasserman TH, Henke M, et al: Phase III randomized trial of amifostine as a radioprotector in head and neck cancer. J Clin Oncol 18:3339–3345, 2000.

4. Calvert AH, Newell DR, Gumbrell LA, et al: Carboplatin dosage: Prospective evaluation of a simple formula based on renal function. J Clin Oncol 7:1748–1756, 1989.
5. Cheng JD, Rieger PT, Von Mehren M, et al: Recent advances in immunotherapy and monoclonal antibody treatment of cancer. Semin Oncol Nurs. 16:2–12, 2000.
6. Donehower RC, Abeloff MD, Perry MC: Chemotherapy. In Abeloff MD, Armitage JO, Lichter AS,
   Niederhuber JE (eds): Clinical Oncology, New York, Churchill Livingstone, 1995, pp 201–218.
7. Dorr RT, Von Hoff DD: Cancer Chemotherapy Handbook. Norwalk, CT, Appleton & Lange, 1994.
8. Early Breast Cancer Trialists' Collaborative Group: Polychemotherapy for early breast cancer: An
   overview of the randomized trials. Lancet 352:930–942, 1998.
9. Erlichman C: Pharmacology of anticancer drugs. In Tannock IF, Hill RP (eds): The Basic Science of
   Oncology, 2nd ed. New York, McGraw-Hill, 1992, pp 317–337.
10. Fishman M, Orlowski MM (eds.): Cancer chemotherapy guidelines and recommendations for practice,
    2nd ed. Pittsburgh, Oncology Nursing Press, 1999.
11. Geels P, Eisenhauer E, Bezjak A, Zee B, Day A: Palliative effect of chemotherapy: Objective tumor re-
    sponse is associated with symptom improvement in patients with metastatic breast cancer. J Clin
    Oncol 18:2395–2405, 2000.
12. Kemp G, Rose P, Turain J, et al: Amifostine pretreatment for protection against cyclophosphamide-in-
    duced and cisplatin-induced toxicities: Results of a randomized control trial in patients with advanced
    ovarian cancer. J Clin Oncol 14: 2101–2112. 1996.
13. Miaskowski C: Oncology Nursing: An Essential Guide for Patient Care. Philadelphia, W.B. Saunders,
    1997.
14. Tannock IF: Biological properties of anticancer drugs. In Tannock IF, Hill RP (eds): The Basic Science
    of Oncology, 2nd ed. New York, McGraw-Hill, 1992, pp 302–316.
15. Tortorice PV: Chemotherapy: Principles of Therapy. In Yarbro C, Frogge M, Goodman M (eds): Cancer
    Nursing: Principles and Practice, 5th ed. Boston, Jones & Bartlett, 2000, pp 352–384.

8. NEW CHEMOTHERAPY AGENTS

Andrea Iannucci, PharmD, BCOP, and Cindy O'Bryant, PharmD

1. What is an FDA-approved indication?

Drugs receive approval from the United States Food and Drug Administration (FDA) based on evidence supporting their safety and efficacy in treatment of a specific disease. The FDA approval process for chemotherapy drugs is rigorous, and new agents often receive initial approval for a limited patient population. For example, paclitaxel (Taxol) was originally approved by the FDA only for treatment of recurrent or refractory metastatic ovarian cancer. In the past 5 years, over 30 new molecules have received FDA approval for cancer indications, not to mention over 20 drugs that received expanded FDA approval for cancer diagnoses. This chapter discusses the chemotherapy drugs that have received FDA approval since 1996.

2. Are chemotherapy drugs used only for their FDA-approved indication?

Frequently chemotherapy drugs are used outside the original FDA-approved indication, usually when evidence, in the form of published clinical trials, supports their use for treatment of a particular disease. Because chemotherapy drugs are associated with so much toxicity, their use outside FDA-approved indications should be reserved for diseases in which there is strong supporting evidence of efficacy.

3. What is an expanded FDA approval?

A drug that is already FDA-approved for one indication receives additional FDA approval for a different disease based on supporting evidence.

TOPOTECAN AND IRINOTECAN

4. How do topotecan and irinotecan work?

Topotecan and irinotecan were the first FDA-approved drugs in the category of topoisomerase I inhibitors. Topoisomerase inhibitors interfere with both types of topoisomerase enzymes, topoisomerase I and topoisomerase II. These enzymes bind to DNA during transcription and replication and form breaks in the DNA strands during the replication process. They help to relieve torsional strain from the complicated, coiled DNA structure, allowing the DNA strands to proceed with transcription and replication more easily. Topoisomerase I produces single-strand breaks in DNA, and topoisomerase II produces double-strand DNA breaks. Topoisomerases also repair the DNA strand breaks once the strands have completed the transcription and replication process. It may be easier to think of the topoisomerases as a kind of "zipper." They zip open the DNA strands during transcription and replication and zip the strands back together once the process is completed. Topoisomerase inhibitors bind to the enzyme while it is bound to DNA. They inhibit the enzyme's ability to repair the DNA strand breaks, which ultimately leads to cell death.

Topoisomerases

ENZYME	FUNCTION	INHIBITORS
Topoisomerase I	Forms single-stranded DNA breaks and repairs during transcription and replication	Irinotecan Topotecan
Topoisomerase II	Forms double-stranded DNA breaks and repairs during transcription and replication	Doxorubicin Daunorubicin Etoposide

5. What is the active metabolite of irinotecan?

Irinotecan is a prodrug that requires activation by carboxylesterases in the liver to SN-38, the major active component. SN-38 is also largely responsible for diarrhea, one of the major side effects of irinotecan.

6. What are the FDA-approved indications for topotecan and irinotecan?

Topotecan (Hycamtin) is FDA-approved for second-line treatment of metastatic ovarian cancer and small-cell lung cancer. Irinotecan (Camptosar; CPT-11) is FDA-approved for treatment of metastatic colon cancer and front-line treatment of colon cancer, in combination with 5-fluorouracil and leucovorin.

7. Are topotecan and irinotecan used for other indications?

Topotecan has shown some promise in the treatment of myelodysplastic syndrome and acute leukemia. Irinotecan has shown some promise in treatment of lung cancer.

8. How are topotecan and irinotecan administered?

Topotecan typically is administered in a dosing schedule of 1.5 mg/m^2 as a 30-minute infusion every day for 5 days. The cycle is repeated every 3 weeks.

Irinotecan may be administered on a weekly or 3-week schedule. When used as a single agent, the typical weekly dose is 125 mg/m^2, administered as a 90-minute infusion for 4 weeks, followed by 2 weeks of rest. Weekly doses are adjusted based on blood counts and symptoms of diarrhea. For the 3-week regimen, irinotecan is typically dosed at 350 mg/m^2 and administered as a 90-minute infusion every 3 weeks.

9. What are the major side effects of topotecan and irinotecan?

Topotecan is generally well tolerated. The major side effect is myelosuppression. Some patients may require use of a colony-stimulating factor while receiving topotecan. Nausea and vomiting are mild; thus, serotonin ($5HT_3$) receptor antagonists (e.g., ondansetron, dolasetron) are generally not required for nausea protection. Some patients, especially those receiving the drug for myelodysplastic syndrome or acute leukemia, may experience mucositis. Alopecia is a common side effect. Fever and flulike symptoms as well as diarrhea occur in some patients.

The most common side effects with **irinotecan** are diarrhea and myelosuppression. Chemotherapy doses may need to be adjusted based on the severity of diarrhea or degree of myelosuppression. Diarrhea from irinotecan can be severe and debilitating, requiring aggressive management. Because irinotecan is more emetogenic than topotecan, patients generally require treatment with a serotonin receptor antagonist to prevent nausea and vomiting.

10. Why is diarrhea such a troublesome side effect of irinotecan?

Diarrhea due to irinotecan typically occurs in two phases, early and late. **Early diarrhea** occurs within the first 24 hours of treatment in as many as one-half of patients who receive the drug and is thought to be related to a cholinergic process. It can occur quickly, even during infusion, and is commonly preceded by facial flushing, nasal congestion, or abdominal cramping.

Late diarrhea occurs in about 90% of patients receiving the drug and is thought to be caused by accumulation of the SN-38 metabolite in the gut due to the high levels of carboxylesterases in the intestinal mucosa. The onset of late diarrhea is typically 11 days after treatment with a usual course of about 3 days. Late diarrhea can be severe and, if not treated aggressively, may prove to be fatal. Complications include electrolyte abnormalities and dehydration.

11. What risk factors predispose patients to developing diarrhea with irinotecan?

Patients over the age of 65 years seem to be at greater risk.

12. How should diarrhea from irinotecan be managed?

Early diarrhea should be managed with the anticholinergic drug atropine, which typically is administered intravenously in doses of 0.25–1 mg at the first sign of symptoms. Most patients respond well to treatment. Patients who have had problems with early-onset diarrhea can be pre-medicated with atropine for subsequent cycles of treatment.

Late diarrhea is much more difficult to treat. The most effective treatment appears to be high-dose loperamide. Patients should be instructed to take 2 capsules (4 mg) of loperamide at the first onset of loose stools or diarrhea and to repeat 1 capsule (2 mg) every 2–4 hours until 12 hours have passed without a bowel movement. If diarrhea recurs, patients should start the loperamide regimen again. The high-dose regimen exceeds the recommended daily dose of loperamide but is well toler-ated. The complications of uncontrolled diarrhea far exceed the complications of the high-dose lop-eramide. Other antidiarrheal agents, such as diphenoxylate-atropine sulfate and octreotide, are not as effective in managing late diarrhea. The antiangiogenesis agent, thalidomide, has shown some promise in decreasing the incidence of irinotecan-induced diarrhea in a small pilot study.

EPIRUBICIN

13. What is epirubicin?

Epirubicin (Ellence), an anthracycline drug similar to doxorubicin, is FDA-approved for ad-juvant treatment of lymph node-positive breast cancer. It was approved after a comparative study demonstrated better efficacy with the CEF regimen (cyclophosphamide, epirubicin, and 5-fluo-rouracil) compared with the CMF regimen (cyclophosphamide, methotrexate, and 5-fluorouracil) in the adjuvant treatment of breast cancer. It was not compared with AC (doxorubicin [Adriamycin] + cyclophosphamide) or AC+T (AC + paclitaxel [Taxol]), which are widely con-sidered the standard regimens for adjuvant treatment of breast cancer in the U.S.

14. How is epirubicin administered?

The FDA-approved dosing regimen is 100–120 mg/m^2, which may be administered all at once on day 1 of each cycle or divided into 2 doses administered on days 1 and 8 of each cycle. Cycles are repeated at 21–28-day intervals. Epirubicin typically is administered as an intravenous push over 3–5 minutes. Extravasation precautions are necessary because epirubicin is a vesicant.

15. How is epirubicin different from doxorubicin?

Epirubicin is similar to doxorubicin in mechanism of action, side-effect profile, and spec-trum of activity. The major advantage is that epirubicin is less cardiotoxic than doxorubicin. Epirubicin doses of 70–90 mg/m^2 are approximately equivalent to doxorubicin doses of 60–75 mg/m^2 in terms of the potential to cause myelosuppression. These doses are considered therapeu-tically equipotent.

16. Does epirubicin cause cardiotoxicity?

Clearly epirubicin can cause the same type of debilitating cardiomyopathy associated with doxorubicin. In fact, the FDA-approved dosing regimen of epirubicin can cause cumulative car-diac toxicity in approximately the same number of cycles as doxorubicin.

Comparative Cardiotoxicity of Epirubicin and Doxorubicin

DRUG	TYPICAL DOSE	CUMULATIVE DOSE ASSOCIATED WITH INCREASED RISK OF CARDIOTOXICITY	NUMBER OF CYCLES TO REACH CUMULATIVE DOSE
Epirubicin	100–120 mg/m^2	900 mg/m^2	8–9
Doxorubicin	50–60 mg/m^2	500 mg/m^2	8–10

17. What is the role of epirubicin in the current treatment of breast cancer?

Limited. Evidence to support the use of epirubicin over doxorubicin in currently accepted stan-dard adjuvant breast cancer regimens (e.g., AC or AC + paclitaxel) is not available. The advantage of epirubicin over doxorubicin in terms of cardiotoxic potential is minimal at the FDA-approved dosing regimen. In addition, the cost of epirubicin is significantly higher than the cost of doxoru-bicin (as much as 7 times the price of generic doxorubicin, according to the 2000 Redbook average wholesale price listing).

CYTARABINE LIPOSOME INJECTION

18. What is cytarabine liposome injection?

Cytarabine liposome injection (Depocyt) is a long-acting, liposomal cytarabine preparation for intraventricular (into a ventricular reservoir) or intrathecal (through a spinal needle) administration. Cytarabine liposome injection is indicated for treatment of lymphomatous meningitis.

19. What advantages does cytarabine liposome injection offer over regular cytarabine?

Cytarabine liposome injection has been compared with cytarabine in the management of cerebrospinal fluid (CSF)-positive lymphoma. Patients were randomized to receive either cytarabine liposome injection 50 mg every 2 weeks or free cytarabine 50 mg twice weekly for 1 month. All patients received dexamethasone, 4 mg orally twice daily, on days 1–5 of each cycle. Patients who responded to treatment received an additional 3 months of consolidation treatment and 4 months of maintenance therapy. Response was defined as conversion from positive to negative CSF cytology at all sites known to be positive plus the absence of neurologic progression. Of 14 randomized patients, the difference in response rate was statistically significant with 41% for cytarabine liposome injection and 6% for free cytarabine (p = 0.04). There was a trend toward increased time to disease progression and increased survival in the cytarabine liposome injection arm, but these outcomes did not reach statistical significance. Approval of cytarabine liposome injection was based on the significant improvements in response rate in comparison to free cytarabine, but it did not demonstrate a clear survival advantage or clinical benefit advantage over free cytarabine.

20. How is cytarabine liposome injection administered?

Cytarabine liposome injection may be administered into an intraventricular reservoir or intrathecally (IT) via a lumbar puncture. Filters should *not* be used in preparing or administering cytarabine liposome injection. The dosing regimen for cytarabine liposome injection is as follows:

Induction   50 mg IT/intraventricular every 2 weeks × 2 doses (weeks 1 and 3)
Consolidation 50 mg IT/intraventricular every 2 weeks × 3 doses (weeks 5, 7, and 9), then
                   one additional dose at week 13
Maintenance   50 mg IT/intraventricular every 4 weeks × 4 doses (weeks 17, 21, 25, and 29)

21. Why do patients need dexamethasone as a premedication with cytarabine liposome injection?

All patients should receive dexamethasone, 4 mg orally or intravenously twice daily for 5 days, beginning on the day of each dose of cytarabine liposome injection. Without dexamethasone, virtually 100% of patients develop arachnoiditis (neck rigidity, neck pain, nausea, vomiting, headache, fever, and back pain). Pretreatment with dexamethasone reduces the incidence of arachnoiditis by about two-thirds.

22. What is the current role of cytarabine liposome injection?

The role of cytarabine liposome injection has been limited by a temporary lapse in availability due to manufacturing issues. In late 2000 the drug was still unavailable, but it is anticipated that it will be available again in 2001. In addition, the high cost and narrow FDA-approved treatment indication further limit its use. Use of the drug outside the FDA-approved indication of lymphomatous meningitis requires prior authorization with insurance providers to ensure proper reimbursement.

GLIADEL WAFERS

23. What are Gliadel wafers? Summarize their clinical benefits.

A Gliadel wafer is a biodegradable polymer "wafer" impregnated with carmustine. The wafers are used for local treatment of recurrent glioblastoma multiforme. Compared with placebo, Gliadel wafers marginally increase survival in patients with glioblastoma multiforme, but survival has not increased in patients with other types of tumors.

24. How are Gliadel wafers administered?

Gliadel wafers are administered directly into the surgical cavity after resection of the brain tumor. Each wafer is about the size of a dime and contains 7.7 mg of carmustine. The recommended dose is 8 wafers, or 61.6 mg of carmustine, inserted directly into the resection cavity. The wafers gradually dissolve, releasing the drug over a period of 2–3 weeks. Local delivery of carmustine ensures adequate concentrations at the site of the tumor, bypassing the blood-brain barrier.

25. What are the side effects of Gliadel wafers?

The major side effects relate to local effects. Some patients may experience an increase in cerebral edema, and the risk of postsurgical intracranial and wound infections may be increased slightly. In addition, there is a slight increase in the incidence of seizures within 5 days of surgery. Systemic side effects, commonly associated with intravenously administered carmustine, including myelosuppression, are not seen with Gliadel wafers.

BUSULFAN INJECTION

26. What is the role of busulfan injection in current oncology practice?

Busulfan injection (Busulfex) is an intravenous preparation of the oral drug busulfan, which has been used for many years in the treatment of chronic myelogenous leukemia and bone marrow transplantation. Busulfan injection is not interchangeable with oral busulfan. The use of intravenous busulfan should be limited to experienced bone marrow transplant centers with the expertise required for adequate dosing and monitoring of intravenous busulfan therapy.

27. What is the rationale for development of an intravenous preparation of busulfan?

Although the oral formulation has been used for many years, its administration is challenging because it is formulated in 2-mg tablets. Dosing of oral busulfan for bone marrow transplant patients is typically 1 mg/kg of ideal body weight for 12–16 doses. For some patients, this regimen may translate into as many as 35–40 tablets per dose. Administration is sometimes made easier by putting several tablets into gelatin capsules. However, high-dose busulfan is also highly emetogenic and may be difficult for patients to tolerate. Oral administration is further complicated when patients experience emesis shortly after receiving a dose. In some instances, emesis necessitates quantifying the number of tablets visible in the vomitus and giving replacement doses.

In addition to problems with administration, the oral bioavailability of busulfan is highly variable. In fact, it can vary as much as two-fold in adults and up to 6-fold in children. Each patient's actual exposure to the drug, based on determination of area under the concentration time curve (AUC), is unpredictable because of variations in bioavailability. Busulfan also has a narrow therapeutic index in the setting of high-dose chemotherapy. Overdosage can lead to fatal liver and lung toxicity. Underdosage can lead to an ineffective chemotherapy regimen and relapse of disease. For a drug with such a narrow therapeutic index, it would be ideal to be able to predict drug exposure.

28. Why do we not administer intravenous busulfan to all patients who receive busulfan?

Even though the administration of busulfan is simplified with an intravenous preparation, it has been difficult to convert all patients and protocols requiring high-dose busulfan to the intravenous formulation. The main reason is that all dosing standards have been based on the oral form. The optimal AUC for busulfan should be < 1500 μmol/L/min to avoid excessive toxicity. However, there is significant variability in the range of AUCs with current oral dosing regimens. For patients receiving the standard 1 mg/kg dose of oral busulfan, the equivalent intravenous dose may be as much as 0.8 mg/kg or as little as 0.5 mg/kg to achieve the same desired AUC. Because there is so much variability in AUCs for patients receiving oral busulfan, global conversion of oral dosing regimens to intravenous dosing regimens has been impossible. Currently, intravenous busulfan is best administered in a setting where busulfan levels can be pharmacokinetically monitored to ensure that levels do not exceed the toxic range.

29. What are the side effects of busulfan injection?

The side-effect profile of busulfan injection is identical to that of oral busulfan, although some of the toxicities may be lessened by more precise dosing and pharmacokinetic monitoring with the intravenous formulation. Toxicities include myelosuppression, veno-occlusive disease of the liver, pulmonary fibrosis, and seizures. All patients receiving intravenous busulfan should receive phenytoin for prevention of seizures during treatment.

ARSENIC TRIOXIDE

30. What is arsenic trioxide? How does it work?

Arsenic trioxide (Trisenox) was approved by the FDA in September 2000 for the treatment of acute promyelocytic leukemia (APL) in patients who have relapsed after treatment with retinoid- and anthracycline-based chemotherapy. The exact mechanism by which arsenic trioxide works is not completely understood. Arsenic trioxide causes intracellular changes and fragmentation of DNA that lead to cell breakdown and death. This process of "programmed cell death " is called apoptosis.

31. How is arsenic trioxide administered?

Arsenic trioxide is administered as an intravenous infusion over 1–2 hours. Administration occurs in two phases, induction and consolidation. For induction therapy, arsenic trioxide is administered in a dosage of 0.15 mg/kg/day until the patient achieves complete remission. The maximal number of induction doses should not exceed 60. For consolidation, arsenic trioxide is administered in the same dosage for 25 doses over a 5-week period.

32. What side effects are associated with arsenic trioxide?

Common adverse reactions in clinical trials include light-headedness during the infusion, fatigue, musculoskeletal pain, and mild hyperglycemia. In addition, patients may experience leukocytosis and retinoic acid syndrome. Features of retinoic acid syndrome include fluid retention, fever, pulmonary infiltrates, and pleural effusions. The cause of the syndrome relates to the elevation in white blood cell counts (leukocytosis), typically > 10,000 cells/ml, that many patients experience during treatment with arsenic trioxide. The leukocytosis is associated with migration of myeloid cells to extravascular tissues, eliciting an immune response. Retinoic acid syndrome is managed with administration of corticosteroids.

BEXAROTENE

33. What is bexarotene?

Bexarotene (Targetin) is a member of a subclass of retinoids that selectively bind and activate retinoid X receptors (RXRs). Once active, the receptors partner with various other receptors to activate the RXR pathway. The activation of this pathway leads to the induction of apoptosis (programmed cell death) by regulating the expression of genes that control cellular differentiation and proliferation. Bexarotene is FDA-approved for the treatment of cutaneous manifestations of cutaneous T-cell lymphoma (CTCL) in patients who are refractory to at least one prior systemic therapy (i.e., psoralen ultraviolent A-range, electron-beam therapy). The exact mechanism of action of bexarotene is unknown.

34. Describe the dose and route of administration of bexarotene.

Bexarotene is available in two dosage forms, 75 mg soft gelatin capsules and 1% topical gel. The initial recommended dose of oral bexarotene is 300 mg/m^2/day, which should be given as a single daily dose with food. The dose may be adjusted downward by 100 mg/m^2/day to a dose of 100 mg/m^2/day or temporarily withheld if necessitated by toxicity. Once toxicity is controlled, the dose may be readjusted upward with close monitoring. If there is no tumor response after 8 weeks of therapy and the drug is well tolerated by the patient, the dose may be escalated to 400 mg/m^2/day. Bexarotene should be continued for as long as the patient benefits from treatment.

The initial recommended topical dose is a generous coating of the gel sufficient to cover the CTCL lesion, which is applied every other day for the first week. The frequency of application may be increased at weekly intervals to once daily, twice daily, 3 times daily, and 4 times daily, as tolerated. If application-site toxicity occurs, the drug may be temporarily withheld or the frequency reduced. The gel should not be applied to unaffected skin or near mucosal surfaces. Occlusive dressings should not be used with gel application.

35. What are the most common side effects of bexarotene?

Lipid abnormalities, hypothyroidism, dose-related neutropenia, and headaches are the most commonly associated side effects with **oral administration** of bexarotene. Complete blood count with differentiation should be performed before therapy and periodically throughout treatment. Liver function test abnormalities have been reported. Elevations in aspartate aminotransferase (AST), alanine aminotransferease (ALT), bilirubin, and alkaline phosphatase appear to be dose-related. Baseline liver function tests should be obtained and monitored weekly for the first 4 weeks of treatment or until stable and every 8 weeks thereafter. If lab values reach > 3 times the upper limit of normal, bexarotene may be withheld or discontinued. Like other retinoids, bexarotene is associated with photosensitivity. Repeated **topical administration** of bexarotene gel has low potential for significant plasma concentrations. Adverse events with the topical administration of bexarotene are limited to the site of application. The most common adverse events are rash, pruritus, and pain.

36. What drugs may interact with bexarotene?

Bexarotene appears to be hepatically metabolized by cytochrome P450 3A4. Therefore, concomitant administration of bexarotene with itraconazole, ketoconazole, erythromycin, gemfibrozil, grapefruit juice, and other inhibitors of cytochrome P450 3A4 is not recommended. The inhibition of this enzyme can potentially increase plasma concentrations of bexarotene. Inducers of cytochrome P450 3A4, such as rifampin, phenytoin, and phenobarbital, may decrease plasma concentrations of bexarotene and are not recommended for concomitant administration. Vitamin A in doses > 15,000 IU should be avoided to prevent potential additive toxicity.

CAPECITABINE

37. What is capecitabine?

Capecitabine (Xeloda) is a prodrug of the antimetabolite 5-fluorouracil (5FU). Capecitabine must be converted enzymatically to 5FU by thymidine phosphorylase to exert its pharmacologic activity. Thymidine phosphorylase is found in many tissues within the body and is expressed in higher concentrations in some human carcinomas. This results in higher tumor concentrations of the drug. Once capecitabine is converted to 5FU, it binds to thymidylate synthetase and thus inhibits the formation of thymidylate from uracil and DNA synthesis. A metabolite of 5FU can also interfere with RNA processing and protein synthesis. Capecitabine is FDA-approved for the treatment of patients with metastatic breast cancer resistant to both paclitaxel and an anthracycline-containing chemotherapy regimen or resistant to paclitaxel alone and when further anthracycline therapy is contraindicated (i.e., patients who have received cumulative doses of 400 mg/m^2 of doxorubicin or doxorubicin equivalents). Capecitabine is also awaiting FDA approval for use in colorectal cancer.

38. Describe the dose and route of administration of capecitabine.

Capecitabine is available in two tablet strengths, 150 mg and 500 mg. The recommended dose of 2500 mg/m^2/day divided into 2 daily doses for 14 days with a 1-week rest period. Each chemotherapy cycle is 21 days. Doses should be administered orally with food. No studies have been performed to ensure the safety and efficacy of capecitabine tablets when crushed. If it is necessary to crush the tablets, appropriate recommendations for safe handling of cytotoxic drugs by health-care personnel should be followed. In patients with moderate renal impairment (creatinine clearance of 30–50 ml/min), a dose reduction to 75% of the starting dose is recommended. Toxicity due to capecitabine therapy may be managed by symptomatic treatment, dose interruptions, and dose adjustments. Recommended dose modifications are shown below.

Recommended Dose Modifications of Capecitabine

TOXICITY*	DURING COURSE OF THERAPY	DOSE ADJUSTMENT FOR NEXT CYCLE (% OF STARTING DOSE)
Grade 1	Maintain dose level	Maintain dose level
Grade 2		
First appearance	Interrupt until resolved or grade 0–1	100
Second appearance	Interrupt until resolved or grade 0–1	75
Third appearance	Interrupt until resolved or grade 0–1	50
Fourth appearance	Discontinue treatment permanently	
Grade 3		
First appearance	Interrupt until resolved or grade 0–1	75
Second appearance	Interrupt until resolved or grade 0–1	50
Third appearance	Discontinue treatment permanently	
Grade 4		
First appearance	Discontinue permanently *or* If it is believed to be in the best interest of the patient to continue, interrupt until resolved to grade 0–1	

* National Cancer Institute of Canada Common Toxicity Criteria, except for hand-foot syndrome, which is defined according to a grading system incorporated by Roche Pharmaceutical and accepted by the FDA.

39. What are the most common side effects of capecitabine?

Diarrhea, neutropenia, and hand-foot syndrome are the most common side effects. Elevated bilirubin, alkaline phosphatase, AST and ALT have been reported in patients taking capecitabine. Close monitoring should be performed in patients with hepatic metastases. Diarrhea is a dose-limiting side effect in about 50% of patients and may be severe. Patients should be monitored closely and given fluid and electrolyte replacement as needed. Standard antidiarrheal treatments such as loperamide are recommended. Nausea and vomiting and stomatitis also may be severe.

Hand-foot syndrome (palmar-plantar erythrodysesthesia) can be characterized by numbness, tingling, painless or painful swelling, paresthesia or dysesthesia, erythema, blistering and desquamation on the palms of the hand or soles of the feet. Symptoms may be managed by dose modification. Hand creams/ointments or oral pyridoxine may provide additional relief.

40. Discuss the drug interactions of capecitabine.

The administration of **antacids** containing aluminum hydroxide or magnesium hydroxide immediately after administration of capecitabine may result in higher drug concentrations and increased toxicity. Patients should be advised to delay the administration of antacids for at least 2 hours after taking capecitabine. **Leucovorin** potentitates the activity and toxicity of 5FU. Deaths from severe enterocolitis, dehydration, and diarrhea have been reported in patients taking leucovorin in combination with capecitabine. Capecitabine may alter prothrombin time (PT) and international normalized ratio (INR) in patients receiving concomitant therapy with **warfarin** anticoagulants. Regular monitoring of PT and INR should be performed. Capecitabine also may interact with **phenytoin**, resulting in elevated phenytoin levels. Phenytoin levels should be monitored closely and doses adjusted as needed as long as a patient is taking both medications.

TEMOZOLOMIDE

41. What is temozolomide?

Temozolomide (Temodar) is a derivative of the alkylating agent dacarbazine. Temozolomide is a prodrug of 5-(3-methyltriazen-1-yl)imidazole-4-carboximide (MTIC). It works by inhibiting DNA replication and inducing apoptosis. Temozolomide is FDA-approved for the treatment of adults with refractory anaplastic astrocytoma and patients who have experienced disease progression on a drug regimen containing a nitrosurea and procarbazine. Temozolomide is 100% absorbed in the gastrointestinal tract and can cross the blood-brain barrier.

42. Describe the dose and route of administration of temozolomide.

Temozolomide is supplied as 5-mg, 20-mg, 100-mg, and 250-mg capsules with a recommended single daily dose of 150 mg/m^2/day for 5 days every 28 days. Each dose should be taken orally on an empty stomach at bedtime to reduce potential side effects. According to manufacturer recommendations, capsules should not be chewed or opened. Subsequent doses are based on nadir platelet and absolute neutrophil counts (ANC) from the previous cycle and day 1 of the next cycle. If both the nadir and day 1 ANC and platelet counts are > 1500/mm^3 and 100,000/mm^3, respectively, temozolomide may be increased to 200 mg/m^2/day for 5 days. Temozolomide should not be administered until ANC and platelet counts exceed 1500/mm^3 and 100,000/mm$_3$, respectively. If at any time during therapy the ANC or platelet count decreases to < 1000/mm^3 or 50,000/mm^3, respectively, the dose of the next cycle should be reduced by 50 mg/m^2/day. The lowest recommended dosage is 100 mg/m^2/day.

Because of the risk of inappropriate dosing, the manufacturer recommends that each daily dose be packaged and dispensed separately and labeled as days 1, 2, 3, 4, and 5. Patients should be advised to take all capsules in each daily dose package.

43. What are the most common side effects of temozolomide?

Nausea and vomiting, fatigue, headache, and myelosuppression are common. Nausea and vomiting usually are mild to moderate and may be controlled with antiemetics. Bedtime administration also may help to control nausea and vomiting. Use with caution in patients with severe renal or hepatic impairment.

44. Discuss the drug interactions of temozolomide.

A pharmacokinetic drug interaction exists between temozolomide and valproic acid. The clearance of temozolomide is slightly decreased with concomitant use of valproic acid. The clinical importance of this interaction is unknown.

DOCETAXEL

45. What is docetaxel?

Docetaxel (Taxotere) is a semisynthetic taxane produced from inactive precursors extracted from the needles of the European yew (*Taxus baccata*). Docetaxel, like paclitaxel, is an antimicrotubule agent. Unlike other antimicrotubule agents, the taxanes promote microtubule assembly and stabilize these organelles to resist disassembly, therefore inhibiting cell replication. Docetaxel possesses a higher binding affinity than paclitaxel for tubulin, the protein subunit of the spindle microtubules. The difference in binding affinity between the two agents results in the formation of microtubules that differ in size and structure. The increased potency of docetaxel may be explained by its higher binding affinity, ability to achieve higher intracellular concentrations, and slower cellular efflux. Docetaxel is FDA approved for (1) treatment of locally advanced or metastatic breast cancer that has progressed during anthracycline-based treatment or relapsed during anthracycline-based adjuvant therapy and (2) treatment after failure of prior chemotherapy. Recently it was approved for treatment of non-small-cell lung cancer (NSCLC) that does not respond to cisplatin-based therapy. Docetaxel is also under study for use in several other types of cancer.

46. Describe the dose and route of administration of docetaxel.

For the treatment of breast cancer, the current recommended regimen is 60–100 mg/m^2 infused intravenously (IV) over 1 hour every 21 days. For NSCLC, docetaxel is most commonly administered at a dose of 100 mg/m^2 infused IV over 1 hour every 21 days. Once-weekly dosing at 30 mg/m^2 may be advantageous in some patients because of the low incidence of hematologic toxicity. Dose modifications should be based on ANC and platelet counts. Doses should be held until the ANC and platelet counts are at least 1500/mm^3 and 100,000/mm^3, respectively. The dosing regimen also should be modified if the patient experiences febrile neutropenia, severe neutropenia, and other severe nonhematologic toxicities. Docetaxel clearance appears to be decreased in patients with liver metastases or abnormal LFTs. Generally it should not be used in patients with a total bilirubin > the upper limit of normal (ULN) or an AST or ALT > 1.5 times ULN with an alkaline phosphatase > 2.5 times ULN.

47. What other precautions relate to the administrastion of docetaxel?

1. To prevent severe hypersensitivity reactions and to reduce the incidence of fluid retention, all patients should be premedicated with oral dexamethasone prior to treatment. Patients are given a prophylactic regimen of oral dexamethasone, 8 mg twice daily for 3 days. Dexamethasone should be initiated 1 day before administration of docetaxel.

2. Docetaxel is an irritant and should be administered with caution. Currently there is no specific treatment for docetaxel-induced extravasation reactions. General conservative measures and avoidance of warm compresses are recommended for treatment.

3. When diluted and undiluted docetaxel solutions come in contact with plasticized polyvinyl chloride materials, substantial leaching of diethylhexyl phthalate (DHEP) occurs in a concentration- and time-dependent manner. To minimize patient exposure to leached DHEP, docetaxel solutions should be dispensed in glass bottles or in nonpolyvinyl chloride (non-PVC) containers, and non-PVC tubing should be used during administration of docetaxel.

48. What are the most common side effects of docetaxel?

Bone marrow suppression. The bone marrow suppression is dose limiting and manifested by neutropenia, anemia, and thrombocytopenia. Neutrophil nadirs generally occur on days 7–10, and neutrophil counts recover by days 15–21. Patients who experience severe neutropenia should receive a dose reduction for the next cycle of chemotherapy. If clinically relevant, packed red blood cell transfusions or erythropoeitin therapy may be used for treatment of anemia.

Hypersensitivity reactions. Docetaxel-induced hypersensitivity reactions usually occur within minutes after initiation of infusion. It is unclear whether these reactions are associated with docetaxel itself or with excipients in the drug formulation. Reactions can range from mild (i.e. flushing and localized skin reactions) to severe (i.e., hypotension and/or bronchospasm). Patients should receive prophylactic oral dexamethasone and also may require diphenhydramine. The infusion rate may be decreased to reduce hypersensitivity reactions. Docetaxel must be discontinued if the hypersensitivity reaction is severe.

Fluid retention. Peripheral edema and weight gain are characteristic of fluid retention in patients treated with docetaxel. Pleural or pericardial effusion and ascites have been reported less frequently. The incidence and severity of fluid retention increases with cumulative dose of docetaxel > 400 mg/m^2. Premedication with oral dexamethasone can delay the onset and decrease the severity of fluid retention. Other measures, such as sodium restriction and diuretics, can be used to treat peripheral edema.

Peripheral neuropathy. Neurosensory effects occur in approximately 50% of patients treated with docetaxel. Peripheral neuropathy generally is characterized by paresthesia or dysesthesia with numbness and tingling in a stocking-and-glove distribution. Dose modifications may be necessary if neuropathy becomes severe and prevents patients from performing activities of daily living. Peripheral motor dysfunction resulting in extremity weakness also may occur.

Other common side effects include mild-to-moderate **nausea and vomiting**. **Alopecia** occurs in approximately 70% of patients but is fully reversible.

49. Discuss the drug interactions of docetaxel.

Docetaxel, like paclitaxel, is a radiosensitizing agent. Increased toxicity may occur with concurrent use of radiation therapy. Docetaxel is metabolized by the cytochrome P450 system. Inhibitors of the P450 system may decrease the clearance of docetaxel, whereas inducers may increase clearance.

GEMCITABINE

50. What is gemcitabine?

Gemcitabine (Gemzar) is a synthetic pyrimidine nucleoside. It was originally synthesized as an antiviral agent. Gemcitabine is an antimetabolite that acts as an inhibitor of DNA synthesis. A phosphorylated form of gemcitabine inhibits DNA polymerase and competes with the physiologic substrate cytidine for incorporation into the DNA. Once incorporated, DNA synthesis is terminated and apoptosis occurs. Gemcitabine is FDA-approved for first-line treatment of locally advanced or metastatic pancreatic cancer and for second-line treatment of pancreatic cancer previously treated with 5FU. It also is approved for use in combination with cisplatin for the first-line treatment of patients with inoperable, locally advanced, or metastatic NSCLC. Gemcitabine is under study for use in several other cancers.

51. Describe the dose and route of administration of gemcitabine.

The current recommended dose of gemcitabine for first- or second-line treatment of locally advanced or metastatic pancreatic cancer is 1000 mg/m^2 given IV over 30 minutes once weekly for up to 7 weeks, as tolerated, followed by a 1-week rest period. Subsequent cycles are 28 days. The dose is 1000 mg/m^2 given IV over 30 minutes once weekly for 3 weeks, followed by a 1-week rest period. In the treatment of NSCL, gemcitabine may be used as a single agent or in combination with other agents. As monotherapy gemcitabine is most commonly dosed at 1000 or 1250 mg/m^2 given IV over 30 minutes once weekly for 3 weeks, followed by 1 week of rest. Similar doses and dosing schedules may be used in combination with cisplatin, vinorelbine, or other chemotherapy agents. When administered in combination with cisplatin, gemcitabine should be infused first, followed immediately by cisplatin. Increased toxicity is seen when gemcitabine infusions are longer than 1 hour in duration. Dose modifications are based on ANC and platelet counts. If the ANC is 500–999/mm^3 or the platelet count is 50,000–99,000/mm^3, 75% of the full dose should be given weekly. If the ANC is < 500/mm^3 or the platelet count < 50,000/mm^3, the weekly dose should be withheld until counts are above these levels. There are no recommended dose adjustments for renal or hepatic impairment.

52. What are the most common side effects of gemcitabine?

Myelosuppression, flulike syndrome, rash, and elevated liver transaminases are the most common side effects. Myelosuppression is dose-limiting; neutropenia is more common than thrombocytopenia. The nadir usually occurs between days 8 and 15. Flulike symptoms are easily treatable with acetaminophen. A generalized rash is common; onset is usually within 48–72 hours of infusion. The rash is erythematous and maculopapular and routinely involves the extremities. Topical corticosteroids can be used for treatment. Other toxicities that may occur are severe hypotension, pulmonary toxicity (i.e., bronchospasm and dyspnea), and proteinuria. The emetogenicity of gemcitabine is very low.

53. Discuss the drug interactions of gemcitabine.

Gemcitabine is a potent radiosensitizer. Safe and effective regimens of combined gemcitabine and radiation have not been established. Caution should be used if the two therapies are use concurrently.

DOXORUBICIN HCL LIPOSOME INJECTION

54. What is doxorubicin HCl liposome injection?

Doxorubicin HCl liposome injection (Doxil) is an anthracycline cytostatic antibiotic encapsulated in long-circulating STEALTH liposomes. Anthracyclines exert their antineoplastic effects by intercalating between DNA strands, causing deformation of DNA with resultant inhibition of topoisomerase II. Inhibition of topoisomerase II, the enzyme responsible for DNA strand breakage and repair, results in increased DNA fragmentation and eventual apoptosis. The STEALTH liposomes are formulated to increase blood circulation time of the drug. At least 90% of the encapsulated doxorubicin is contained in the liposome during circulation. It is hypothesized that because of small size and length of time in circulation, the liposomes are able to penetrate the altered vasculature of tumors. Once distributed to tissue, the encapsulated doxorubicin is released by an unknown mechanism. Doxorubicin HCl liposome injection is FDA-approved for (1) metastatic ovarian carcinoma that is refractory to both paclitaxel- and platinum-based chemotherapy regimens and (2) AIDS-related Kaposi's sarcoma that has progressed during prior combination chemotherapy or in patients who are intolerant of prior therapy.

55. Describe the dose and route of administration of doxorubicin HCl liposome injection.

The recommended dosing for treatment of ovarian cancer is 50 mg/m^2 given IV at an initial rate of 1 mg/minute once every 28 days. If no infusion-related adverse events are observed during the initial dose, the rate of subsequent infusions can be increased to complete administration of the drug over 1 hour. A minimum of 4 courses is recommended because the median time to response in clinical trials was 4 months. The recommended dose for the treatment of Kaposi's sarcoma is 20 mg/m^2 given IV over 30 minutes once every 21 days for as long as the patient responds and tolerates treatment. Dose modifications may be based on hematologic and non-hematologic toxicities. Doxorubicin HCl liposome injection is not a vesicant but should be considered an irritant. Precautions should be used to avoid extravasation. Do not use doxorubicin HCl liposome injection with in-line filters.

Recommended Dosing in Patients with Elevated Bilirubin Levels

SERUM BILIRUBIN	PERCENT OF NORMAL DOSE ADMINISTERED
1.2–3.0 mg/dl	50
> 3.0 mg/dl	25

56. What are the common side effects of doxorubicin HCl liposome injection?

Neutropenia, anemia, hand-foot syndrome, and nausea are the most common side effects. Myelosuppression is generally moderate and reversible. Cytokine support may be used during treatment if the patients experiences severe hematologic toxicity. Hand-foot syndrome occurs in about 40% of patients and is generally seen after 2–3 cycles. Symptoms may be managed by dose modification. Hand creams/ointments or oral pyridoxine (150 mg orally 2 or 3 times/day) may provide additional relief. Patients should be advised to keep the affected area moisturized, clean, and dry; to avoid pressure on the skin (including tight clothing and shoes, tape, and jewelry); and to avoid heat, hot water, and sun exposure for 3–5 days after administration. Nausea should be treated by premedication with and/or concomitant use of antiemetics. Other less frequent adverse events are infusion-related reactions, stomatitis, and secondary acute myelogenous leukemia. The use of doxorubicin HCl liposome injection is contraindicated in patients who have a hypersensitivity to conventional doxorubicin.

It appears that doxorubicin HCl liposome injection reduces the risk of anthracycline-induced cardiotoxicity, but adequate studies have not been done. At present the manufacturer recommends that warnings related to the use of conventional doxorubicin be observed.

57. Discuss the drug interactions of doxorubicin HCl liposome injection.

No formal drug interaction studies have been conducted with doxorubicin HCl liposome injection. However, the doxorubicin in the injection may potentiate the toxicity of other anticancer therapies.

THALIDOMIDE

58. Summarize the history of thalidomide.

Thalidomide has an infamous history. In the late 1950s and early 1960s it was used as a sedative agent and as an antiemetic agent for nausea and vomiting associated with pregnancy. Although it was not FDA-approved in the United States at that time, it was approved and widely used in other countries. In 1961 thalidomide was withdrawn from the world market when it was found to be a teratogen; its use was associated with severe congenital malformations, most notably phocomelia.

Investigational use in the U.S. for treatment of graft-vs.-host disease in bone marrow transplant patients and for various uses in the management of AIDS began in the early 1990s. Thalidomide also was shown to be extremely beneficial in treatment of the painful erythematous lesions associated with leprosy. In 1998, the FDA approved thalidomide for treatment and maintenance therapy of leprosy amid great controversy. Because of its known teratogenic effects, it is the most heavily regulated drug in the U.S. Thalidomide is available only through physicians and pharmacies registered in the System for Thalidomide Education and Prescribing Safety (STEPS) Program. Registration in the STEPS program is done through the manufacturer, Celgene.

59. How does thalidomide work?

Various mechanisms of action have been proposed. Thalidomide is thought to inhibit the process of angiogenesis, or formation of new capillaries from existing blood vessels. Inhibition of angiogenesis may disrupt tumor growth and spread. Thalidomide is also thought to modulate cytokines that mediate and regulate immunity and inflammation. In that capacity it is effective in treatment of graft-vs.-host disease and cachexia and wasting associated with AIDS.

60. What is thalidomide's role in cancer treatment?

Thalidomide is not currently FDA-approved for use in cancer treatment. It has shown promise in multiple myeloma and is currently under further investigation for this indication. Thalidomide is also used investigationally in the treatment of various other malignancies, such as breast cancer, brain tumors, head and neck cancer, sarcomas, prostate, and lung cancers. One small pilot study suggested a benefit to thalidomide in management of diarrhea due to irinotecan therapy.

61. What are the side effects of thalidomide?

The most common side effects are sedation and constipation. Sedation can be minimized by administering the drug at bedtime or by using an antisedative such as methylphenidate. Tolerance to daytime sedation may develop after a patient has been stabilized at a particular dose for several weeks. Good hydration and a stool softener are useful in managing the constipation. Some patients may require stimulant laxatives to relieve constipation. Particular caution for this side effect should be observed in patients who are receiving opiate analgesics and may already be experiencing constipation. Some patients may experience dizziness and orthostatic hypotension. These side effects can be minimized if patients are instructed to sit up and stand from a supine position gradually. An erythematous rash can occur in patients receiving thalidomide. Thalidomide should be discontinued in patients with rash because progression to more serious skin reactions, such as Stevens-Johnson syndrome, has been reported. Peripheral neuropathy and neutropenia also have been reported.

62. How is thalidomide administered?

Thalidomide is available orally in 50-mg capsules. The optimal dosing regimen for treatment of cancer has not been determined. In the treatment of multiple myeloma, the most common dosing regimen is 200 mg/day orally for 14 days; the dose is increased by 200 mg as tolerated, approximately every 14 days. The maximal dose is typically 800 mg/day. The minimal effective dose in multiple myeloma is thought to be 400 mg/day. The optimal duration of therapy is not well established. It is thought that treatment of multiple myeloma should continue for a minimum of 100 days before response is evaluated. Toxicity may limit duration of treatment.

GLUTAMINE

63. What is glutamine? How is it useful for treating side effects related to chemotherapy?

Glutamine is not a chemotherapy agent but is under study for treatment of side effects associated with chemotherapy. It is the most abundant of the body's 20 amino acids involved in protein synthesis. Cancer and/or its treatments can lead to glutamine depletion. Clinical trials are under way in NCI-sponsored Cooperative Groups and academic/hospital-based cancer centers to investigate the efficacy of supplemental glutamine in protecting normal tissues from chemotherapy and radiotherapy. Recent data suggest that glutamine may be beneficial in preventing and treating various side effects and toxicities, such as diarrhea, mucositis, arthralgia, myalgia, and peripheral neuropathy. Of interest, glutamine supplementation also may decrease tumor growth by upregulation of the immune system, enhancing tumor cell susceptibility to chemotherapy.

The optimal dose and duration of glutamine therapy have not been determined. However, anecdotal and clinical experiences suggest that the following dose and schedule has resulted in symptom reduction: glutamine powder, 10 gm orally 3 times/day, beginning on the day of chemotherapy or 24 hours after chemotherapy for 3–5 days.

Cambridge Nutraceuticals, Boston (800-265-2202; web site: www.cambridgenutra.com) recommends the following dose for patients undergoing chemotherapy and radiation therapy: Glutamine powder, 10 grams orally 3 times/day, beginning on the day of therapy and for 4 days after treatment. The cost for 480-gram jar of glutamine powder is about $45.

REFERENCES

1. Anderson BS, Madden T, Tran HT, et al: Acute safety and pharmacokinetics of intravenous busulfan when used with oral busulfan and cyclophosphamide as pre-transplantation conditioning therapy: A phase I study. Biol Blood Marrow Transplant 6(5A):548–554, 2000.
2. Anderson PM, Schroeder G, Skubitz KM: Oral glutamine reduces the duration and severity of stomatitis after cytotoxic cancer chemotherapy. Cancer 83:1433–1439, 1998.
3. Baker DE: Epirubicin. Drug Link Special Edition (Facts and Comparisons Newsletter) June, 2000.
4. Camacho LH, Soignet SL, Ho R, et al: Leukocytosis and the retinoic acid syndrome in patients with acute promyelocytic leukemia treated with arsenic trioxide. J Clin Oncol 18:2620–2625, 2000.
5. Chabner BA, Longo DL (eds): Cancer Chemotherapy and Biotherapy: Principles and Practice. Philadelphia, Lippincott-Raven, 1996.
6. Dooley Km, Goa KL: Capecitabine. Drugs 58:69–76, 1999.
7. Dorr RT, Von Hoff DD: Cancer Chemotherapy Handbook, 2nd ed. East Norwalk, CT, Appleton & Lange, 1994.
8. Finley RS, Balmer C (eds): Concepts in Oncology Therapeutics, 2nd ed. Bethesda, MD, American Society of Health-System Pharmacists, 1998.
9. Gliadel wafers for treatment of brain tumors. Med Lett 40:92, 1998.
10. Govindarajan R, Heaton KM, Broadwater R, et al: Effect of thalidomide on gastrointestinal toxic effects of irinotecan [letter]. Lancet 356:566–567, 2000.
11. Howell SB, Glantz MJ, LaFollette S, et al: A controlled trial of Depocyt for the treatment of lymphomatous meningitis. Proceedings of ASCO 18:10a, 1999 [abstract 34].
12. Hvizdos KM, Goa KL: Temozolomide. CNS Drugs 12:237–243, 1999.
13. Klimberg VS, McClellan JL: Glutamine, cancer, and its therapy. Am J Surg 172:418–424, 1996.
14. Miller RM: Docetaxel: A taxoid for the treatment of metastatic breast cancer. Am J Health Syst Pharm 55:1777–1791, 1998.
15. Miller VA, Benedetti FM, Rigas JR, et al: Initial clinical trial of selective retinoid X receptor ligand, LGD1069. J Clin Oncol 15:790-795, 1997.
16. Nirenberg A: Thalidomide: When everything old is new again. Clin J Oncol Nurs 5:15–18, 2001.
17. Olavarria E, Hassan M, Eades A, et al: A phase I/II study of multiple-dose intravenous busulfan as myeloablation prior to stem cell transplantation. Leukemia 14:1954–1959, 2000.
18. Ryberg M, Nielsen D, Skovsgaard T, et al: Epirubicin cardiotoxicity: An analysis of 469 patients with metastatic breast cancer. J Clin Oncol 16:3502–3508, 1998.
19. Savarese D, Boucher J, Corey B: Glutamine treatment of paclitaxel-induced myalgias and athralgias. J Clin Oncol 16:3918–3919, 1998.
20. Soignet SL, Maslak P, Wang ZG, et al. Complete remission after treatment of acute promyelocytic leukemia with arsenic trioxide. N Engl J Med 339:1341–1348, 1998.
21. Stomiolo AM, Allerheiligen SR, Pearce HL: Preclinical, pharmacologic, and phase I studies of gemcitabine. Semin Oncol 24(2 Suppl 7):S7-2–S7-7, 1997.
22. Stucky-Marshall L: New agents in gastrointestinal malignancies. Part 1: Irinotecan in clinical practice. Cancer Nurs 22:212–219, 1999.
23. Tardi TG, Boman NL, Cullis PR: Liposomal doxorubicin. J Drug Target 4(3):129–140, 1996.
24. Thomas M: Glutamine and cancer therapy symptom management. Network News: An Update for Community-based Oncology Professionals. Oncology Therapeutics Network (OTN), May, 2000, pp 1–2.
25. Xeloda (capecitabine) package insert: Roche Pharmaceuticals, Nutley, NJ, 2000.

9. TIPS FOR ADMINISTERING CHEMOTHERAPY

Jennifer Petersen, RN, MS, OCN, *and Carol Blendowski,* RN, BS, OCN

1. What qualifications are needed to administer chemotherapy?

Patients with cancer receive complicated drug regimens and schedules with the potential for severe side effects and reactions. Only nurses and physicians with advanced educational preparation should administer chemotherapy. Such preparation includes certification in chemotherapy administration, which consists not only of didactic instruction but also of clinical application and skill supervision. The practitioner also should be knowledgeable about the proper procedures for drug preparation, handling and alternate methods of drug delivery, including various vascular access devices and ambulatory infusion pumps and their associated complications.

Since 1998 the Oncology Nursing Society (ONS) has developed an official credentialing program for cancer chemotherapy certification. The course consists only of didactic instruction using the second edition of the *Cancer Chemotherapy Guidelines* as a textbook. For more information contact the Oncology Nursing Society (ONS) and visit the ONS website: www.ons.org.

2. What are the most important precautions for preventing errors in chemotherapy administration?

Serious errors in chemotherapy administration are relatively rare considering the number of patients treated. Although even the most knowledgeable practitioner can make mistakes, errors most likely occur when untrained personnel are asked to perform tasks beyond their expertise or when an order is written in an unclear way that allows misinterpretation. Important precautions include the following:

1. Administration of chemotherapy should be delayed until a properly trained practitioner is available. With rare exceptions (e.g., high-grade lymphoma), administration of chemotherapy is not an emergency procedure.

2. Only qualified personnel should write orders or administer chemotherapy.

3. A documented double-check mechanism should be used by personnel preparing and administering the drugs.

4. The patient should be cared for by only one or two nurses who communicate and work together to chart which drugs have been given and repeatedly check that they have the right dose of the right drug for the right patient via the right route according to the right schedule.

5. Nurses need to question any aspect of the order that is contrary to customary practice or to what has been done for the patient in the past, especially when unusually high doses or unusual schedules are involved.

6. Nurses should be careful not to permit distractions while checking an order or administering treatment. Too often the nurse is treating 4 or 5 patients at one time and forgets to check an order or to identify a patient properly. Distractions such as telephones, pagers, and physicians' requests for assistance should be kept to a minimum in the treatment area.

7. Nurses working in a solo practice may have to prepare and administer chemotherapy. In this setting, the physician should be responsible for double-checking all chemotherapeutic agents before they are administered.

8. Two nurses should double-check and document the proper volume, dose, and programmed rate of all ambulatory pumps when patients are connected and discharged on continuous infusion chemotherapy.

3. Who should write chemotherapy orders? How should they be written?

Only the attending physician or oncology fellow (not the resident or intern) responsible for the patient's care and most familiar with the drug regimen and dosing schedule should write the order for chemotherapy. Orders should be written according to the following guidelines:

1. The order should be written clearly and without abbreviations.

2. Any dose modification requires a new written order. The original order should *not* be erased, crossed out, or tampered with in any manner.

3. The dose should be written first as it is to be calculated (mg/m^2 or mg/kg), and the total dose should be indicated along with route and length of time of the injection or infusion.

4. If one drug in a combination is to be given for 1 day only and the other(s) for more than 1 day, this distinction should be clearly indicated.

Many oncology clinics have converted to chemotherapy software ordering programs. Such programs guide thorough and legible ordering of chemotherapy. Although the treatment plan can be easily accessed and implemented by many members of the health care team, the original order remains the responsibility of the attending physician or oncology fellow.

4. Give an example of an appropriately written chemotherapy order.
Patient is 72 cm tall and weighs 150 lb; m^2 = 2.
Order: Cisplatin 75 mg/m^2 = 150 mg in 250 ml normal saline IV over 1 hour (day 1 only)
Etoposide 75 mg/m^2 = 150 mg in 250 ml normal saline IV over 1 hour on days 1, 2, 3.
Etoposide total dose = 450 mg over 3 days.

5. How is dosing of carboplatin different from dosing of most chemotherapeutic agents?
The dose of carboplatin is based on area under the curve (AUC). It is expressed as total milligrams, not milligrams per square meter (mg/m^2), and correlated with the desired AUC level. AUC dosing for carboplatin correlates better with toxicity than dosing based on body surface area (BSA) and is calculated with the Calvert formula:

$$\text{Total dose} = \text{target AUC} \times (\text{glomerular filtration rate} + 25)$$

6. Should a nurse take a verbal order for chemotherapy?
No. *Verbal orders for chemotherapy should not be given or taken.* The risk of confusion about drug names and dosages is too great. People unfamiliar with chemotherapy may mistake carboplatin for cisplatin, vincristine for vinblastine, or Taxol for Taxotere. Mitoxantrone may be easily mistaken for mitomycin because both have a similar dosage range, both are used for breast cancer, both have an unusual color (mitomycin is light purple, mitoxantrone is dark blue), and both can be given by intravenous push. However, mitoxantrone is given more commonly as an infusion over 15 minutes; it is potentially dangerous to give mitomycin as an infusion because it is a vesicant. An error such as giving the wrong drug or wrong dose can be fatal.

7. Can small, frail veins that may have been adequate for methotrexate and 5-fluorouracil be used for doxorubicin, a known vesicant?
Small veins do not necessitate use of a vascular access device (VAD) to administer a vesicant. However, the vein must be properly selected and prepared before venipuncture is attempted. The nurse should take time, avoid distraction, and be focused on the patient.

8. Give guidelines for selecting the proper arm vein.
1. Begin your exam at the dorsum of the hand and move upward.
2. Avoid the antecubital fossa for vesicant administration.
3. The distal forearm is the best site to avoid nerve and tendon damage.
4. Avoid veins that have been used in the past 24 hours.
5. Avoid veins with compromised circulation.
6. Evaluate the need for a VAD if multiple cycles of chemotherapy are planned.

9. What steps should the nurse follow before attempting venipuncture?
- Apply warm compresses.
- Use gravity.
- Have the patient squeeze a handball.
- Offer a hot drink.

10. How can you distinguish among extravasation, irritation, and flare reaction?

Extravasation, although rare, is probably one of the most worrisome findings that a nurse encounters. It is characterized by swelling, erythema, pain at the IV site, and inability to obtain blood return (usually). Vein **irritation** manifests as complaints of achiness and tightness along the vein accompanied by redness and darkness. Blood return usually is present. **Flare reaction** almost always has blood return and is not characterized by pain; it is associated with immediate blotches around the needle site and streaking or itching along the vein.

11. True or false: As long as you have blood return, you do not need to worry about extravasation.

False. Extravasations of vesicant agents may occur in the presence of perfect blood return. Evidence of good blood return is not the only measure of safe and trouble-free injection of a vesicant. If pain, swelling, or tension is evident in the surrounding tissue, the drug probably has infiltrated despite adequate blood return. Do not ignore the patient's complaint of pain—it may be the first sign of extravasation.

12. What should you do if you are giving a vesicant and lose blood return?

The main problem with small veins is that blood return may be intermittent during drug injection. The saying, "If in doubt, pull it out," is appropriate but sometimes not practical. Because presumably the best vein already has been chosen, removal of the needle without cause is not only unnecessary but also may diminish the chance of safe delivery of the drug. If any of the cardinal symptoms of extravasation (pain or swelling at the site) is present, the nurse should stop injecting the drug and attempt to aspirate. If it is not possible to aspirate blood or drug, the needle is removed and the site is treated as an extravasation (see question 13).

In cases involving flare at the site (redness or itching along the vein) and loss of blood return, the nurse should stop injecting the drug, switch to saline, and give 10–30 ml of saline through the line while observing for swelling and symptoms of discomfort. If the vein is determined to be patent, the vesicant is again connected and injected slowly. The blood return again may be evident as the drug is given. The nurse should not try to reposition the needle or press down on the cannula to obtain a blood return. This strategy may result in damage to the vein and seepage of the drug out of the vein (i.e., extravasation).

13. If extravasation is suspected, what should the nurse do?

1. Stop the drug.
2. Aspirate and leave the needle in place.
3. Call the physician.
4. Give an antidote (when appropriate) through the needle or by subcutaneous injection if the needle is already removed.
5. Remove the needle, and avoid undue pressure.
6. Apply cold or heat (depending on the extravasated drug) for 15 minutes 4 times/day for 24 hours.
7. Arrange consultation with a plastic surgeon.
8. Photograph the IV site.
9. Document the incident (see form on following page).

14. How often should a VAD be checked during continuous infusion of a chemotherapeutic agent or vesicant?

Extravasations with VADs are rare but may occur. Exit sites need to be inspected frequently for signs of edema, erythema, or fluid drainage. The site should be checked every 1–2 hours or more often, according to the patient's condition. Many nurses focus on checking blood return to ascertain catheter tip and needle placement; however, there is no consensus about how often this procedure should be done. It is probably reasonable to check blood return less frequently (every 4–8 hours) because of concerns about infection risk, catheter clotting, or needle dislodgements in implanted ports.

Documentation Record for Suspected or Actual Chemotherapy Drug Extravasation

Patient: _____   **Date** infiltration occurred: _____

Drug: _____ Dilution mg/ml _____   Vesicant _____   Irritant _____

Amount of drug infiltrated: < 1 ml _____   1–3 ml _____   3–5 ml _____   5–10 ml _____   > 10 ml _____

Method of drug administration:
_____ Two-syringe technique IV push
_____ Side-arm with IV freely running
_____ Continuous infusion: Rate ___ cc/hour   Peristaltic pump: ____ Yes ____ No
_____ VAD: ____ Port ____ Tunneled catheter   Type of needle _____
_____ Other: _____

Description of site:
Size _____   Color _____   Texture _____
(Indicate site on diagram)

Process documentation: Describe the events   Right arm   Left arm
that occurred during the drug administration   (Attach photograph)
S (patient's symptoms): _____
_____
_____

O (clinical symptoms): _____
_____
_____

A (assessment): _____ Suspected extravasation _____ Definite extravasation _____

P (plan of care):   Initial actions: _____
_____

Physician notified _____   Instruction _____
_____

Follow-up instructions: ____ _____
_____

Additional comments: _____
Consultations: _____   Plastic surgery _____   Physical therapy _____   Other _____
Date of referral: _____   Follow-up _____
Return appointment: _____   Written instructions for site care reviewed with patient _____
RN signature: _____
Follow-up visit no. 1 (date _____)   Describe site and care instructions (attach photo): _____
_____

Follow-up visit no. 2 (date _____)   Describe site and care instructions (attach photo): _____
_____

Follow-up visit no. 3 (date _____)   Describe site and care instructions (attach photo): _____
_____

Source: Goodman M: Rush Cancer Institute, Chicago.

15. A patient with breast cancer needs only one more dose of doxorubicin. She has absolutely no usable veins in her good arm. Is it safe to use her other arm, even though she has had a node dissection?

If the patient has no evidence or history of swelling, if she is fully informed about the risks, and if an excellent vein is available, it is often safe to proceed, after you have consulted with a physician. More breast surgeons are now performing sentinel lymph node dissections (removal of only the first few nodes in the lymphatic chain), which significantly limit the incidence of lymphedema and other complications. Therefore, the risk in using the operative arm for treatment may be lessened. If the integrity of the vein appears questionable, a temporary central line may be considered.

16. What can be done to minimize the pain of needlestick?

For many patients the pain of the needlestick (e.g., an implanted port, peripheral line, or Zoladex injection) is the most dreaded part of treatment. For some patients, an ethyl chloride spray, ice cubes, or intradermal lidocaine is adequate to partially numb the site. Many institutions have cautiously limited their use of ethyl chloride because it is flammable and dispensed in pressurized glass spray bottles that shatter forcefully if dropped on a hard surface. In addition, it must be stored in a special temperature-sensitive cabinet.

The most effective solution is a topical anesthetic cream (e.g., Emla), which is placed over the port site 1–2 hours before the needle puncture. The topical anesthetic cream also may be used over peripheral veins. Patients often can identify their best veins by running the hand or forearm under warm water and placing the topical anesthetic cream on the site before they come for treatment. An exception is the patient receiving a vesicant or irritant agent; the topical anesthetic cream may numb the site sufficiently to mask the discomfort associated with extravasation or infiltration.

17. Outline the safest way to administer a vesicant agent through a peripheral vein.

1. Select the best vein, preferably one in the forearm, where soft tissue density is greater. However, a straight, supple, easily cannulated vein in the hand is preferable to a smaller, deeper vein in any other location that is more difficult to cannulate.

2. Select a method of administration—either the two-syringe technique or infusion through the side-arm of a freely running IV line. The two-syringe technique is used most often when fluids are not needed to hydrate the patient. A 23-gauge butterfly needle is large enough to permit adequate dilution but causes minimal trauma to the vein. Both methods are equally safe.

3. Flushing with a minimum of 3–5 ml of saline before and after vesicant administration is mandatory to ensure venous access and safe vesicant administration. When the two-syringe technique is used, the nurse should aspirate immediately if extravasation is suspected.

4. Injecting a vesicant through the side-arm of a freely running IV line (angiocath) is preferred when hydration is also needed or when the drug is known to cause vein irritation (e.g., nitrogen mustard).

18. What is the main problem with side-arming?

The nurse has less control over fluid flow in the event of an extravasation. Gravity propels the vesicant into the patient as the nurse clamps off the IV line and then attempts to aspirate the vesicant. The potential result is a greater amount of drug infiltration.

19. Define irritant.

An irritant is a chemotherapeutic agent that can cause a tissue reaction characterized by pain, venous irritation, and chemical phlebitis.

20. What special precautions should you take during administration of an irritant via a peripheral IV?

Infusional pain may be relieved by slowing the drip rate, diluting the drug with extra fluids, or application of warm or cold compresses. For administering an irritant peripherally, angiocaths are preferred over butterfly needles because they offer more stability and reduce the risk for infiltration. The patient should be instructed to report any pain, redness, or swelling around the IV site at any time. Only presssure-sensitive infusional pumps should be used to avoid unecessary delivery of the irritant in the case of an IV infiltration. Infiltration into surrounding tissue during an infusion may result in pain, inflammation, erythema and possibly blistering, all of which resolve with time.

21. Why is the antecubital fossa avoided for chemotherapy administration?

The antecubital fossa is an extremely difficult site to heal in the event of infiltration or extravasation. Infiltrations are also more difficult to detect in the antecubital fossa. Many nurses reserve this area for drawing blood or emergency use. Chemotherapy may cause venous thrombosis or fibrosis, making the antecubital fossa unusable for other purposes.

22. Define hypersensitivity reaction.

A hypersensitivity reaction (HSR) occurs when the immune system is overstimulated by a foreign substance (e.g., chemotherapy) or antigen and forms antibodies that cause an immune response. Sensitization results, and subsequent exposures to the antigen cause a type I allergic reaction. HSRs may occur during the initial or subsequent administration of a chemotherapeutic agent.

23. Describe the symptoms of a hypersensitivity reaction.

Most HSRs occur within the first 15 minutes of infusion or injection, but they are not limited to this time frame. HSRs have been more commonly reported after several exposures. They may present as one or more of the following signs and symptoms: dizziness, flushing, nausea, generalized itching, hives, rash, rhinitis, abdominal cramping, chills, hypotension, dyspnea, bronchospasm, cyanosis, and feelings of agitation, uneasiness, or impending doom.

24. Which drugs are most often associated with HSRs?

Paclitaxel (Taxol). The vehicle in which the drug is mixed (Cremophor EL) rather than the drug itself appears to cause allergic reactions. Most reactions occur with the first or second treatment. Patients are pretreated with corticosteroids and antihistamines with each course of paclitaxel. Diphenhydramine may be used, if needed, but is not given routinely after the third uneventful course.

Etoposide (VP-16). Administration over a minimum of 45–60 minutes prevents a hypotensive episode. Bronchospasm with severe wheezing and flushing also has been observed and generally responds to antihistamines and corticosteroids. More HSRs occur with the generic formulation than with the brand-name drug. Pharmacists need to inform the nurse administering the drugs if the generic form is used.

Cisplatin. Cisplatin and its analogs may cause a type I allergic reaction. Although most clinicians expect HSRs to occur with the first or second use, many reported cases required repeated exposure (4 or 5 times).

Commonly Used Agents That May Cause Hypersensitivity Reactions

AGENT	OVERALL INCIDENCE (%)	CLINICAL PRESENTATION	COMMENTS
L-Asparaginase	20–35	Fevers, aches, chills, urticaria, hypotension, diaphoresis, edema, asthma, laryngeal constriction, loss of consciousness	Incidence may increase with each subsequent administration. Emergency medications and equipment should be readily available during administration. Consider substitution of a similar drug (e.g., *Erwinia* L-asparaginase instead of *Escherichia coli*
Paclitaxel (Taxol)	3–28	Bronchospasm, dyspnea, stridor, facial flushing, edema, hypotension, urticaria, rash	Most patients are premedicated with dexamethasone, 20 mg orally 12 and 6 hr before infusion, as well as diphenhydramine, 25–50 mg IV, and cimetidine, 300 mg, famotidine, 20 mg IV 30 min before infusion.
Docetaxel (Taxotere)	Undetermined	Flushing, rash, pruritus, dyspnea, chest discomfort, bronchospasm, angioedema, hypotension	Currently patients receive dexamethasone, 8 mg orally 2 times/day on day before, day of, and day after treatment. Patients also may receive diphenhydramine, 25–50 mg IV 30 min before infusion
Etoposide (VP-16)	1–3	Rash, facial flushing, angioedema, pruritus, urticaria, hypotension, diaphoresis, wheezing, and dyspnea. Usually occurs with first dose	Etoposide is formulated in solution (Tween 80 and benzyl alcohol) that may contribute to HSR. Generic brands may be associated with higher incidence of HSR. Cross-hypersensitivity between paclitaxel and etoposide appears to be more likely with repeated exposures.

Table continued on following page

Commonly Used Agents That May Cause Hypersensitivity Reactions (Continued)

AGENT	OVERALL INCIDENCE (%)	CLINICAL PRESENTATION	COMMENTS
Teniposide (Vumon)	5 overall 13 in cancers of central nervous system	Rash, facial flushing, angio-edema, pruritus, urticaria, hypotension, wheezing, dyspnea Usually occurs with first dose	Teniposide is formulated in Cremophor EL, which may contribute to HSR
Cisplatin (Platinol), Carboplatin	5	Anxiety, pruritus, cough, dyspnea, diaphoresis, angio-edema, vomiting, rash, urticaria, hypotension	HSRs have been observed with intravenous and intravesicular administrations. HSRs have been reported with mannitol, which can be used as pre-medication for cisplatin.
Procarbazine (Matulane)	15	Maculopapular rash, urticaria, angioedema, toxic epidermal necrolysis Rare type II reactions of interstitial pneumonitis and eosinophilia	Rechallenge is usually unsuccessful, despite pretreatment with cortico-steroids or antihistamines.
Anthracycline antibiotics (doxorubicin, daunorubicin)	1–15	Urticaria, pruritus, angioedema, dyspnea, bronchospasm, hypotension Local flare reaction may manifest as erythema, pruritus, and urticaria around injeciton site.	Cross-reactivity among anthracyclines has been demonstrated

25. How can you tell who may develop an HSR?

Although any patient may experience a serious reaction, people who say that they are "allergic to everything" give cause to pause. Take the extra time to elicit a medical/allergy history. Make note of the drugs to which the patient is allergic. Inquire about HSRs to past chemotherapy. Instruct the patient to report any symptoms to you immediately. Patients who are treated in a private room should have family or staff present to monitor for a possible reaction. First infusions of new chemotherapy regimens should be started slowly and increased gradually to the desired rate.

26. How should an HSR be managed?

A policy and procedure for management of HSRs should be readily available; emergency drugs and emergency equipment should be in good working condition and located in the immediate work area. Posting a quick reference list of medications commonly associated with HSRs, along with management guidelines that include the doses and methods of emergency drug administration, is helpful. In the event of an HSR, the first step is to call for help; then implement the following guidelines:

1. Stop the infusion immediately, stay with the patient, and have the physician notified. Reassure the patient and family.
2. Maintain the IV line with normal saline.
3. Obtain all emergency drugs and oxygen therapy that may be needed to treat the patient.
4. Monitor vital signs, pulse oximetry, and maximize rate of IV fluid infusion if the patient is hypotensive.
5. Administer emergency drugs according to policy and procedure or physician order.
6 Put the patient in supine position to promote adequate perfusion of vital organs.
7. Monitor vital signs every 2 minutes until the patient is stable, every 5 minutes for 30 minutes, and every 15 minutes until a determination of the patient's condition is made.
8. Document the incident and patient reaction in the chart.

9. Pharmaceutical companies make note of incidents such as an HSR; therefore, it is important to provide information to the company about drug lot numbers, diluents, preservatives, and other factors contributing to the cause of the reaction. Adverse events and reactions to medications should be reported to MedWatch at www.fda.gov/medwatch/.

27. What emergency drugs may be used to treat HSRs?

- Epinephrine, 0.1–0.5 mg (1:10,000 solution) by IV push or subcutaneously every 10 minutes as needed.
- Diphenhydramine HCL, 25–50 mg IV.
- Albuterol inhaler to promote bronchodilation.
- Solu-Medrol, 30–60 mg IV, Solu-Cortef, 100–500 mg IV, or dexamethasone, 10–20 mg IV, to ease bronchoconstriction.
- Aminophylline, 5 mg/kg (average dose: 300–500 mg) over 30 minutes if the patient has evidence of bronchospasm or wheezing.
- Dopamine (Intropin), 2–20 μg/kg/min, to maintain blood pressure and organ perfusion.

28. Can patients who have had an HSR receive the causative drug again?

In most cases, patients should not receive the remainder of the drug on the day of the reaction or at any future time, especially if the reaction was significant (bronchospasm, severe hypotension, or generalized urticaria). If the reaction is mild (rash that resolves with diphenhydramine), the physician may choose to continue the drug once the patient stabilizes. If the drug is absolutely necessary and no suitable substitute is available, rechallenge may be appropriate and safe. With subsequent dosing, the patient may require preparation with antihistamines and corticosteroids; emergency drugs and personnel should be in attendance during the rechallenge. The drug also may be further diluted during rechallenges to minimize an HSR.

29. Summarize the guidelines for the administration of trastuzumab (Herceptin).

Patients beginning Herceptin, a monoclonal antibody, are given an initial IV loading dose of 4 mg/kg administered as an infusion over 90 minutes. This is followed by a 60-minute observation period. Patients are monitored for adverse reactions, such as fever, chills, pruritus, urticaria, wheezing, angioedema, and (in rare cases) anaphylaxis. If a reaction occurs, stop the infusion, consult the physician, and/or follow standing orders for HSRs. This reaction is common only in the initial dose and usually subsides in 20–30 minutes. Once symptoms have subsided, reinstitute the infusion at a slower rate. If the patient is strongly HER-2 positive (3+), consider administering acetaminophen (1000 mg) and diphenhydramine (50 mg) orally 30 minutes before beginning the infusion of Herceptin. The subsequent dosing of Herceptin is 2 mg/kg over 30 minutes weekly.

30. Does pain occur at tumor sites during infusions of anticancer agents?

Pain at the tumor site has been observed during infusions of both vinorelbine tartrate (Navelbine) and Herceptin. The incidence is low; however, when it occurs it may be sudden, dramatic, and worrisome to patients. After ruling out more serious problems, patients need assurance that this reaction has been observed and is temporary. At this time the mechanism of tumor site pain is not understood.

31. What different types of drug interactions may occur in the oncology setting?

A true drug interaction occurs when the effects of one drug are altered by concomitant administration of other medications. Drug interactions may be advantageous by producing synergy between drugs or detrimental by causing antagonism, enhanced toxicity, or inhibition of effects. Pharmacokinetic drug interactions are characterized by alteration in the absorption, distribution, metabolism, bioavailability, and elimination of a particular medication. Such interactions may occur directly at the cellular level; for example, coadministration of aspirin and methotrexate causes displacement of methotrexate from its protein-binding site, which results in a higher blood level of methotrexate, decreased elimination of methotrexate, and increased toxicity.

Physical and chemical incompatibilities may occur when multiple drugs are mixed or administered together. A physical incompatibility occurs when the mixture of two or more agents results in a change in appearance of solution (e.g., color, precipitation, or turbidity). Chemical incompatibility results in drug degradation, thereby diminishing its effectiveness. Interactions are not always visibly detectable in an IV bag or tubing; thus, it is crucial to refer to compatibility data before administering IV chemotherapy.

For continuously updated references of all drug interactions, see www.gsm.com.

Compatibility Guidelines for Drugs Commonly Used*

DRUG	LASIX	MANNITOL	K+	MG	HEPARIN	DECADRON	ZOFRAN	KYTRIL
Carboplatin							C	C
Carmustine							C	
Cisplatin	C	C	C	C for 48°	C	C	C	C
Cyclophosphamide	C	C in D5 ½ normal saline for 48°			C	C	C	C
Cytarabine	C		C		I	C	C	C
Dacarbazine					I		C	C
Doxorubicin	I				I	I	C	C
Etoposide			C				C	C
5-Fluorouracil	C		C	C	C		I	C
Ifosfamide							C	C
Methotrexate	C				C	C	C	C
Mitomycin	C				C		C	
Mitoxantrone			C		I		C	
Paclitaxel			C	C	C	C	C	C
Vinblastine	I				C		C	
Vincristine	I				C		C	C
Zofran	I	C	C	C	C	C		
Kytril	C		C	C				

* Compatibilities apply to Y site of infusion or injection unless otherwise specified.
K = potassium, MG = magnesium, C = compatible, I = incompatible.

32. What should be said to a patient who asks, "Can I drink alcohol while receiving chemotherapy?"

The ingestion of alcohol may be contraindicated in certain patients while receiving chemotherapy. For example, patients who drink alcohol while taking procarbazine may experience an Antabuse-like reaction with facial flushing, headache, nausea, and hypotension. Similarly, the incidence of methotrexate-induced hepatotoxicity is increased in patients who consume alcohol. However, patients may be reassured that with other chemotherapeutic agents, alcohol in moderation is allowed.

33. What special precautions should a health care professional take to minimize exposure while mixing, administering, or handling chemotherapeutic agents?

All chemotherapeutic agents should be admixed in a biologic safety cabinet (BSC). While mixing chemotherapy, personnel should wear protective clothing, including surgical latex gloves and a disposable, lint-free, nonabsorbent gown. Careful hand washing is essential. Gloves should be replaced immediately if punctured. Spills should be cleaned up as expediently as possible, and exposed garments should be replaced. If a BSC is not available, protective eye gear and a respirator mask should be worn in addition to the gloves and gown. An absorbent, disposable pad should be placed under the arm or body part to which chemotherapy is given to catch any spills. For handling excreta, surgical latex gloves should be worn; a disposable gown should be added if splashing is possible. See your institution's policy and procedure manual for staff with latex sensitivity.

34. Can a nurse administer chemotherapy through an Ommaya reservoir?

Yes—if she or he has demonstrated competency. An Ommaya reservoir is a small plastic, domelike device placed beneath the scalp. An attached catheter is threaded into the lateral ventricle for administration of chemotherapy intrathecally in patients with central nervous system leukemia or into the spinal fluid in patients with metastatic disease and for obtaining samples of cerebrospinal fluid for examination. The following sterile procedure should be followed:

1. Wear a mask and sterile gloves.
2. Prepare the scalp area with Betadine or chlorhexidene scrub (parting the hair or shaving the area if necessary). Dry with sterile gauze.
3. Use a small-gauge or butterfly needle attached to a syringe, and insert gently into the Ommaya reservoir. (Local anesthetic is usually not needed before puncturing.)
4. Withdraw the spinal fluid (the amount should equal the volume of the infusate).
5. Inject preservative-free chemotherapeutic agent slowly into the reservoir.
6. Remove the needle, and gently pump the reservoir several times.
7. Place a Bandaid over the site, and ask the patient to lie supine for 15 minutes.

Patients should be instructed to notify the physician of signs and symptoms of infection, such as fever > 101°F, tenderness, erythema or swelling at the site, neck stiffness, or headache.

REFERENCES

1. Berg DT: New chemotherapy options and implications for nursing care. Oncol Nurs Forum 24(Suppl): 5–12, 1997.
2. Chapman D, Goodman M: Breast cancer. In Groenwald S, Frogge M, Goodman M, Yarbro C (eds): Cancer Nursing: Principles and Practice, 5th ed. Boston, Jones & Bartlett, 2000, pp 994–1047.
3. Fishman M, Mrozek-Orlowski M (eds): Cancer Chemotherapy Guidelines and Recommendations for Practice. Pittsburgh, Oncology Nursing Society, 1999.
4. Frankel C: Nursing management considerations with trastuzumab (Herceptin). Semin Oncol Nurs 16 (4):23–28, 2000.
5. Goodman M: Her-2, Herceptin, and Breast Cancer. Oncol Nurs Updates 7(1), 2000.
6. Goodman M: Principles of chemotherapy administration. In Groenwald S, Frogge M, Goodman M, Yarbro C (eds): Cancer Nursing: Principles and Practice, 5th ed. Boston, Jones &Bartlett, 2000, pp 385–443.
7. Oncological Nursing Society: Access Device Guidelines: Recommendations for Nursing Education and Practice. Pittsburgh, Oncology Nursing Society, 1996.
8. Oncology Nursing Society: Safe Handling of Cytotoxic Drugs, 2nd ed. Pittsburgh, Oncology Nursing Society, 1997.
9. Trissel LA: Handbook on Injectable Drugs, 8th ed. Bethesda, MD, American Society of Hospital Pharmacists, 1994.
Websites
10. http://www.fda.gov/medwatch/
11. http://www.ons.org
12. http://www.gsm.com

10. BLOOD AND MARROW STEM CELL TRANSPLANT

Beth E. Mechling, RN, MS, AOCN, APN, *and* Mark Brunvand, MD

1. What is a bone marrow transplant?

A bone marrow transplant (BMT) is the intravenous administration of hematopoietic stem cells from the bone marrow. Patients often have the misconception that bone is being transplanted rather than the liquid bone marrow that resembles blood. Hematopoietic stem cells are capable of long-term proliferation and differentiation into all of the blood cells (red and white blood cells and platelets). Although they dwell primarily in the bone marrow, hematopoietic stem cells are also found in the peripheral blood stream, spleen, and umbilical cord. Because hematopoietic stem cells are commonly harvested from the peripheral blood circulation using peripheral blood stem cells (PBSC) for transplantation, bone marrow transplantation is generally called stem-cell transplantation.

2. What are the types of bone marrow or hematopoietic stem-cell transplants?

The different types of transplants reflect the donor sources of stem cells:

Autologous transplant. The stem-cell donor is the patient, whose stem cells are harvested, processed, frozen, and then reinfused after the patient receives chemotherapy and/or radiation therapy.

Allogeneic transplant. The stem cells come from a donor who may be related (sibling or other close relative) or unrelated to the patient. This is the most common type of transplant.

Syngeneic transplant. The stem-cell donor is the patient's identical twin.

3. How common are bone marrow and blood cell transplants?

Statistics from the International Bone Marrow Transplant Registry (IBMTR) indicate continued annual growth in the number of transplants. It is estimated that more than 17,000 allogeneic BMTs and 37,000 autologous (including blood cell and bone marrow) transplants have been performed between 1978 and 1998. In 1998, 7,000 allogeneic transplants were performed. In addition, 16,500 autologous transplants were performed in 1998, with breast cancer (7,500) being the most common indication for autologous PBSC.

4. How is a hematopoietic stem-cell donor selected?

Family members are the most common source of stem cells for allogeneic transplantation. The risk of complications is lowest if the donor is an identical tissue match to the patient. The immune system is designed to reject tissue seen as "foreign," and patients transplanted from donors that are not HLA (human leukocyte antigen)-identical family members almost always have more complicated clinical courses. Each sibling has a 25% chance of being HLA-identical with the patient. If a matched donor is unavailable, unrelated and mismatched related donors can be used as alternatives. The potential unrelated donor must be in good health and between 18 and 55 years of age.

The donor for an allogeneic transplant is chosen by determining the identity of major histocompatibility genes for donor and host. These genes are located on chromosome 6 and encode the HLA. HLAs are proteins located on cell surfaces that have evolved to present antigens to the immune system, defining self vs. non-self. Two classes of genes have been identified within the major HLA locus on chromosome 6. The transplant-relevant class I molecules consist of HLA-A, B and Cw, which are on many cell types in the body that present antigen to CD8-positive T cells. The transplant-relevant class II molecules, HLA-DR and DQ, are present on professional antigen presenting cells and present antigens to CD4-positive T cells.

When siblings are used as donors, the transplant survival rate is similar if the donor and patient are matched at all six loci or mismatched at no more than one class I locus. The greater the degree of histocompatible mismatch between donor and patient, the higher the risk of graft vs. host disease (GVHD) and graft rejection.

5. How does a patient find a compatible unrelated donor?

If partially mismatched family members are included, only 35% of patients have a suitable donor within their family. To address the paucity of family member donors, the National Marrow Donor Program (NMDP), established in 1986, maintains a registry of millions of volunteer marrow donors around the world. The NMDP also administers the various collection, transplant, and donor centers around the world and maintains institutional standards. The NMDP conducts donor drives, similar to blood drives, to attract more potential donors into the pool of volunteers. Blood is collected from the volunteer donors for molecular HLA typing. Special efforts are ongoing to recruit minority donors, particularly African Americans, Hispanics, and Asians, who are currently underrepresented in the U.S. registry. Interested donors should contact the NMDP at 800-MARROW-2.

If a patient does not have a suitable family member as a transplant donor, the physician may initiate a search for volunteer donors from the NMDP registry. It takes an average of 4 months from the initial search request until the transplant can be scheduled. If a suitable unrelated donor is located, he or she is cleared medically for surgery, undergoes an informed consent procedure, and has additional blood drawn for testing. All donor expenses are paid by the NMDP, then billed to the patient and/or transplant center.

6. What is an umbilical cord-blood transplant?

An umbilical cord-blood transplant refers to the harvesting and transplant of progenitor cells (cells capable of differentiating into hematopoietic cells) from the umbilical cord, similar to peripheral and bone marrow stem-cell transplantation. Research is ongoing to determine the role and effectiveness of this type of transplant to enlarge the donor pool for unrelated transplants.

In response to the limited minority donors in the NMDP and the length of time required to harvest stem cells from an unrelated donor, umbilical cord blood registries have been developed. The first umbilical cord blood banks to open in the United States were the Cord Blood Registry Bank at the University of Arizona, Tucson and the New York Blood Center Placental Blood Program. Umbilical cord blood is collected immediately after the delivery of a fetus. The PBSCs are harvested with a syringe from the umbilical cord and then cryopreserved by the collection center. The umbilical cord PBSCs are listed in the registry and available for immediate use (1–2 weeks) by a potential patient. The limitations of PBSCs from an umbilical cord donor are twofold: (1) there is a restricted number of viable hematopoietic progenitors available for infusion into the recipient, and (2) the donor may not be recalled for further PBSC donations required by the patient in the future.

7. When are hematopoietic stem-cell transplants indicated?

The purpose of a stem-cell transplantation is to reestablish marrow and immune function in dysfunctional or damaged bone marrow. The most common indications for allogeneic transplants are hematologic disorders and malignancies, including myelodysplasia/myelofibrosis, leukemias (acute and chronic), lymphomas, multiple myeloma, and severe aplastic anemia. Certain rare genetic and immunologic disorders also are treated with hematopoietic stem-cell transplantation. Autologous stem-cell transplantation is used in patients with solid tumors such as breast, testicular, and some sarcomas and brain cancers. Preliminary data indicate that patients with lymphoma, leukemia, myelodysplasia, sarcomas, and renal cell cancer also may benefit from nonmyeloablative allogeneic hematopoietic stem-cell transplantation.

8. What criteria must be met for a disease to be treated by autologous BMT?

In addition to consideration of the patient's age and general physical condition, the disease under treatment must meet four criteria for an effective transplant:
1. The tumor must be responsive to chemotherapy.
2. Myelosuppression must be the dose-limiting toxicity of effective chemotherapy.

3. Stem-cell transplantation can be performed when tumor burden is low and drug resistance is minimal.

4. The source of stem cells is free of tumor cells.

9. Why are stem-cell transplants performed for breast cancer and other solid tumors?

Research has shown that many solid tumors cannot be cured by standard-dose chemotherapy. Stem-cell transplants enable the use of potentially curative high-dose chemotherapy and/or radiation therapy by reconstituting the hematopoietic and immunologic systems. Patients whose tumors respond to chemotherapy and who relapse (often in sites of initial bulk disease) after complete response are often considered for autologous stem-cell transplantation. The stem cells are collected from the patient and stored before therapy is administered and then returned to the patient after high-dose chemotherapy is delivered.

10. Does autologous stem-cell transplantation improve survival in women with breast cancer?

The data from prospective studies performed in the U.S. and Europe are too immature to define whether autologous transplantation improves overall survival. A prospective, randomized study, performed at multiple sites in the Netherlands, has shown that autologous hematopoietic stem-cell transplantation improved survival and disease-free survival compared with standard-dose therapy in high-risk patients with primary breast carcinoma who presented with at least four positive nodes. These data are currently at 4 years of follow-up in the first 285 patients. Studies in the U.S. have not shown a significant improvement in survival with autologous transplant; however, these studies are plagued with methodologic problems such as high patient drop-out rates, high transplant mortality rates, and prolonged standard chemotherapy.

11. How is harvesting done?

The stems cells are harvested from the bone marrow or peripheral blood of a donor at an approved collection center and then transported to the transplantation center by a trained courier. The donor harvest must be carefully timed with the recipient's treatment schedule.

12. Describe the technique for harvesting marrow stem cells.

Marrow stem cells are collected by repeated bone marrow aspirations from the posterior and/or anterior iliac crests and occasionally the sternum of the donor in an operating room under general anesthesia. The amount of marrow collected is based on patient weight (10 ml marrow per kg patient weight). An average collection is 1–2 liters of marrow. The procedure takes an average of 1–3 hours. In the operating room, the marrow is filtered to remove bone particles and large fat globules and then poured into transfusion bags for further processing and freezing (autologous marrow) or immediate infusion into the recipient (allogeneic marrow).

13. How are PBSCs obtained?

PBSCs are collected from the patient/donor's peripheral blood through a technique called **apheresis**. The machine used in apheresis operates by differential centrifugation to select and separate stem cells based on their density. The remainder of the blood elements are reinfused into the patient.

14. What is mobilization or priming? How is it done?

Before stem cells are collected, a procedure called mobilization or priming is used to increase the number of primitive progenitor cells in the peripheral bloodstream. Mobilization is done by administering chemotherapy and/or colony-stimulating factors (CSFs). Timing the collection of stem cells to coincide with blood cell recovery after chemotherapy decreases the number of hemaphereses required to collect an adequate numbers of stem cells. Granulocyte CSF (G-CSF) also is used before hemapheresis to increase stem cell numbers in the peripheral blood. Protocols vary, but daily G-CSF is commonly given by subcutaneous injection. Stem-cell collections begins on the fourth or fifth day of injections. (Some institutions also choose to prime bone marrow-derived stem cells). Three to four collections, each lasting 2–4 hours, usually are required to collect enough stem cells for transplantation. The stem cells are then processed and frozen for autologous transplantation. Often they are infused immediately into the patient in an allogeneic donation.

15. What are the advantages of PBSCs compared with bone marrow stem cells?

Peripheral stem-cell collection obviates the need for a bone marrow harvest with the attendant risks of anesthesia. A theoretical benefit is less tumor contamination of peripherally derived stem cells. Data from apheresis collection of autologous stem cells in patients with low-grade B-cell lymphoma have documented a 2–3 log decrease in tumor cell contamination with collection of PBSCs. In addition, marrow recovery is more rapid with the use of primed peripheral stem cells, probably because mobilization stimulates committed progenitor cells in addition to stem cells.

16. What is "purging"? How is it done?

The aim of purging is to remove contaminating malignant cells while leaving stem cells intact to reconstitute the hematopoietic system. Purging can be accomplished either in vivo or in vitro. Methods of eliminating malignant cells include the use of chemical agents and antibody purging (monoclonal antibodies combined with complement, cytocidal agents, or magnetic microspheres). Antibody or chemical purging has the potential to damage stem cells and delay engraftment, resulting in prolonged neutropenia and delayed return of T- and B-cell function after transplantation. Research is ongoing to clarify the role and efficacy of purging in transplantation.

17. What is the role of CSFs in transplant?

CSFs, also known as hematopoietic growth factors, are cellular proteins (cytokines) that occur naturally in the body and are responsible for the proliferation, differentiation, and maturation of all hematopoietic cells. The discovery of CSFs and their availability clinically through recombinant DNA techniques have changed the transplant process by significantly decreasing neutropenia and its sequelae. Before the availability of growth factors, neutropenia-related fatal infections had thwarted attempts to improve survival and reduce toxicity of this potentially curative therapy.

Growth factors have been used before transplant to increase the number of stem cells harvested from the periphery and to stimulate neutrophil recovery after transplant. The use of growth factors in transplant for leukemia raised some concern. The growth factor receptors are found on normal progenitor cells as well as on leukemic blast cells. The initial concern was that administration of growth factors may increase leukemia relapse rates by stimulating proliferation of residual leukemia cells. Therefore, growth factors were initially used only after transplantation for solid tumors. Studies using growth factors in patients with leukemia, however, showed no increase in relapse and improved survival in select situations. Growth factors are now used for priming before harvest of stem cells from leukemia patients in remission as well as after induction therapy. Growth factors also are used in an attempt to stimulate functional cells to repopulate the marrow in patients experiencing delayed engraftment or graft failure.

18. Discuss the timing of CSF use.

Time of initiating and using CSFs after PBSC infusion varies from center to center. The CSF is often continued until the patient has engrafted—i.e., has achieved three consecutive daily absolute neutrophil counts of at least 500.

19. How are blood or marrow stem cells returned to the patient?

In allogeneic BMT the donor's marrow is harvested, filtered, and infused through a central line, much like a blood transfusion. With related, HLA-identical donors, the stem cells can be infused immediately if stem-cell processing is not required. If the recipient is not at the same center as the donor, the donor's marrow is transported by courier to the transplant center immediately after collection.

In autologous transplants, previously harvested marrow and/or blood stem cells are frozen in liquid nitrogen. Dimethyl sulfoxide (DMSO) is added before freezing to protect the cell membranes during freezing and thawing. At transplant, the frozen bags of blood or marrow stem cells are rapidly thawed in a 37°C water bath. They are infused directly by bag or syringe into a central venous catheter. This procedure is usually well tolerated by the patient.

20. What side effects are related to the preservation and storage of stem cells?

Premedication with an antiemetic and an antihistamine helps to alleviate many of the following side effects related to DMSO: nausea, vomiting, flushing, chest discomfort, abdominal pressure, occasional hypotension/bradycardia, and an unpleasant taste. DMSO is highly volatile and has an unpleasant odor, but the most troubling side effect is a decrease in the partial pressure of oxygen in arterial blood (PaO_2). The odor often can be detected on the patient's breath for up to 24 hours after infusion of cells. Patients should be well hydrated before and after the infusion of stem cells to prevent renal complications from the DMSO load. Most centers limit the infusion of stem cells so that the patient receives < 10 ml/kg/day DMSO. Storage of the stem-cell product may cause some red cell lysis, and patients may note hemoglobinuria for 24 hours after the infusion.

21. What is the role of the conditioning regimens for allogeneic and autologous transplantation?

Stem-cell transplantation is preceded by a preparative or conditioning regimen of chemotherapy with or without total body irradiation (TBI). In allogeneic and autologous transplants, the purpose of conditioning is to eradicate malignant cells and decrease the risk of relapse. In allogeneic transplants, conditioning regimens are used for immunosuppression to block the patient's remaining immune cells from rejecting the infused donor hematopoietic cells, i.e., primary graft rejection. The conditioning regimen does not "create space" within the marrow, as previously postulated.

The theory behind the development of myeloablative conditioning regimens is to increase doses of chemo-radiotherapy beyond marrow toxicity to nonhematologic toxicity, in hopes of killing the cancer cells that remain in patients with diseases that have high relapse rates. The intent of myeloablative therapy followed by hematopoietic cell transplant is to effect a dose escalation of therapy. In transplantation, the high doses of chemo-radiotherapy required for maximal kill of cancer cells inherently result in irreversible marrow damage.

In theory, conditioning regimens can eliminate the residual tumor cells after response to standard-dose treatment. In fact, several trials have shown that more stringent conditioning results in lower relapse rates. However, these results usually come at a cost of increased toxicity at the time of transplant. After myeloablative chemo-radiotherapy, stem-cell rescue—either autologous or allogeneic—must be administered to ensure hematopoietic function after transplant.

22. What types of drugs are used for conditioning regimens?

The drugs in most conditioning regimens have a log-linear relationship as drug doses are escalated. For example, alkylator chemotherapy agents have a log-linear cell-kill as doses are increased. Each time the chemotherapy dose is doubled, a 10-fold increase in tumor cell kill is achieved. Thus, with a regimen including three drugs, doubling of each drug gives a 10^3-fold increase in cancer cell killing.

23. Discuss nonmyeloablative conditioning regimens.

Two drug classes, purine analogues (fludarabine or 2CDA) and mycophenolate mofetil (MMF), have been integrated in the conditioning and GVHD prophylaxis regimens used for allogeneic transplantation. These drugs have increased the immunosuppression inherent in allogeneic transplantation regimens without the degree of damage to the patient's hematopoietic system seen with classical conditioning. MMF is approved for treatment of solid organ transplant rejection.

The integration of these drugs with nonmyeloablative doses of busulfan, melphalan, cyclophosphamide, or TBI (200–400 cGy) has allowed delivery of conditioning with 2–10% 100-day mortality rates and enough immunosuppression to allow engraftment of donor hematopoietic cells. Transplantation of allogeneic stem cells after one of these regimens is known as a nonmyeloablative or "mini" transplant. If engraftment fails after one of these regimens, the patient's autologous marrow function will return; hence, the designation of nonmyeloablative conditioning. Models of GVHD indicate that GVHD rates may be lower after a nonmyeloablative transplant. This finding, however, does not appear to be the case with initial follow-up of 3–4 years.

24. Discuss the role of TBI in transplantation.

TBI is the exposure of the entire body to gamma radiation and is an important component of many BMT conditioning regimens. The LD_{50} (lethal dose) of a single dose of radiation is about 600 cGy, and death often results from myeloablation. Doses of radiation in myeloablative regimens are usually 2–3-fold higher than the single-dose LD_{50}. Dose responses to malignancy occur up to 1575 cGy of fractionated total body irradiation. Data from the treatment of relapsed severe aplastic anemia transplants have confirmed that TBI is profoundly immunosuppressive. TBI doses in nonmyeloablative regimens typically are in the range of 200–400 cGy as one or two fractions. Coupled with fludarabine and post-transplant MMF, this dose of TBI is enough to allow engraftment of donor hematopoietic cells after transplant. TBI has two additional advantages: (1) it remains effective even in cancers that have become resistant to chemotherapy, and (2) it treats sanctuary sites, such as the central nervous system and testes.

25. What are the side effects and complications of TBI?

Many normal tissues are affected by TBI. Potential acute side effects include nausea and vomiting, diarrhea, enlarged salivary glands, mucositis, and dry mouth. The most critical areas affected are the lung (idiopathic interstitial pneumonia), gastrointestinal tract, reproductive system, central nervous system, and lens of the eye. As a result, some long-term side effects of TBI include sterility, cataracts, chronic pulmonary disease, leukoencephalopathy, endocrine dysfunction, sterility, and secondary malignancies. In addition to sterility, problems with sexuality, both physiologic (vaginal dryness, and ejaculatory problems) and psychologic (body image and cancer survivor issues), may occur.

Data from yeast experiments indicate the presence of genes that stop progression through the cell cycle to facilitate DNA repair after radiation exposure. These genes may have human homologs that facilitate resistance to radiation in human malignancies.

26. What are the major problems in the early posttransplant period?

The major effects of conditioning and marrow infusion for both autologous and allogeneic transplant are similar despite differences in preparative regimens and disease. GVHD and interstitial pneumonia are the major causes of death after allogeneic BMTs. The chemotherapy and/or radiation conditioning regimen causes the following major side effects and complications in the immediate posttransplant period:

Hematologic effects: neutropenia, thrombocytopenia, anemia, hemolytic uremic syndrome

Infection due to neutropenia is the major cause of death during intensive chemotherapy. Bacterial and fungal infections and reactivation of viruses (herpes simplex and cytomegalovirus) are the most common problems immediately after BMT. Ninety percent of first fevers during the neutropenia of transplantation are caused by bacteria. Historically gram-negative bacteria accounted for the highest morbidity and mortality rates. However, since the widespread use of long-term indwelling catheters, gram-positive organisms are the major pathogens responsible for most cases of bacteremias in the first 60 days after transplant.

Gastrointestinal effects: nausea, vomiting, mucositis, esophagitis, and severe diarrhea. Nausea and vomiting may result from the conditioning therapy as well as antibiotics. The combination of mucosal damage and nausea and vomiting can make eating difficult or impossible, necessitating parenteral nutrition.

Pulmonary effects: noncardiogenic pulmonary edema, infection, and diffuse alveolar hemorrhage (serious).

Cardiac effects (less common): cardiac arrhythmias, myocardial edema or fibrosis, and congestive failure.

Renal effects: hemorrhagic cystitis, renal insufficiency, and renal failure. Renal failure may result from chemotherapeutic agents with or without antibiotics, immunosuppression, and liver damage.

Neurotoxicity (carmustine, thiotepa, busulfan): seizures, dementia, confusion, and diplopia.

Dermatologic toxicity, ranging from mild rashes to severe blisters and bullae (due to multitude of medications).

Veno-occlusive disease (VOD) of the liver, an obstructive disease of the hepatic venules resulting in portal hypertension and liver failure, may occur in 10–60% of patients. Time of occurrence is usually between day 7 and day 28. VOD is a clinical syndrome consisting of hepatomegaly, right upper quadrant discomfort, fluid retention and weight gain, and elevated serum bilirubin. Treatment is primarily supportive; 70% of patients recover spontaneously.

27. What causes GVHD?

GVHD, which is seen primarily in allogeneic transplants, results when the infused donor PBSCs recognize the recipient as foreign tissue.The donor's T lymphocytes mediate this response. The greater the degree of immunologic HLA disparity between donor and recipient, the more common and more severe the GVHD reaction. Donor-host sex mismatching, donor parity, and patient age also play a role in the incidence and severity of GVHD.

28. List the triad required for diagnosis of GVHD.

1. The graft must contain immunologically competent cells.

2. The host must possess important transplantation alloantigens that are lacking in the donor graft; therefore, the host appears foreign to the graft.

3. The host must be incapable of mounting an effective immunological reaction against the graft.

29. What is the difference between acute and chronic GVHD?

Acute GVHD (aGVHD) occurs between engraftment and day 100 and is mediated by lymphokines. The organ systems targeted in aGVHD are the skin (dermatitis: ranging from minor rash to desquamation), gut (enteritis: severe diarrhea to painful ileus), and liver (hepatitis with elevated bilirubin and alkaline phosphatase).

Chronic GVHD (cGVHD) occurs after day 100 and may be mediated by cellular immune cells such as natural killer cells. Chronic GVHD affects the skin (scleroderma-like syndrome), liver (elevated transaminases/bilirubin), oral mucosa (ulcerations, xerostomia, lichenoid changes), lungs (bronchiolitis obliterans), and gut (dysphagia, pain, and weight loss). Sicca syndrome (decreased eye lacrimation and vaginal vault ulceration, strictures, and atrophy) also may occur.

30. How is the severity of GVHD graded?

Staging of Graft-vs.-Host Diease

	CLINICAL STAGE			CLINICAL GRADE OF SEVERITY	
STAGE	SKIN	LIVER	GUT	GRADE	DEGREE OF ORGAN INVOLVEMENT
+	Maculopapular rash < 25% body surface	Bilirubin 2–3 mg/dl	Diarrhea 500–1000 ml/day	1	+ to ++ skin rash; no gut involvement; no decrease in clinical performance
++	Maculopapular rash 25–50% body surface	Bilirubin > 3–6 mg/dl	Diarrhea > 1000–1500 ml/day	2	+ to +++ skin rash; + gut or liver involvement (or both); mild decrease in clinical performance
+++	Generalized erythroderma	Bilirubin > 6–15 mg/dl	Diarrhea > 1500 ml/day	3	++ to +++ skin rash; ++ to +++ gut or liver involvement (or both); decrease in clinical performance
++++	Desquamation and bullae	Bilirubin > 15 mg/dl	Pain or ileus	4	Similar to grade 3 but with ++ to ++++ organ involvement and extreme decrease in clinical performance

From Oncology Nursing Society: Manual for Bone Marrow Transplant Nursing: Recommendations for Practice and Education. Oncology Nursing Press, 1994, with permission.

31. What is the graft-vs.-leukemia effect?

Graft-vs.-leukemia effect refers to the potentially beneficial immunologic effect of mild GVHD in eliminating residual leukemia in the host. In allogeneic patients experiencing grade II acute GVHD with mild chronic GVHD, the relapse rate is one-third the rate in patients without detectable GVHD. The lack of a GVHD reaction in autologous or syngeneic stem-cell transplantation is suspected to play a role in the higher relapse rate in autologous/syngeneic transplants. Thus, some groups are attempting to induce GVHD in autologous marrow recipients.

32. How is GVHD prevented?

The first and most important way to prevent GVHD is by finding an identically matched donor. Even in this case, however, prophylactic immunosuppressive drugs (cyclosporine, FK506, methotrexate, MMF, antithymocyte globulin, and steroids) are used singly or in combination to minimize the recipient's immunologic response to donor marrow. All of these drugs have side effects and toxicities. Another preventive method is T-cell depletion of the graft. Because T cells are believed to be responsible for the recognition and immunologic reaction in GVHD, reducing their numbers in the donor marrow may reduce the incidence and severity of the problem. However, because T cells also seem to play a role in engraftment of the marrow, this procedure has potential risks. To date, T-cell depletion studies have reported lower GVHD rates but higher rejection and relapse rates so that overall survival has not improved.

33. How is GVHD treated?

Intensive nursing interventions are needed to manage GVHD toxicities such as skin (erythroderma, bullous formation, desquamation), gut (e.g., severe diarrhea, mucositis), and other organ toxicities. Patients with GVHD are even more susceptible to infections than during the period of neutropenia because of the immunosuppressive effects of both GVHD and the drugs used to treat it.

34. Are the infectious problems after BMT different from the infectious problems after standard chemotherapy?

Different degrees of immunosuppression are associated with autologous and allogeneic transplants; immunosuppression is less after autologous BMT, but immunologic compromise may last over a year. The type of infectious problems after BMT differ from those normally encountered after standard chemotherapy because of the more severe and prolonged immunologic insult caused by the intensive chemotherapy and radiation treatment of transplant. In patients receiving bone marrow without growth factors or after T-cell depletion or cord blood transplants, profound neutropenia (absolute neutrophil counts < 100) may last for approximately 2–4 weeks. The white blood cell count slowly and gradually increases toward normal if engraftment of the infused PBSCs occurs on schedule. During the period of profound neutropenia, patients are extremely vulnerable to serious, potentially life-threatening infections and sepsis. This threat is increased by the disruptions that chemotherapy, radiation therapy, and invasive procedures inflict on the body's first line of defense, the skin and mucous membranes. The presence of indwelling venous catheters also increases the risk for acute infections during the period of neutropenia. Immunologic defects are intensified and further prolonged in the allogeneic patient with GVHD. The chemo-radiotherapy used in transplantation can cause detectable abnormalities of T- and B- cell function for at least 1 year after transplantation. This immunosuppression can be longer if GVHD is present.

35. How can infections be prevented?

Protective isolation procedures remove the threat from body flora and latent viral invaders. Many transplant centers also institute prophylactic antibiotic, antiviral, and antifungal therapy when patients become neutropenic. This coverage is broadened if the patient develops a first fever. Ganciclovir has improved survival rates in cytomegalovirus-positive patients who develop viremia.

36. What isolation precautions are needed during BMT?

Protective isolation procedures are intended to minimize the transmission of microbes from the external environment to the immunosuppressed patient. Although protocols and definitions vary among institutions, protective isolation usually refers to a private room, visitor restrictions, low microbial diet, and handwashing. Because several studies examining the benefits of protective isolation in BMT centers have not supported the use of strict protective isolation, many centers have relaxed restrictions and allow patients to leave their rooms without masks, relying on handwashing as the main protective technique. The advent of early-discharge and outpatient BMTs also has contributed to the reexamination of protective isolation procedures.

Some centers use special air-filtering systems called high-efficiency particulate air filters (HEPA). Laminar airflow isolation is used by some centers with HLA-matched unrelated donor transplants or partially matched transplants because of the greater risk of GVHD and its associated immunosuppression. This level of isolation is difficult for patients to cope with during the stresses of the transplantation. In strict laminar airflow isolation, contact with caregivers and visitors is limited, and all persons must gown, glove, and mask before entering the patient's room.

37. Do patients need to be hospitalized for BMT?

For patients who have undergone autologous and nonmyeloablative stem-cell transplants, there are three patterns of care:

1. **Traditional approach.** The patient is hospitalized for the conditioning regimen and throughout the period of pancytopenia until blood counts have recovered. Most patients undergoing myeloablative allogeneic transplants remain in the hospital from the initiation of conditioning therapy through recovery of blood counts.

2. **Early-discharge approach.** The patient is hospitalized for the conditioning regimen and then discharged from the hospital with daily follow-up in the outpatient clinic. Care provided in the outpatient clinic includes physical assessment, bone marrow and progenitor cell infusion, parenteral antibiotics, electrolytes, and blood transfusions.

3. **Outpatient model.** The patient receives both conditioning therapy and post-chemotherapy care in the outpatient setting. Nonmyeloablative allogeneic transplants, with lower toxicity in the first 2 months, may be performed in the outpatient setting. In both the early-discharge and outpatient models, a caregiver must be present to care for the patient outside the hospital. Usually patients are housed in a "medical-motel" type of facility. Patients receiving BMT in the outpatient setting have reported increased acceptance and independence, decreased isolation, and improved physical conditioning. Organized education for patient and caregiver is crucial to the success of outpatient transplantation.

38. How often is readmission necessary with the early-discharge approach?

Data from the Duke University Transplant Program, which began a pilot program of early discharge after BMT in 1991, indicate that approximately 35% of patients are readmitted to the hospital. Reasons for readmission include new-onset fever, dehydration, protracted nausea and vomiting, uncontrolled diarrhea and/or caregiver respite. Some centers that formerly required myeloablative transplant patients to receive care from the transplant center for the first 100 days now allow earlier return to the care of referring physicians.

39. How does a patient choose a transplant center? What questions should the patient ask?

Depending on the type of disease and treatment, nurses can advocate for patients to be knowledgeable consumers about the quality of the program in which they seek treatment. Patients should be encouraged to ask some or all of the following questions:

• What types of diseases are treated and what types of transplants are performed?
• Are nurses and doctors specially trained to perform transplants?
• How long has the program been in existence, and how many BMTs have been performed?
• What are the outcomes of other patients treated for the same disease?
• Does the staff at the center perform investigational treatments and report results to a transplant registry?

       • Can the patient talk to previous patients at the center?
       • What support resources and housing are available for patients and family?

40. What type of follow-up care do BMT patients require?

Important aspects of follow-up care in the early recovery period are the prevention and management of complications from the conditioning regimen and PBSC reinfusion. Blood counts may not have fully recovered, resulting in the possibility of fatigue, fever, and/or bleeding. Close assessment and administration of antibiotics, blood products, and GVHD therapy also may be required. The gastrointestinal tract may not be fully recovered, necessitating antiemetics, antidiarrheals, fluids, electrolytes, and nutritional support. The intensity of needs depends largely on how early the patient is discharged after the conditioning therapy and bone marrow/stem-cell reinfusion. Initially, the patient may be seen in clinic 3–7 days/week for physical and laboratory assessment.

As the acute toxicities of BMT resolve, outpatient follow-up is less frequent. Most transplant centers request follow-up visits annually to evaluate disease response, survival, disease free survival, toxicities related to transplant, and quality of life.

41. How does cGVHD complicate follow-up?

Patients with cGVHD may require follow-up care at a transplant center for several years after BMT. Attention to immunosuppressive therapy, evaluation of response of GVHD, management of acute and chronic infections, and psychosocial and nutritional support require supervision from a multidisciplinary transplant team. Patients may be seen in the clinic setting as often as every day if GVHD is not well controlled.

42. What psychosocial issues are involved in follow-up care?

Psychosocial care is an important aspect of BMT follow-up. Patients often experience ambivalence at hospital discharge. Consistent caregivers, ongoing contact with a social worker, and support groups are helpful. As patients make the transition from inpatient to outpatient settings, it is also important to monitor and assess the needs of the caregivers because their role is vital to the success of outpatient care.

43. Describe the expected long-term physical effects of BMT.

Most physical effects occur within the first year and include toxicities or side effects from chemotherapy, radiation therapy, immunosuppressive drugs, or relapse of the original disease. Other potential delayed complications include immunodeficiency, autoimmune disorders, dental problems, and aseptic bone necrosis (steroid-induced). The rate of second malignancies appears to be 10–15% at 20 years after transplant.

44. Describe the long-term physical effects of cGVHD.

Effects from cGVHD may occur 5 years or more after transplant. Examples include skin changes, dry eyes and mouth, diarrhea, weight loss, anorexia, and pulmonary and liver involvement. The skin is involved in 95% of patients who develop cGVHD. Symptoms consist of dryness, itching, and absence of sweating; skin tightness and contractures may develop later. The mouth and eyes are also frequently affected with symptoms of dryness and pain. Extensive cGVHD can cause disability as a result of contractures, skin disfigurement, weight loss, and malaise. Patients with GVHD are also at risk for developing late infectious complications from encapsulated bacteria, varicella zoster virus, and *Pneumocystis carinii*.

45. How long does it take for patients to return to normal after BMT? How does BMT affect a person's quality of life?

The trauma of undergoing transplant usually affects all aspects of well-being and quality of life (physical, social, psychological, and spiritual domains). The first year after transplant often is characterized by great emotional intensity and fear as patients cope with continued treatment of transplant-related complications, including GVHD and infections. Many of the physical effects lessen over time, and most patients can resume a more normal function within 1 year after the procedure. A few patients (5–15%) experience lasting physical effects that may not improve and require permanent adaptation or significant rehabilitation. Chronic GVHD, pulmonary problems, reproductive effects, and second malignancies are among the most devastating complications.

Many patients do not experience a linear recovery from the psychological, social, and existential effects of transplant. Most BMT survivors report only mild-to-moderate psychological distress. Survivor guilt, changed relationships with family and friends, and changes in employability and insurability are unpredictable nonphysical effects. Because some patients encounter difficulties in returning to work, vocational retraining may be an important element in full recovery.

Long-term survivors may be reluctant to share seemingly "minor" issues with health care providers because they do not want to appear ungrateful for a second chance at life. Informing patients of survivor groups and celebrations, networks, newsletters, and on-line computer resources is a first step to providing good follow-up care to the growing number of long-term survivors.

46. Describe the beneficial effects of BMT.

Despite the physical, psychological, and social difficulties that BMT patients face, the majority indicate that, given the same circumstances, they would still elect to undergo BMT. Beneficial effects reported by transplant patients include a renewed sense of purpose and meaning in life and reprioritizing what is important. Most report they are "glad to be alive" or to have a "second chance" at life. With regard to social functioning, the ability to resume pre-BMT roles has a positive impact. Studies suggest that follow-up services and resources allowing patients to talk about their stories and to share long-term emotional challenges are important aspects of the nurse's tasks.

47. Is it difficult to get insurance coverage for BMT?

Because BMT is costly (approximately $50,000–$175,000), obtaining insurance coverage is a complex and dynamic process. Of interest, studies at the University of Washington indicate that when the cost of transplantation is analyzed, the cost of transplant per year of life prolongation is the same as for treating moderate hypertension. Patients without insurance are not eligible for transplant unless they are able to pay for the procedure upfront out of their own pocket.

Insurance policies vary widely in language about transplant. Some policies may be vague about coverage, whereas others specifically deny coverage for transplant based on the perception that it is "experimental treatment/therapy."

Collaborations between insurance companies and specific institutions or "centers of excellence" have evolved in parallel with other changes in health care economics. In some cases, transplant centers in close geographic proximity compete in terms of which center can offer an insurance company the lowest capitated fee. If patients' expenses for care exceed the agreed-upon price, the transplant center assumes the additional cost. The financial issues surrounding transplant can create significant ethical dilemmas for patients, providers, and insurers.

48. What educational and support resources are available to patients and families to help cope with the stresses of BMT?

BMT programs often have extensive patient education and support resources. Books, monographs, and videos for and by patients are now available. The topics range from description of the procedure to specific care practices (e.g., Hickman catheter) and long-term effects and care. Active newsletters are sent out by some centers, and one patient-developed newsletter has a regular subscription list. Most transplant centers have implemented websites in the past 5 years. The websites vary in information and often include survival statistics, patient and caregiver education, resource links, virtual tours of the center, and biographies of the transplant team. The sites are easily accessible on the worldwide web and offer patients the ability to view potential transplant sites without traveling to the location.

Support and survivor groups can be contacted through the larger BMT programs as well as the Internet. Many programs offer formalized psychosocial consultations with social workers, nurses, or psychologists to all patients.

49. What are the likely directions for BMT in the future?

Hematopoietic stem-cell transplantation is an ideal vehicle for gene therapy. Multiple strategies are under development to facilitate gene therapy to treat inborn errors of metabolism such as sickle cell anemia. In vitro models are being developed to remove stem cells from animals with inborn errors of metabolism, replace the damaged gene, and transplant the stem cells. These strategies may allow autologous transplant with the patient's own stem cells, in which the damaged gene has been replaced. If the disease is manifested in hematologic cells or if small amounts of the gene product can correct the phenotype, autologous stem cells in which the defective gene is replaced may be used to correct the defect. With time, the modified autologous stem cells may take over a greater portion of hematopoiesis, correcting the gene defect for the life of the patient.

The use of nonmyeloablative transplants is an example of the power of immune-mediated antineoplastic treatment, i.e. graft-vs.-malignancy. Many centers are working to decrease the toxicity of conditioning by substituting immunosuppression for high-doses of myeloablative chemoradiotherapy. These regimens decrease the toxicity of the transplantation conditioning regimen, allowing the graft to eliminate the remaining malignant cells. We are finally entering a time when targeted chemotherapy (monoclonal antibody with conjugated chemo or radiotherapy) will allow treatment of patients with less damage to normal cells. Such new agents can be used to condition patients before transplant, allowing older patients to be treated with less toxicity.

Acknowledgments

The authors acknowledge Mary Roach MS, RN, OCN, and Marie Whedon MS, RN, AOCN, FAAN, for their contributions in the first edition of *Oncology Nursing Secrets*. The authors also thank Peggy Russell, Penny Odem, and Karrie Witkind for assistance with data gathering for this manuscript.

REFERENCES

1. Antman K: High-dose chemotherapy in breast cancer: The end of the beginning? Biol Blood Marrow Transplant 6:469–475, 2000
2. Appelbaum F, Fay J, Herzig G, et al: American Society for Blood and Marrow Transplantation Guidelines for Training. Biol Blood Marrow Transplant 1:56, 1995.
3. Crouch MA, Ross JA: Current concepts in autologous bone marrow transplantation. Semin Oncol Nurs 10:12–19, 1994.
4. Cronk JW, Ross M: Bone marrow transplantation. In Wood ME (ed): Hematology/Oncology Secrets, 2nd ed. Philadelphia, Hanley & Belfus, 1999, pp 210–215.
5. Horowitz MM: New IBMTR/ABMTR slides summarize current use and outcome of allogeneic and autologous transplants. International Bone Marrow Transplant Registry Website, 2000.
6. Oncology Nursing Society: Manual for Bone Marrow Transplant Nursing: Recommendations for Practice and Education. Pittsburgh, PA, Oncology Nursing Press, 1994.
7. Phillips G, Armitage, J Bearman S, et al: American Society for Blood and Marrow Transplantation Guidelines for Clinical Centers. Biol Blood Marrow Transplant 1:54–55, 1995.
8. Stadtmauer EA, O'Neill A, Goldstein LJ, et al: Conventional dose chemotherapy compared with high-dose chemotherapy and autologous hematopoietic stem cell transplantation for metastatic breast cancer. Philadelphia Bone Marrow Transplant Group. N Engl J Med 342:1069–1076, 2000.
9. Stewart S: Bone Marrow Transplants: A Book of Basics for Patients. BMT Newsletter, Highland Park, IL, 1992.
10. Thomas ED, Blume KC, Forman SJ: Hematologic Cell Transplantation, 2nd ed. Malden, MA, Blackwell Science, 1999.
11. Whedon MB, Ferrell BR: Quality of life after bone marrow transplantation:Beyond the first year. Semin Oncol Nurs 10:42–57, 1994.
12. Whedon, MB, Wujcik D: Blood and Marrow Stem Cell Transplantation: Principles, Practice and Nursing Insights, 2nd ed. Boston, Jones & Bartlett, 1997.
13. Whedon MB, Stearns D, Mills L: Quality of life of long-term adult survivors of autologous bone marrow transplantation. Oncol Nurs Forum 22:1527–1537, 1995.

11. BIOLOGIC THERAPY

Heidi Mahay, PharmD

1. What are biologic response modifiers?

A biologic response modifier is defined as any substance capable of altering (modifying) the immune system with either a stimulatory or a suppressive effect. This definition includes agents that restore, augment, or modulate the host's immunologic mechanisms. Biologic agents produce direct antitumor activities as well as other effects; they may interfere with the ability of tumor cells to survive, metastasize, or differentiate. Biologic therapy involves the use of the following agents: monoclonal antibodies, hematopoietic growth factors, interleukins, interferons, and tumor necrosis factor.

2. What are monoclonal antibodies?

Monoclonal antibodies (MABs) are antibodies generated against a specific antigen. Hybridoma technology, developed in the mid 1970s, fuses an antibody-secreting cell with a malignant cell, resulting in a single antibody that can recognize a single antigen. This technology allows the production of unlimited amounts of pure MABs that are highly specific for a single antigen. The use of antibodies as carriers to deliver drugs and toxins to tumor cells was proposed in the early 1900s and was given the name "magic bullets. Today MABs tailored to recognize specific antigenic determinants on tumor cells can be used diagnostically to detect cancer cells or therapeutically to enhance or cause the destruction of cancer cells.

3. What MABs are currently available?
• Trastuzumab (Herceptin)   • Gemtuzumab ozogzmicin (Mylotarg)
• Rituximab (Rituxan)

4. How does trastuzumab work?

Trastuzumab is a monoclonal antibody approved for the treatment of metastatic breast cancer. It binds to the protein, HER2/*neu*, which is overexpressed in 25–30% of human breast cancers and associated with poor prognosis and poor chemotherapy response. Trastuzumab may be used as a single agent or in combination with chemotherapy, and can be administered in the outpatient setting.

5. What is the recommended regimen for trastuzumab?

The recommended regimen consists of a 4 mg/kg loading dose given as a 90-minute infusion and a weekly maintenance dose of 2 mg/kg given as a 30-minute infusion if the loading dose is well tolerated. Both infusions can be given in the outpatient setting.

6. What are the side effects of trastuzumab?

The major side effects are infusion-related chills and fevers in 40% of patients with the first infusion. These symptoms can be treated with acetaminophen, diphenhydramine, and meperidine with or without reduction in the rate of the infusion. Other side effects include nausea, vomiting, and pain at the tumor site. Caution must be used in patients who have a history of cardiac dysfunction because trastuzumab may exacerbate or result in cardiotoxicity.

7. How does rituximab work?

Rituximab is indicated for treatment of refractory or relapsed low-grade or follicular, CD20-positive, B-cell non-Hodgkin's lymphoma. It binds to the CD20 antigen on the surface of the lymphoma cells and prevents cell growth, resulting in cell lysis.

8. What is the recommended regimen for rituximab?

Rituximab may be used as a single agent or in combination with chemotherapy and is well tolerated. The recommended dose is 375 mg/m^2 once weekly for 4 weeks. Retreatment is based on clinical judgment. The loading dose is infused at 50 mg/hr, and the rate is increased by 50 mg/hr every 30 minutes to a maximum of 400 mg/hr if no adverse effects occur. Subsequent doses can be infused at 100 mg/hr, increasing the rate by 100 mg/hr to a maximum of 400 mg/hr.

9. Discuss the major side effects of rituximab.

The major side effects are infusion-related fever, chills, and aches, which typically occur during the first infusion. These side effects resolve with slowing of the infusion and premedication with acetaminophen and diphenhydramine.

10. What is the indication for gemtuzumab?

Relapsed acute myeloid leukemia (AML) expressing the CD33 antigen.

11. What is the recommended regimen for gentuzumab?

The recommended dose is 9 mg/m^2 given as two intravenous infusions separated by 14 days. Infuse over 2 hours; do *not* administer as an IV push or bolus.

12. What are the major side effects of gentuzumab?

Infusion-related complex with fever, chills, nausea, and vomiting. Myelosupression is a major toxicity.

13. What are colony-stimulating factors?

Colony-stimulating factors (CSFs) or hematopoietic growth factors (HGFs) are hormone-like proteins endogenous to the human body. They are essential to the hematopoietic system for proliferation, differentiation, and maturation of blood cells. CSFs bind to receptors on the hematopoietic cell membrane and regulate the growth and maturation of the specific stem and precursor cells. Granulocyte colony-stimulating factor (G-CSF), granulocyte-macrophage colony-stimulating factor (GM-CSF), erythropoietin-alpha (EPO), and interleukin-11 (oprelvekin, Neumega) are the CSFs commercially available for clinical use.

Pharmaceutical Characteristics of Colony-Stimulating Factors

CYTOKINE	GENERIC NAMES	COMMERCIAL SOURCE	BRAND NAMES	NORMAL ENDOGENOUS SOURCES
C-GSF	Filgrastin Lenograstin	*E. coli*	Neupogen Neutrogin	Monocytes, macrophages, fibroblasts, endothelial cells, keratinocytes
GM-CSF	Sargramostin Molgramostim Regramostin	*E. coli* Yeast	Leukine Leucomac Prokine	T-lymphocytes, monocytes, macrophages, fibroblasts, endothelial cells, osteoblasts, epithelial cells
EPO	Epoeitin-α		Epogen Procrit	Renal cells, hepatocytes
IL-11	Oprelevkin	*E. coli*	Neumega	Renal cells, hepatocytes

14. What is the difference between G-CSF and GM-CSF?

G-CSF: Commercially available G-CSF is derived from *Escherichia coli*. The main biologic and pharmacologic effect of G-CSF is to increase proliferation and differentiation (maturation) of neutrophils from their precursors, the committed progenitor cells. G-CSF enhances both function and endurance of neutrophils.

GM-CSF: Unlike G-CSF, GM-CSF affects multiple hematopoietic stem cells, including the precursors for granulocytes, macrophages, eosinophils, and megakaryocytes. The major effect of GM-CSF is to stimulate production of mature neutrophils and macrophages. GM-CSF potentiates the survival and function of mature neutrophils and also may increase microbial killing by enhanced phagocytosis and superoxide production.

15. Describe the dose and route of administration of G-CSF and GM-CSF.

The recommended dose is 5 µg/kg/day of G-CSF or 250 µg/m²/day of GM-CSF. The effect of G-CSF is dose-related; doses of 5–10 µg/kg/day have little effect on cell lines other than neutrophils. However, higher doses of G-CSF are associated with a 25% decrease in platelets. G-CSF is given at a higher dose (10 µg/kg/day) for mobilization of progenitor cells and after bone marrow transplant. G-CSFs can be administered subcutaneously or intravenously. Subcutaneous self-administration is convenient and can be taught to most patients. If intravenous administration is preferred, infusions given over approximately 15–20 minutes are suggested. Side effects are sometimes increased with intravenous administration. Dosage escalation of the CSFs is not recommended. Currently available data suggest that rounding the dose to the nearest vial size may improve patient convenience and decrease costs without affecting clinical efficacy.

16. What special considerations apply to Neupogen?

1. Neupogen is contraindicated in patients with hypersensitivity to *E. coli*-derived proteins.

2. Neupogen is available in premeasured syringes.

3. Do *not* dilute Neupogen in any solution containing saline because the product may precipitate.

4. Neupogen should not be exposed to dry ice or frozen. If it is inadvertently frozen, it is stable up to 24 hours; however it should not be used beyond 24 hours. When patients are traveling, they should be advised to wrap Neupogen in newspaper or bubble wrap to prevent direct contact with frozen gel refrigerant packs.

17. What uses of G-CSF and GM-CSF are approved by the Food and Drug Administration (FDA)?

The FDA has approved the use of G-CSF and GM-CSF to decrease the incidence of infection in patients undergoing myelosuppressive chemotherapy and bone marrow transplant. Both agents also are approved for use in patients with HIV infection, myelodysplastic syndromes, aplastic anemia, and congenital, cyclic, and acquired neutropenia. The use of CSFs in AML has been shown to improve morbidity, shorten hospital stays (about 2–5 days), and reduce infectious complications in adults, especially those > 55 years of age. Clinical studies in patients < 55 years of age are limited.

18. What are the general indications for using G-CSFs to support chemotherapy?

G-CSFs are used primarily to decrease anticipated morbidity (infections) and possibly mortality from the severe neutropenia that accompanies myelosuppressive chemotherapy. Primary prophylaxis, the use of G-CSFs after the first cycle of chemotherapy before the occurrence of febrile neutropenia, is indicated for patients receiving first-time chemotherapy in which the incidence of severe neutropenia is > 40% (e.g., adults with leukemia, patients undergoing bone marrow transplant). Generally, since most standard chemotherapy regimens do not result in severe neutropenia, G-CSFs are not recommended with the initial cycles of chemotherapy; however, they are administered after subsequent cycles of chemotherapy with a documented occurrence of febrile neutropenia in an earlier cycle. This practice is termed secondary administration. Other circumstances for secondary administration of G-CSFs include prolonged neutropenia that may delay chemotherapy or cause inappropriate dose reductions. G-CSFs also are recommended to stimulate hematopoietic progenitor cells and reconstitute bone marrow elements after high-dose chemotherapy.

19. When should G-CSF and GM-CSF be initiated? How long should they be continued?

G-CSFs should not be given within 24 hours before and no earlier than 24 hours after cytotoxic therapy, because they may enhance the myelotoxicity of chemotherapeutic agents by increasing cell turnover rate. Clinical data have shown that beginning G-CSF or GM-CSF 24–72 hours after the completion of chemotherapy provides optimal neutrophil recovery. G-CSF should be administered daily for up to two weeks, until the absolute neutrophil count (ANC) has reached 10,000/mm^3 after the expected chemotherapy-induced neutrophil nadir. The appropriate ANC is still debated among physicians. G-CSF therapy should be monitored by obtaining complete blood and platelet counts at least once to twice weekly. G-CSF should be discontinued after the neutrophil count is >10,000/mm^3.

20. Define ANC. How is it calculated?

The ANC is the absolute neutrophil count and is the same as the absolute granulocyte count (AGC). It is a measure of the mature white blood cells within the total white blood cell (WBC) count. Neutrophils are responsible for the phagocytosis and digestion of bacteria. Neutropenia generally is defined as an ANC < 1000. The ANC is calculated by multiplying the percent of granulocytes (neutrophils + bands) by the total WBC:

Total WBC = 3.5 (3,500)
Neutrophils = 28%
Bands = 3%
28% (neutrophils) + 3% (bands) = 31% (0.31)
ANC = 3.5 × 0.31 = 1,085

21. Is timing crucial in drawing blood levels after G-CSF and GM-CSF are given?

An initial transient leukopenia occurs about 1 hour after injection of G-CSF because of the transient decrease in circulating neutrophils and monocytes. This effect occurs with every dose and is followed by an increase in neutrophils. Blood samples for monitoring the hematologic effects of G-CSF, therefore, should be drawn before rather than after the daily dose. A CBC and platelet count should be obtained weekly during Neupogen therapy.

Transient leukopenia resulting in disappearance of circulating neutrophils, eosinophils, and monocytes also occurs with each dose of GM-CSF. The leukopenia may be accompanied by pulmonary sequestration of neutrophils. GM-CSF prolongs the half-life of circulating neutrophils from 8 to 48 hours. The proliferation of eosinophils is enhanced, and neutrophilia is also seen.

22. What are the side effects of G-CSF and GM-CSF?

The most frequent adverse effect of **G-CSF** is bone pain characterized by a transient mild, dull ache; this effect occurs in approximately 20% of patients. Bone pain is usually mild and can be managed with analgesics such as acetaminophen or other nonsteroidal anti-inflammatory drugs (NSAIDs). Occasionally, the bone pain may be severe enough to require opioids. A rare complication is leukocytoclastic vasculitis, which is manifested as a rash. Patients receiving G-CSF for longer than 1 year may experience hair thinning, splenomegaly, persistent bone pain, and, in rare cases, thrombocytopenia. Minor elevations of lactate dehydrogenase (LDH) and alkaline phosphatase also have been reported.

GM-CSF has been reported to cause a first-dose effect in certain patients within 3 hours of administration. This effect is characterized by flushing with hypotension, tachycardia, arterial oxygen desaturation, musculoskeletal pain, shortness of breath, and nausea; it is more common after intravenous than subcutaneous administration. Fortunately, intravenous administration of GM-CSF is relatively uncommon. GM-CSF can also induce fever and chills at doses > 3 µg/kg. Doses > 20 µg/kg/day are not well tolerated. The major dose-limiting side effects are weight gain with fluid retention, pleural and pericardial inflammation and effusions, and venous thrombosis.

23. What is erythropoietin?

Erythropoietin (EPO) was the first hematopoietic growth factor approved for clinical use. EPO, a glycoprotein hormone produced by the kidney, stimulates the production of red blood cells. EPO primarily regulates the production of the red blood cell line with little effect on other cells. It is currently approved for the treatment of anemia associated with chronic renal failure, chemotherapy, and use of zidovudine. Recent studies have shown that EPO also may be of benefit for other chronic anemias, including anemia associated with neoplastic infiltration of the bone marrow, and in the treatment of myelodysplastic syndromes.

24. What are the side effects of erythropoietin?

Side effects of EPO include flulike symptoms, occasional headache, and hypertension. It is not clear whether the incidence of vascular access thromboses is increased with the use of EPO.

25. What is the role of erythropoietin in patients with cancer?

Many factors cause anemia in patients with cancer; however, the predominant causes are related to the cancer itself or to cytotoxic chemotherapy. The anemia results from both increased destruction and decreased production of red blood cells. Studies evaluating the effectiveness of EPO in patients with cancer receiving chemotherapy report substantial rises in hemoglobin levels with decreased transfusion requirements, subjective improvement in anemia-related symptoms (fatigue), improvement in performance status and ability to work, and increased quality of life (QOL). Patient-reported functional capacity and QOL were enhanced independently of tumor response.

26. What is the dose of EPO for cancer patients receiving chemotherapy? How is it given?

According to prescribing information, the recommended starting dose of EPO for treatment of anemia due to cancer chemotherapy is 150 U/kg subcutaneously 3 times/week. However, once weekly doses of 600 U/kg are used in the surgical setting, and many oncologists now use once-weekly doses of EPO in patients with cancer, starting at 40,000 U per week.

27. How is EPO therapy monitored?

If an adequate response (hemoglobin > 1 g/dl from the patient's baseline value) does not occur after 4 weeks of therapy, the dose can be increased to 300 U/kg 3 times/week or 60,000 U once weekly. Further dosage increases are unlikely to improve response. The subsequent dose can be titrated based on the rate of hemoglobin or hematocrit rise and should be decreased when hematocrit reaches the target range of 30–36%, hemoglobin reaches the target range of > 12 g/dl, or hematocrit increases by more than 4 points during 2 weeks. At 8 weeks of therapy, an assessment is done to determine whether to continue the EPO. If there has been an increase in the hemoglobin or hematocrit from the baseline value *or* a decrease in red blood cell transfusions, the EPO may be resumed at about 75% of the previous dose. If hemoglobin is > 13 g/dl or if the hematocrit rises above 40%, EPO should be held or discontinued. If there has been no improvement in symptoms and hemoglobin/hematocrit values, the physician may consider discontinuing the EPO. Iron supplementation should be provided because stimulation of erythropoiesis by EPO causes a state of relative iron deficiency.

28. What is interleukin-11?

Interleukin-11 (IL-11, oprelvekin) is a thrombopoietic growth factor that stimulates megakaryocyte progenitor cells and hematopoietic stem cells. IL-11 also increases platelet production by inducing megakaryocyte maturation. Commercially available IL-11 (Neumega) is derived from *E. coli.*

29. Describe the dose and route of administration of IL-11.

The recommended dose in adults is 50 μg/kg subcutaneously once daily. Treatment with IL-11 begins 6–24 hours after completion of chemotherapy and is continued until the post-nadir platelet count is ≥ 50,000/mm^3. Dosing beyond 21 days is not recommended. Treatment should be discontinued at least 2 days before starting the next planned chemotherapy cycle.

30. What are the side effects of IL-11?

The most frequent adverse effect of IL-11 is mild to moderate fluid retention, which may manifest as peripheral edema and/or dyspnea. Caution should be used in patients with preexisting pleural or pericardial effusions or ascites because IL-11 may cause worsening. Decreases in hemoglobin values also have been observed, but they are thought to be due to a dilutional effect. Flu-like symptoms (fever, chills, arthralgia, myalgia, bone pain) have not been observed.

31. What is interleukin-2?

Interleukin-2 (IL-2) is a glycoprotein produced by helper T-cells after stimulation by antigens and IL-1. The primary function of interleukins (between leukocytes) is immunomodulation and immunoregulation of leukocytes. IL-2 promotes proliferation and differentiation of B- and T-cells as well as monocytes and also has many immunologic effects. The IL-2 receptor is present mainly on activated T-cells. The effects of IL-2 include proliferation of various cytotoxic cells, including natural killer (NK) cells, lymphokine-activated killer (LAK) cells, and tumor-infiltrating lymphocytes (TIL), which aid in the destruction of tumor cells without damaging normal cells. FDA-approved aldesleukin (Proleukin) or IL-2 is produced by recombinant DNA technology (placement of human genes inside bacteria or yeast cells to produce large quantities of highly purified protein).

32. What are the uses of IL-2?

IL-2 causes tumor regression in metastatic renal cell cancer, malignant melanoma, and colorectal cancer resistant to conventional chemotherapy agents. Responses in patients with renal cell cancer have been ~ 20%. When used as a single agent in patients with malignant melanoma, IL-2 has shown response rates of ~ 15%. The overall response rate for colorectal cancer is 10%. Regimens using IL-2 in combination with other agents continue to be investigated.

33. How should IL-2 be administered?

IL-2 is administered most commonly by intravenous infusion; it also has been administered subcutaneously. The dosage of IL-2 should be adjusted carefully according to patient tolerance, response, and route of administration. The potency of aldesleukin usually is expressed in international units (IU). Other units also have been reported, including Cetus units (CU) and Roche units (RU), but they are not equivalent (1 RU = 3 IU; 1 CU = 6 IU).

34. Discuss the toxicities associated with IL-2.

Most IL-2-induced toxicities appear to be dose-related and are reversible or manageable with appropriate supportive care. IL-2 has the potential to cause side effects in nearly every organ system. The most common dose-limiting toxicities of IL-2 are hypotension, fluid retention, and renal dysfunction. IL-2 causes a decrease in peripheral vascular resistance with peripheral vasodilatation and tachycardia, thus producing hypotension. Most patients receiving intense therapy with IL-2 require blood pressure support with pressors such as dopamine.

A problematic side effect is vascular leak syndrome (VLS), which presents as peripheral edema and weight gain (often > 10% of body weight). Ascites with or without pleural effusions and pulmonary edema may accompany VLS. Patients with underlying cardiovascular or renal abnormalities may be more susceptible to these side effects. VLS is managed with vasopressors (e.g., dopamine), albumin, fluid support, diuretics, and oxygen.

A major side effect is a flulike syndrome 4–6 hours after initiation of therapy. Another significant side effect is fatigue, which may be due to cytokine release. Other adverse effects include nausea, vomiting, and diarrhea, which can be managed with adequate antiemetic therapy and antidiarrheals. Patients receiving IL-2 also may experience thrombocytopenia, anemia, eosinophilia, and a skin erythema with burning and pruritus. Skin erythema can be managed with a moisturizing cream such as Eucerin. Neurologic changes, hypothyroidism, and bacterial infections are also common.

35. What are the interferons?

The interferons (IFNs) are proteins belonging to the cytokine family. Three types have been described in humans: alpha (IFN-α), beta (IFN-β), and gamma (IFN-γ). Each type originates from a distinct cell and has different biologic and chemical properties.

36. Discuss the biologic effects of IFNs.

The IFNs have antiviral, immunomodulatory, and antiproliferative properties. Type A IFNs are clinically useful in oncology and are potent immunostimulants with antiproliferative and antiangiogenic qualities. The antiviral effects of the IFNs include inhibition of intracellular replication of viral DNA as well as protection of cells from viral attack. The immunomodulatory effects include augmenting natural killer (NK) cell function, upregulating cytotoxic T-cell function, enhancing macrophage activity, and indirectly increasing B-cell immunoglobulin production by enhancing T-cell activity. IFNs directly inhibit DNA and protein synthesis in tumor cells and increase tumor cell recognition by stimulating expression of human lymphocyte antigens (HLAs) and tumor-associated antigens on tumor cell surfaces. In addition, IFNs increase all cell phases, prolonging the overall generation time and thus inhibiting the rate of cell growth.

37. What are the therapeutic uses of the interferons?

Most of the trials to date have used recombinant IFN-α. Labeled indications in cancer include hairy cell leukemia and acquired immunodeficiency disease (AIDS)-associated Kaposi's sarcoma, chronic myelogenous leukemia, follicular non-Hodgkin's lymphoma, and malignant melanoma. Other uses of IFN-α include multiple myeloma and renal cell carcinoma. Nononcologic indications for use of IFN-α include condylomata acuminata, chronic hepatitis B, and hepatitis C. IFN-β is used for multiple sclerosis and IFN-γ for chronic granulomatous disease.

38. How are the interferons administered?

Recombinant IFN-α-2a and IFN-α-2b are administered by intramuscular or subcutaneous injection. Induction therapy for malignant melanoma requires intravenous administration for the first 4 weeks of treatment.

39. Discuss the adverse effects associated with interferon use. How can they be managed?

Pharmacologic doses of IFNs have been associated with various side effects, including an acute flulike syndrome with fever, chills, malaise, myalgias, and headache that begins 2–8 hours after the first subcutaneous injection. Flulike symptoms may be prevented or at least alleviated with administration of acetaminophen 650 mg before the IFN injection and every 4 hours thereafter for a total of 24 hours. Adequate hydration is important to decrease many of the flulike symptoms. Administration of IFN at bedtime enables the patient to sleep through the flulike symptoms of initial therapy. Tolerance (tachyphylaxis) to the flulike effects develops over several days to weeks.

Other side effects include fatigue and depression, which are the most common dose-limiting and dose-related side effect of IFN-α. Bedtime administration may help to minimize the fatigue, along with strategies to reduce activities and conserve energy. Severe fatigue, however, may require dosage decreases or discontinuation of therapy. Assessment of depression and use of selective serotonin reuptake inhibitors (SSRIs) often improve both fatigue and depression. Gastrointestinal symptoms such as anorexia, nausea, vomiting, and diarrhea are rare at low doses but increase in frequency and severity as the dose increases. Antiemetics and antidiarrheals help to control some of these symptoms. Hydration levels influence tolerance of therapy. Neurologic effects such as vertigo, decreased mental status, confusion, depression, and paresthesias occur at low doses but may increase in severity and incidence at increased doses. Hematologic effects can include decreased leukocytes, granulocytes, and thrombocytes.

40. What is tumor necrosis factor? What are its effects?

Tumor necrosis factor (TNF-α), also called cachexin, is a natural substance produced by activated macrophages, monocytes, and lymphocytes after exposure to endotoxin. As a type of cytokine, TNF causes tumor and healthy tissue necrosis by decreasing or stopping blood flow. In vitro studies in mice and other animal models have shown that TNF has cytotoxic or cytostatic effects on tumor cells with virtually no effect on normal cells. TNF is released in the bloodstream and binds to receptors on tumor cell membranes, where it produces cell arrest and cell lysis. TNF has been studied for the treatment of melanoma, colorectal carcinoma, AIDS-related Kaposi's sarcoma, B-cell lymphoma, non-small cell lung cancer, ovarian cancer, and glioma. To date, however, TNF has not shown significant palliative or curative therapy for any type of cancer. The clinical use of TNF has been limited by its severe systemic toxicities (coagulopathy, cytopenia, and pulmonary failure). Clinical investigations are ongoing to determine the utility and efficacy of TNF in oncology. Current investigations involve the use of TNF and melphalan in isolated limb perfusion in patients with nonresectable soft-tissue sarcoma.

41. List resources for use of biologic therapy.

The following pharmaceutical companies offer excellent instruction books, monographs, and videotapes for staff and patient education as well as professional advice from clinical support specialists. They usually provide financial reimbursement/assistance programs as well:

Amgen, Inc.	800-77-AMGEN (Neupogen, Infergen)
Chiron Therapeutics	800-244-7668 (IL-2)
Genentech/IDE8	800-626-3553 (Herceptin, Rituxin)
Genetics Institute	888-4463344 (Neumega)
Immunex Corporation	800-IMMUNEX (Leukine)
Ortho Biotech	800-325-7504 (Procrit)
Roche Laboratories	800-7ROFERON (Interferon)
Schering Corporation	800-526-4099 (Interferon)
Wyeth Laboratories	800-544-9871 (Mylotarg)

ACKNOWLEDGMENT

The author thanks Deborah Nelson, RN, BSN,OCN, for her thoughtful review and contributions to this chapter.

REFERENCES

1. Andavolu MVS, Logan LJ: Leukocytoclastic vasculitis as a complication of granulocyte colony-stimulating factor (G-CSF): A case study. Ann Hematol 78:79–81, 1999.
2. Anderson CM, Rasool HJ: Biologic therapy of cancer. In Wood, ME (ed.): Hematology/Oncology Secrets, 2nd ed. Philadelphia, Hanley & Belfus, 1999, pp 206–210.
3. Bociek RG, Armitage JO: Hematopoietic growth factors. Cancer 46:165–187, 1996.
4. Chabner BA, Longo DL (eds): Cancer Chemotherapy and Biotherapy. Philadelphia, J.B. Lippincott, 1996.
5. Demetri GD, Kris M, Wade J, et al: Quality of life benefit in chemotherapy patients treated with epoetin alfa is independent of disease response or tumor type: Results from a prospective community oncology study. J Clinl Oncol 16:3412–3425, 1998.
6. Georgetown University Medical Center, Lombardi Cancer Center: Clinical pathway for epoetin alfa in chemotherapy-induced anemia for patients with non-myeloid malignancies. In Oncology Critical Pathways. Rockville, MD, Association of Community Cancer Centers, 1998.
7. Kaye JA: Clinical development of recombinant human interleukin-11 to treat chemotherapy-induced thrombocytopenia. Curr Opin Hematol 3:209–215, 1996.
8. Kim B, Litton GJ: Biological therapy: Interferons, interleukins, and monoclonal antibodies. In Pazdur R, Coia LR, Hoskins WJ, Wagman LD (eds.): Cancer Management: A Multidisciplinary Approach, 3rd ed. Melville, NY, PRR, 1999, pp 677–691.
9. Rieger PT (ed): Biotherapy: A Comprehensive Overview. Boston, Jones & Bartlett, 1995.
10. Rosenberg SA: Principles of cancer management: Biologic therapy. In DeVita VT Jr, Hellman S, Rosenberg SA: Cancer: Principles and Practices of Oncology, 6th ed. 2001, pp 307–328.
11. Smith TJ: Economic analysis of the clinical uses of the colony-stimulating factors. Curr Opin Hematol 3:175–179, 1996.
12. Snead RB, Harker LA: Preclinical studies and potential clinical applications of c-mpl ligand. Curr Opin Hematol 3:197–202, 1996.
13. Srivastava A, Purdy M: Colony-stimulating factors. In Wood ME (ed.): Hematology/Oncology Secrets, 2nd ed. Philadelphia, Hanley & Belfus, 1999, pp 198–205.

12. CLINICAL TRIALS

Pamela A. Rossé, RN, MS, CRA, and Mary T. Garcia, RN, MPH, CCRA

1. Describe how a clinical trial differs from a protocol.

A **clinical trial** is a planned investigation involving patients. It is designed according to accepted scientific methods and is intended to determine the most effective treatment for future patients with a given medical condition.

A **protocol** is the written form of a clinical trial; it outlines the objectives of the study and summarizes research information currently available relative to the treatment under study. In addition, a protocol explicitly delineates criteria for inclusion and exclusion of participants. It also provides a detailed description of the treatment involved and specifies parameters for evaluating outcomes.

2. What types of clinical trials is the oncology nurse likely to encounter?

Studies may be designed as therapeutic or preventive, or they may address biologic or genetic questions and involve tissue/specimen collection and testing. Therapeutic studies may include one or several modalities, such as chemotherapy, radiation therapy, surgery, hormonal therapy, immunotherapy, gene therapy, or alternative therapies for symptom management.

3. How does an institutional review board (IRB) function?

An IRB is entrusted with the task of protecting the rights and welfare of human participants in research by asking the following questions:
1. Do the benefits outweigh the risks?
2. Is there adequate protection for the participants, including informed consent?
3. Is the selection of participants equitable?

4. How are the members of an IRB selected?

Membership requirements for IRBs in the United States are established by the Office for the Protection of Human Research (OPHR), which is a branch of the National Institutes of Health. Other government agencies, such as the Food and Drug Administration (FDA), also regulate IRB activities. A minimum of five members of varied backgrounds, gender, and racial and cultural perspectives is required. A typical IRB may include physicians, pharmacists, nurses, scientists, lawyers, clergy, and community representatives. At least one nonmedical person and one person with no direct affiliation to the reviewing institution are mandated. Special expertise is required by regulation when studies involving vulnerable populations (e.g., children, prisoners, cognitively impaired people) are considered. All studies must be approved by an IRB before any patients or subjects may be enrolled. The IRB also must be kept abreast of changes and informed of adverse events related to the studies. IRBs have the authority to suspend and close studies that previously have been approved if regulations are not adhered to by the investigators and study personnel.

5. How can informed consent be ensured?

To inform potential participants adequately about the study, specific points must be covered:
- Reason for the study (and clear recognition that it is research)
- Specific procedures that will be used for both diagnosis and treatment
- Alternative treatments
- Potential risks and benefits of participation (including the right to refuse without consequence)
- Assurance of confidentiality
- Clarification of compensation (or lack thereof)
- Voluntary participation

The consent process involves discussion of all of the preceding points with a potential subject. Information about the study may be provided by the physician, research nurse/data manager, pharmacist, or others knowledgeable about the clinical trial. Researchers are strongly encouraged to provide consent forms written at a 6th-grade reading level; however, the abundance of medical terms is often confusing. Frequently patients have just learned of their diagnosis; although seemingly aware of what they have heard and agreed to do, they have many questions later that require further clarification of the study process. Federal regulations require evidence that consent is provided in a manner that allows maximal comprehension and assessment of the subjects' understanding of the study.

6. Under what special circumstances may informed consent be waived?
Sometimes the only access to a new therapy is through a clinical trial. In an emergency in which the patient may be not be capable of giving consent, the study treatment may be considered. In cases involving minors or legal guardianship, the patient may not be the person providing consent.

7. How is informed consent obtained from non–English-speaking participants?
When non–English-speaking subjects are enrolled in a study, it is permissible to present an oral presentation, followed by a "short form" stating that the elements of consent were presented orally in the subject's native language. A translator, fluent in the subject's native language as well as English, must provide the consent information to the patient or patient representative and obtain appropriate signatures on the short form.

8. Under what circumstance may eligibility criteria be waived?
On occasion, the IRB may approve participation in a study for a single patient on a compassionate basis, usually when no alternative treatment is available.

9. Must subjects participate in all aspects of a study once they sign a consent form?
With the advent of multiple components requiring consent, IRBs are faced with the challenges of maximizing participation while preventing coercion. For example, a subject may be willing to participate in the treatment but unwilling to undergo extra tests or biopsies. Previously, subjects in many studies were required to participate in special testing if they desired to participate in the treatment portion. Some IRBs now insist that, when feasible, the consent form be divided into sections so that the subject has the opportunity to agree or refuse to participate in separate testing, additional follow-up, release of information, or other aspects of the study. While attempting to offer participants maximal autonomy, IRBs must remain cognizant of situations in which refusal to participate in additional testing may compromise the integrity of the study.

10. Are subjects reimbursed for participation in a study?
Studies may be sponsored by government sources, pharmaceutical companies, or individual institutions and investigators, and funding varies accordingly. Usually, patients participating in cancer treatment studies do not receive money for participation, although study costs or drugs may be provided. In special circumstances reimbursement may be approved by the officiating IRB. Typically, if the patient is insured, routine health care costs and standard-of-care costs are billed; remaining expenses are absorbed by the funding source. However, some costs may have to be paid by the patient. Recent findings indicate that, for the most part, insurance agencies are reluctant to cover expenses associated with clincial trials. Some experts speculate that this reluctance is a major contributing factor to the low accrual rate of adults (approximately 3%) for cancer clinical trials in the United States. For-profit, not-for-profit, and charitable organizations may wish to contribute financially and help to defray patients' costs. Meanwhile, professional organizations such as the Oncolgy Nursing Society and Institute of Medicine are working diligently to institute policies that expand clinical trial reimbursement.

With increasing frequency, payment incentives are offered to subjects who participate in prevention and early detection studies. These studies involve a healthier group of subjects than cancer treatment studies. Payments and other types of incentives, such as restaurant coupons, are often minimal compensation compared with the degree of involvement required of the subject. Like reimbursement, such compensation or incentives must be approved by an IRB.

11. How are therapeutic studies characterized?

Every new chemotherapy drug is tested in three subsequent trials called phase I, phase II, and phase III before it is approved by the FDA for general use. It is becoming more common for studies to combine objectives associated with the different phases (e.g., phases I and II or phases II and III). However, not all studies fall within the phase classification system (e.g., prevention, early detection, quality-of-life studies, cost-of-treatment studies). On the other hand, additional characteristics may be used to classify a trial, such as adjuvant or neoadjuvant.

12. Explain the purpose of phase I studies.

Phase I studies are dose-escalating clinical trials designed to determine the maximum tolerated dose (MTD) of a new drug, alone or in combination with another drug or modality. The phase I trial also helps to establish an optimal therapy schedule, to determine pharmacokinetic properties, and to identify toxicities associated with therapy. It is not a primary goal of phase I trials to determine efficacy. Frequently, phase I involves patients who have had extensive treatment, and different types of cancer may be included. Because the study is concluded once the MTD is reached, the numbers are often small (e.g., 20 patients) but may include 100 or more.

13. What are the goals of phase II studies?

Phase II studies evaluate antitumor activity in specific tumors and further define toxicities. The number of patients frequently ranges from 100–200, but several hundred may be involved.

14. Describe the primary goal of phase III studies.

Phase III studies compare a promising new treatment with established therapy in clinical practice to determine whether one is superior for treating a specific disease. Large numbers of participants are required.

15. What are adjuvant and neoadjuvant studies?

Adjuvant studies are designed to provide additional therapy to patients who have been deemed free of disease after treatment. The goal is to prevent recurrence.

Neoadjuvant studies are designed to treat patients before as well as after surgery, with the belief that the surgery resulted in no further evaluable disease. The goals are to optimize the success of surgery and to prevent recurrence.

16. Define eligibility and evaluability. Why are they important?

Eligibility refers to meeting the qualifications stipulated in the protocol for participation in the study. **Evaluability** refers to how well the protocol was followed once the patient was enrolled; essentially, it determines how usable the patient's data are.

Both concepts are crucial to the integrity of the study. For example, if a patient does not have the same type, grade, or stage of cancer as required in the protocol, the progress of disease may not be affected by the proposed therapy. Significant differences among patient characteristics make it difficult to include them in the same pool for analyses. Similarly, if patients are not treated for their disease in a standardized manner, it is difficult to generalize about the results. Of equal importance, if a patient does not meet one of the criteria (e.g., adequate renal or cardiac function), serious toxicities may occur.

17. In clinical trials with multiple treatment regimens, who decides which regimen a particular patient will receive?

In studies with multiple treatment regimens, each regimen is called an arm. Patients are often randomized to specific arms of a study or assigned to different treatments by a process similar to flipping a coin. Usually, the randomization schedule is generated by a computer. For some studies assignment may be blinded (that is, the patient does not know which treatment he or she is receiving) or double-blinded (neither the patient nor the healthcare team knows which drug is administered). At times, failure to achieve complete or partial response (CR or PR) to one treatment results in crossover (switching) to another arm of treatment.

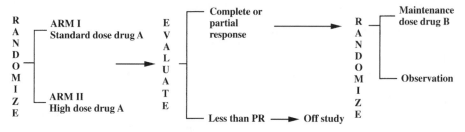

Example of randomization.

18. Define equipoise and explain its significance in clinical trials.

Equipoise means "even balance." In relationship to clinical trials, it refers to approaching studies from an unbiased perspective. The concept of equipoise is fundamental in conducting clinical research and is particularly relevant during presentation of a clinical trial to subjects. Because of the investigational nature of a study, it is important to impress on subjects that they may receive no direct benefit. It is also paramount, in studies with more than one treatment option, to present all treatments with equal enthusiasm. Sometimes this task is difficult for the healthcare team because, based on professional experience, they may believe that one therapy is more promising than others.

Studies that compare therapy with no therapy (observation) are particularly challenging. It is often difficult to do nothing when a patient is faced with the diagnosis of cancer. In such cases it may be beneficial to remember that many investigational cancer therapies ultimately have been deemed ineffective, while at the same time they are associated with numerous and significant toxicities.

19. What role does pharmacokinetics play in clinical trials?

Often the drug tested in a clinical trial is reviewed for its pharmacokinetic properties. To measure absorption rates, duration of action, distribution within the body, and excretion, blood or other types of samples are collected at specifically designated intervals before and after administration of therapy. Sometimes no samples or perhaps only one or two samples are required. In other cases, samples may be required only when a patient experiences significant untoward side effects.

Timing in obtaining samples is often critical to the validity and reliability of data. Every effort should be made to adhere to established blood-draw or other sampling times. The study coordinator should be informed of instances in which the schedule cannot be maintained in case other arrangements are needed; special notation should be documented in the patient's clinical trial record.

20. In general, what kinds of information do investigators look for once a study has ended?

At the conclusion of a clinical trial the primary investigators pay particular attention to data that answer the following questions:

1. Were the original study questions (usually found in the objectives section of the protocol) answered? Most commonly these questions are related to endpoints such as survival time, types of tumor responses, and time to recurrence.

2. What were the toxicities (in detail)? Do they outweigh the benefits?

3. Was each patient eligible and evaluable? If not, it may be difficult to generalize about the data.

21. What are the implications if the treatment schedule stipulated in the protocol is not followed?

Obviously, clinical trials are designed with specific scientific questions in mind. The schedules of treatments are typically based on previously conducted trials (animal, human, or both). The primary treatment schedules may be discontinued if significant toxicities result. Many protocols provide a schedule for modification of therapy based on specific toxicities and their severity. When no modification schedule is provided or in unique patient situations, the primary investigator should be contacted to discuss whether the patient should remain in the study.

As a general rule, the protocol schedule should not be violated because it is inconvenient or because the treating physician does not agree with the way the protocol is written. Such issues should be taken into consideration before the patient enters a clinical trial. Deviation from the stipulated protocol may be dangerous, because the alternative treatment may not have been studied at great length. Furthermore, deviation may make the patient's data unevaluable. Compromise of treatment may jeopardize timely completion of select studies and even preclude some patients from participating in an innovative study.

22. Give an example of why it is important to follow the treatment schedule.
In a phase I study, drug X is tested on a limited sample size. Additional patients were hopeful of entering the study, but only 20 patients were accepted before the study was closed for analyses. During the analyses it is discovered that patient 18 did not receive drug X on days 1, 7, and 21 as stipulated in the protocol. Instead, the patient received the drug on days 1, 10, and 42 because she was out of town. If the investigators had known this information before beginning the analyses, they might have chosen to allow an additional patient to enter the study as a replacement for patient 18. The unfortunate patient who would have been number 21 was precluded from joining the study because the investigators believed that all previous patients were eligible and evaluable. Furthermore, a lack of evaluable data may preclude meaningful results.

23. What if a patient decides to discontinue treatment earlier than the protocol stipulates?
Every patient has the right to discontinue participation in a clinical trial at any time, and this right should be clearly stated in the consent form. In such cases, the patient, family, and healthcare team should thoroughly discuss appropriate alternatives, including no treatment. Even though the patient discontinues therapy, some of the early data may still be useful. Examples include toxicities and perhaps tumor response. In the final analysis, the primary investigators and biostatisticians decide whether the patient is evaluable.

Many clinical trials require follow-up of the patient's status until death to determine whether long-term survival was affected by the treatment tested (otherwise known as survival curve information). If the patient has chosen to discontinue participation, the type of long-term follow-up (i.e., the degree of intrusiveness) that may be continued must be clarified with and approved by the patient. In such cases, even if the patient has discontinued active participation in a clinical trial, the study remains open at an institution until all patients have died.

24. How much information is shared with the patient whose condition precludes treatment at the full dose specified by the protocol?
A patient's condition may deteriorate once he or she has entered in a study. Rather than dropping the patient from the study, provisions may be instituted to allow the patient to remain in the study at a reduced treatment dose. This situation poses the question of whether it is worthwhile for the patient to remain in the study. At the heart of this question is the patient's right to know about his or her treatment. At the same time, the healthcare team must struggle with other fundamental questions: Will a modified investigational therapy be any better or worse than the originally proposed investigational therapy—or, for that matter, than standard therapy? Do the benefits outweigh the risks? Because it is mandated that patients be adequately informed about participation in research studies, it seems logical to provide them with the facts necessary to make a truly informed decision. Therein lies the difficulty: all of the facts are not typically known to the healthcare team. If they were, there would be no need for an investigational study. One of the most honest approaches is to provide the facts that are known and to discuss issues for which the answers remain unknown.

25. How can the oncology nurse contribute to the validity of clinical trials?
1. **Identification of potential study patients.** Oncology nurses are in a critical position for fostering clinical trial research. They possess knowledge of cancer disease processes and understand

the rationale for treatment. They frequently have unique insights into whether a patient is likely to be able to comply with a protocol.

2. **Protecting the integrity of the study.** Most participants in an oncology clinical trial believe that in some way they are contributing to cancer research. If information about their cases is compromised by the heathcare team, the patients' efforts have been undermined. Thus, adherence to a protocol is paramount. Because the nurse is frequently responsible for coordinating patient care, the nurse should be aware of protocol guidelines and remain in contact with the coordinators of the trial. The treatment plan must be followed exactly, including drug administration, pre- and posthydration guidelines, antiemetic therapy, specified antibiotics, and use of cell-stimulating factors. Various tests must be performed at specified times, and radiotherapy and/or surgery must be synchronized accordingly. The nurse may be able to make suggestions that promote feasibility and ensure adherence.

3. **Documentation in the medical record.** In addition to routine requirements, it is of great value to those who review the data for study purposes to find notations relative to (1) the patient's current performance status; (2) dose modifications or schedule changes and reasons for them; (3) specific symptoms of toxicity, including onset and duration; and (4) supportive care, particularly as related to symptom management.

4. **Patient advocacy.** Often the oncology nurse is in a position to support patients' decisions to begin, continue, or discontinue treatment. Similarly, in investigational studies the nurse may need to help patients verbalize their decision to participate or not to participate to family or other healthcare team members. The nursing staff also can help patients to feel comfortable with their informed decision or even to change their decision, if circumstances permit.

26. **List websites that are relevant to oncology clincial trials.**
Specific cancer trial information
- cancernet.nci.nih.gov/trialsrch.shtml
- cancertrials.nci.nih.gov/finding/centers/index.html
- dcs.nci.nih.gov/trials/index.html
- ctep.info.nih.gov
- centerwatch.com

Many universities with medical schools provide websites that link to clinical trials. Type in the university's name followed by key words such as "cancer trials," "cancer studies," or "cancer research." Also try substituting the word oncolgy for cancer. In addition, cooperative oncology groups have a website of their current trials (e.g., SWOG.org).

General cancer trial information
- cancer.org
- cancertrials.nci.nih.gov/finding/centers/index.html

Detailed information about current news related to clinical trials/patient safety
- nci.nih.gov/aboutnci/pressrelease.html

REFERENCES

1. Berry DL, Dodd MJ, Hinds PS, Ferrell BR: Informed consent: Process and clinical issues. Oncol Nurs Forum 23:507–512, 1996.
2. Ehrenberger H: TechTalk: Clincial trials are just a click away. ONS News 15(4):7, 2000.
3. Information Sheets: Guidance for Institutional Review Boards and Clinical Investigators 1998 Update. Rockville, MD, Office of Associate Commissioner for Health Affairs, Food and Drug Administration, 1998.
4. Jassak P, Ryan MP: Ethical issues in clinical research. Semin Oncol Nurs 5(2):102–108, 1989.
5. Meier E: Groups support insurance coverage for clinical trials. ONS News 15(4):7, 2000.
6. Protection of Human Subjects and Institutional Review Board Requirements: Food and Drug Administration Regulatory Primer. Rockville, MD, Office of AIDS and Special Health Issues, U.S. Department of Health and Human Services, 1996.
7. Rosse PA, Krebs LU: The nurse's role in the informed consent process. Semin Oncol Nurs 15(2):1–9, 1999.
8. Varricchio CG, Jassak PF: Informed consent: An overview. Semin Oncol Nurs 5(2):95–98, 1989.
9. Wager E, Tooley PJH, Emanuel MB, Wood SF: Get patient consent to enter clinical trials. BMJ 311:27–30, 1995.
10. White-Hershey D, Nevidjon B: Fundamentals for oncology nurse/data managers: Preparing for a new role. Oncol Nurs Forum 17:371–377, 1990.
11. Wujcik D: Insurance coverage concerns may limit participation in clinical trials. ONS News 15(4):3, 2000.

13. BLOOD COMPONENTS

Rocky Billups, RN, Tonya P. Cox, RN, BSN, OCN, and
Marcia L. Maxwell, RN, BSN, CCRN

1. What are the four ABO blood types?

The four blood types are A, B, AB, and O. A and B are antigens present on the RBC membrane. A person may have both antigens and be AB or neither antigen and be O. Individuals who lack these antigens on their RBC membranes may make antibody to the antigens when exposed to the A, B, or AB antigens. Individuals with a particular antigen on their RBC membrane will not make antibody to that antigen. Thus, people with the blood type O are known as universal donors. Conversely, people with the blood type AB are universal recipients. The population distribution in the United States is as follows:

BLOOD TYPE	PERCENT	BLOOD TYPE	PERCENT
A positive	34%	AB positive	3%
A negative	6%	AB negative	1%
B positive	9%	O positive	38%
B negative	2%	O negative	7%

2. What is the Rh system?

The Rh system refers to the presence or absence of Rh antigens. The six most common Rh antigens are C, D, E, c, d, and e. Presence of the D antigen means that a person is Rh-positive. Absence of the D antigen denotes an Rh-negative person. Expression of the Rh D antigen can occur by transfusion of an Rh-positive blood product in an Rh-negative person or through pregnancy in an Rh-negative woman carrying an Rh-positive fetus. Such exposure of an Rh-negative person to Rh-positive RBCs will result in the production of antibodies to the Rh antigen. The main difference between the two classes A, B, O, and Rh is that antibodies may randomly develop to A and/or B in a person who lacks these antigens, but the Rh-negative person will not develop antibodies to Rh without exposure to Rh.

3. What are the acceptable donor blood types for the eight ABO/Rh blood types?

PATIENT BLOOD TYPE	ACCEPTABLE DONOR BLOOD TYPE							
	A POSITIVE	A NEGATIVE	B POSITIVE	B NEGATIVE	AB POSITIVE	AB NEGATIVE	O POSITIVE	O NEGATIVE
A positive	X	X					X*	X*
A negative		X						X*
B positive			X	X			X*	X*
B negative				X				X*
AB positive	X*	X*	X*	X*	X	X	X*	X*
AB negative		X*		X*		X		X*
O positive							X	X
O negative								X

* If plasma is incompatible, reduce volume to 200 ml.

4. **What are the primary components of whole blood?**
Whole blood components include red blood cells, platelets, fresh frozen plasma, cryoprecipitate, factor concentrates, and white blood cells.

5. **What are the common indications for transfusion of whole blood and primary components?**
Whole blood—historically used for intravascular volume expansion in patients experiencing hypovolemic shock. Whole blood is not commonly used for transfusions because sound resource management requires that it be divided into its various components (e.g., RBCs, platelets, plasma) and utilized appropriately.

Packed red blood cells (PRBCs)—usually administered to oncology patients for intravascular volume expansion, support during hemorrhage, and treatment of symptomatic anemia.

Platelets—transfused for significant thrombocytopenia or hemorrhage. A platelet count of < 10,000 or active bleeding with a platelet count < 50,000 are commonly accepted transfusion thresholds. Platelets may also be transfused to boost a platelet count to > 50,000 immediately prior to or during a procedure.

Fresh frozen plasma (FFP)—contains clotting factors, albumin, globulins, and antibodies and is administered to reverse the effects of coumadin, to correct coagulation abnormalities due to a deficiency of factors II, V, VII, IX, X, and XI or massive blood transfusions, and as treatment for thrombotic thrombocytopenic purpura. FFP is no longer recommended for primary intravascular volume expansion because there are other more readily available products which may be used for this purpose.

Cryoprecipitate—portion of the plasma which is rich in certain clotting factors, including factors VIII and XII, von Willebrand factor, and fibrinogen. It is most commonly used to prevent or control bleeding in patients with disseminated intravascular coagulation (DIC) or those with inherited coagulation abnormalities.

Factor concentrates—concentrates of individual plasma proteins which are used to replace specific factor deficiencies.

White blood cells (WBCs)—granulocytes are most commonly collected via apheresis and must be transfused within 24 hours. They are used in patients with prolonged neutropenia who have active infections, especially gram-negative or fungal infections, that are unresponsive to antibiotics or antifungal therapy. They are generally irradiated and commonly cause febrile nonhemolytic reactions. Patients may be premedicated with acetaminophen and diphenhydramine, and meperidine is used to manage chilling. They should be ABO compatible and infused via standard blood tubing without a leukocyte filter. Some studies have indicated benefit with granulocyte transfusions, but the effectiveness is still debated.

6. **Why do PRBC transfusion requirements vary among oncologic patients?**
The reasons for transfusing are multifactorial. Experience of the practitioner, understanding of the literature, and individual patient presentations guide medical and nursing judgment about transfusion decisions. Religious and personal patient preferences must also be discussed in regard to transfusion of blood products. Where possible, reducing exposure to banked blood is the goal, which may be accomplished in some patients through the use of erythropoietin.

7. **Which intravenous solution is used to prime blood tubing for administration of all products?**
Normal saline, 0.9%, is the only intravenous solution that is compatible with blood products. Agglutination or hemolysis may occur with use of other intravenous solutions.

8. **Are premedications commonly administered before infusion of PRBCs and platelets? Why?**
Pretransfusion medications that were once given to prevent febrile and allergic reactions are now considered unnecessary unless the patient has experienced a reaction in the past. When necessary, acetaminophen (650–1000 mg) and diphenhydramine (25–50 mg) are used as premedications.

Occasionally, Solu-Cortef also may be administered as a premedication. The doses prescribed vary depending on the patient's clinical status. These drugs are used to prevent nonhemolytic febrile and allergic transfusion reactions.

9. What are the acceptable parameters for transfusion time of blood products?

Generally, PRBCs are infused over 90–120 minutes or 3–4 ml/kg/hr. The time of infusion depends on the age of the patient as well as clinical status. In the critical care unit, PRBCs may be infused in as little as 5–10 minutes to treat massive blood loss. To reduce the risk of bacterial contamination and sepsis, PRBCs must be transfused within 4 hours of leaving the blood bank.

Platelets are infused over 20–60 minutes or 10 ml/min. In emergent situations such as exsanguination in a thrombocytopenic patient, platelets can be infused in less time. The longer platelets hang after being dispensed from the blood bank, the less effective they become. For patients that are platelet refractory, some institutions give platelets by a continuous infusion but for no longer than 4 hours per unit.

FFP is usually infused over 15–30 minutes or 10 ml/min. Cryoprecipitate is infused over 3–15 minutes or 10 ml/min.

Granulocyte transfusions begin slowly and increase to the rate ordered by the physician. The recommended length of infusion is 1–4 hours. Since granulocytes are suspended in plasma and will settle to the bottom of the bag, it is recommended that the bag be agitated every 10–15 minutes during infusion. Do not administer amphotericin B within 4–6 hours of the granulocyte infusion, as cumulative pulmonary insufficiency has been reported.

Factor concentrates may be given as an intravenous bolus or as a continuous infusion.

Note: It is important to evaluate the pulmonary status of each patient before rapid infusion of any blood product.

10. What parameters should be followed for monitoring vital signs during a patient's transfusion?

The frequency of vital sign monitoring depends on your facility's blood administration policy. According to common guidelines, complete vital signs should be monitored before beginning administration, 15 minutes into the administration, and immediately after infusion is complete. The rationale for such standards is the increased risk of transfusion reactions associated with blood products. Remember that clinical symptoms, not changes in vital signs, are often the first indication of a transfusion reaction. Remain with the patient for the first 10–15 minutes, and monitor for fever or chills, hypotension, dyspnea, headache, or hives.

11. Why should PRBCs and platelets be leukocyte-reduced for patients who receive multiple transfusions?

The benefits of transfusing leukocyte-reduced products include reducing febrile nonhemolytic transfusion reactions and decreasing cytomegalovirus (CMV) risk. Leukocyte-reducing blood products also decrease the risk or lengthen the time in which a patient becomes alloimmunized. Alloimmunization is a disorder that results when human leukocyte antigen (HLA) on the surface of leukocytes or human platelet antigen on the surface of platelets triggers antibody formation in the recipient. When subsequent units of products containing these antigens are transfused at a later time, the antibodies destroy the leukocytes or platelets, reducing the benefit or "bump" expected from the product. Patients with hematologic malignancies and bone marrow transplant recipients should receive leukocyte-reduced PRBCs and platelets.

12. What are two methods of collecting platelet concentrates?

The two methods of obtaining platelet concentrates are random-donor and single-donor collections. Random-donor platelets are obtained from each unit of whole blood during processing. Platelets from several different donors are then pooled into a single pack for administration. Single-donor platelets are collected via apheresis from an individual donor and dispensed for administration.

HLA-matched platelets are obtained from a single donor who has a partial HLA match with the recipient.

13. What are the advantages of using single-donor platelets?

Use of single-donor platelets decreases sensitization (alloimmunization) of the recipient and the risk of transfusion-transmitted diseases.

14. What are two strategies for overcoming platelet refractoriness due to alloimmunization?

Two strategies used are crossmatching the single donor platelet unit and HLA-matching of the platelet unit to the recipient. A crossmatched platelet unit is less expensive and may be more readily available than an HLA-matched platelet unit.

15. What techniques are used for leukocyte reduction?

The most common techniques available for leukocyte reduction are washing, centrifugation, freezing, and filtration. Currently, leukocyte filtration is the most common method of leukocyte reduction. Depending on the method, leukocyte reduction can occur at the blood center shortly after or during collection, after storage but before the unit is released from the blood center, or at the bedside. At the bedside, leukofiltration is accomplished during transfusion with the addition of a commercially available filter that is attached to the blood product and intravenous tubing. Several commercially available filters consistently remove 95–99% of the leukocytes. Although bedside filtration is effective, it has some drawbacks. For example, as blood warms during transfusion, filtration becomes less efficient. The FDA permits blood products to be labeled "leukocyte-reduced" if they contain less than 5.0×10^6 WBCs.

16. Why are blood products irradiated?

Gamma radiation of blood products is currently the most efficient and reliable method to decrease the incidence of developing transfusion-associated graft-vs.-host disease reactions (TA-GVHD). Irradiation of blood products, usually exposing them to 1500 to 3500 cGy, will interrupt lymphocytic mitosis and prevent TA-GVHD through inhibition of lymphocytic proliferation. The following patients are at greatest risk for developing TA-GVHD: BMT recipients; patients with Hodgkin's or non-Hodgkin's lymphoma; patients with congenital immunodeficiency syndromes; patients with certain solid tumors such as neuroblastoma and glioblastoma; granulocyte transfusion recipients; and patients receiving transfusions from relatives.

17. Name the different types of transfusion reactions.

With the transfusion of any blood or blood component, patients may experience an adverse reaction. Transfusion reactions can be placed into two categories: acute reactions and delayed reactions (see tables on following pages).

Acute reactions may be seen within minutes to hours after the blood product is infused.

Delayed reactions may occur days to years after the transfusion. Symptoms may be mild to severe, and diagnosis may be complicated by the long incubation period between transfusion and reaction. All patients who have received blood and blood product transfusions must be informed of the potential for delayed reactions.

18. What is the most common transfusion reaction in the oncologic setting?

Nonhemolytic febrile transfusion reaction. Patients with cancer often require frequent transfusions to maintain adequate blood counts. The greater the number of antigens a person is exposed to through multiple transfusions, the higher the risk of reactions. As a result of antigen exposure, patients may develop allergic or febrile reactions to all erythrocyte and platelet transfusions. Hemolytic transfusion reactions present similarly to nonhemolytic febrile transfusion reactions in the early stages. Hemolytic transfusion reactions account for 0.5–1% of all transfusion reactions and contribute to 70% of transfusion-related deaths. It must be assumed that any recipient of blood products is prone to any reaction at any time during a transfusion. Therefore proper recognition and management of all acute, adverse effects may be lifesaving for some patients.

Acute Transfusion Reactions

ACUTE REACTION	CAUSE AND TIME TO ONSET	SIGNS AND SYMPTOMS	TREATMENT	PREVENTION
Allergic/ anaphylaxis	Sensitivity to plasma protein or donor antibody, which reacts with recipient antigen Onset: 5–15 minutes after initiation of transfusion	• Flushing • Itching, rash • Urticaria, hives • Asthmatic wheezing • Hypotension • Laryngeal edema • Nausea, vomiting • Possible cardiac arrest	• Stop transfusion immediately. • Maintain IV access with normal saline. • Notify physician and blood bank. • Give antihistamine as directed. • Observe for anaphylaxis (may need epinephrine if respiratory distress is severe). • If hives are the only clinical symptom, the transfusion can sometimes continue at a slower rate.	• Ask patient about past transfusion reactions. • May need emergency medications at bedside.
Febrile, non-hemolytic	Possible sensitivity to donor WBCs, platelets, or plasma proteins. Recent evidence demonstrates that cytokines released by donor WBCs during storage play a significant role. Onset: 30 minutes after initiation and up to 6 hours after completion of blood product.	• Sudden shaking, chills • Rise in temperature >1°C from baseline • Headache • Flushing • Anxiety • Muscle pain	• Stop transfusion immediately. • Keep vein open with normal saline. • Notify physician and blood bank. • Send blood samples to lab for testing. • Check temperature frequently. • Give antipyretics as ordered—treat symptomatically.	• May need to premedicate with antipyretics before transfusion. • Leukocyte-reduced blood products should be considered for future transfusions.
Bacterial sepsis reactions	Transfusion of bacteria-contaminated blood product. Onset: Anytime during or 2 hours after transfusion.	• Rapid onset of chills • High fever • Vomiting, diarrhea • Abdominal pain • Severe hypotension • Nausea	• Stop transfusion immediately. • Keep vein open with normal saline. • Notify physician and blood bank. • Obtain cultures of patient's blood and return unit with administration set to blood bank for culture. • Treat septicemia as ordered—IV fluid resuscitation, antibiotics, vasopressors, and steroids.	• Aseptic technique with initial collection of unit. • Proper storage and handling. • Complete infusions within 4 hours; change administration set and filter after 4 hours of use.

(Table continued on next page)

Acute Transfusion Reactions (Continued)

ACUTE REACTION	CAUSE AND TIME TO ONSET	SIGNS AND SYMPTOMS	TREATMENT	PREVENTION
Volume overload	Fluid administered at a rate or volume greater than what the cardiovascular system can tolerate. Onset: Any time during or 1–2 hours after transfusion	• Tachycardia • Hypertension • Increase in CVP and pulmonary arterial wedge pressure (PAWP) • Jugular venous distention • SOB, cough • Crackles • Sudden severe headache	• Slow or stop transfusion. • Notify physician. • Place patient upright with feet dependent. • Administer as ordered diuretics, oxygen, and morphine.	• Administer PRBCs instead of whole blood when possible. • Minimize saline when possible. • Monitor pulmonary status during transfusion.
Acute hemolytic transfusion reaction (AHTR)	Transfusion of incompatible ABO blood products causing intravascular destruction of RBCs resulting in massive hemolysis. Improper infusion with D5 solution. Incorrect processing of unit. Onset: 5–15 minutes after initiation of transfusion.	• Shaking, chills • Fever • Lower back pain • Chest tightness • Heat and pain along vein • Tachycardia • SOB • Hypotension, cardiac arrest • Hemoglobinuria • Hemoglobinemia • Bleeding • Acute renal failure • DIC	• Stop transfusion immediately. • Disconnect blood tubing from IV site. • Keep IV open with normal saline. • Notify physician and blood bank. • Treat shock if present with fluid resuscitation. • Draw blood samples and collect urine sample. • Give diuretics (mannitol). • Monitor I & O. • Maintain good urine output (> 1 ml/kg/hr). • May require dialysis if renal failure occurs. • Low-dose dopamine may be used. • Platelets, FFP, and cryoprecipitate may be used to reverse DIC.	• Carefully verify patient ID from sample collection to product infusion. • Begin transfusion slowly and closely monitor vital signs. Note: Consequences are in proportion to the amount of incompatible blood transfused.

Delayed Transfusion Reactions

DELAYED REACTION	CAUSE AND TIME TO ONSET	SIGN AND SYMPTOMS	TREATMENT	PREVENTION
Delayed hemolytic reaction	The destruction of transfused RBCs by an antibody not detectable during crossmatch but formed rapidly after transfusion. Onset: 2–14 days after transfusion.	• Fever • Mild jaundice • Gradual fall in hematocrit	• Hemoglobinuria is rare. Generally, no acute treatment is required. Recognition of reaction is important as subsequent infusions may cause an acute hemolytic reaction.	• The crossmatched blood sample should be drawn within 3 days of blood transfusion. • Antibody formation may occur within 90 days of transfusion and/or pregnancy.
Hemosiderosis (Iron accumulation)	Consequence of chronic RBC transfusions. Excess iron is deposited in the tissues, particularly affecting the heart, endocrine system, liver, and spleen.	• Diabetes • Compromised thyroid function • Arrhythmias • CHF • Other symptoms related to specific organ failure	• Treat symptomatically. • Administer deferoxamine (Desferal), which binds iron and promotes iron excretion via the kidneys. Administer IV, IM, or SC. • Monitor ferritin levels (goal is < 2500 µg/L).	• Reduce transfusion requirements using erythropoietin if recommended.
Transfusion associated graft-versus-host disease (TA-GVHD)	Donor lymphocytes recognize the transfusion recipient as foreign, setting up an immune response and attacking the host tissues. Onset: Days to weeks after the transfusion	• Erythematous skin rash • Liver function test abnormalities • Profuse, watery diarrhea • Fever	• Immunosuppression • Symptomatic management of pruritus, and pain • Fluid and electrolyte replacement for diarrhea Note: This disease process has a high mortality rate.	• Transfuse with irradiated blood products.
Hepatitis B	Transmitted from blood-donor to recipient via infected blood products	• Elevated liver enzymes (ALT/AST) • Nausea and vomiting • Poor appetite • Abdominal pain • Fever (rare)	• Symptoms usually resolve in 4 weeks–4 months or longer. • Can result in permanent liver damage. • Treat symptomatically with fluids, rest, and restricted protein diet.	• Screen blood donors. • Those who have a history of viral hepatitis are permanently deferred. • Hepatitis B vaccine for high-risk populations.

(Table continued on next page)

Delayed Transfusion Reactions (Continued)

DELAYED REACTION	CAUSE AND TIME TO ONSET	SIGNS AND SYMPTOMS	TREATMENT	PREVENTION
Hepatitis B (cont.)		• Dark urine/jaundice • Enlarged, tender liver • Increased risk for cirrhosis and hepatocellular carcinoma.		
Hepatitis C (non-A, non-B hepatitis)	Hepatitis C virus transmitted from blood donor to recipient via infected blood products.	• Similar to hepatitis B but usually less severe. • Significant risk of chronic liver disease • Increased risk of cirrhosis and liver cancer.	• Symptoms usually mild and require no treatment.	• Screen blood donors (ALT, anti-HBc antibody, anti-hepatitis C antibody).
Epstein-Barr virus (EBV) Cytomegalovirus (CMV) Malaria Chagas' disease	Transmitted through infected blood products.	• Refer to signs and symptoms related to specific disease processes.	• Refer to treatment recommendations for specific disease processes.	• Question prospective blood donors regarding cold, flu, sore throat, foreign travel.
Human immunodeficiency virus (HIV)/acquired immunodeficiency syndrome (AIDS)	HIV virus transmitted from blood donor to recipient via infected blood products. Onset: 4–12 weeks after transfusion serologic marker may be detected.	• Fever, chills • Muscle/joint aching • Diarrhea • Maculopapular rash • Fatigue/malaise • Unexplained weight loss • Lymphadenopathy • Decreased number of T-helper cells	• Treatment of HIV-associated infections and malignancies. • AZT may delay onset of AIDS symptoms. • Other antiviral agents are being trialed. • Active disease is treated symptomatically.	• Test each donor for HIV antibody.

(Table continued on next page)

Delayed Transfusion Reactions (Continued)

DELAYED REACTION	CAUSE AND TIME TO ONSET	SIGNS AND SYMPTOMS	TREATMENT	PREVENTION
Human T-lymphotropic virus, types I & II (HTLV I/II)	Transmitted from blood donor to recipient via blood products. Onset: A few months to 2 years after transfusion.	• HTLV-I-associated myelopathy (tropical spastic paraparesis) involves progressive spastic weakness of lower body. • Risk of lymphoma/leukemia	• HTLV-I-infected individuals have a 4% risk of developing neurologic or neoplastic disease. • If disease occurs, treat symptomatically.	• Screen all prospective blood donors for anti-HTLV-I and II antibodies.
Syphilis	Spirochetemia caused by *Treponema pallidum.* Incubation 10–90 days. No transfusion-related infections reported since 1976.	• Three stages of disease. • Early stage is most infectious and is characterized by the appearance of a chancre (primary sore).	• Penicillin therapy	• Test blood for spirochetes. • Organism is fragile and will not remain viable in blood stored 24–48 hours at 4°C.

Tables adapted from Nettina SM (ed): The Lippincott Manual of Nursing Practice, 6th ed. Philadelphia, Lippincott Williams & Wilkins, 1996.

19. What are the appropriate steps when a transfusion reaction is suspected?

1. Stop the blood component infusion immediately and notify the physician and blood bank.

2. Disconnect and save the blood and tubing from the IV site.

3. Maintain intravenous access with 0.9% normal saline solution.

4. Maintain adequate airway.

5. Monitor blood pressure and heart rate. Notify physician of systolic blood pressure changes > 20 mmHg or heart rate change of > 20 beats/minute.

6. Administer antihistamine.

7. Institute diuresis.

8. Perform a blood-bank work-up according to institutional policy. This commonly includes rechecking paper work; repeating cross-match, direct antiglobulin test, and urine test for hemoglobinuria; and returning the unused portion of the blood product to the laboratory or blood bank for evaluation.

9. Monitor renal status for hemoglobinuria. The patient may require hydration to ensure adequate renal perfusion.

10. Monitor coagulation status. This may entail drawing a screening panel for disseminated intravascular coagulopathy.

11. Monitor for signs of hemolysis. Serial laboratory tests may be ordered, including a complete blood count, full chemistry panel, urinalysis, and bilirubin with fractionation to evaluate levels of indirect and direct bilirubin.

12. Culture the patient for a septic event.

20. Is it necessary to test blood products for cytomegalovirus (CMV)?

Yes. The transmission of cytomegalovirus via any blood product is of particular concern for patients with suppressed T-lymphocyte function. About 1% of the blood donor population tests positive for antibodies to the virus, and less than 1% of donors appear able to transmit the infection. Clinical disease in patients with healthy immune systems is rare and usually limited to mononucleosis syndromes or mild hepatitis. However, for patients with compromised immune systems, CMV infections may lead to life-threatening, multisystem disease. Clinical manifestations include hepatitis, pneumonitis (the most fatal complication), retinitis, central nervous system disease, gastrointestinal tract disease, and hematologic abnormalities. The risk of transfusion-associated CMV infection may be essentially eliminated by the use of leukocyte-reduced blood products or CMV seronegative blood products. Either alternative is recommended for patients at risk for severe CMV disease.

21. What is the risk of transfusion-associated transmission of hepatitis C virus (HCV), hepatitis B virus (HBV), human T-cell lymphotropic virus, type-1 (HTLV-1) and human immunodeficiency virus (HIV)?

HCV	1:103,000
HBV	1:63,000
HTLV-1	1:641,000
HIV	1:430,000

22. What potential adverse effects may be seen when massive blood products are transfused?

Compromised patients with an underlying potential for bleeding disorders may experience extreme loss of red cells and coagulation factors. Replacement requirements may range from 2–20 products daily. When massive transfusions are required, the nurse must be aware of the potential adverse effects of massive transfusions.

Adverse Effects of Massive Blood Product Transfusions

ADVERSE EFFECT	CAUSE	CLINICAL MANIFESTATIONS	TREATMENT
Hypocalcemia	Sodium citrate is a commonly used anticoagulant for most blood products. With massive transfusions there is the potential for the excess citrate to bind to calcium in the recipient's blood.	• Perioral or acral numbness • Tensing of muscles • Nausea, vomiting, diarrhea, and abdominal cramping • Myocardial depression • Seizure activity • EKG shows prolonged Q-T interval and bradycardia • Tetany seen with Chvostek's and Trousseau's signs	• Monitor plasma ionized calcium levels. • If calcium replacement is necessary, administer 10 ml of 10% calcium gluconate IV for every 2 units of blood transfused.
Hypothermia	The rapid transfusion of large volumes of refrigerated blood products via a central line may decrease the body's core temperature and induce a hypothermic state: 34°C–36°C = Mild hypothermia 30°C–34°C = Moderate hypothermia < 30°C = Severe hypothermia	• Shaking, chills, hypotension • Impulses that stimulate the heart are delayed or withheld • An Osborne wave or J wave may be seen at the end of the QRS complex • Widening of all EKG complexes into ventricular fibrillation	• For rapid infusion, use of a blood warmer is indicated. • The blood warmer should not warm to more than 38°C. • Overheating can cause hemolysis.
Hyperkalemia	Plasma potassium levels in stored blood increases by approximately 1 mEq/L per day due to passive leakage of potassium out of red cells. An insidious rise in serum potassium levels is generally well tolerated; however, a rapid rise in potassium due to rapid transfusions of multiple units may be serious or even fatal.	• Generalized muscle twitching, cramps, and diarrhea • EKG changes, including tall peaked T waves, widened QRS interval, prolonged PR interval, and flat P waves progressing to ventricular fibrillation and cardiac arrest	• For emergency treatment, administer hypertonic dextrose (D50), regular insulin 10–20 units IV, and sodium bicarbonate.

23. How should the nurse respond to the patient who is fearful of receiving blood products?

The nurse should clarify the patient's fears and reinforce why the patient needs a transfusion, what monitoring procedures will be done, and how long it will take. If the patient is concerned about the risk of infection, the nurse should inform the patient that all donor blood products in the United States are screened for infectious diseases to minimize risk and provide current statistics about the incidence of infection after receiving blood products. Reassure the patient that most transfusions proceed without problems. However, if the patient develops signs and symptoms of a transfusion reaction, the patient should immediately report them to a healthcare provider. Many institutions and some states require that a patient give informed consent for blood product transfusions. In the process of informed consent, a patient has the right to refuse any treatment or procedure.

24. Are there any benefits to receiving blood products from relatives?

The only benefit to receiving blood products from family members is psychological well-being. Although a family member may have the same blood type as the patient, the cross-match may not be compatible. Patients who are platelet-refractory sometimes get a significant response with related donor platelets. However, no published data support the use of related donor platelets vs. HLA-matched unrelated donors.

25. Can patients donate autologous red cells before a scheduled procedure?

Yes. Policy governing these donations varies among institutions. Usually 1 week is required between donated units, although two units may be donated 72 hours apart in some circumstances. Each institution sets its own standard regarding the minimum hemoglobin or hematocrit required before autologous donation may be performed. PRBCs can be stored for 42 days without freezing.

26. What do the patient and family need to know about donating PRBCs or platelets for a relative?

The above criteria for donating autologous PRBCs also apply to family members wishing to donate blood for a patient. Platelets can be donated by family members every 72 hours. There is often an additional charge to the patient for designated donations.

27. What factors may render a person ineligible for donating blood?

Every blood bank has general guidelines for assessing blood donor eligibility. These vary depending on the institution. The following persons may not be eligible to donate blood:

- Persons who have had acupuncture, electrolysis, ear/body part piercing, and tattoos (for 12 months) unless sterile, disposable needles were used
- Persons on antibiotics (may be eligible 48 hours after completion or if using for acne)
- Persons with hepatitis or HIV
- Persons receiving hepatitis A and B vaccines are deferred for 24 hours after injection
- Persons with Lyme disease
- Persons with malaria (eligible 3 years after becoming symptom-free)
- Women who are pregnant or who have delivered within 6 weeks
- Persons with diarrhea if associated with flu symptoms (30-day deferral)
- Persons who have received a transfusion of blood or blood products (deferred for 12 months)
- Persons with diabetes controlled with insulin (may be acceptable, if free from infection and have physician permission)

The following risk factors represent a 12-month deferral for the donor: use of street or illicit drugs through the nose, accidental contact with another person's blood/body fluid or an accidental needle stick, and incarceration for more than 72 hours. Additionally, persons taking the following medications may be deferred: Accutane, Proscar, Propecia, Coumadin, flu shots, and allergy vaccines (24-hour deferral).

(Bonfils Blood Center Medical Guidelines for Volunteer Blood Donors. Denver, Colorado, revised May 2000.)

28. Can PRBCs be infused through an infusion pump?

Infusion pumps must be designated as compatible with infusion of blood products. If information cannot be found about pump compatibility with blood products, the pump should not be used for infusion because it may cause lysis of blood cells.

29. Can blood products be administered in the home setting?

Yes. Home care agencies with blood product infusion services have policies and procedural guidelines that direct blood product administration in the home. Common criteria for home administration of blood products include the following: (1) the patient has received a previous uncomplicated transfusion with no history of allergic, life-threatening reactions. (2) The patient has a physical limitation that makes leaving the home a taxing effort. (3) The patient is alert, cooperative, and able to respond to bodily symptoms. (4) The patient's medical condition allows safe transfusion at home. (5) The patient has access to a telephone. (6) The patient has a hemoglobin < 10 gm/dl and a platelet count < 20,000.

Reimbursement of blood product administration in the home depends on the patient's insurance policy.

30. Can blood products be administered in an outpatient setting?

Yes. Follow your facility's blood administration policy for blood processing and transfusion. Detailed discharge instructions must be given to the patient and family covering the signs and symptoms of adverse reactions, both immediate and delayed, and notification of physician. It is often very helpful to provide patients with educational materials to supplement the verbal information they have received.

31. How much of an increase in hemoglobin should be expected in the patient who is not losing blood following a transfusion of 1 unit of PRBCs? How long after a transfusion do you need to wait before an accurate post-transfusion hemoglobin can be obtained?

In the patient who is not losing blood by bleeding or destruction, an increase in the hemoglobin of approximately 1 gm/dl and an increase of 3–4% in the hematocrit for each unit of PRBCs transfused can be expected. Contrary to what might be intuitively expected, the fluid that is administered with PRBCs quickly equilibrates with the extravascular space. Thus, a post-transfusion hemoglobin can be obtained 15 minutes after the completion of the transfusion. The value will be comparable to a hemoglobin obtained 24 hours later, and the time saved in not bringing the patient back for a follow-up post-transfusion hemoglobin is obvious.

32. What are "incompatible crossmatch" blood transfusions?

Patients who have been heavily transfused over a period of years, such as those with sickle cell disease, have been exposed to many RBC antigens and have therefore developed numerous antibodies. There are circumstances under which crossmatch compatible RBCs are not available, and the least incompatible units may be transfused with an order from the patient's attending physician. The units are blood type compatible. A baseline plasma hemoglobin is usually drawn before administering these units, 15 minutes into the infusion, and after the infusion. An increase in the plasma hemoglobin from baseline indicates a hemolytic reaction is occurring. Each institution should have a policy issued by the blood bank governing plasma hemoglobin results and the circumstances under which the unit must be discontinued.

33. What size IV access is necessary for infusion of blood products?

Blood products can be administered to patients through a peripheral or central catheter. Large catheters such as an 18- or 19-gauge catheter facilitate faster flow rates. A 22-gauge catheter may be used in an adult; however, the flow rate will be slow. Using small gauge catheters will not cause hemolysis of RBCs unless you try to increase the infusion rate by applying pressure to the product bag. Always check the patency of your access before obtaining the blood product from the blood bank.

34. What educational resources regarding blood product transfusions are available on the internet?

The American Association of Blood Banks has an excellent internet site that offers educational information to both patients and healthcare providers. It can be accessed at www.aabb.org. Additionally, most local and regional blood centers have internet sites where educational information can be obtained.

REFERENCES

1. American Association of Blood Banks: Circular of Information for the Use of Human Blood and Blood Components. Available at www.aabb.org

2. American Association of Blood Banks: Facts About Blood and Blood Banking. 2000. Available at www.aabb.org
3. Armitage JO, Atman KH (eds): High-Dose Cancer Therapy: Pharmacology, Hematopoietins, Stem Cells, 2nd ed. Baltimore, Williams & Wilkins, 1995.
4. Cook LS: Nonimmune transfusion reactions: When type and cross match aren't enough. J Intraven Nurs 20:15–22, 1997.
5. Cook LS: Blood transfusion reactions involving an immune response. J Intraven Nurs 20:5–14, 1997.
6. Cummings RO (ed): Advanced Cardiac Life Support. Dallas, American Heart Association, 1997.
7. Dennison, RD (ed): Pass CCRN. St. Louis, Mosby, 1996.
8. Ewald G, McKenzie C (eds): Manual of Medical Therapeutics: The Washington Manual, 28th ed. Boston, Little, Brown, 1995.
9. Fitzpatrick L, Fitzpatrick T: Blood transfusions: Keeping your patient safe. Nursing97 27:34–42, 1997.
10. Friedman MM: Risk management strategies for home transfusion therapy. J Intraven Nurs 20:179–187, 1997.
11. Huh YO: Leukocyte-reduced, cytomegalovirus-screened and irradiated blood components: Indications and controversies. Curr Issues Transfus Med April/June: 1993. Available at www.mdanderson.org.
12. Jetter EK, Spivey MA: Noninfectious complications of blood transfusion. Hematol Oncol Clin North Am 9:187–203, 1995.
13. Nettina SM (ed): The Lippincott Manual of Nursing Practice, 6th ed. Philadelphia, J.B. Lippincott, 1996.
14. Perry AG, Potter PA (eds): Clinical Nursing Skills & Techniques, 4th ed. St. Louis, Mosby, 1998.
15. Rinder HM, Arbini AA, Snyder EL: Optimal dosing and triggers for prophylactic use of platelet transfusions. Curr Opin Hematol 6:437–441, 1999.
16. Schreiber GB, Busch MP, Kleinmann SH, Korelitz JJ: The risk of transfusion–transmitted viral infections. N Engl J Med 334:1685–1690, 1996.
17. Suzama K, DeChristopher PJ, et al: Practice parameter for the recognition, management and prevention of adverse consequences of blood transfusion. Arch Pathol Lab Med 124:61–70, 2000.
18. Wallas CH: Massive blood transfusion. 2000 UpToDate [serial online] Feb 1998; 8(2). Available at www.uptodate.com
19. Walter-Coleman S, Shelton BK: Transfusion therapy for patients critically ill with cancer. AACN Clin Iss 7:37–45, 1996.
20. Wiesen AR, Hopenthal DR, Byrd JC, et al: Equilibration of hemoglobin concentration after transfusion in medical inpatients not actively bleeding. Ann Intern Med 121:278–280, 1994.

14. VASCULAR ACCESS DEVICES

Charlene Trouillot, RN, MS, ANP, OCN, and
Deborah DeVine, RN, MS, AOCN, CRNI

1. What is a central line?

A central line, commonly called a vascular access device (VAD) or central venous catheter (CVC), is a temporary or long-term intravenous catheter inserted into one of the major veins of the neck or chest (subclavian, superior vena cava, internal or external jugular) or peripherally through the basilic or cephalic vein. The distal tip of a central line terminates in or near the superior vena cava, just above the right atrium. The femoral venous system (leading to the proximal inferior vena cava) may be used if the superior vena cava cannot be catheterized.

2. How soon can a CVC be used after placement?

A central line may be used after the position of the radiopaque catheter tip in the superior vena cava is confirmed by fluoroscopy or radiography. Implanted ports may be used immediately after placement, perhaps even accessed during surgery. Some surgeons may request that the port not be accessed until postoperative swelling has decreased.

3. What are the advantages of a central line?

- The high blood flow of the vena cava promotes rapid dilution of intravenous (IV) fluids and concentrated solutions, thereby preventing an inflammatory response and the rapid thrombosis that occurs in smaller peripheral veins.
- A central line provides more stable access to the venous system, decreasing the risk of infiltration and tissue damage when irritating agents are administered.
- Central lines are capable of infusing incompatible solutions at the same time, through two or more separate lumens.
- CVCs shorten hospital stays by providing access for therapy in an outpatient setting.
- Central venous access also may be used to overcome physical or psychological factors associated with repeated venipuncture.

4. Summarize the various uses of central lines.

CVCs can be used for administration of IV fluids, antibiotics, chemotherapy, blood products, total parenteral nutrition, and analgesics. They also may be used for performing laboratory blood sampling, dialysis/pheresis, continuous arterial venous hemodialysis (CAVHD), and continuous venous venous hemodialysis (CVVHD). Acute or intensive care (ICU) management may require central venous or pulmonary capillary wedge pressure measurement, cardiac output determination, or rapid infusion of crystalloids, blood products and other solutions. Central lines are commonly inserted in patients whose condition requires large-volume infusion (e.g., bleeding, trauma, surgery, sepsis) or hemodynamic monitoring. Nonacute indications for insertion of central lines include patients with human immunodeficiency virus (HIV), cancer, sickle cell disease, Crohn's disease, and osteomyelitis.

5. What materials are used to make central lines?

Central lines are made of several different materials, including polyvinyl chloride, polyurethane, and silicone. The stiffer nature of polyvinyl chloride catheters allows easier insertion but also may damage the tunica intima, leading to platelet aggregation and thrombus formation. Silicone is biocompatible, extremely soft and pliable, inexpensive, and hydrophobic (offering protection from bacterial growth). Polyurethane catheters are indicated for short-term use and placed percutaneously; they are stronger than silicone but become softer and longer after insertion when warmed by blood.

Newer catheters, such as hydromer-coated polyurethane, have higher success rates on insertion and are designed to prevent bacterial growth and adherence (more common on rougher surfaces) as well as platelet deposition and aggregation. Bonded catheters are impregnated with antimicrobial substances such as silver sulfadiazine and chlorhexidine. Bonded catheters may substantially reduce the incidence of catheter-related infection and extend dwell time, thereby proving their cost effectiveness.

6. What are the major types of central lines?
- Nontunneled catheters
- Tunneled catheters
- Peripherally inserted central catheters (PICCs)
- Implanted ports

7. Which type is most commonly used? List its major advantages and disadvantages.
Nontunneled catheters (Fig. 1) are the most commonly used central lines. Available with 1–4 lumens, they are easily inserted into the subclavian, internal, or external jugular vein; the right internal jugular is preferred, because it forms a straight line to the SVC. Optional features include heparin, antibiotic, or antiseptic coatings along the catheter and addition of a Dacron cuff. Nontunneled catheters are associated with the highest incidence of catheter-related infections. Other disadvantages include daily flushing, routine sterile dressing changes, and restrictions on activities such as swimming, contact sports, and rough play for adolescents or children.

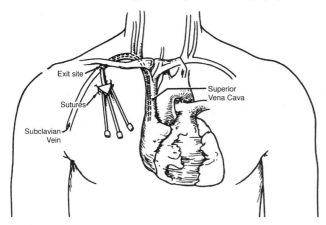

FIGURE 1. Nontunneled catheter. (Drawing by Mel Drisko; courtesy of Educational Support Services, University of Colorado Health Services Center.)

8. Discuss the advantages and disadvantages of tunneled catheters.
Tunneled catheters (Hickman, Broviac, Leonard, and Groshong) are indicated for long-term therapy (more than several months) (Fig. 2). Single-, double-, and triple-lumen catheters are available. Insertion costs are high (approximately $2500–3000) if anesthesia and the operating room are used; however, most tunneled catheters can be placed safely under fluoroscopy in the radiology department. After insertion in a central vein, the catheter is tunneled several centimeters under the skin and brought out through the skin to a suitable exit site (anterior chest between the sternum and nipple, upper abdominal wall). Unlike most nontunneled catheters, the subcutaneous portion of the tunneled catheter includes a Dacron cuff that adheres to scar tissue, forming an internal anchor and barrier against the inward spread of microorganisms. A second antimicrobial cuff also may be present (e.g., Vita Cuff, which releases silver ions as a deterrent to infection). The tunneling of the catheter offers the theoretical advantage of reducing the rate of infection. CVCs may be placed with minimal risk of catheter infections outside the operating room if maximal barrier precautions are used (e.g., sterile gloves, gown, drape, masks). Disadvantages include site care with dressing changes for the first few weeks, activity restrictions, and regular flushing. Once the exit site of a tunneled catheter has healed (approximately 3–4 weeks), the sterile dressing change is modified to a clean technique, which decreases cost and time.

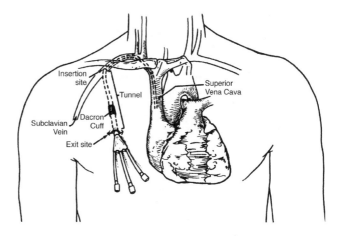

FIGURE 2. Tunneled catheter. (Drawing by Mel Drisko; courtesy of Educational Support Services, University of Colorado Health Services Center.)

9. Discuss the advantages and disasdvantages of PICCs.

PICCs (Fig. 3) generally are indicated for short-term use (> 5 days but usually < 1 year). Insertion costs are lowest (about $300) of all CVCs. PICCs are easily placed by a trained nurse or physician into the cephalic or basilic veins of the antecubital space and are available with one or two lumens. The basilic vein provides the straightest, most direct route into the central venous system. Advantages include reduced insertion risks (e.g., pneumothorax) and decreased rates of infection in comparison to other nontunneled CVCs. Disadvantages include daily flushing (weekly for the outpatient Groshong PICC), sterile dressing changes, and activity restrictions. Self-care may be difficult or impossible because the patient is required to change the dressing and flush the catheter with one hand. PICC placement requires adequate peripheral antecubital access, which may be difficult to locate in some patients.

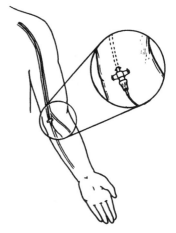

FIGURE 3. Peripherally inserted central catheter. (Drawing by Mel Drisko; courtesy of Educational Support Services, University of Colorado Health Services Center.)

10. Describe the appropriate use of implanted ports. What are their advantages and disadvantages?

Implanted ports (e.g., Mediport, Portacath, Infusaport, Cathlink) are made of stainless steel, titanium, or plastic (Fig. 4). They are indicated for long-term use. Port implantation is usually done under fluoroscopy in the interventional radiology suite or in the operating room at costs similar to those for tunneled catheters. Single- or double-lumen and low-profile (preferable in thin patients) ports are available. Ports are implanted entirely under the subcutaneous tissue and attached to a catheter that is threaded into the SVC. Smaller ports also may be implanted peripherally, like a PICC, in the forearm with the catheter threaded into the SVC. Advantages of the port include minimal site care with no dressing and infrequent flushing (once per month) when not accessed, which may decrease costs and infection rates. Implanted ports are associated with the lowest rate of infectious complications of all CVCs. Many patients prefer ports because they preserve bodily image and require no restrictions on activities, such as bathing or swimming. Disadvantages include discomfort related to accessing the port with a noncoring needle and the need for a surgical procedure for removal when the port is no longer needed or becomes infected. Ports are not recommended for patients undergoing treatment who will have prolonged nadirs, such as bone marrow transplant recipients or leukemia patients.

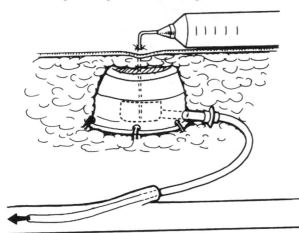

FIGURE 4. Implanted port. (Drawing by Mel Drisko; courtesy of Educational Support Services, University of Colorado Health Services Center.)

11. Can a nurse assume that any line resembling a PICC is a central line?

No. If you do not have documentation of line placement, you should question the patient carefully. The line may be midline (with the tip resting in a vein below the shoulder) or midclavicular (with the tip resting in the subclavian vein). If the position of the line cannot be reliably obtained through history or documentation, a chest radiograph should be performed.

12. How is a Groshong catheter different from other catheters?

A Groshong catheter (Fig. 5) is a silastic catheter with a two-way valve at the tip. Infusion of fluid opens the valve outward, and aspiration of blood opens the valve inward. When not in use, the pressure-sensitive two-way valve remains closed to prevent backward flow of blood or air into the catheter. The closed valve results in a potentially lower incidence of fibrin sheath formation and eliminates the need to clamp the catheter when injection caps are removed. Groshong valves are available for tunneled catheters, PICC lines, and implanted ports. Because blood clotting may be of less concern, normal saline is used instead of heparin for flushing; however, heparin is not incompatible with the material used to make Groshong catheters and can be infused, if needed, in patients with deep vein thrombosis.

13. What factors should be considered in choosing a central line?

- Costs
- Length of therapy
- Treatment schedule (daily, continuous, intermittent)
- Type of drug or fluids to be infused (e.g. vesicant, pH < 5 or > 9, serum osmolality > 500 Osm/L)
- Frequency of blood tests
- Benefits and risks
- Patient preference (cosmetic appearance, activity/work limitations, anxiety associated with needlesticks)
- Site care and flushing requirements
- Capability of patient or significant other to care for a central line at home

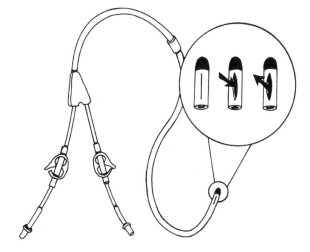

FIGURE 5. Groshong catheter and valves. (Drawing by Mel Drisko; courtesy of Educational Support Services, University of Colorado Health Services Center.)

14. What risks are involved with insertion of central lines?
- Bleeding and hematoma
- Malpositioned tips and migration
- Pneumothorax
- Catheter embolism
- Air embolus
- Nerve injury
- Dysrhythmias
- Introduction of bacteria

Rare complications of PICC placement are nerve injury and arterial puncture, most commonly of the ulnar artery.

15. The nurse observes bloody drainage at the insertion site of a newly placed central line. Is this a worrisome finding?
It is common for blood to saturate the dressing of a new exit site. Patients with a low platelet count should be monitored for increased bleeding, and bloody dressings should be changed as frequently as needed to prevent infection. Application of manual pressure or use of a sandbag helps to prevent development of a hematoma.

16. What are the signs and symptoms of malpositioned tips?
Malpositioned tips are common and may be especially problematic with PICCs (4–38%). Catheters may be coiled in the superior vena cava, malpositioned in the jugular vein when the basilic vein is used, or malpositioned in the axillary vein when the cephalic vein is used. If the tip is malpositioned in the jugular vein, wait for 24 hours to allow gravity to assist with catheter reposition or flush with a steady stream of 20 ml normal saline. The catheter also can be repositioned with the use of a guidewire.

SITE OF MALPOSITIONED CATHETER	SYMPTOMS
Internal jugular vein (ipsilateral or contralateral)	Sensation of ear gurgling, headache, swelling, or neck pain
Axillary vein	Hand and arm swelling, with arm and shoulder pain
Azygos vein	Vague back discomfort
Innominate or contralateral subclavian vein	Shoulder pain or swelling of contralateral arm
Internal thoracic vein	Anterior chest pain or tenderness
Right atrium or ventricle	Thrombosis, arrhythmia, or perforation of catheter, leading to pulmonary embolus

17. Should a PICC be removed for signs of phlebitis?

No. Immediate removal is not necessary. Sterile postinsertion phlebitis is the most common complication of PICCs (12.5–23%), occurring within 24–48 hours after insertion. It may be caused by trauma to the endothelial lining of the vein during insertion and consequent vasoconstriction. Powdered gloves also may irritate the vein and should be avoided. A warm pack should be applied at the first sign of redness and swelling along the vein, palpable venous cord, skin temperature change, or tenderness. Rest, elevation of the affected arm, and nonsteroidal anti-inflammatory drugs (NSAIDs) may be of benefit. If symptoms do not improve within 24 hours or resolve in 72 hours, the catheter may need to be removed.

18. How can the risk of malpositioned PICCs be decreased?

A technique that may reduce the incidence of misplaced PICCs by up to 13% involves pulling the guidewire back a few centimeters during insertion. This technique makes the tip more pliable and allows blood flow from the subclavian and jugular veins to push the tip downward into the SVC. The patient should be sitting or semireclining to take advantage of gravity while the PICC is advanced slowly. The patient is instructed to turn his or her chin toward the insertion site while the catheter is threaded. The guidewire is reinserted gently, if needed, to determine placement by radiograph, provided that the guidewire tip cannot penetrate the catheter.

19. What is considered routine care and maintenance of a central line?

Routine care of a central line catheter includes cleansing the exit site, changing dressings and caps, and flushing the lumens to prevent clotting. Cleansing solutions, type of dressing, and frequency of dressing changes or flushing are controversial issues. Site care protocols vary from hospital to hospital. Hemodialysis catheters should be used solely for hemodialysis and manipulated by trained hemodialysis personnel.

Common Maintenance Procedures

VAD	DRESSING	FLUSHING (EACH LUMEN)*	CAP CHANGE†
Central (sub-clavian)	Transparent dressing every 5–7 days; gauze dressing on alternate days or with catheter change	Heparin 100 U/ml, 1–3 ml/day	Weekly
PICC lines	24 hr after insertion, then transparent dressing every 5–7 days or gauze dressing on alternate days	Heparin 100 U/ml, 3 ml/day	Weekly
Tunneled	Transparent dressing every 5–7 days; gauze dressing on alternate days, then clean technique unless myelosuppressed	Heparin 100 U/ml, 3 ml/day	Weekly
Implanted port	For continuous access, change non-coring needle and transparent dressing every week or gauze dressing on alternate days	Heparin 100 U/ml, 3–5 3–5 ml/month when not in use; daily flush-otherwise	Weekly
Groshong (tunneled or PICC)‡	Transparent dressing every 5–7 days; gauze dressing on alternate days, then clean technique unless myelosuppressed	Normal saline, 5–10 ml/week as outpatient; daily flush as inpatient	Weekly

* Heparin solution may be 10 U/ml concentration.
† Change caps more often if damaged or used frequently.
‡ Bard Access Systems, Salt Lake City, UT.

20. How should the exit site be cleaned?

Common features of all protocols include removal of the old dressing, inspection of the exit site for signs of infection, cleansing the skin, and covering with a sterile dressing. The site should be cleaned with an appropriate antiseptic, using friction, and working outward in a circular pattern from the exit site (Fig. 6). Tunneled catheters have two incisions requiring care. The site where the catheter was inserted appears as a closed incision with sutures. Hospital personnel should wear gloves when cleaning the site or changing dressings. Sterile gloves and mask should be considered during dressing changes. Clean technique may be used by the patient at home.

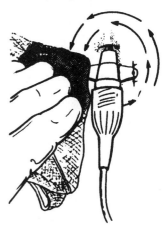

FIGURE 6.   Proper technique for cleansing the exit site. (Courtesy of University Hospital Biomedical Services, Denver, CO.)

21. What solutions or agents are recommended for cleaning the exit site?

Isopropyl alcohol (70%) removes skin oils and squamous skin cells and provides the most rapid and greatest reduction in microbial counts on the skin. However, it has no residual antimicrobial activity. Alcohol should be applied before iodine.

Povidone-iodine (10%) or **tincture of iodine** (1–2%) should be allowed to remain on the skin for at least 2 minutes to enhance antimicrobial activity while drying. To prevent skin irritation, it may need removal with alcohol after drying. It is effective for use before catheter insertion but has not been thoroughly evaluated in decreasing catheter colonization and infection.

Aqueous chlorhexidine (2%) has the advantage of residual antibacterial activity (up to 6 hours). One study showed that it was superior to alcohol or povidone-iodine in prevention of CVC infections and bacteremia; however, this concentration is not commercially available in the United States. A recently introduced, sustained-release chlorhexidine gluconate patch for use in dressing the catheter insertion site holds promise for decreasing VAD infections.

22. Should antimicrobial ointments be used?

The Centers for Disease Control and Prevention (CDC) does not recommend routine use of topical ointments. Iodophor ointments have been proved ineffective; polymicrobial ointments have some benefit but may increase the frequency of candidal infection.

23. Are gauze dressings better than transparent dressings?

Ideal dressings should minimize the build-up of skin microorganisms, provide protection against external contamination, keep the exit site dry, be nonirritating and easy to apply and remove, and permit convenient examination of the site. A gauze and tape dressing, in which tape should cover the entire gauze surface securing all edges, may be preferred for diaphoretic or fragile skin. However, visualization of the site is limited. In addition, gauze and tape dressings do not provide a bacterial and water barrier for the site, with an increased risk of potential contamination. Transparent semipermeable membrane dressings permit continuous inspection of the site, adhere well, provide protection against external moisture, and assist in stabilizing the catheter. One limitation of the transparent dressing is moisture retention beneath the dressing, which can significantly increase colonization of the site. Newer, more moisture-permeable transparent dressings move moisture away from the site and appear to reduce colonization below the dressing.

24. How often should dressings be changed?

The frequency of dressing changes is controversial and variable (see table with question 19). Gauze and tape dressings need to be changed every 24–48 hours. Transparent dressings usually are changed every 72 hours or once weekly. (It is not known how long a transparent dressing can remain safely in place.) All types of dressings should be changed after showering or when damp, loose, or soiled. Tunneled catheters may not need a dressing after several weeks of healing. It may be preferable not to use a dressing for tunneled catheters because of a lower risk for infection. If gauze is used under a transparent dressing because of increased secretions or drainage, the dressing is considered a gauze and tape dressing and should be changed accordingly.

25. How are central lines usually flushed?

Heparin, in concentrations of 10–1,000 U/ml, is the accepted flush solution for all CVCs except the Groshong, which uses saline. Frequency of flushing ranges from once weekly to as often as twice daily. The Intravenous Nursing Society (INS) recommends that the flushing volume be equal to two times the internal volume of the catheter and any add-on devices. Clamp the catheter or remove the syringe while maintaining positive pressure. Every effort should be made to remove blood from the injection cap. New positive-pressure devices designed to prevent backflow and eliminate the use of needles are replacing the traditional heparin lock. CVCs are designed to withstand various infusion pressures, but the pressure should not exceed 25–40 PSI (pounds/square inch). Smaller sized syringes generate pressures in excess of this limit. Avoid using syringes smaller than 5 ml or needles longer than 1 inch. Flush heparin-locked devices with saline before and after administering medications. A different syringe and needle should be used for each lumen that is flushed. Neonates and infants may require flushing with preservative-free saline only.

26. Is saline as effective as heparin for routine flushing?

CVCs usually are flushed once daily with heparin with intermittent flushes of normal saline (e.g., between antibiotics). Recent studies report that 0.9% saline solution is as effective as heparin in preventing phlebitis and maintaining patency in peripheral lines; however, it is not yet routine practice to use only saline. Flushing the catheter with heparin not only prevents thrombosis but also may reduce infection because thrombi and fibrin deposits are potential sites of microbial growth. Even low doses (250–500 U) of heparin may be associated with thrombocytopenia and bleeding problems. Heparin-induced thrombocytopenia, which affects 1–2% of patients receiving heparin, is an immune allergic response in which the patient develops an antibody to platelets. The clumped platelets can cause clotting events such as deep vein thrombosis or pulmonary embolism. Normal saline is more cost-effective than heparin and may cause less interference with laboratory tests. If only saline is used as a flush for central lines, the potential for occlusion, phlebitis, and formation of small clots or fibrin strands may be increased. Low-dose warfarin, 1 mg/day orally, may be used prophylactically to decrease the incidence of thrombus. Preservative-free saline may be used for infants and neonates.

27. Can a registered nurse remove a central line?

In accordance with hospital policy and specific State Board of Nursing Practice Acts, nurses may discontinue a central venous catheter with a physician's order. The nurse should remember the following points when removing a catheter:

1. To prevent pulmonary embolus, instruct the patient to perform a Valsalva maneuver while the catheter is withdrawn, or pull the line during end expiration if the patient is on mechanical ventilation or during expiration for patients unable to bear down.

2. Because air may enter a subcutaneous tract into a vein, apply ointment and an occlusive dressing for at least 24 hours.

3. Contact the physician immediately if difficulty is encountered with removing the catheter or Dacron cuff. A cutdown procedure by the physician may be indicated to remove the cuff, particularly if a tunnel infection is suspected. A chest radiograph or venogram is recommended if there is any question about incomplete catheter removal.

28. What should be done if a PICC is resistant to removal?

Resistance to removal may be caused by thrombus, fibrin sheath, or venospasm. The following tips may facilitate removal of a resistant PICC:

1. Remove the catheter at a moderate rate, using gentle traction. Position the patient in an upright/sitting position with the arm at 90°. *Aggressive pulling is contraindicated.*
2. Do not apply pressure at or near the course of the vein.
3. Use warm compresses to distend the vein.
4. Attempt removal again in 20–30 minutes after the spasm has abated.
5. If spasm is still present, wait an additional 12–24 hours.
6. Infuse warm normal saline over 5–15 minutes via a distal IV line to increase blood flow.
7. A warm or alcoholic beverage also may help to relieve the spasm.

29. How are implanted ports accessed?

Using sterile procedures, locate the port by palpation. Clean the site with povidone-iodine or chlorhexidine 2%, starting over the port and moving outward in a circular motion. Using the fingers of one hand to stabilize the port, insert the needle through the skin, and push through the septum until the needle lightly touches the bottom of the port. Needle position is verified by blood return. If neither irrigation nor aspiration is possible, the needle may need to be pushed further into the septum or repositioned.

30. Are Huber needles necessary to access implanted ports?

Except in emergencies, a Huber (noncoring) needle should be used to access an implanted port because it preserves the life of the septum. A port septum is good for 1,000 (using a 19-gauge needle) or 2,000 (using a 22-gauge needle) punctures. The gauge and length of the needle are determined by the viscosity of the infused solution, depth of port placement, and type of implanted port. Huber needles (90°) with extension tubing, wings, and foam pad attached are frequently used for continuous infusion. The cathlink, however, is accessed with a straight angiocath. A straight Huber needle may be used for withdrawing blood samples or giving bolus injections. All needles and extensions should be primed with normal saline before use.

31. How often should Huber needles be changed?

To prevent skin breakdown, change the needle at least every 7 days. In the case of intermittent injections, some patients prefer that the port be accessed daily. Before needle removal at the end of the infusion, flush with normal saline followed by heparin.

32. How is discomfort decreased when ports are accessed?

Topical anesthetics, such as Emla cream (lidocaine 2.5%, prilocaine 2.5%) covered with a transparent dressing, may be applied to the skin over the port at least 1 hour before needle placement. Application of ice over the site or ethyl chloride spray also may be helpful.

33. How much blood should be discarded before blood is sampled?

Approximately 5 ml of blood from adults and 3 ml from children are discarded before drawing the sample. There is no need to discard any blood when drawing blood cultures. All infusions should be stopped for at least 1 minute, and blood should be drawn through the proximal lumen via the catheter hub or through the injection cap. Clamp all lumens not in use. Pulling back slowly on the syringe prevents catheter collapse. A vacutainer may be used to decrease needle-stick risk, except in the case of Groshong catheters and PICCs. Flush with 10–20 ml (20 ml for Groshong) of normal saline after blood withdrawal. Heparin adheres to the catheter wall and can result in prolonged prothrombin time or partial prothrombin time. Consider drawing these particular tests from a peripheral vein if the CVC has been flushed with heparin.

34. What complications are associated with central lines?

• Infection	• Occlusion	• Pinch-off
• Sepsis	• Migration	• Extravasation

35. What are the signs of central line infection?

Erythema, pain, and purulence at the exit site or along the tunnel are the most consistent indicators of infection. Immunosuppression may diminish or completely mask these signs. Infection of central lines may present as sepsis without another apparent source or as thrombosis alone. Risks for infection include:

- Type of catheter material
- Longer duration of use
- Emergent vs. elective placement
- Skill of the operator
- Absence of maximal barrier precautions during placement (sterile gloves, gown, drape, masks)
- Increased number of lumens
- Age (< 1 year or > 60 years)
- Failure to maintain sterile technique during routine care
- Altered host defenses (dermatitis, burns, HIV infection, neutropenia)
- Sepsis at time of placement

36. What is the difference between local and systemic infections?

Local infections may occur at the exit site, port pocket, or tunnel. An **exit-site infection** is suggested by erythema that extends approximately 2 cm from the exit site, with warmth, tenderness, swelling, or purulence. A **tunnel infection** is defined as inflammation along the subcutaneous tract of the catheter, extending > 2 cm from the exit site. A **port pocket infection** is characterized by inflammation or necrosis of the skin over an implantable device or purulence in the pocket containing the device. Port pocket infections closely resemble tunnel infections in treatment and response to therapy. Do not cannulate an implanted port if a port pocket infection is suspected.

A **systemic catheter-related infection** may or may not involve the soft tissue around the catheter and refers to the presence of signs and symptoms of bacteremia (presence of bacteria cultured from the blood) or sepsis. A **systemic catheter-related bloodstream infection** (CR-BSI) is defined as isolation of the same organism from a catheter segment culture and a peripheral blood culture with clinical symptoms of a bloodstream infection and no other apparent source of infection. Criteria that implicate the catheter as the source of infection include semiquantitative cultures showing > 15 colony-forming units (CFUs) of the same organism or quantitative cultures showing that the number of organisms cultured from the central line is 5–10 times the number cultured from the peripheral blood.

37. What are the four sources of catheter-associated infection?

1. Skin insertion site (most common)
2. Catheter hub
3. Secondary catheter infection from bloodstream seeding
4. Infusate contamination (rare)

38. How is infection in central lines treated?

Management depends on the causative organisms and extent of infection. Empiric treatment consists of an antimicrobial effective against gram-positive and gram-negative organisms. Specific antibiotic therapy is directed against organisms recovered from culture. Local site infections may be treated by aggressive site care and oral antibiotics (e.g., a quinolone) in the absence of neutropenia. Outpatient management may be successful for people with intact immune systems whose infection is localized to the exit site without fever or hypotension. Tunnel infections may require catheter removal. An untreated port pocket infection can develop into an abscess requiring removal and surgical drainage. Sepsis requires parenteral antibiotics and possible catheter removal.

39. What organisms commonly cause catheter-related infections? Which infections require catheter removal?

The most common organisms have been coagulase-negative staphylococci, *Staphylococcus aureus*, enterococci, and *Candida* spp. Exit-site infections, tunnel infections, and even bacteremia due to coagulase-negative staphylococci usually can be treated without catheter removal, although the rate of recurrence is decreased if the catheter is removed. Because *S. aureus* is associated with serious complications, removal of the catheter is suggested. Fungal infections occur less frequently but require catheter removal. Exit-site infections with gram-negative organisms, including *Pseudomonas* spp., *Klebsiella* spp., *Acinetobacter* spp., and *Serratia* spp., may respond to antibiotic therapy, but involvement of the tunnel usually requires catheter removal. Catheter removal is indicated for infections with gram-positive bacilli and atypical mycobacteria.

40. What can be done to prevent catheter infections?

Prevention strategies include hand-washing, strict aseptic technique, and patient education. Special catheter designs include antimicrobial substances to prevent colonization, heparin coatings that may decrease formation of fibrin sleeves and thereby colonization of bacteria, or use of a collagen cuff impregnated with silver ions, which exerts an antimicrobial effect for 4–6 weeks and serves as a barrier to organisms that migrate down the catheter. Prophylactic use of antibiotics as a flush solution in combination with heparin shows promise.

41. What should be done if there is no blood return with aspiration?

If there is no blood return, the catheter may no longer be in the venous system. The site should be assessed for:
- Drainage due to catheter rupture, obstruction, or fibrin sheath
- Subcutaneous swelling due to catheter damage or infusate exiting backward out of the vein
- Stricture of sutures, kinking of the catheter
- Swelling of the neck, throat, or arm
- Loops of tunneled catheter under the skin

Ask the patient to change position (e.g.. Trendelenburg position), to increase venous flow, and to cough or breathe deeply to help move the catheter away from the vein wall. Remove the injection caps and attempt to aspirate. Vigorously infuse 10–20 ml of normal saline while assessing for swelling. For implanted ports, try to reposition the needle. If catheter placement is still questionable, confirm position in the SVC by chest radiograph and/or dye study. Do not infuse chemotherapy until tip placement is confirmed.

42. What causes central line occlusion?

Occlusion should be considered when the ability to infuse fluids is lost and blood return is absent with aspiration. Partial obstruction is indicated by resistance to flushing and/or absence of blood return with aspiration. Causes include the following:
- **Intraluminal thrombus** may result from injury to the vein wall during insertion, contact with the catheter tip, or hardened blood in the catheter lumen.
- **Extraluminal fibrin sleeve** formed at the catheter entry site into the vein may impair ability to flush but not to withdraw, because it acts as a flap that blocks the tip when withdrawal is attempted but opens with injection.
- **Drug precipitate** may be formed by incompatible solutions, inadequate flushing, or calcium phosphorus complexes (as with total parenteral nutrition).
- **External occlusion** may occur when a catheter is clamped, twisted, or constricted by sutures or a nonpatent Huber needle.

43. How is an occluded line treated?

Instillation of **urokinase** into a central line used to be the treatment of choice to dissolve clots. Urokinase is currently unavailable by mandate of the Food and Drug Administration (FDA).

Alteplase (tissue-type plasminogen activator) is currently the agent of choice for clearing catheter-related thrombosis. It restores function in 60–80% of thrombosed catheters. The standard concentration is 1 mg/ml. Instill an adequate volume (usually 2 ml), and allow a dwell time of 30–120 minutes. Repeat if catheter function is not restored.

Streptokinase also may be used. It is approved by the FDA but is highly antigenic. The recommended procedure is to inject 250,000 U of streptokinase into an occluded line and allow it to dwell for 1–2 hours before attempting to aspirate the dissolved clot. Patients with a recent history of streptococcal infection or repeated use of streptokinase may have developed antibodies that render streptokinase ineffective.

44. What should you do if you are uncertain whether the occlusion is due to blood clotting or drug precipitation?

A **thrombolytic agent** is recommended as the first choice for treatment. If it fails, alternative approaches include prolonged thrombolytic infusion, transfemoral stripping of the fibrin sheath, or catheter exchange over a guidewire.

Although limited information is available, **hydrochloric acid** (HCl) 0.1% has been reported to dissolve mineral deposits without serious adverse effects. The recommended procedure is to dissolve 0.2–1 ml of 0.1% HCl in normal saline (amount determined by catheter volume), allow to dwell for 1 hour, and then aspirate. Febrile reactions have been reported if large amounts are used.

Sodium bicarbonate may be used to dissolve clots due to medications with a high pH, such as phenytoin sodium. In addition, 70% **ethyl alcohol** can be used to dissolve fat associated with lipid occlusion. The alcohol is left in the catheter for 1–32 hours, and the procedure is repeated if the first trial is not successful. Side effects include dysgeusia.

45. Of what serious complication should nurses be aware during use of declotting agents or even during routine flushing?

Potential release of an infected clot or septic emboli. Patients have demonstrated signs of hemodynamic instability (hypotension) and sepsis within a few minutes after flushing.

46. Is extravasation a common complication of CVCs?

Although more common in peripheral IV access, extravasation is a potential complication of CVCs. Symptoms of extravasation may include pain, burning or stinging, and perhaps swelling or leaking. Blood return may or may not be present. If extravasation is suspected during infusion of a vesicant, the nurse should stop the infusion and aspirate the residual. If symptoms are present, a chest radiograph or dye study should be performed to confirm placement in the venous system.

47. What are the major causes of extravasation?

1. Needle dislodgement from ports.

2. Formation of a fibrin sheath along the catheter tract, starting from the exit site and extending toward the catheter tip. When fluid infuses from the catheter tip, it backtracks along the catheter and leaks out of the exit site.

3. Catheter damage. Overvigorous flushing may weaken or even perforate the catheter wall, resulting in catheter separation and embolism.

4. Dislodgement or migration of a catheter tip from the venous system. Although the mechanism for spontaneous migration is unclear, coughing or sneezing may be factors, especially with softer catheters.

48. What is "pinch-off syndrome"? How is it recognized?

Pinch off results from compression and shearing of the catheter between the clavicle and first rib in about 1% of patients. It should be suspected with intermittent lack of blood return or intermittent inability to infuse. It is made worse by sitting and relieved by raising the arms overhead. Pinch off is recognized on chest radiograph by a narrowing of the catheter between the clavicle and first rib. It may result in embolization and is an indication for catheter removal and replacement. It may not be discovered until after catheter fracture when the catheter fragment must be retrieved from the central veins, pulmonary artery, or heart.

49. Can a central line be repaired?

A leaking catheter must be repaired or removed to prevent infection and air embolus. Catheter lumens are damaged by overvigorous flushing, which weakens the catheter wall and eventually causes a hole. Instruct patients that, if a catheter tears or breaks, they should fold the remaining end of the catheter in half, cover it with gauze, and secure it tightly with a rubber band. If a clamp is available, the patient should clamp the catheter above the leak and consult a doctor or nurse immediately. Some damaged central lines can be repaired, including tunneled catheters and PICCs. Using sterile technique, follow the manufacturer's instructions provided with the repair kit.

REFERENCES

1. Baranowski L: Central venous access devices: Current technologies, uses and management strategies. J Intraven Nurs 16:167–194, 1993.
2. Blum AS: The role of the interventional radiologist in central venous access. J Intraven Nurs 22(Suppl 6):S32–S39, 1999.
3. Brandt B, DePalma J, Irwin M, et al: Comparison of central venous catheter dressings in bone marrow transplant recipients. Oncol Nurs Forum 23:830–836, 1996.
4. Brown JM: Polyurethane and silicone: Myths and misconceptions. J Intraven Nur 18:120–122, 1995.
5. Camp-Sorrell D (ed): Access Device Guidelines: Recommendations for Nursing Practice and Education. Pittsburgh, Oncology Nursing Society, 1996.
6. Dearborn P: Nurse and patient satisfaction with three types of venous access devices. Oncol Nurs Forum 24:34–40, 1997
7. Delisio N: Revised intravenous nursing standards of practice. J Intraven Nurs 21(Suppl 1):S1–S85, 1998.
8. Eastridge BJ, Lefor AT: Complications of indwelling venous access devices in cancer patients. J Clin Oncol 13:233–238, 1995.
9. Held-Warmkessel J: Catheter malfunction. Clin J Oncol Nurs 4(5):239–241, 2000.
10. Intravenous Nursing Society Position Paper on PICC Lines. 1998.
11. Krzywada EA: Predisposing factors, prevention and management of central venous catheter occlusions. J Intraven Nurs 22(Suppl 6S):S11–S37, 1999.
12. Larue GD: Improving central placement rates of peripherally inserted catheters. J Intraven Nurs 18:24–28, 1995.
13. Macklin D: How to manage PICCs. Am J Nurs 97(9):30, 1997.
14. Maki DG, Ringer M, Alvarado CJ: Prospective randomised trial of povidone-iodine, alcohol, and chlorhexidine for prevention of infection associated with central venous and arterial catheters. Lancet 338:339–342, 1991.
15. Moureau N: Vascular access education and training. PICC Excellence 1:5–30, 1998.
16. National Association of Vascular Access Networks: The use of alteplase (t-PA) for the management of thrombotic catheter dysfunction. Guidelines from a consensus conference of the national association of vascular access networks. Clinician 18(2):1–14, 2000.
17. Pearson ML, for the Hospital Infection Control Practice Advisory Committee: Guideline for prevention of intravascular device-related infections.Infect Control Hosp Epidemiol 17:438–473, 1996.
18. Peripherally inserted central catheters; selection, insertion and management. In Bard Access Training Manual. Salt Lake City, Bard, 1996.
19. Ray CE: Infection control principles and practices in the care and management of central venous access devices. J Intraven Nurs 22(Suppl 6):S18–S25, 1999.
20. Ryder MA: Peripherally inserted central venous catheters. Nurs Clin North Am 28:937–971, 1993.
21. Winslow MN, Trammel L, Camp-Sorrell D: Selection of vascular access devices and nursing care. Semin Oncol Nurs 11(3):167–173, 1995.
22. Young LS: Sepsis syndrome. In Mandell GL, Bennett JE, Dolin R (eds): Principles and Practice of Infectious Disease, 4th ed. New York, Churchill Livingstone, 1995, pp 690–705.

15. GENETIC ADVANCES

Constance Engelking, RN, MS, OCN, and Rita Wickham, RN, PhD, AOCN

1. What is the significance of genetics in human disease?

It has been said that all diseases have a genetic basis, which is generally obscured by time and environmental factors, and that most people die of genetic diseases—but few notice. The science of molecular genetics is rapidly expanding to identify and clarify the role of genes involved in many adult-onset chronic, multifactorial conditions. Approximately 5–8% of the population have disorders that can be directly attributable to the inheritance of a mutation in a single gene. Recessive mutations are implicated in many conditions. Thus, the affected person has to inherit a copy of the mutation from both parents to develop cystic fibrosis or sickle cell anemia. On the other hand, Huntington's disease, hereditary hemochromatosis, inherited cancer syndromes, and familial hypercholesterolemia are among the autosomal dominant disorders.

2. Is cancer a genetic disease?

Yes. Most malignancies are sporadic, that is, the initial transforming event occurs in some somatic cell after birth. Frank malignancy results from the accumulation of mutations in several genes (multi-hit theory), and still other mutations are necessary for metastasis to occur. Only 5–10% of all cancers result because of an inherited (germline) mutation in a cancer susceptibility gene. Furthermore, because the mutated gene is found in all body cells, carriers are at increased risk for cancers in other organs. This mutation alone is not sufficient to cause cancer and a second, acquired mutation in the normal copy (allele) of the gene inherited from the unaffected parent later in life sets off the chain of genetic events that leads to cancer (the two-hit hypothesis).

3. How many people are carriers of cancer susceptibility genes?

Estimates vary. For instance, approximately 1 in 500 women is predisposed to developing breast or ovarian cancer because of inheritance of a mutation in *BRCA1* (breast cancer predisposition gene 1) or *BRCA2*, which are tumor suppressor genes. Women who carry an abnormal copy of one of these genes have a 50–85% risk of developing breast cancer by age 85, whereas an 85-year-old woman without a *BRCA1* or *BRCA2* mutation has an 11% risk of breast cancer. The risk for ovarian cancer is also higher, particularly in women with mutations in *BRCA1*. Inherited mutations in cancer susceptibility genes have been implicated in almost every type of cancer, but these cases represent the minority of all cancers. Understanding the genetic mechanisms of tumorigenesis for inherited cancer predispositions is greatly aiding in the understanding of sporadic cancer development.

4. What benefits will advances in genetic science bring to oncology?

Understanding the genetic basis for cancer will open doors for prevention, early detection, and new management options. The clarification of identifiable genetic characteristics associated with high risks for particular malignancies will facilitate more accurate prediction of personal cancer risk and targeted preventive interventions for at-risk people. In fact, better understanding of the interaction of genetics and environment will permit us to tailor programs of total cancer risk management to people with cancer-prone genetic profiles.

5. Discuss the potential effects of genetic science on diagnosis and treatment.

Gene trials are investigational at present, but advances in genetic science have led to novel diagnostic and treatment options. In the future, DNA-based diagnostic approaches that further subcategorize various malignancies according to molecular prognostic indicators will make it possible to customize treatment recommendations based on more accurate probabilities of response to therapy and risk for recurrence. Pharmacogenetics is an advancing science and will be useful in developing new therapeutic strategies that involve repair or replacement of missing or malfunctioning genes or, more likely, gene products. Genetically targeted pharmaceuticals will allow treatment interventions specific to the genetic status of the tumor, with better tumor eradication and fewer side effects.

6. What is the Human Genome Project (HGP)?

Officially launched in 1990 under the aegis of the National Institutes of Health (NIH) and the Department of Energy (DOE), the HGP is a federally-funded, multibillion-dollar international initiative. The goal of the HGP is to map fully the regions of the human genome known to contain most genes as well as the genomes of selected model organisms by the year 2005. New technologies were developed to meet the HGP goal. For instance, in the 1970s a scientist might have to work an entire year to sequence 15–20 nucleotides. Despite some technologic advances in the 1980s, many people doubted that we would be able to sequence the huge number of nucleotides by 2010. However, with currently available computerized automatic sequencing technology, approximately 12,000 nucleotides are decoded every second. The HGP goal is being accomplished by systematically mapping the genomes of several anonymous men and women of varying ethnic backgrounds.

7. What two groups are working to map the human genome?

Two groups with competing interests have been working to develop the technology and map the genome: scientists at institutions that are part of the HGP consortium and privately based commercial companies. The goal of the HGP is to make information about identified sequences immediately available to scientists by publishing it on the Internet; commercial companies patent their discoveries and intend to sell their databases to pharmaceutical companies. In June 2000, both groups jointly announced that a "working draft" of the human genome had been completed. Although 97% of the genome was mapped and > 38,000 genes positively identified, only 24% was "completely" finished. It is anticipated that the project will be completed in 2002 or 2003.

8. Once the map is completed, what next?

Once the map is completed, we will have all of the letters of the code that makes the human blueprint. This extraordinary achievement, however, is just the beginning. We still have to identify the genes, what they produce or control, and how gene products are involved in the thousands of biochemical processes of the body. Thus, ongoing work in the HGP will be to translate this progress to therapeutic use in medicine.

9. How are the ethical and legal issues addressed?

Since its inception the HGP has attempted to define and address the most critical ethical, legal, and social concerns that will emerge as the genome is unveiled and clinical applications of genetic science become more common. To address such issues, a part of each HGP budget is dedicated to the Ethical, Legal, and Social Implications branch (ELSI). ELSI seeks to develop strategies that will ensure (1) confidentiality and fair use of genetic information, (2) appropriate presentation of genetic information in clinical settings, and (3) effective education of providers and consumers of health care.

10. How are genes and the genome mapped?

Gene mapping consists of three interdependent map construction methods. The primary difference among the three types of genetic maps is the level of detail. In general, linkage mapping is a method of identifying the location of specific genes, whereas physical and sequence maps describe the overall and specific DNA sequencing of the genome.

11. What are the major uses of linkage maps?

Linkage maps are useful to identify disease-causing genes by their proximity to known polymorphic DNA markers, which usually are inherited together. Polymorphisms are alternative forms (alleles) of a gene that occur in at least 2% of the population. Only 0.02% of human DNA is polymorphic—and this tiny amount accounts for genetic differences in populations and genetic individuality in people.

12. How are physical and sequence maps used?

Physical maps identify an actual gene or genes within an area of interest. New scientific and computer-based technologies have increased the ability to search for disease-causing genes and corresponding disease-associated mutations as well as to generate sequence maps. Sequence maps are the most detailed of the maps, providing the actual order of the base pairs in a specific gene. Knowing a gene sequence is essential to identify gene expression and functions.

13. Define genome.

An organism's genome is composed of all genetic material necessary for the development and functioning of that organism. All organisms, plant and animal, have a genome. Analyzing a genome is analogous to dissecting the body. Just as the body can be separated into organs, and organs into tissues, so the genome can be reduced to molecular components that are progressively less complex.

14. What are the largest and most complex elements of the human genome?

Chromosomes. Human beings have 23 pairs of chromosomes: 22 pairs of autosomes and 1 pair of sex chromosomes (X and Y). Chromosomes are located in the cell nucleus and are rodlike structures composed of deoxyribonucleic acid (DNA) wrapped around proteins.

15. Describe the structure of DNA.

DNA, the cornerstone element of the genome, is a double-stranded helical structure that has a "twisted ladder" appearance. A single rung, or building block, of DNA is two nucleotides, which constitute one base pair (bp). Each nucleotide consists of a nitrogenous base, one sugar (deoxyribose) group, and one phosphate group. There are four nitrogenous bases: two purines (adenine [A] and guanine [G]) and two pyrimidines (thymine [T] and cytosine [C]). These always bind selectively to form four complementary base pairs: AT, TA, GC, and CG. The base pairs are the rungs that connect the two sidebars of the ladder.

16. What are genes?

Genes are the DNA protein-coding sequences spaced along the chromosomes. They include the sequences that regulate when and how much of a protein is made.

17. Discuss the function and types of RNA.

For a cell to synthesize a protein, DNA must be transcribed into ribonucleic acid (RNA), a single-stranded nucleic acid in which uracil replaces thymine and ribose is the sugar. Three different types of RNA—messenger RNA (mRNA), ribosomal RNA (rRNA), and transfer RNA (tRNA)—are involved in transcription of DNA to mature RNA (some noncoding sections, called introns, are excised out) and translation of exons (expressed sections) to protein. The genetic code for all organisms accounts for 20 different amino acids that are strung together to make a vast array of proteins. Each amino acid is assembled from one codon (or codons, because there is some redundancy in the code) that consists of three nitrogenous bases (or nucleotides) along the mRNA. The "reading frame" along the RNA thus consists of each group of three nucleotides. Flanking regions occur at each end of the gene code for starting and stopping gene expression.

18. What is the relationship among genotype, phenotype, and karyotype?

These three terms are descriptors of an individual's genome. **Genotype** encompasses the inheritable traits (and disorders) of an individual that distinguish one species from another (i.e., man or mouse). **Phenotype** refers to the expression of genes (physical, morphologic, and biochemical manifestations of an individual) and results from the interaction between the genotype and the environment. **Karyotype** is a figure that displays a specific individual's complement of chromosomes, in which the autosomes are numbered, shown in pairs, and arranged from largest to smallest and followed by the sex chromosomes. Karyotypes are derived by cytogenetic techniques and show characteristic banding, depending on the type of stain used.

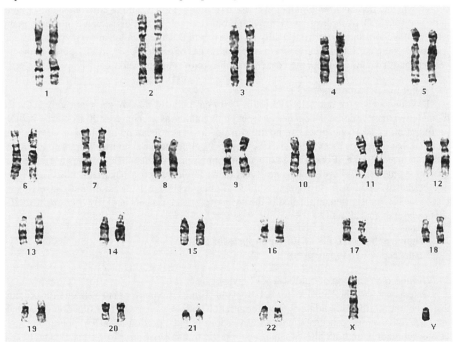

Normal human karyotype of a male. Note 22 pairs of autosomes and sex chromosomes X and Y. (Courtesy of the Clinical Cytogenetics Laboratory, Rush Presbyterian St. Luke's Medical Center, Chicago, IL.)

19. Discuss the relationship of DNA to genes.

Genes are functional subsections of the DNA chain and are highly variable in size. For instance, a small gene that codes for a globulin is 1,500 bp or 1.5 kilobases (kb) long, whereas a dystrophin gene consists of 3,000,000 bp (or 3000 kb). Genes are the smallest functional units of DNA and hold the instructions that guide cellular production of specific protein products necessary for an organism's function and replication. There are slight variants of some genes. These alternate forms of the alleles for particular genes are polymorphisms and account for observable (or otherwise detectable) differences in individuals. Polymorphisms arose by the process of mutation, which may have caused a variation that is harmless (i.e., eye color, blood type), helpful (i.e., mutation in a particular receptor that makes an individual resistant to HIV infection), or harmful (i.e., mutation in a cancer susceptibility gene or in a gene causing another Mendelian [single gene] disorder). Harmful mutations are more common events in large genes than in small genes.

Each gene is an ordered sequence of nucleotides found at a certain location on a specific chromosome. For example, *BRCA1*, a breast cancer susceptibility gene, is located on the long (q) arm of chromosome 17 in the 12-21 interval (17q12-21). *BRCA1* is approximately 100 kb and codes for a protein of 1863 amino acids. *BRCA2*, another breast cancer susceptibility gene, is located at 13q (long arm)12-13. The short arm of each chromosome is termed the p (for petite) arm.

20. How many genes do humans have?

The actual number of human genes is unknown, but it is estimated to range from 50,000 to 115,000, scattered among approximately 3.15 billion bp located on 46 chromosomes. Genes are estimated to constitute about 3–30% of the total DNA, or 90–900 million bp; the remaining DNA has structural integrity, regulatory, and other unknown functions.

21. Discuss the role of gene mutations in cancer.

Cancer can occur because of deleterious mutations in genes involved with the regulation of cell growth and division. Such mutations arise in response to exposure to environmental carcinogens or errors in DNA replication. Genes that promote or inhibit cell division are most important, whereas mutations in genes that normally repair errors in DNA replication allow mutations to persist and accumulate. Thus, the two most important types of cancer susceptibility genes in the development of sporadic and inherited cancer include protooncogenes and tumor suppressor genes.

22. What are protooncogenes?

Protooncogenes are normally genes that "turn on" cell division. When incorrectly activated by mutation, they become oncogenes and can be thought of as accelerators of neoplastic cellular proliferation. A protooncogene can be transformed to an oncogene by insertion of viral genetic material that increases its expression (i.e., human T-cell leukemia) and by chromosome translocation or inversion (i.e., Burkitt's and other lymphomas, many leukemias, Ewing's and other sarcomas). At the cellular level, oncogenes function as dominant genes. That is, a mutation in only one of the two alleles is sufficient to turn on uncontrolled cell division and cause cancer. Oncogenes are most often implicated in the onset of sporadic cancers and play roles in the malignant progression of all tumors.

23. What are the two types of tumor suppressor genes?

"Gatekeepers" and "caretakers."

24. Discuss the function of "gatekeeper" genes.

Gatekeepers are the "brakes" for cell division. Tumor suppressor genes encode for proteins that function in growth regulatory or differentiation pathways. Loss of one functioning copy is not sufficient to cause cancer. Deletions or insertions of large portions of DNA, point mutations, or other mutations in both alleles lead to neoplastic transformation. Most persons who have a germline mutation in a cancer susceptibility gene carry an altered tumor suppressor gene that functions as a gatekeeper. Over 100 of such genes have been identified, including *BRCA1*, *BRCA2*, retinoblastoma (*RB1*), Wilms' tumor (*WT1*), and familial adenomatous polyposis (*APC*). One tumor suppressor gene that is commonly mutated in most advanced cancers is p53, which has been termed the "watch-dog" of the human genome. That is, p53 is a mediator between environmental mutagens and development of cancer; it prevents a cell from progressing from G1 to S phase unless the damage can be repaired. When both copies of p53 are normal, irreparable mutations are recognized and the cell undergoes apoptosis (programmed cell death). When both copies are inactivated by mutations, there is no "stop" signal for cell division.

25. Discuss the function of "caretaker" genes.

Neoplastic transformation of caretaker tumor suppressor genes does not act directly to promote tumor growth but leads to genetic instability and accumulation of genetic errors. This process accelerates the development of cancer. Under normal circumstances, DNA that has been incorrectly replicated during the S phase of cell division is repaired, or the cell undergoes apoptosis. Mutations in caretaker genes cause DNA repair mechanisms to become dysfunctional—a rare event compared with other malignant changes associated with inherited cancer risk. Mutations in DNA repair genes are implicated in hereditary nonpolyposis colorectal cancer (HNPCC) and other rare malignancies, such as xeroderma pigmentosum.

26. What genetic mutations may lead to the development of cancer?

Mutations are stable (or unstable, as in cancer), heritable changes in a gene or DNA sequence. As mentioned, mutations are expected events that occur infrequently but predictably and usually result in polymorphisms of the most common allele (termed the "wild type"). Harmful mutations cause disease, and may be spontaneous, or result from physical, chemical, biologic, or genetic factors. Cancer may result from the mutation of a single copy of an oncogene or mutations in both alleles of a tumor suppressor gene.

Mutations are categorized as somatic or germ line. A somatic mutation occurs in one gene in a particular body (somatic) tissue, is acquired through carcinogenic exposure, and causes a sporadic malignancy. Germline mutations are present in all body cells, including gametes, and can be passed to children (each child has a 50% chance of inheriting the mutated allele). It is likely that three to seven mutations must occur before the development of solid tumors, whereas fewer mutations are necessary for the development of leukemias. Several different types of genetic changes are found in cancer cells, including gross structural changes in chromosomes and subtle changes in genes.

27. What gross changes may be seen in chromosomes?
1. Change in the number of chromosomes (aneuploidy)
2. Chromosome translocations
3. Gene amplifications
4. Incorporation of exogenous genetic sequences from viruses that contribute to abnormal cell growth
5. Point mutations and frameshift mutations

28. What types of aneuploidy may be seen?
Monosomy, absence of, trisomy, or multiple copies of particular chromosomes. Aneuploidy is usually a later change in the progression from less to more malignant disease and can be detected by cytogenetic analysis.

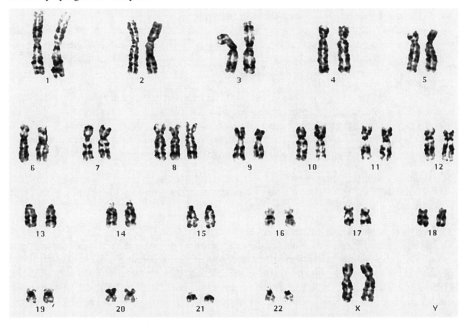

Karyotype of a female showing trisomy 8, a common cytogenetic abnormality found in hematologic malignancies. (Courtesy of the Clinical Cytogenetics Laboratory, Rush Presbyterian St. Luke's Medical Center, Chicago, IL.)

29. What are the two types of chromosome translocations?
Balanced translocations refer to chromosomal material exchanged between at least two nonhomologous (different) chromosomes. **Unbalanced translocations** occur when a fragment or an entire chromosome joins with another chromosome, resulting in aneuploidy in daughter cells. Translocations may result in fusion proteins that have different functions. For example, if an oncogene is inserted next to and fuses with a protooncogene, the activated complex is expressed as one gene. This process is common in many sporadic malignancies, including solid

tumors and leukemias (e.g., the appearance of the Philadelphia chromosome in chronic myelo-cytic leukemia [CML]).

30. Define gene amplification.

A gene amplification consists of 5–100-fold multiplication of a small region of a chromo-some. Gene amplifications are common in advanced malignancies.

31. Which cancers are known to be associated with incorporation of viral genetic sequences?

Cervical cancer (human papillomavirus), Burkitt's lymphoma (Epstein-Barr virus), hepato-cellular carcinoma (hepatitis viruses), and T-cell leukemia (retroviruses).

32. What are point mutations and frameshift mutations?

Point mutations are very small and subtle changes that affect a single base pair. They can result in a harmless polymorphism, a missense mutation, or a nonsense mutation. **Frameshift mutations** affect two or more base pairs and most often result in nonsense mutations.

33. Explain the three mechanisms that cause point mutations.

1. Deletion: loss or removal of one or more nucleotides.
2. Insertion: the gain or addition of one or more nucleotides.
3. Substitution: one nucleotide is substituted for another, changing the base pair.

34. What mechanisms cause frameshift mutations?

In frameshift mutations, two or more base pairs are deleted or inserted into the protein coding region of the gene (an exon), which changes the reading frame. Frameshift mutations alter the pro-tein sequence, often leading to a truncated, nonfunctional protein product (see question 36).

35. What is a missense mutation?

A point mutation (change in a single base pair) that results in a change in a single codon and thus in a single amino acid, which results in a structurally different protein. It cannot always be deter-mined whether this change is harmless (i.e., does not alter the functionality of the protein coded) or disease-causing. For example, a single point mutation in sickle cell disease is sufficient to change the conformation of the hemoglobin molecule in people who inherit a mutated copy from both parents.

36. What is a nonsense mutation?

A point or frameshift mutation that alters an important amino acid and thus changes the structure, stability, or function of the protein.

37. Why are nonsense mutations especially harmful?

Because they change a base pair or the reading frame so that one of the codons that signal "stop" is reached much earlier than in a normal protein. For example, in the Ashkenazi Jewish population, a common mutation in *BRCA1* is the deletion (del) of two nucleotides at position 185 (185delAG)—in a gene that is 100,000 base pairs long. This mutation results in truncation and nonfunctionality of the protein product for which it codes and is present in > 20% of Jewish women who develop breast cancer before the age of 40.

38. How does genetic redundancy affect mutations?

Because of redundancy in the genetic code, a change in one nucleotide may code for the same amino acid. For instance, a change in the DNA triplicate TGT to TGG results in a corre-sponding change in the RNA codons from UCU to UCC, but both code for the amino acid serine.

39. Is DNA testing or risk factor assessment a reliable means of predicting cancer?

The genetic profile has been characterized as a person's "future diary"—a blueprint describ-ing the person's possible physiologic destiny. Genetic information is indeed unique, but it is based on a code that has been deciphered only partially; the encoding of proteins and their functions is still largely unknown. Consequently, the full implication of an individual's genetic profile is still to be defined. It is not yet known, for example, what percentage of people will actually develop malignant diseases for which genetic risk has been identified. Furthermore, the development of cancer also depends on exposure to environment factors over a long period. Although risk factors for many cancers have been identified, none is entirely predictive. Even cigarette smoking, the major risk factor, does not predict lung cancer: 90% of people with lung cancer have a significant pack-year history, but only about 15% of such smokers develop lung cancer. Thus, the identification of a mutated cancer susceptibility gene predicts only increased risk—not certainty for cancer. For instance, the woman who carries a mutation in *BRCA1* or *BRCA2* may never develop breast cancer, whereas the woman who does not have a germline mutation in one of these genes may develop breast cancer because 85–90% of breast cancers are sporadic.

40. What are the psychologic concerns about DNA testing?
Gaps in knowledge place the value of personal genetic information about cancer risk in question and raise the psychosocial dilemma of revealing risks with no clear knowledge about management approaches (with a few exceptions). Knowledge about genetic status may produce high levels of anxiety, which may motivate the person to follow lifestyle, self-care, and routine screening recommendations. Conversely, a sense of fatalism may interfere with preventive health care.

41. What are the social concerns about DNA testing?
The uniqueness of genetic information raises concerns that if such data become "public," they may give rise to genetic discrimination. For example, an insurer or employer who becomes aware of a genetic predisposition for cancer may offer reduced health benefits or higher cost premiums or eliminate the person for promotional opportunities. At the worst, discrimination based on projections of bad health outcomes may result in denial of health insurance or employment, despite the lack of clear data to confirm that genetic discrimination is occurring.

42. How can DNA testing affect families?
Positive results of genetic tests reveal information not only to the person who underwent the test but also, at least potentially, to family members. They may have health implications for future generations. Because most germline cancer susceptibility gene mutations are transmitted in an autosomal dominant fashion, affected people know that they inherited the mutation from one of their parents (as is usually evident in the family pedigree). Similarly, each child of an affected person has a 50% chance of inheriting the mutation. Information about the genetic status of one family member cannot be shared without the permission of the tested person and the consent of the family members. Obvious ethical issues are raised in relation to rights, autonomy, privacy, and choice. Moreover, family secrets (e.g., paternity issues) that have far-reaching effects on interpersonal relationships and emotional well-being may be exposed when DNA testing is undertaken. In addition, transmitter and survivor guilt, as well as depression and overprotection or abandonment of a child, may result when people learn that they may have passed a genetic disorder to their offspring.

43. Describe the rationale for genetic screening programs with some degree of public access. How is individual privacy protected?
Such information will enable scientists to gain knowledge about genetic disorders and the effects of specific therapies. Because the availability of personal genetic information is a relatively new phenomenon, there are no clear solutions to protect genetic privacy. Recommendations for genetic screening have been proposed through various groups (e.g., National Advisory Council for Genomic Research, American Cancer Society), but guidelines that regulate the privacy of information in DNA databanks have not yet been established. Currently, the best efforts to maintain confidentiality are found in the "shadow medical records," which are shared only with the geneticist or genetics care team and the individual.

44. What organizations have issued position statements about genetic testing for cancer?
Although commercial tests are available for some cancer susceptibility genes and other tests are available in research settings, relatively few position papers have addressed important questions

such as "Who should undergo a genetic test?" Groups that have published position papers include the National Advisory Council for Human Genome Research (NACHGR), the American Society of Clinical Oncology (ASCO), the National Breast Cancer Coalition (NBCC), and the National Society of Genetic Counselors (NSGC).

45. Summarize the position statements of NACHGR and NBCC.

Both groups have taken more restrictive approaches than ASCO. In 1994, for example, NACHGR concluded that it was premature to offer cancer genetic risk testing outside a carefully monitored research setting and raised crucial questions that should be answered about DNA testing for presymptomatic identification of cancer risk. Examples relate specifically to gene mutations (i.e., defining the number, determining actual incidence in the general population, and predicting the actual risk of cancer) and relevant laboratory and technical issues related to cancer gene tests, such as quality control. NACHGR also raised other areas of concern, including those of determining what methods are most effective and feasible for educating large numbers of at-risk people, how to ensure informed consent, how to provide culturally sensitive genetic counseling, and how to avoid genetic discrimination. NBCC also recommended limiting *BRCA1* testing to research settings until more is known about the mutation and called for a written plan to manage potentially discriminatory consequences and to establish therapeutic options before widespread testing is permitted.

46. Summarize the position of ASCO.

In 1996, ASCO took a more permissive stance, stating that cancer risk counseling is a legitimate function of clinical oncologists, who should receive the necessary education to assume such a role. ASCO's position is that cancer predisposition testing should be offered to selective patients when (1) the person has a strong family history of cancer or early age of cancer onset; (2) the test can be adequately interpreted; and (3) test results will influence medical management of the affected person or family member(s). Genetic testing in research settings was recommended but not mandated. ASCO defined three categories of indications for genetic testing. Genetic testing is clearly indicated for patients in category one, which includes families with well-defined hereditary syndromes for which either a positive or negative result will change medical care (e.g., families with familial adenomatous polyposis, MEN2A or 2B, retinoblastoma, and Von Hippel-Lindau syndrome). Genetic testing may be offered to families in category two, who have hereditary syndromes for which the medical benefit of identification of a carrier (heterozygote) is presumed but not proved (e.g., hereditary breast ovarian syndrome, nonpolyposis colon cancer, Li-Fraumeni syndrome). Genetic testing is not indicated for patients in category three, which includes people with a family history of cancer, but the significance of detecting a germline mutation is not known (e.g., melanoma-associated syndromes, ataxia telangiectasia-associated susceptibilities).

47. What is the position of NSGC?

NSGC did not take an explicit stance on testing but sought to educate clinicians about the complexities of genetic testing for adult-onset conditions and to increase their awareness about the importance of a multidisciplinary approach that will ensure appropriate pretest education, genetic counseling, and posttest follow-up.

48. What is the position of commercial entities that offer screening tests?

Commercial entities that offer screening tests for various types of cancer (e.g., breast, ovarian, and colorectal cancers) argue that genetic testing is an individual choice and that availability will force the refinement of such testing and bring potentially life-saving diagnostic tests to the public.

49. What are the primary sources of genetic information?

Various data sources are available for collecting genetic information, including family history, physical examination, selected laboratory studies, and molecular genetic studies. Family history is most important as a case-finding tool and provides the clues for disease that provide the basis for a decision to pursue more in-depth genetic screening and potentially to recommend a genetic test. Physicians and nurses who are not genetics specialists can gather data regarding at least three generations of blood relatives. Such historical data permit construction of a pedigree (also called a family tree or genogram) that may illuminate the existence of a possible trait or disorder across generations.

50. What findings in the family history raise suspicion of inherited susceptibility risk?

- Family members diagnosed with cancer at unusually young ages (15–20 years earlier than predicted).
- High rate of the same type of cancer in the family (especially rare tumors).
- Family members who have had more than one tumor in the same organ (i.e., multicentric foci) or cancer in both paired organs (i.e., bilateral breast cancer).
- Family member with primary cancers diagnosed in multiple different organs.

Physical examination and other diagnostic tests that reveal characteristics associated with genetic disorders (i.e., polycystic kidneys in patients with familial adenomatous polyposis) and thus provide another piece in the genetic puzzle.

51. What should be done if the family contains clues to cancer susceptibilty?

If such clues are evident, the patient should be informed of the possibility of familial or inherited cancer predisposition and should be referred to a multidisciplinary cancer risk clinic. Specialist physicians, nurses, genetic counselors, psychologists, and others are educated to understand complex genetic information and to teach and counsel patients. One or more of these team members will gather another family history. Because recalled information about family members (particularly second- and third-degree relatives) may be inaccurate, actual medical records, pathology reports, cancer registry data, and copies of death certificates are gathered. Before any genetic test is considered, the proband (the person seeking genetic testing) should receive extensive teaching about the type of familial cancer that is suspected and the predictive value of a genetic test. Because the association between a mutation identified in a laboratory test and actual development of cancer is imperfect, the predicted likelihood that someone with a positive test will develop cancer is expressed as a range. In addition, the risks (psychological and social), benefits, and limitations (i.e., a test result may be uninformative because the significance of some mutations is not known) of a gene test are discussed. The genetic specialist also explores and explains other areas and presents alternatives to gene testing. Patients who choose to undergo a gene test must give written, informed consent and must receive face-to-face posttest education and genetic counseling as well as psychosocial and medical follow-up. Thus, an actual gene test is undertaken only after careful assessment, education, deliberation, and patient support.

52. How may advances in genetic science be applied to early diagnosis of cancer?

Increased understanding about genes, coupled with advances in laboratory technology, is leading to new ideas for diagnostic measures and gene therapies for cancer. At least 10 years of development are needed before gene therapies become widely used. One new application of genetic knowledge to cancer screening is examining stool for mutations in *K-ras*, which is a protooncogene. Point mutations in *K-ras* occur early in the process of carcinogenesis and precede mutations in other tumor suppressor genes that are necessary for frank cancer to develop. This investigational test is undergoing large clinical trials and appears to be highly sensitive and specific for cancers and adenomas. Another investigational diagnostic measure is gene marking, which entails inserting an identifiable gene into a patient's cells to "label" the gene for future recognition. One application of gene marking under study is to establish whether bone marrow cells labeled with a marker gene that confers neomycin resistance (i.e., *NoeR*) are the source of relapse after autologous blood cell transplant.

53. Describe the potential role of genetic advances in the treatment of cancer.

Gene therapy encompasses correcting genetic errors by manipulating or altering abnormal genes to replace faulty DNA with corrected, functional versions; by sensitizing tumor cells so that they are more likely to be destroyed; by providing a cell with a new phenotypic function; and by supporting other drug therapies. Gene therapy recently was shown to be effective in curing severe combined immunodeficiency (SCID) in two children. However, this feat was relatively easy because bone marrow stem cells were the defective cells harvested from the children. The cells were bathed in a growth factor, infected with a retrovirus carrying a normal replacement gene, and reinfused into the children. This type of gene therapy will never be as straightforward for cancer because of the number of gene mutations that have occurred and subsequent immunologic differences in tumor cells, lack of knowledge about which genes or gene products are critical, technical difficulties of getting the corrected gene into all tumor cells, and other problems. Nonetheless, there is a great deal of enthusiasm for the potential value of gene therapy in cancer, and approximately 70–75% of all clinical trials of these therapies involve cancer patients.

54. List different techniques for clinical application of gene addition or alteration therapy.

1. Delivering normal genes to restore tumor suppressor or protooncogene function. This approach may be feasible when tumors are small and is likely to be used as adjuvant therapy or in conjunction with chemotherapy or other treatments.

2. Antisense therapy, whereby a nucleotide sequence that complements and inactivates tumor RNA binds with it and prevents translation of defective protein. This method of suppressing tumor growth is under study in leukemias and other tumors.

3. Stimulation or reconstitution of immune responses against cancer by attacking tumor genes through tumor cell vaccination with a genetically modified immunostimulatory cytokine gene (e.g., IL-2 or TNF in neuroblastoma, melanoma, renal cell carcinoma).

4. Injection of a foreign HLA gene (e.g., *HLA-B7* to heighten tumor immunogenicity in melanoma).

5. Insertion into neoplastic cells of a "suicide gene" that encodes an enzyme that converts a prodrug to toxic metabolites. For example, a gene for herpes simplex thymidine kinase [TK] is inserted into brain tumor cells and followed by a course of ganciclovir to destroy tumor cells that have taken up the TK gene.

6. Introduction of a multidrug resistance gene into bone marrow (e.g., to protect normal hematopoietic cells from myelosuppression induced by dose-intensive chemotherapy).

7. Introduction of tumor suppressor gene to "turn off" tumor cell proliferation (e.g., *p53* gene into colorectal cancer cells).

8. Monoclonal antibody therapy to counter the effect of altered tumor suppressor gene activity. One currently available therapy is herceptin, which is effective in blocking the effect of HER-2/*neu* when it is overexpressed in breast cancer (and perhaps other tumors) and makes the tumor more aggressive.

55. Summarize the current status of gene transfer therapy.

Currently all gene transfer is investigational and involves only somatic cell techniques. That is, genetic alterations are achieved in individual patients and cannot be passed along to their offspring. However, the technology for germline gene transfer does exist. Although currently considered unethical, future technologic advances may make germline gene transfer feasible to prevent cancer in high-risk people.

56. What is pharmacogenetics?

Pharmacogenetics is the study of how a patient's genes determine response to drugs. This exciting application of gene therapy is being used to develop customized drugs and is likely to speed up new drug development. Pharmacogenetics provide a means for drugs to interact more specifically with protein products.

57. What safety considerations are associated with gene transfer therapy?

Safety concerns include both patients and health care providers. There may be both immediate and long-term complications for patients, which are largely unknown because of the early stage of gene therapy science. For instance, publicity about the negative effects of gene therapy and the death of a young man in a gene therapy trial have led to greater controls.

As in the development of other anticancer therapies, safety concerns for health care providers are related to potential occupational hazards associated with the administration of gene therapies, especially with the use of retroviruses. Specific regulations have been enacted to protect clinicians. For example, FDA regulations do not permit clinical use of retroviral vectors until they have been modified to eliminate their replicating ability. Accordingly, protocols involving retroviral vectors cannot begin until confirmatory quality control testing has been conducted. In addition, compliance with universal precautions is considered adequate protection against any viral hazards that may exist, although none have been demonstrated to date.

58. How will advances in genetic science affect cancer nursing?

The amount of information about genetics and genetic advances in the lay media is astonishing. Every day information from just published scientific papers is translated into plain English and finds its ways to local newspapers, television, tabloids, and news magazines—often before the scientific publication reaches the medical library. Patients, therefore, are armed with a great deal of information and questions. As oncology nurses, we cannot afford to wait until current investigational diagnostic and therapeutic strategies are part of everyday practice to become informed about basic genetics and to take a more active role in cancer genetics in particular. Furthermore, the Oncology Nursing Society (ONS) has taken the position that generalist and advanced practice oncology nurses must be educated and partner with other healthcare providers to provide care to high-risk individuals. Two position statements, *Genetic Counseling* and *Genetics: Testing and Risk Assessment,* are available at the ONS website.

59. How should nurses educate themselves about genetic science?

Nurses are the largest group of health care providers and must take the responsibility for their own educational needs. As Lashley says, nurses need to be able to "think genetically" in clinical situations. Nurses should understand basic mechanisms of genetic inheritance, have information about common single-gene and complex genetic disorders, understand how genetics contributes to human diversity, recognize how genetic and environmental factors interact in health and disease, and be able to provide nursing care for patients with genetic diseases. In addition, nurses should be able to interpret genetic risks to patients (i.e., when a patient is told that the risk for inheriting a mutated cancer susceptibility gene is 50%, it means that each child has a 50% risk—not that half of the children will inherit the mutation), and understand some nursing implications arising from the social, legal, and ethical issues. Fortunately, there are many opportunities for nurses to increase their knowledge about genetics, including basic textbooks, continuing education courses, formal genetics courses, and genetics websites.

Genetics Websites

RESOURCE	WEB ADDRESS
Robert Lurie Cancer Center, Cancer Genetics Site	www.cancergenetics.org
Human Genome Project	www.ornl.gov/hgmis/medicine.html
International Society of Nurses in Genetics	www.nursing.Creighton.edu/isong
Clinical Genetics: Self Study for Health Care Providers	www.vh.org/Providers/Textbooks/ClinicalGenetics/Contents/html
Online Mendelian Inheritance in Man	www.ncbi.nlm.nih.gov/Omim/
CancerNet (National Cancer Institute [NCI])	http://cancernet.nci.hih.gov/clinpdq/cancer_genetics/
Myriad Laboratories (commercial site)	www.myriad.com

Table continued on following page

Genetics Websites (Continued)

RESOURCE	WEB ADDRESS
Yahoo Human Genetics	www.yahoo.com/Science/Biology/Genetics/Human_Genetics/
Secretary's Advisory Committee on Genetic Testing (SACGT)	http://www4od.nih.gov/oba/sacgt.html
Centers for Disease Control Genetics and Disease Prevention Update	http://www.cdc.gov/genetics.html
Online Journal of Issues in Nursing, September 30, 2000 issue on genetics	http://www.ana.org/ojin/topic13_6.htm
Genetics and Your Practice, 3rd ed.	http://mchneighborhood.ichp.edu/wagenetics/906317266.html
Oncolink: Genetics and Cancer	http://oncolink.upenn.edu/causeprevent/genetics
Understanding Gene Testing (publication from NCI)	http://www.gene.com/ae/AE/AEPC/NIH/

60. What questions should nurses ask to obtain a fairly comprehensive family history that includes the patient's siblings, parents, grandparents, and children?

- Have you ever had cancer? What type, age at diagnosis, treatment?
- Have you had more than one kind of cancer?
- Have you been told that you have precancerous lesions (i.e., cervical dysplasia, atypical moles, colon polyps, breast carcinoma in situ)?
- Have any of your closest (first-degree) blood relatives (mother, father, brothers, sisters, or children) ever had cancer? What kind(s), ages at diagnosis, treatments?
- Have any of your grandparents, aunts and uncles, nieces or nephews (second-degree relatives) had cancer? (Ask same questions.)

Nurses can then construct a pedigree to look for patterns that may indicate health problems with a familial component. The "picture" provided by a pedigree can help the nurse design and implement teaching plans that help patients address (and perhaps decrease) environmental risk factors (e.g., increasing exercise, weight loss, and smoking cessation in the person who has a strong family history of cardiac disease or hypertension). In addition, the pedigree may identify patients who would benefit from consultation at a cancer genetics risk clinic.

61. What does the future hold for oncology nursing?

Although all implications of the "genetic revolution" are as yet unknown, such advances certainly will contribute significantly to the already transforming paradigm of cancer nursing practice and care. The current emphasis on disease management will be increasingly replaced by attention to cancer prevention and screening for high-risk indicators. Thus, nursing practice and care will be transformed from a short-term, episodic approach to a longer-term, continuous approach. The current concentration on symptom management and palliative care is likely to shift toward wellness promotion and preventive lifestyle behaviors, which will affect patient education. Patient profiles will change because of the point on the health/illness continuum at which patients present to the health team. Rather than seeking medical care because of symptoms that lead to diagnoses, patients will be followed proactively based on identified genetic and environmental risks for developing cancer (and other diseases). This may mean that people have less certain outcomes than in the past, because at this point we cannot predict who will actually develop cancer. Thus, people may be at significant and sustained risk for anxiety, and may adopt a fatalistic attitude about the inevitability of cancer and not engage in preventive behaviors. Nurses are key health care providers who can anticipate such responses to genetic information and respond with targeted teaching and counseling for at-risk families. In addition, although few nurses are involved in clinical trials of gene therapies, successes will rapidly move to the general clinical arena. Oncology nurses will be, once again, in a strategic position to become part of the expanding genetics care team, to pioneer new gene therapies and screening approaches, and to define human responses to these new strategies.

ACKNOWLEDGMENT

The authors thank Jeffrey Shaw, MS, for his thoughtful review of this chapter.

REFERENCES

1. American Society of Clinical Oncology: Statement on the genetic testing for cancer susceptibility. J Clin Oncol 14:1730–1736, 1996.
2. Engelking C: The human genome exposed: A glimpse of promise, predicament, and impact on practice. Oncol Nurs Forum 22(Suppl):3–9, 1996.
3. Engelking C: Genetics in cancer care: Confronting a Pandora's box of dilemmas. Oncol Nurs Forum 22 (Suppl):27–34, 1996.
4. Lashley FR: Genetics in nursing education. Nurs Clin North Am 35:795–805, 2000.
5. Lea DH: Gene therapy: Oncology nursing implications. Semin Oncol Nurs 13:115–122, 1997.
6. Lewis R: Human Genetics, 4th ed. New York, McGraw-Hill, 2001.
7. Lessick M, Wickham R, Rehwaldt M: Breast and ovarian cancer: Genetic update and implications for nursing. MEDSURG Nurs 6:341–349, 1997.
8. Loescher L: The family history component of cancer genetic risk counseling. Cancer Nurs 22: 96–102, 1999.
9. McKinnon WC, Baty BJ, Bennett R, et al: Predisposition genetic testing for late-onset disorders in adults: A position paper of the National Society of Genetic Counselors. JAMA 278: 1217–1220, 1997.
10. Offit K: Clinical Cancer Genetics. New York, Wiley-Liss, 1998.
11. Rothenberg KH: Genetic information and health insurance: State legislative approaches. J Law Med Ethics 23:312–319, 1995.
12. Scanlon C, Fibison W: Managing Genetic Information: Implications for Nursing Practice. Washington, DC, American Nurses Association, 1995.
13. Vogelstein B, Kinzler KW (eds): The Genetic Basis of Human Cancer. New York, McGraw-Hill, 1998.
14. Weber C: Cytokine-modified tumor vaccines: An antitumor strategy revisited in the age of molecular medicine. Cancer Nurs 21:167–177, 1998.
15. Wheeler VS: Gene therapy: Current strategies and future applications. Oncol Nurs Forum 22:20–26, 1995.

16. COMPLEMENTARY AND ALTERNATIVE MEDICINE THERAPIES

Georgia M. Decker, MS, RN, CS-ANP, AOCN,
and Mary Jo Cleaveland, RN, MS

1. How are complementary and alternative therapies defined?

The interchangeable use of the terms "complementary" and "alternative" by clinicians has caused confusion and miscommunication. Alternative medicine is an umbrella term that was used to describe therapies not taught in U.S. medical schools or provided in U.S. hospitals. Because many medical schools now include these therapies in their curricula and some are now provided in hospitals, the term is no longer appropriate. Complementary and alternative do not describe a particular therapy but rather the intent with which it is used. When a therapy is used as alternative it is used "instead of; " when a therapy is complementary, it is used "with" a conventional therapy.

2. What other words have been used to describe complementary or alternative therapy?

The following terms are sometimes used inappropriately to describe complementary and alternative medicine (CAM) therapies:

Quackery: term used by some healthcare professionals and others to describe any therapy with which they disagree. Proof of quackery requires scientific and legal documentation.

Unproven: the therapy has not been proved to be effective or ineffective.

(W)holistic:the whole person is treated, not just a symptom or condition.

3. How are CAM therapies characterized?

The National Center for Complementary and Alternative Medicine (NCCAM), formerly known as the Office of Alternative Medicine (OAM), was established within the National Institutes of Health (NIH) to seek data about the efficacy of alternative health care and to establish an information clearinghouse on CAM therapies. NCCAM describes seven categories of CAM therapies: (1) alternative systems of medical care, (2) mind-body medicine, (3) bioelectromagnetic therapy, (4) herbal medicine, (5) pharmacologic and biologic therapies, (6) manual healing methods, and (7) diet, nutrition, and lifestyle changes.

4. List examples in each of the CAM categories and describe the major controversies.

CATEGORY	DESCRIPTION	EXAMPLES	CONTROVERSIES/COMMENTS
Alternative system of medical care	Stresses prevention of disease and promotion of health, including emphasis on personal responsibility and self-healing	Traditional Chinese medicine Naturopathy Ayurvedic medicine	These systems are a way of being and a way of living. They are not meant to be parceled into individual or separate modalities. Western medicine has begun to incorporate various aspects of these modalities.
Mind-body medicine	Known as behavioral medicine; unites bio-medical, behavioral, and psychological strategies for promotion of health	Meditation Guided imagery Visualization Relaxation Spirituality Art therapies Music therapy Biofeedback Yoga	Controversies exist over whether mind-body interventions prolong survival or merely enhance quality of life and sense of being healed. Imagery and visualization have been used by patients with cancer for relief of treatment- and disease-related symptoms, including pain control. Concerns have been raised about use of guided imagery in

Table continued on following page

CATEGORY	DESCRIPTION	EXAMPLES	CONTROVERSIES/COMMENTS
Mind-body medicine (*cont.*)			patients with a psychiatric history. The idea that mental efforts can alter the course of cancer has not been proved by research and may induce feelings of guilt and inadequacy in patients whose disease progresses despite best efforts.
Bioelectromagnetic therapies	Based on use of energy as healing modality	Acupuncture Magnet therapy Cymatics	The contemporary use of magnets has stimulated discussion and research regarding claims that magnets reduce pain and may have health-promoting benefits. Acupuncture (taken from traditional Oriental medicine) has proved to be helpful for various symptoms and is now accepted for pain relief.
Herbal medicine	Based on Doctrine of Signatures, which states that a plant's appearance or characteristics provide a clue to medicinal implications	Herbs may be used as single agents or in combination Herbs used to treat cancer include essiac and pau d'arco tea	Patients believe that "natural means safe" and that "if a little is good, a lot is better." The concern for all patients is possible herb-drug interactions. More information about this issue will become available. To report an adverse event, call 1-888-SAFE-FOOD or access website at http://www.fda.gov/ medwatch/partner.htm. Because herbs are not regulated or standardized, safety issues must be scrutinized.
Pharmacologic and biologic therapies	Most often used as alternatives and have been described as having the "lure of cure"[23]	Laetrile Shark cartilage Oxidative therapies Antineoplastons PC-SPES (combination of 14 herbs for prostate cancer)	The concern has always been that patients will use these therapies instead of conventional therapies. Because we do not know many of the components of these therapies, any risk associated with use as single agent or in combination has yet to be identified.
Manual healing methods	Usually involve touch and often are viewed as complementary therapies	Reiki Chiropractic Reflexology Massage Therapeutic touch (misnomer because actual touch is not involved)	Although touch is usually desirable, especially in our culture, the kind of touch has important implications. Controversies related to effect of therapeutic touch have arisen, but it remains a popular complementary therapy.
Diet, nutrition, and lifestyle changes	Use of food or other supplements to prevent and treat illness Appeal to patients because they can be initiated immediately and patients have control over them	Macrobiotics Kelley-Gonzalez High-dose vitamin therapies Antioxidants	Some controversies are related to risk of malnutrition with restrictive dietary programs, effects of antioxidants and/or vitamins during certain therapies, and effects of soy in certain cancers.

5. How often do patients with cancer seek CAM therapies?

In a 1990 survey of over 5,000 patients with cancer, Lerner and Kennedy found that 9% reported having used at least one of these therapies. In 2000, Richardson and colleagues reported an 83% rate of CAM therapy use in 453 people treated at a major cancer center. In a small Canadian survey, 75% of 30 patients with cancer reported using some form of CAM in conjunction with biomedical treatments. Other research reveals CAM therapy use ranging from 50–72%.

6. Do certain patients use CAM therapies more often than others?

Patient demographics revealed by Eisenberg and associates show that women (57%) use CAM therapies more often than men. Younger age (51% > 50 years), more education (77% had > 13 years of education), and higher economic factors (60% > $35,000 annual income) are linked to the use of CAM therapies; certain ethnic and lower socioeconomic groups are reported to use spiritual healing and herbs.

7. Which CAM therapies have been helpful to patients?

The following CAM therapies have been identified as helpful by cancer patients participating in clinical trials:

Spiritual	94%
Imagery	86%
Massage	80%
Lifestyle/diet	60%
Relaxation	50%
Herbal/botanical	20%
High-dose vitamins	14%

8. What political and social factors affect the use of unproven CAM therapies?

A person with cancer often receives information about CAM therapies from well-meaning family members and friends. In an effort to be helpful and supportive, the community often presents the layperson's view of the many choices of therapies. The media (news reports and magazine articles) provide another source, sometimes fraught with misinformation. Many people turn to pamphlets, magazines, and journals. A recent study revealed that most patients obtain information about CAM therapies at health food stores. Most health food store workers made product recommendations (e.g., shark cartilage and essiac) without adequate knowledge of the patient's medical condition and use of other drugs. In addition, some healthcare practitioners promote themselves as having the cure for cancer. Such promotion is seductive and can be misleading to vulnerable patients.

With the widespread interest in CAM therapies in conjunction with conventional treatment for cancer, the National Institutes of Health established the NCCAM. Further national interest in CAM therapy was demonstrated in recent testimony about integrative oncology before the House Committee on Government Reform, which led to the appointment of the White House Commission on Complementary and Alternative Medicine.

9. What research protocols or studies are under way to determine the effects of CAM therapies?

NCCAM has reviewed some CAM therapies in their best-case series. Research in the early 1990s showed that acupuncture was helpful in the management of nausea secondary to chemotherapy. Clinical trials are under way to investigate several approaches, such as the use of oral shark cartilage for patients with advanced lung cancer, pancreatic enzymes and dietary supplements for patients with pancreatic cancer, and PC-SPES for patients with prostate cancer. The Osher Center for Integrative Medicine at the University of California in San Francisco has active studies investigating how lifestyle changes may affect patients with breast and prostate cancer. Spiegel and colleagues reported a beneficial effect of support group intervention in women with metastatic breast cancer. Follow-up studies by Spiegel are under way at the University of Rochester. Examples of research centers and projects are listed in the table on the following page.

PROGRAM	INSTITUTION
NIH-NCCAM-funded research and research centers	
Gonzalez regimen (randomized clincal trial)	Columbia University
Pediatric Center for Complementary and Alternative Medicine	University of Arizona
Botanical Dietary Supplements for Women's Health	University of Illinois, Chicago
Nonpharmacologic Analgesic for Invasive Procedures	Beth Israel Deaconess Medical Center
Neuroprotective Agents from Oriental Medicine	University of Maryland
Neurobiology of Acupuncture Analgesics	Beijing University
Self-transcendence in Breast Cancer Support Groups	University of Texas, Austin
Antioxidant Effects of Herbs on Pain in Cancer Patients	Johns Hopkins University
Method for Making an Improved St. John's Wort	Aphios Corporation
NIH-NCCAM cooperative agreements	
Shark Cartilage Trial	Community Clinical Oncology Program
Shark Cartilage Trial	University of Texas/M.D. Anderson Cooperative Research Base
Center to Assess Alternative Therapy for Chronic Illness	Beth Israel Deaconess Medical Center
UT Center for Alternative Medicine Research in Cancer	University of Texas Health Science Center, Houston
Center for the Study of Complementary and Alternative Therapies for Pain	University of Virginia

10. Do cancer patients use more CAM therapies than patients with other life-threatening or chronic illnesses?

A 1990 Harvard survey found that 1 in 3 (36%) Americans used "unconventional" therapies with visits to providers of alternative therapies exceeding visits to primary care providers. In addition, 70% of those reporting use did not inform their allopathic physician. Respondent demographics are familiar: younger age, female gender, high level of education, and affluence. The most frequent consumers were people with non–life-threatening conditions such as back problems, allergies, asthma, arthritis, anxiety, and depression. More recently, 15 million American adults reported using prescription medications concurrently with herbs and/or high-dose vitamins. Contemporary use of CAM therapies has dramatically increased in persons with cancer by 50–83% in comparison to the previous rate of 46% in a national survey of all Americans.

11. Is there a particular point along the continuum of care when patients with cancer use CAM therapies?

In the past, it was believed that most patients with cancer turned to CAM therapies only when the disease did not respond to conventional therapies or no further therapies were available. Reportedly, they rarely chose alternatives in lieu of conventional therapies. However, given what we now know about lack of disclosure to allopathic practitioners, much of this information is questionable. We know that patients with cancer turn to CAM therapies as complementary to conventional therapies. Many report that their experiences with CAM therapies help to alleviate side effects of conventional therapies and increase their sense of control and well-being. Patients contemplate CAM therapy as a way of avoiding passivity and coping with feelings of hopelessness. A small number of patients report using CAM therapies instead of conventional therapies, even in the face of progressive disease.

12. What complementary and alternative therapies do patients with cancer most frequently use?

Recent surveys report that prayer and spiritual practices are the most commonly used CAM therapies. Mind-body therapies, including relaxation and imagery, and movement (physical therapies) are followed by vitamins, herbal medicine and diet, nutrition, and lifestyle.

13. Which mind-body technique can be used effectively in clinical practice?

Relaxation is a frequently used mind–body therapy that is simple for nurses to use and teach patients and family caregivers. Relaxation is an alert, hypometabolic state of decreased sympathetic nervous system arousal that can be achieved in various ways from simple breathing exercises to hypnosis and biofeedback. The effects of relaxation exercises are gradual and cumulative.

14. Describe the steps of Benson's relaxation technique.

1. Select a focus word or phrase that is comforting to you.
2. Assume any comfortable position and close your eyes. (If preferred, eyes may be open.)
3. Relax your muscles.
4. Breathe slowly and naturally. As you exhale, silently repeat your focus word or phrase to yourself. (If you cannot think of a focus phrase, you can also count slowly from 1 to 10.)
5. If thoughts come to mind, let them go and return to the focus words. Continue for 10–20 minutes.
6. When you are finished, do not stand up immediately. Sit quietly for a minute or two, allowing the return of other thoughts. Then open your eyes and continue sitting for another minute before standing up.
7. Practice once or twice each day.

15. Describe Weil's relaxation/breathing exercise.

1. Place your tongue in the yogic position. Touch the tip of your tongue to the inner surface of the upper front of your teeth, then slide it just above your teeth until it rests on the alveolar ridge, the soft tissue between the teeth and the roof of the mouth. Keep it there during the whole exercise.
2. Exhale completely through the mouth, making an audible whoosh.
3. Close your mouth and inhale quietly through your nose to a (silent) count of four.
4. Hold your breath for the count of seven.
5. Exhale audibly through the mouth to a count of eight.
6. This entire process is one breath cycle. Repeat four times, then breathe normally.
7. If you have difficulty exhaling with your tongue in place, try pursing your lips.

16. Are there any contraindications to massage therapy in patients with cancer?

Because massage stimulates lymphatic drainage and improves circulation, there is concern that it may support the spread of cancer. The general rule is to use gentle massage and to avoid sites of lymphatic drainage around the tumor. An exception is the use of a specific type of massage technique to treat lymphedema after mastectomy. No pressure massage should be used in patients with low platelets (e.g., patients with leukemia or severe marrow depression). Gentle, slow-stroke massage may enhance relaxation and increase feelings of well-being. (For further information about massage in patients with cancer, refer to the *Journal of the American Massage Therapists Association*, Part I, vol. 39(3), Fall 2000, and Part II, vol. 39(4), Winter 2001.)

17. What is therapeutic touch?

Derived from ancient practices of laying on of hands, therapeutic touch is a systematic method for promoting healing or comfort through the use of hands. As described by Krieger, it involves the intentional use of the hands to direct energy to the patient. The three steps in the 15–20 minute therapeutic touch process are (1) centering oneself, letting go of busy thoughts and activities, and intending to be with the person; (2) scanning the person's body with the hands a few inches away from the body to assess personal energy and identify areas of heat or cold or other differences; and (3) moving the hands over the person ("unruffling") and then directing energy with the hands to places within the body that feel tense or distressed.

18. Is therapeutic touch effective?

Research has shown that therapeutic touch is effective in reducing pain, relieving anxiety, reducing behavioral distress in infants and toddlers, and decreasing headache pain. For patients with cancer, therapeutic touch may be used when massage is contraindicated for the general relief of anxiety and stress and for management of pain. Nurses throughout the United States can learn therapeutic touch in nursing schools, through continuing education classes, or from a video produced by the National League for Nursing.

19. What are the Gerson and Kelley-Gonzalez Programs?

Restrictive dietary programs that claim to have therapeutic benefit for patients. Gerson suggests that cancer growth is supported by a potassium and sodium imbalance. Thus, the Gerson program focuses on detoxification, cleansing, and juicing with specific supplementations (low sodium and high potassium). The Kelly-Gonzalez program involves the use of restrictive diet, vitamin and mineral supplementation, pancreatic enzymes, and coffee enemas. Both programs are under investigation in patients with various types of cancer.

20. What controversies surround the use of soy?

Some herbs (e.g., dong quai, ginseng) and soy contain phytoestrogens that may increase the risk of cancer and/or recurrence in women with estrogen-responsive tumors. Soy should not be consumed as a supplement but as a whole food. The American Dietetic Association recommends that soy intake should be limited to 2 servings/week in women who have an estrogen-responsive breast cancer treated with tamoxifen. Further research is needed to determine the risks and benefits of phytoestrogen use.

21. Why should oncology nurses be concerned about the use of herbs by their patients?

The increased use of herbs has magnified the potential for herb-herb and herb-drug interactions and adverse events. Patients should be particularly cautioned not to take an herbal remedy and drug for the same condition. Accurate diagnosis is imperative before using any drug or herb. No one should take any treatment based on what condition they think they have.

22. List some precautions about use of herbs.[15]

1. Patients should be asked about herbal use.
2. "Natural" does not mean safe.
3. Combined use of herbal and pharmaceutical can cause interactions.
4. Herbal content and efficacy are not standardized among manufacturers.
5. Lack of quality control and regulation may result in contamination during manufacture.
6. Herbs are contraindicated for women who are trying to become pregnant, who are pregnant, or who are lactating.
7. Herbal treatments should not be used in larger than recommended doses.
8. Herbal remedies should not be used for more than several weeks.
9. Herbal treatments with known adverse effects and toxicities should be avoided.
10. Infants, children, and elderly people should not use herbal treatments without professional advice.

23. Which herbs can affect platelet aggregation or increase the risk of bleeding?

Patients undergoing surgery or cancer therapies and/or taking anticoagulants should be aware that the following herbs may increase the risk of bleeding or interfere with platelet development: alfalfa, angelica, anise, arnica, Asa Foetida, bogbean, boldo, capsicum, celery, chamomile, clove, danshen, feverfew, garlic, ginger, gingko, horse chestnut, horseradish, licorice, meadowsweet, onion, papain, passion flower, poplar, prickly ash, quassia, red clover, turmeric, wild carrot, wild lettuce, and willow.

24. Which herbs are approved by the Food and Drug Administration?

Aloe (laxative)	Psyllium (laxative)
Capsicum (topical analgesic)	Senna (laxative)
Cascara (laxative)	Witch Hazel (astringent)

25. What herbs are listed as unsafe by the FDA?

American mistletoe, arnica, bittersweet nightshade, bloodroot, broom, chapparal, deadly nightshade, Dutch tonka bean, English tonka bean, ephedra, European mistletoe, heliotrope, horse chestnut, Jimson weed, lily of the valley, lobelia, Madagascar periwinkle, mandrake, Mayapple, morning glory, periwinkle, snakeroot, spindle tree, St. John's wort, sweet flag, true alap, wahoo, wormwood, and yohimbine.

26. Which herbs have sedative properties?

Calamus, calendula, California poppy, catnip, capsicum, celery, couch grass, elecampane, Siberian ginseng, German chamomile, goldenseal, gotu kola, hops, Jamaican dogwood, kava, lemon balm, sage, St. John's wort, sassafras, skullcap, shepherd's purse, stinging nettle, valerian, wild carrot, wild lettuce, and Withania root yerba mansa.

27. How do I know when a CAM therapy practitioner is properly credentialed?

Begin by contacting the state office responsible for professional licensing. The credentialing of each type of practitioner, as well as scope of practice, may vary from state to state. For example, some states license massage therapists and acupuncturists, whereas other states may license only acupuncturists who are physicians or nurses.

28. Can nurses provide CAM therapies as nursing interventions?

Scope of practice issues must be addressed through each state's Nurse Practice Act. In some states, certain interventions may be practiced only under the supervision of a medical doctor. Nurses are responsible for knowing the regulations in their state as well as the policies in their institutions. Before offering therapies to patients, it is important to know whether your institution has a policy about the provision of CAM therapies and to practice accordingly to avoid liability.

Many nurses are trained in massage and therapeutic touch. Some nurses have private practices and often are listed in the directories of their professional organizations. To find nurses trained in massage therapy, contact the National Association of Nurse Massage Therapists (800-336-2668). Nurses experienced in therapeutic touch are often members of the Nurse Healers-Professional Associates (412-355-8476) or the American Holistic Nurses Association (919-787-5181).

29. What should patients with cancer expect from oncology nurses in relation to CAM therapies?

Patients must feel comfortable about confiding in nurses and other health care providers about the use of CAM therapies. A safe, nonjudgmental, caring atmosphere may facilitate this exchange of information. A primary wish of all patients with cancer is that doctors and nurses listen to their struggles with the diagnosis and treatment choices. Many patients look for guidance that makes them a full partner in designing their treatment. Patients may turn first to a nurse to explore his or her thoughts. The ethical dilemma facing nurses is to balance the patient's rights of free choice and personal control with the duty to protect the patient from harm. Nurses need to be knowledgeable about various CAM therapies or able to refer patients to appropriate, reliable references.

30. Where can the person with cancer obtain information about CAM therapies?

Many resources are available. However, not all provide reliable information. Public libraries and bookstores have a variety of resources. The following resources provide dependable and different information about complementary and alternative therapies:

- American Cancer Society: 1-800-ACS-2345; website: http://www.cancer.org.
- National Cancer Institute's Cancer Information Service: 1-800-2422-6237.
- National Institutes of Health National Center for Complementary and Alternative Medicine: 1-888-644-6226.; websites: http://nccam.NIH.gov/nccam; http://altmed.od.nih.gov/nccam; and http:// nccam.nih.gov/nccam/research/grants/rfb/fy99.html
- Alternative Medicine Foundation, Bethesda, MD: 301-581-0116. website: http://www.AMFoundation.org or http://www.herbmed.org.

- Center for Alternative Medicine Research and Education at Beth Israel Deaconess Medical Center, Boston: 617-632-7770; website: http://www.compmed.caregroup.org.
- HealthWorld Online, Culver City, CA: http://healthy.net/wlcome/story/p2htm.
- National Medicines Comprehensive Database: *Pharmacist's Letter*, Stockton, CA. 209-472-2244; website: http://www.naturaldatabase.com
- Review of Natural Products Facts and Comparisons, St. Louis: 800-223-0554; website: http://www.drugfacts.com
- Richard and Hilda Rosenthal Center for Complementary and Alternative Medicine, Columbia, University, College of Physicians and Surgeons, New York: 212-543-9550; website: http://Cpmcnet.columbia.edu/dept/rosenthal
- Onebody.com offers direct communication with providers of holistic care, integrated care, and research.
- www.amtamassage.org offers information about massage therapy.

31. What journals or books are helpful for nurses as well as patients?

Scientific Review of Alternative Medicine: www.hcrc.org/stram

Focus on Alternative and Complementary Therapies (FACT): www.fact@exeter.ac.com

Alternative Therapies in Health and Medicine: www.alternative-therapies.com

Nutrition after Cancer: A Guide for Informed Choices. American Cancer Society, publication pending.

Blumenthal M (ed): The Complete German Commission E Monographs. Austin, TX Botanical Council, 1998.

Geffen J: The Journey through Cancer: An Oncologist's Seven Level Program for Healing and Transforming the Whole Person. New York, Crown Publishers, 2000.

Decker G (ed): An Introduction to Complementary and Alternative Therapies. Pittsburgh, Oncology Nursing Press, 1999.

Foster S, Tyler VE: The Honest Herbal. Binghamton, NY, Pharmaceutical Products Press 1999.

Gordon J: Manifesto for a New Medicine: Your Guide to Healing Partnerships and the Wise Use of Alternative Therapies. New York, Addison-Wesley, 1996.

Gordon J: Comprehensive Cancer Care. Cambridge, MA, Perseus Publishing, 2000.

Lerner M: Choices in Healing: Integrating the Best of Conventional and Complementary Approaches to Cancer. Cambridge, MA, MIT Press, 1994.

Pelton R, Overholser L: Alternatives in Cancer Therapy: The Complete Guide to Non-traditional Treatments. New York, Simon & Schuster, 1994.

Physicians' Desk Reference for Herbal Medicine, 2nd ed. Montvale, NJ, Medical Economics Company, 2000.

REFERENCES

1. Acupuncture. NIH Consensus Statement. Bethesda, MD, National Institutes of Health, 1997, pp 1–34.
2. Bennet M, Lengacher C: Use of complementary therapies in a rural cancer population. Oncol Nurs Forum 26:1287–1294.
3. Benson H, Stark M: Timeless Healing: The Power and Biology of Belief. New York, Simon & Schuster, 1997.
4. Blumenthal M (ed): The Complete German Commission E Monographs. Austin, TX Botanical Council, 1998.
5. Burstein HJ, Gelber S, Guadagnoli E, Weeks JC : Use of alternative medicine by women with early stage cancer. N Engl J Med 340:1733–1739.
6. Cassileth BR: Evaluating complementary and alternative therapies for cancer patients. CA Cancer J Clin 49:362–375, 1999.
7. Cassileth B, Chapman C: Alternative and complementary cancer therapies. Cancer 77:1026–1034, 1996.
8. Cannistra SA (ed): Can the mind fight cancer? Cancer Smart 4:9, 1998.
9. Decker GM, Myers J: Commonly used herbs. Can J Oncol Nurs [in press].
10. Eisenberg DM, Davis RB, Ettner SL, et al: Trends in alternative medicine in the United States, 1990–1997: Results of a follow-up national survey. J AMA 29:1569–1575. 1998.

11. Eisenberg DM, Kessler RC, Foster C, et al: Unconventional medicine in the United States. N Engl J Med 328:246–252, 1993.
12. Fletcher DM: Unconventional cancer treatments: Professional, legal and ethical issues. Oncol Nurs Forum 19:1351–1355, 1992.
13. Geffen J: The Journey Through Cancer: An Oncologist's Seven-Level Program for Healing and Transforming the whole Person. New York, Crown Publishers, 2000.
14. Gotay CC, Dimitriu D: Health food store recommendations for breast cancer patients. Arch Fam Med 9:692–699, 2000.
15. Heinerman J: Heinerman's Encyclopedia of Healing Herbs and Spices. Englewood Cliffs, NJ, Prentice-Hall, 1996.
16. Kao GD, Devine P: Use of complementary health practices by prostate cancer patients undergoing radiation therapy. Cancer 88:615–619, 2000.
17. Lerner IS, Kennedy BJ: The prevalence of questionable methods of cancer treatment in the US. Cancer 42:181–191, 1992.
18 Montbriand MJ: Freedom of choice: An issue concerning alternative therapies chosen by patients with cancer. Oncol Nurs Forum 20:1195–1200, 1993.
19. National Institutes of Health National National Center for Complementary and Alternative Medicine Website:http://nccam.nih.gov/nccam/research/grants/rfb/fy99.html.
20. Oncology Nursing Society Position on Complementary and Alternative Therapies. Pittsburgh, Oncology Nursing Press, 2000.
21. Physicians' Desk Reference for Herbal Medicine, 2nd ed. Montvale, NJ, Medical Economics Company, 2000.
22. Richardson MA, Sanders T, Palmer JL, et al: Complementary/alternative medicine use in a comprehensive cancer center and the implication for oncology. J Clin Oncol 18:2505–2514.
23. Rosenfeld I: Dr. Rosenfeld's Guide to Alternative Medicine. New York,: Random House, 1996.
24. Ryder BG: The Alpha Book on Cancer and Living. Alameda, CA, Alpha Institute, 1997.
25. Sollner W, Maislinger S, DeVries A, et al: Use of complementary and alternative medicine by cancer patients is not associated with perceived distress or poor compliance with standard treatment but with active coping behavior: A survey. Cancer 89:873–880, 2000.
26. Sparber A, Bauer L, Curt G, et al: Use of complementary medicine by adult patients participating in cancer clinical trials. Oncol Nurs Forum 27:623–630, 2000.
27. Spiegel D, Morrow GR, Classen C, et al: Group psychotherapy for recently diagnosed breast cancer patients: A multicenter feasibility study. Psychooncology 8:482, 1999.
28. Strasen L: The silent healthcare revolution: The rising demand for complementary medicine. Nurs Econ 17:246–256, 1999.
29. Vandecreek L, Rogers E, Lester J: Use of alternative therapies among breast cancer outpatients compared with the general population. Altern Ther Health Med 5:71–76, 1999.
30. Weil A: Eight Eeeks to Optimum Health. New York, Alfred Knopf, 1997, p 108.
31. White JD: Complementary, alternative, and unproven methods of cancer treatment. In DeVita VT, Hellman S, Rosenberg SA (eds): Cancer: Principles and Practive of Oncology, 6th ed. Philadelphia, Lippincott Williams & Wilkins, 2001, pp 3147–3157.

III. Hematologic Malignancies

17. HODGKIN'S DISEASE

Robert Avery, MD, FACP, and Elder Granger, MD, FACP

Quick Facts—Hodgkin's Disease

Incidence	In the United States, it is estimated that Hodgkin's disease will be diagnosed in 7400 people in 2001 (< 1% of all new cancers). Rare in children under 10 years of age. Bimodal age distribution: first peak at 25–30 years (5 cases per 100,000) and second peak at 75–80 years (7 per 100,000). Sex distribution nearly equal in adults (before age 10, more frequent in boys).
Mortality	Estimated 1300 deaths in 2001.
Etiology	Unknown; possibly related to Epstein-Barr virus.
Risk factors	Increased parental education and small family size (delayed-infection); 90% of cases in Caucasians

Rye's Histologic Classification

TYPE	INCIDENCE (%)	PRESENTATION	PROGNOSIS
Lymphocyte-predominant	5	Healthy young male, stage I–II	Excellent
Mixed cellularity	30	Any stage, often retroperitoneum, HIV cases	Fair
Nodular sclerosis	60	Female predominance; neck or mediastinum	Good
Lymphocyte-depleted	2	Wasting syndrome, febrile, liver +, marrow +	Poor

Signs and symptoms	Asymptomatic cervical, supraclavicular, and mediastinal nodes Enlarged superficial nodes (70%) Mediastinal adenopathy (50–60%) Involvement of spleen and paraaortic nodes (25–40%) Infradiaphragmatic presentations (about 15%) Unexplained weight loss Unexplained fever with temperatures above 38.5°C (101°F) Drenching night sweats Pruritus (10–15%) Lymph node pain with alcohol ingestion (1–10%)
Metastases	Liver and bone marrow (5–10%)
Ann Arbor staging system	Stage I Involvement of single lymph node region (I) or single extralymphatic organ or site (I_E)
	Stage II Involvement of 2 or more lymph node regions on same side of diaphragm (II) or localized involvement of extralymphatic organ or site (II_E)
	Stage III Involvement of lymph node regions on both side of diaphragm (III), possibly with an extralymphatic organ or site (III_E), involvement of spleen (III_S), or both (III_{SE})
	Stage IV Disseminated involvement of 1 or more extralymphatic organs, with or without associated lymph node involvement, or isolated extralymphatic organ site with distant nodal involvement
	All stages are subclassified as A (asymptomatic) or B (fever, night sweats, loss of > 10% of body weight).

Table continued on following page

153

Quick Facts—Hodgkin's Disease

Treatment	Stages I, IIA		Chemotherapy for 4 months + limited radiation therapy or full-field radiation therapy alone
	Stages IB, IIB, IIIA, IIIA$_1$		Chemotherapy for 6 months ± radiation therapy
	Stages IIIA$_2$, IIIB		Chemotherapy for 6 months ± radiation therapy
	Stage IVA, IVB		Chemotherapy for 6 months ± radiation therapy
	Bulky mediastinal disease		Chemotherapy for 6 months + radiation therapy
5-year	Stages I, IIA	85–95%	Stages IIIA$_2$, IIIB 60–80%
disease-free	Stages IB, IIB	80–85%	Stages IVA, IVB 30–50%
survival rate	Stages IIIA, IIIA$_1$	60–85%	

1. What is Hodgkin's disease?

Hodgkin's disease (HD) is a malignancy of unknown etiology usually arising in lymph nodes. It often affects young adults and is one of the most curable cancers. The histologic pattern and anatomic distribution vary with age. HD is a histologic diagnosis based on the recognition of multinucleated Reed-Sternberg (RS) cells surrounded by a background of benign-appearing host inflammatory cells composed of lymphocytes, plasma cells, and fibroblasts.

2. Describe a Reed-Sternberg cell.

The RS cell, which is considered malignant, is diagnostic of HD. It may have one or more nuclei or nuclear lobes and two or more large nucleoli. A variant called the L&H cell has a nucleus that resembles a popped kernel of corn and is called a popcorn cell. The origin of the RS cell is unknown, but it is thought to be an altered B lymphocyte. In rare instances, cells resembling RS cells are found in benign illnesses and other malignancies.

3. How is Hodgkin's disease related to a viral cause?

Although the cause of HD is unknown, a viral association is implicated by occasional case clusterings, immune defects, and the presence of Epstein-Barr virus (EBV) genome in involved lymph nodes.

4. Compare the four histologic types of HD.

Lymphocyte-predominant (nodular and diffuse). Nodular lymphocyte-predominant HD is essentially B-cell lymphoma. Most patients present with early-stage disease; systemic symptoms are infrequent (10%). The 5-year survival rate is approximately 90%; relapses after 5 years may be seen.

Mixed cellularity. RS cells are rare and may be mistaken for T-cell or diffuse large cell lymphomas. It often presents in older patients with more advanced-stage disease and is most common among patients with acquired immunodeficiency syndrome (AIDS). The 5-year survival rate for all stages is 50–60%.

Nodular sclerosis. The most common histopathologic type, nodular sclerosis, is found more often in women and young adults. It is associated with the lacunar cell variant of the RS cell. Patients often present with neck or mediastinal lymphadenopathy. The incidence of systemic symptoms is about 30%. Prognosis is good, with a high 5-year survival rate.

Lymphocyte-depleted. This rare form of HD was earlier mistaken for large-cell lymphoma. It presents primarily in older patients with advanced-stage disease and has the worst prognosis of the four types. The 5-year survival rate is < 50%.

5. What are the Cotswolds staging modifications?

In 1989 an international conference in Cotswolds, England recommended the following modifications of the Ann Arbor staging system:

- Suffix X should be added to patients with bulky disease (maximal dimension of nodal mass > 10 cm or mediastinal mass > $\frac{1}{3}$ of the chest wall diameter).

- The number of anatomic regions involved should be indicated by a subscript (e.g., II_3).
- A new category of response to therapy, unconfirmed/uncertain complete remission (CRu), should be used to designate patients achieving > 90% partial response with stable adenopathy.

6. What signs and symptoms are associated with HD?

Cervical, supraclavicular, and mediastinal nodes are involved in 50–70% of cases. In contrast to non-Hodgkin's lymphoma, HD can be isolated and exhibits more orderly or contiguous lymph node spread. Generalized pruritus occurs in 10–15% of cases and lymph node pain with alcohol ingestion in 1–10% of the cases. Patients also may be anergic (i.e., they do not react to allergy skin testing). B symptoms (indicative of larger tumor burden) consist of unexplained loss of > 10% of body weight in the previous 6 months, unexplained fever with temperatures above 38.5°C (101°F), and drenching night sweats. Common laboratory findings include elevated sedimentation rate and elevated levels of lactate dehydrogenase (LDH).

7. What are the poor prognostic factors in HD?

The stage or extent of disease is the most important prognostic variable. Other factors indicative of a poorer prognosis include bone marrow, lung, or liver involvement; bulky disease (nodal diameter > 10 cm); B symptoms; high erythrocyte sedimentation rate; low hematocrit and high LDH (higher rate of relapse); large mediastinal mass; and age over 65 years. Extensive splenic involvement has a poor prognosis if treated with primary irradiation. Elderly patients tend to present with more advanced stages, a worse prognostic histology, and other medical problems that cause difficulty in tolerating chemotherapy.

8. How is the diagnosis of HD usually established?

In addition to adequate surgical biopsy of involved tissue, the following procedures for staging are recommended:

- Detailed history recording duration and presence or absence of B symptoms and unexplained pruritus
- Detailed physical examination with special attention to all node-bearing areas
- Radiologic studies: chest radiograph; computed tomography (CT) of thorax, abdomen, and pelvis; bipedal lymphangiogram (optional)
- Hematologic studies: complete blood count (CBC); erythrocyte sedimentation rate; bilateral bone marrow biopsy
- Biochemistry: liver function tests; renal function test; serum LDH, albumin, calcium, and alkaline phosphatase
- Other procedures: gallium and technetium isotope scanning; multiple-gated acquisition blood-pool scan (MUGA); magnetic resonance imaging (MRI); staging laparotomy (optional)

9. How does stage affect treatment choice?

Radiation therapy is highly effective for early-stage disease, whereas chemotherapy is more effective for late-stage disease.

10. When is staging laparotomy indicated?

Diagnostic staging laparotomy has been one of the most controversial areas in HD management. Few randomized trials have fully assessed its necessity. Of note, 40% of patients with clinical stage IA or IIA disease require extended courses of chemotherapy, 20% due to upstaging and 20% due to relapse. For this reason, recent trials have evaluated the use of short-course chemotherapy followed by involved-field radiation. Sufficient data now available demonstrate that short-course chemotherapy followed by radiation therapy is a highly effective means to treat early-stage HD and has eliminated the need for staging laparotomy.

Some patients with early-stage HD have a low risk of disease below the diaphragm, do not require staging laparotomy, and are candidates for radiation therapy alone. The most favorable prognostic group includes women younger than 40 years with lymphocyte-predominant HD or nodular sclerosing HD, stage I disease, no B symptoms, normal erythrocyte sedimentation rate, and only 1 lymph node group involved. Other favorable groups include patients with clinical stage I disease and mediastinal disease only, men with clinical stage I disease and lymphocyte-predominant histology, and women with clinical stage II disease with only 2–3 sites of involvement.

Patients with high-risk early-stage disease require combined chemotherapy and radiation therapy. High risk factors include age > 49, large mediastinal mass, B symptoms, erythrocyte sedimentation rate > 30, or more than 3 sites of involvement.

11. How is HD treated?
More than 75% of cases are curable, and more than 50% of recurrent disease after primary therapy can be cured. HD responds to radiation therapy alone, combination chemotherapy, or radiation and chemotherapy combined.

12. What chemotherapy regimens are effective in treating HD?
The most common regimens are MOPP and ABVD (see table below). Each regimen is given over 28 days, and most patients receive 6 cycles. If tumor burden is reduced between the fourth and sixth cycles, two more cycles are given. Patients are treated over 6–8 months (2 months after best response). Hybrid variations of these regimens include combined MOPP/ABV and alternating MOPP/ABVD. ABVD and the hybrid regimens have been proved more effective than MOPP alone, and ABVD has fewer long-term side effects, such as risk of leukemia and azoospermia. Therefore, ABVD is the current regimen of choice for advanced HD.

Chemotherapy for Hodgkin's Disease

DRUGS	DOSE (MG/M^2)	ROUTE	DAYS
MOPP			
Mechlorethamine (nitrogen mustard)	6	IV	1, 8
Oncovin (vincristine)	1.4	IV	1, 8
Procarbazine	100	PO	1–14
Prednisone	40	PO	1–14
ABVD			
Adriamycin (doxorubicin)	25	IV	1, 15
Bleomycin	10	IV	1, 15
Vinblastine	6	IV	1, 15
Dacarbazine	375	IV	1, 15

IV = intravenously, PO = orally.

13. Discuss the common complications of chemotherapy.
Complications and side effects include nausea, vomiting, alopecia, sterility in men and women, myelosuppression, neuropathy, cardiomyopathy, and aseptic necrosis of femoral heads (related to prednisone). Although secondary malignancies (acute nonlymphocytic leukemia and non-Hodgkin's lymphoma) are associated with chemotherapy alone, they are more common after radiation plus chemotherapy. ABVD is not associated with an increased risk of myelodysplasia or acute leukemia, nor does it cause sterility. However, it is associated with more cardiac and pulmonary toxicity.

14. What is the most common complication of radiation therapy?
Hypothyroidism is the most common complication of mantle radiation therapy. It can be treated with thyroid replacement therapy. Other complications include myelosuppression, pericarditis, pneumonitis, myelopathy, and transient azoospermia. Secondary cancers related to radiation therapy include solid tumors (e.g., breast, lung, thyroid cancer), sarcomas, salivary cancer, and skin cancers. The risk of breast cancer is high in women who have received radiation therapy before the age of 20, and the risk of lung cancer is increased 9 times if the patient smokes.

15. What is Lhermitte's syndrome?
From 6–12 weeks after mantle radiation therapy, approximately 15% of patients develop a shocklike sensation radiating down the back of the extremities when the head is flexed. This is

due to radiation causing temporary demyelinization of the spinal cord. The symptoms resolve spontaneously and do not cause any permanent neurologic damage.

16. Describe the role of bone marrow transplantation in the present and future treatment of HD.

The results of clinical studies of high-dose chemotherapy (HDC) with autologous bone marrow or peripheral stem cell infusion have been promising. Although the results vary because of diverse patient populations, multiple studies have shown complete remission rates of 40–70% with 5-year relapse-free survival rates of 20–40%. Randomized studies comparing standard- dose salvage chemotherapy with HDC are lacking. Current data support the use of HDC for patients who are resistant to or have relapsed from primary chemotherapy. Peripheral blood stem cells can be used instead of autologous bone marrow for patients with inadequate marrow.

17. Discuss the most important nursing considerations in caring for patients with HD.

In addition to providing patient education and support through a long and highly toxic regimen of primary therapy, nurses need to pay particular attention to information about potential long-term effects and development of secondary cancers. In addition, higher levels of chronic fatigue, anxiety, and depression requiring psychosocial support are found in survivors of HD.

The patient must be educated about the prolonged period of appropriate follow-up for possible recurrence after therapy. The patient must understand that a small foci of Hodgkin's disease may cause no symptoms but still lead to relapse or recurrence. All members of the multidisciplinary team should be sensitive to the patient's fear of recurrence. The patient may interpret every word or facial expression of the treatment team as a likely clue that the HD has recurred. The risk of relapse is greatest within the first 2 years and decreases with time. Follow-up should include physical examinations, radiographs, and appropriate blood work (e.g., LDH, CBC, alkaline phosphatase) every 3 months for the first 2 years, every 6 months for the third through fifth years, and then annually. Generally, patients are considered cured if they remain in remission for 5 years.

18. What is the effect of pregnancy on HD? Of HD on pregnancy?

Pregnancy has no documented adverse effect on the natural history of HD, and HD has no effect on the course of gestation, delivery, or incidence of prematurity or spontaneous abortions. The management of HD during pregnancy must be individualized. Therapeutic abortion is not mandatory, and many patients have been successfully treated while pregnant with no adverse effect on the fetus. The greatest risk to the fetus is in the first trimester. A therapeutic abortion may be medically indicated if treatment with chemotherapy or irradiation is required because of evidence of rapid disease progression, visceral involvement, or systemic symptoms. If treatment cannot be delayed, modified supradiaphragmatic irradiation or chemotherapy can be used safely. Survivors of HD may have an increased risk of miscarriage as a result of chemotherapy and radiation therapy.

19. Are patients with AIDS at increased risk of developing HD?

HIV-positive patients are at increased risk of developing HD and usually present with aggressive, advanced-stage disease and B symptoms. HD is not an AIDS-defining cancer at this time. Treatment with standard chemotherapy may produce long-term remissions, but 50% of patients die within 15 months, one-half due to HD and one-half due to opportunistic infections.

20. Discuss future directions for HD.

Investigations are being conducted for administration of less toxic regimens, use of biologic response modifiers, and administration of high-dose chemotherapy with bone marrow transplantation. Because of the high chance of cure, efforts are under way to reduce the long-term effects of therapy.

The views expressed in this chapter are those of the author and do not necessarily reflect the views of the Department of Defense or any of its agencies.

REFERENCES

1. Bhatia S, Robison LL, Ooberlin O, et al: Breast cancer and other second neoplasms after childhood Hodgkin's disease. N Engl J Med 334:745–751, 1996.
2. Brain MC, Carbone PP (eds): Current Therapy in Hematology-Oncology, 5th ed. St. Louis, Mosby, 1995.
3. Cabanillas FF, Rodriguez MA, Waxman L: MD Anderson lymphoma practice guidelines. www.oncology.com/pg/LymphomaAndAidsRelated/Group-Lymphoma.pdf
4. Canellos G, Anderson JR, Propert KJ, et al: Chemotherapy of advanced Hodgkin's disease with MOPP, ABVD, or MOPP alternating with ABVD. N Engl J Med 327:1478–1484, 1992.
5. Connors J, Reece DE, Diehl V, Engbert A: Hodgkin's lymphoma: New approaches to treatment. American Society of Hematology, Educational materials, 1998, www.hematology.org/education/hema98/connors.pdf
6. Diehl V, Mauch P, Connors JM: Hodgkin's lymphoma. American Society of Hematology, Educational materials 1999, www.hematology.org/education/hema99/diehl.pdf
7. Diehl V, Mauch PM, Harris NL: Hodgkin's disease. In DeVita VT, Hellman S, Rosenberg SA (eds): Cancer: Principles and Practice of Oncology, 6th ed. Philadelphia, Lippincott-Raven, 2001, pp 2339–2387.
8. Diehl V, Josting A: Hodgkin's disease. Cancer J Sci Am 6(Suppl. 2):S150–S158, 2000.
9. Fleming ID, Cooper JS, Henson DE, et al: AJCC Cancer Staging Handbook, 5th ed. Philadelphia, Lippincott-Raven, 1998, pp 259–261.
10. Greenlee RT, Hill-Harmon MB, Murray T, Thun M: Cancer statistics, 2001. CA Cancer J Clin 51:15–36, 2001.
11. Klasa R, Connors JM, Fairey R, et al: Treatment of early stage Hodgkins's disease: Improved outcome with brief chemotherapy and radiation without staging laparotomy. Ann Oncol 7:10, 1996.
12. Loge JH: Fatigue and psychiatric morbidity among Hodgkins's disease survivors. J Pain Symptom Manage 19 (2):91–99, 2000.
13. Murphy GP, Lawrence W, Lenhard RE: Hodgkin's disease and non-Hodgkin's lymphomas. In American Cancer Society Textbook of Clinical Oncology, 2nd ed. Atlanta, GA, American Cancer Society, 1995, pp 451–469.
14. Peleg D, Ben-Ami M: Cancer complicating pregnancy: Lymphoma and leukemia complicating pregnancy. Obstet Gynecol Clin North Am 25:366–383, 1998.
15. Prior E, Goldberg AF, Conjalka MS, et al: Hodgkin's disease in homosexual men: An AIDS-related phenomenon? Am J Med 81:1085–1088, 1986.
16. Santoro A, Bonfante V, Viviani S, et al: Subtotal nodal (STNI) vs. involved field (IFRT) irradiation after 4 cycles of ABVD in early stage Hodgkin's Disease (HD). Proce Am Soc Clin Oncol 15:A1271, 415, 1996.
17. Strauss DJ: Human immunodeficiency virus-associated lymphomas. Med Clin North Am 81:495–510, 1997.
18. Van Leeuwen FE, Klokman WJ, Stovall M, et al: Roles of radiotherapy and smoking in lung cancer following Hodkin's disease. J Natl Cancer Inst 87:1530–1537, 1995.

18. LEUKEMIA

Lowell Anderson-Reitz, RN, MS, ANP, AOCN, and Jeff Matous, MD

1. Define leukemia.

Leukemia is a group of hematologic diseases of bone marrow and lymph tissue. It includes abnormalities of proliferation and maturation of both myeloid and lymphoid cell lines. The effect of leukemia is proliferation of abnormal white cells, which overcrowd the bone marrow and cause decreased function of normal hematopoietic stem cells.

2. List the four primary types of leukemia.

1. Acute myelogenous leukemia (AML)
2. Acute lymphocytic leukemia (ALL)
3. Chronic myelogenous leukemia (CML)
4. Chronic lymphocytic leukemia (CLL)

3. What are the less common diseases of blood-forming cells?

Hairy cell leukemia, myelodysplastic syndrome, myeloproliferative disease, polycythemia vera, and plasma cell dyscrasias (e.g., multiple myeloma, Waldenstrom's macroglobulinemia).

4. How do acute leukemias differ from chronic leukemias?

Acute leukemias are malignancies of hematopoietic stem cells. The diagnosis is based on the cell of origin with attention to morphologic features as well as cytochemical, immunophenotypic, and cytogenetic information. The acute leukemias are aggressive diseases with a short natural history.

Chronic leukemias are myeloproliferative or lymphoproliferative disorders. CML is a clonal disease of myeloid stem cells. CLL is characterized by proliferation of mature-appearing lymphocytes in marrow, blood, spleen, and lymph nodes. The chronic leukemias also are characterized by unique immunophenotypic, cytogenetic, and molecular changes. Their natural history is progressive and marked by indolent periods.

5. Describe the classification system for AML.

AML is classified most often according to the French-American-British (FAB) system, which consists of subtypes based on cell origin and morphology as well as flow cytometric and immunohistochemic differences. In the future, AML probably will be classified by molecular and cytogenetic differences rather than cell morphology.

French-American-British Classification of Acute Myelogenous Leukemia

M0	Acute myeloblastic leukemia, minimally differentiated
M1	Acute myeloblastic leukemia without maturation
M2	Acute myeloblastic leukemia with differentiation
M3	Acute promyelocytic leukemia
M4	Acute myelomonocytic leukemia
M5	Acute monocytic leukemia
M6	Erythroleukemia
M7	Acute megakaryoblastic leukemia

6. How is the prognosis of AML determined?

Prognosis is based primarily on age and identified chromosomal translocations as opposed to FAB subtypes. The translocations associated with better prognosis are t(8;21), t(15;17), and inversion 16.

7. Describe the classification system for ALL.

The FAB subtypes are **L1, L2,** and **L3**. They are based on cell size, nuclear shape, amount and appearance of cytoplasm, and number and prominence of nucleoli. Further differentiation of ALL subtypes is based on morphology, immunophenotypic typing of malignant cells, and clinical features such as age, tumor burden at diagnosis, presence or absence of splenomegaly, and presence or absence of central nervous system involvement.

8. How is CML classified?

CML is characterized by a chromosomal rearrangement known as the Philadelphia chromosome and has three distinct phases. The **chronic phase** usually lasts 3–5 years and normally is associated with few symptoms. The **accelerated** and **blast phases** resemble acute leukemias and have a poor prognosis.

9. How is CLL classified?

Classification is based on clinical presentation. A modified version of the Rai system consists of three stages: low risk, intermediate risk, and high risk. Prognosis is directly related to each stage. The **low-risk group** is associated with isolated lymphocytosis; the **intermediate-risk group** exhibits lymphocytosis with lymphadenopathy and/or splenomegaly; and the **high-risk group** is identified by lymphocytosis with anemia and/or thrombocytopenia. Survival usually is measured in years.

10. Discuss the incidence of AML.

AML occurs more frequently in industrialized countries and has an overall incidence of 2.25 cases per 100,000 population. The incidence increases with age; the median age at diagnosis is 64 years. AML is more common in men than in women. In 2001, new cases of AML are estimated at 10,000, with 7,200 deaths.

11. What causes AML?

AML, also known as acute nonlymphocytic leukemia (ANLL), is a malignancy of the myeloid or monocytic stem cell. The exact cause is unknown. Several genetic disorders are associated with development of AML, suggesting a genetic link. Chromosomal abnormalities associated with AML probably result from acquired genetic mutations over the person's lifetime. Environmental exposures have been implicated, including smoking, solvents (e.g., benzene), rubber and paint manufacturing, radiation exposure, and alkylating chemotherapy agents.

12. What is the cure rate for AML?

AML is an aggressive disease that, if left untreated, results in death within months. Current treatments provide a cure rate near 40%.

13. Describe the presenting signs and symptoms of AML.

The signs and symptoms at the time of diagnosis result from abnormal hematopoiesis. Because of the increased production of immature, nonfunctioning leukemic cells and decreased numbers of other white cells, infection with fever is one of the most common signs. Platelet production also is limited by overcrowding of bone marrow space with leukemic cells. Associated signs include increased bruising, petechiae, bleeding gums, and epistaxis. Patients often experience significant malaise and fatigue as a result of severe anemia. Less common signs and symptoms include swollen gums, bone pain, sweats, weight loss, skin lesions, adenopathy, and involvement of the central nervous system.

14. What are the common treatment courses for AML?

AML is treated most commonly with an intense chemotherapy induction and consolidation plan. Cytarabine and anthracycline-type agents (e.g., mitoxantrone, idarubicin, daunorubicin) are generally accepted treatments in the **induction phase**, which often is called the 7 and 3 treatment course. A common example follows:

Cytarabine, 100 mg/m^2/day, as a continuous intravenous (IV) infusion for 7 days
and
Idarubicin, 12 mg/m^2, as an IV push (IVP) on days 1, 2, and 3

A bone marrow biopsy often is performed on day 14 to determine the status of the leukemia. If the bone marrow is free of disease, the first consolidation course is initiated in 3–4 weeks. If residual disease is seen, the patient often undergoes an additional induction phase with the same drugs or a new combination. The **consolidation phase** most commonly consists of 2–4 cycles of high-dose cytarabine (HIDAC):

Cytarabine, 3 gm/m^2 IV every 12 hours for 6 doses over 3–5 days

15. Discuss the role of bone marrow transplant in patients with AML.

Allogeneic bone marrow transplantation during the first remission has become more accepted over time. Currently it offers a cure rate of 50–60%. Success depends on dose intensity in conjunction with the graft vs. leukemia effect of the donor's lymphocytes. Because morbidity and mortality rates are higher (20–30%) with bone marrow transplantation, risk vs. benefit must be discussed before choosing among treatment options.

16. What is the graft vs. leukemia effect?

An allogeneic bone marrow transplant provides the recipient with a new immune system. The active T cells recognize the malignant leukemic cells as foreign and abnormal. The desired effect is that the T cells will be vigilant in ridding the body of abnormal leukemic cells.

17. How is acute promyelocytic leukemia (APL) treated?

The treatment of APL (subtype M3 of AML) includes the use of all-transretinoic acid (ATRA) for many months. This regimen, in addition to standard induction therapy, has improved the cure rate for APL.

18. Describe the treatment of relapsed AML.

Relapsed AML is curable only with stem-cell transplantation. Traditionally, a course of chemotherapy is administered in an attempt to induce a second remission before transplantation. The current approach uses chemotherapy with or without monoclonal antibody treatment.

19. How is relapsed AML treated in patients who have undergone allogeneic bone marrow transplantation?

The first line of treatment is donor lymphocyte infusion (DLI), which is intended to enhance the graft vs. leukemia effect and eradicate leukemic cells. Monoclonal antibodies also may be used.

20. Discuss the role of monoclonal antibodies in the treatment of relapsed AML.

Monoclonal antibodies may be used for both transplant and traditionally treated patients. The most promising example is CMA-676 (Mylotarg), also known as anti-CD33 antibody. Mylotarg is complexed with calicheamicin, an antitumor antibiotic. Nearly 90% of AML cells express CD33 on their surface. When Mylotarg is infused, it specifically seeks out cells expressing CD33, and the calicheamicin generates double-stranded DNA breaks that lead to cell death. Complete remission has been seen in nearly 30% of patients treated with Mylotarg. New treatments using monoclonal antibodies are under development and probably will become first-line therapies as well as mainstays of treatment for relapsed AML.

21. What other treatments are under investigation?

Trials using arsenic for treatment of relapsed M3 APL are under way. Several studies are examining the use of both ATRA and arsenic for first-line therapy as well as treatment of relapsed leukemia.

22. Discuss the incidence of ALL.

In 2001, approximately 3500 new cases will be diagnosed in the United States, and approximately 75% of all cases are in children younger than 15 years. ALL is more common in boys and Caucasians than in girls and other races. It is the most common childhood malignancy.

23. What causes ALL?

The cause is unknown.

24. What is the cure rate for ALL?

ALL is an aggressive malignancy of lymphoid stem cells that, if left untreated, leads to death within months. Before the availability of intense chemotherapy regimens, it was always fatal. With current therapies the cure rate is 70–80%.

25. How does ALL differ from AML?

The malignant lymphoid clone of ALL originates in bone marrow, thymus, and lymph tissue. The lymphoblasts have a propensity for tissue infiltration and often sequester in sanctuary sites such as the central nervous system (CNS) and testicles.

26. Describe the presenting signs and symptoms of ALL.

The most common signs and symptoms are associated with abnormal hematopoiesis or organ infiltration by leukemic cells. Malaise, fatigue, fever, and bone pain are the most common symptoms at diagnosis. Malaise and fatigue result from anemia, whereas fever most often is associated with the disease itself and often resolves with therapy. Bone pain is associated with bone erosion or infiltration of the periosteum with leukemic cells. Pain may result from organ involvement (e.g., hepatomegaly, splenomegaly). Patients with CNS involvement may experience nausea, vomiting, or headaches.

27. How is ALL treated?

The general treatment for ALL is divided into three phases: (1) the **induction phase**, which is intended to eradicate the disease; (2) the **intensification phase**, which has dramatically improved survival rates; and (3) the **maintenance phase**, which begins once remission has been achieved and is continued for 2–3 years to preserve remission. The most active chemotherapeutic agents are vincristine, prednisone, an anthracycline, and L-asparaginase. The L3 type of ALL is morphologically identical to Burkitt's lymphoma and requires a more aggressive therapy course. Diagnostic lumbar punctures are required. Even in the absence of disease, prophylactic intrathecal chemotherapy or radiotherapy is needed.

28. Describe the three phases of the Linker regimen for ALL.

1. **Induction**
   Vincristine, 2 mg by IVP on days 1, 8, 15, and 22
   Daunorubicin, 50 mg/m^2 IV on days 1, 2, and 3
   Prednisone, 60 mg/m^2 orally (PO) on days 1–28
   L-Asparaginase, 6000 U/m^2 intramuscularly (IM) on days 17 and 28
2. **Intensification**
   Cycles 1, 3, 5, and 7
     Vincristine, 2 mg by IVP on days 1 and 8
     Daunorubicin, 50 mg/m^2 IV on days 1 and 2
     Prednisone, 60 mg/m^2 PO on days 1–14
     L-Asparaginase, 6000 U/m^2 IM on days 2, 4, 7, 9, and 11–14
   Cycles 2, 4, 6, and 8
     Cytarabine, 300 mg/m^2 IV on days 1, 4, 8, and 11
     Teniposide (VM-26), 165 mg/m^2 IV on days 1, 4, 8, and 11

Cycle 9
  Methotrexate, 690 mg/m^2 by continuous IV infusion for 42 hours
  Leucovorin, 15 mg/m^2 IV every 6 hours for 12 doses, starting 42 hours after initiation
    of methotrexate
3. **Maintenance**
  6-Mercaptopurine, 75 mg/m^2/day PO
  Methotrexate, 20 mg PO every week

29. Describe the Linker regimen for CNS therapy.
Radiotherapy, 1800 Gy during weeks 5–7
  or
Intrathecal methotrexate, 12 mg/week for 6 weeks

30. Is bone marrow transplantation a useful option in ALL?
Allogeneic bone marrow transplantation as part of initial therapy has not been shown to change significantly the disease-free survival rates in patients with ALL when compared with conventional chemotherapy. This is most likely due to a less significant graft vs. leukemia effect.

31. How is relapsed ALL treated?
CNS relapse heralds systemic relapse. Usually relapse is treated with the same regimen used for initial therapy or with a combination of different chemotherapeutic agents. In adults, allogeneic bone marrow transplant is considered the best treatment for systemic relapse when a suitable donor is available.

32. Discuss the incidence of CML.
CML occurs more frequently in the older population. The median age at diagnosis is 53 years. The incidence is 1 in 100,000, with an estimated 4700 new cases in 2001. CML is more common in men than in women.

33. What causes CML?
CML is one of the myeloproliferative diseases; other examples include essential thrombocytopenia, polycythemia vera, and idiopathic myelofibrosis. CML is associated with the Philadelphia chromosome or (9;22) translocation. The *ABL* proto-oncogene on chromosome 9 is translocated near the *BCR* (breakpoint cluster region) gene on chromosome 22. The exact cause is unknown, but there appears to be a link with radiation exposure.

34. What is the prognosis for CML?
CML has an insidious onset with a progressive pattern and inevitable conversion to an aggressive acute leukemia. The median survival time is 4–5 years. Once the disease has converted into the accelerated or blast phase, it becomes much more difficult to treat; survival usually is measured in months.

35. Describe the presenting signs and symptoms of CML.
Nearly 30% of patients are diagnosed before they experience any symptoms. Presenting signs and symptoms are related to abnormal hematopoiesis. The most common are fever, sweats, bone pain, weight loss, malaise, and fatigue. Fever and sweats, as in ALL, often are related to progressive disease as opposed to infection. Malaise and fatigue often are related to anemia associated with decreased red cell production. Some patients also experience left upper quadrant pain or early satiety due to splenomegaly. Less common signs and symptoms, such as bleeding, thrombosis, arthralgias, and priapism, usually are associated with late disease.

36. How is CML treated?
The most commonly used chemotherapeutic agent is hydroxyurea, which alleviates symptoms but does not prolong survival. The other option is alpha-interferon, which is associated with increased morbidity compared with hydroxyurea but provides some patients with both hematologic

and cytogenetic responses. Hematopoiesis is normalized, and the Philadelphia chromosome is reduced or eradicated, resulting in longer survival. Treatment regimens include the following:

Hydroxyurea, 500–3000 mg/day PO

or

Alpha-interferon, 2 million U/m^2 3 times/week subcutaneously (SQ),
increasing to 5 million U/m^2/day SQ

Once the disease progresses to the accelerated phase, treatment mirrors that of acute leukemia. Recently an investigational drug (ST1-571), designed specifically to treat the unique *BCR/ABL* translocation, has shown great promise.

37. What is the role of bone marrow transplantation in treatment of CML?

For many patients in the first chronic phase, allogeneic bone marrow transplant is the best treatment option. When an HLA-matched sibling is available as donor, the cure rate is 60%.

38. Discuss the incidence of CLL.

CLL is the most common leukemia in North America, with an estimated 8100 new cases in 2001. The incidence is higher in men than in women and occurs most frequently with advancing age.

39. What causes CLL?

CLL is identified by accumulation of lymphocytes in marrow, blood, and lymph tissue, but the exact cause is unknown. The incidence is increased among farmers and rubber and asbestos workers, and a familial link in as many as 8.8% of cases indicates the possibility of genetic factors. However, no chromosomal abnormalities have been identified in association with CLL.

40. What is the prognosis of CLL?

Patients diagnosed in the low-risk stage with significant progression have a normal life expectancy without treatment. CLL can convert into more aggressive diseases, such as prolymphocytic leukemia, diffuse large-cell lymphoma (Richter syndrome), acute leukemia, or multiple myeloma. Once this progression occurred, treatment is much more difficult, and mortality rates rise significantly.

41. Describe the presenting signs and symptoms of CLL.

CLL is a slow, insidious disease that often is diagnosed on routine hematologic evaluation. Nearly 40% of cases are diagnosed before symptoms are experienced. The most common presenting symptom is fatigue, which probably is related to disease progression rather than anemia. Patients also may present with diffuse adenopathy and pain due to splenomegaly, which results from infiltration of lymphocytes in the spleen. Less common signs and symptoms are weight loss, fevers, bruising, and tonsilar swelling.

42. How is CLL treated?

Treatment is based on stage and progression of disease. Because CLL is considered incurable, treatment generally is reserved for symptomatic patients. Patients in the low-risk stage who do not have progression are placed under close observation. Patients with intermediate- and high-risk stages are treated if symptoms are present. The most commonly used agent is the alkylating agent, chlorambucil (0.4 mg/kg IV every 2 weeks). Cyclophosphamide with or without prednisone has been used with similar response rates. The nucleoside analogs also have excellent activity against CLL. Allogeneic bone marrow transplantation is considered in some patients who are nonresponders to conventional therapy if the disease continues to progress. Once CLL has converted to a more aggressive disease, therapy is the same as for the new disease type.

43. What diagnostic tests and procedures are commonly used during the evaluation and treatment of leukemias?

1. Complete blood count (CBC)
2. Full chemistry panels

3. Coagulation studies (prothrombin time, partial thromboplastin time, D-dimer, fibrin split products, fibrinogen)
4. Bone marrow biopsy and aspirates (to evaluate morphologic evidence of disease)
5. Cytogenetic testing (to evaluate chromosomal abnormalities)
6. Flow cytometry (to evaluate immunohistochemical evidence of disease; more specific than morphology)
7. Computed tomography (CT) scans
8. Node biopsies

44. What are the common complications of leukemia?
Infection and bleeding. Most complications are associated with abnormal hematopoiesis and caused by the disease itself. Some complications are associated directly with the treatment for leukemia, including mucositis, diarrhea, anorexia, nausea and vomiting, and alopecia. These secondary complications can be serious and do not always have well-defined treatment plans.

45. What is the leading cause of death in leukemic patients?
Infectious complications, which are common and serious in patients with leukemia. Many patients with acute leukemias have an infectious process at the time of diagnosis. Because treatment regimens cause prolonged neutropenia, such infections may worsen even as new opportunistic infections begin.

46. How are the symptoms of infection different in leukemic patients?
Healthcare providers must be vigilant because patients may not have the usual signs of infection, such as fever, erythema, or pus, in the presence of a low granulocyte count.

47. How are infections treated?
Broad antibiotic therapy along with antiviral coverage is required. Aggressive antifungal treatment should be considered in persistently febrile patients, who are at risk for atypical fungal infections.

48. How can infections be prevented?
Neutropenic precautions vary by institution. Basic precautions, such as handwashing, avoidance of contact with sick people, impeccable personal hygiene, and careful preparation of fresh fruits and vegetables, should be upheld.

49. List the common causative organisms and sites of infection in neutropenic patients.
The most common causative organisms in myelosuppressed patients are gram-positive and gram-negative bacteria. Nearly 80% of infections are caused by gram-positive bacteria and are related to indwelling central catheters. Most infections, whether caused by gram-positive or gram-negative bacteria, are self-induced. Common organisms are *Escherichia coli, Pseudomonas* spp., *Klebsiella* spp., and *Staphylococcus aureus*.

SITE	ORGANISMS
Skin	*Staphylococcus aureus, Pseudomonas aeruginosa, Klebsiella pneumoniae, Escherichia coli*, herpes zoster
Pharynx	*S. aureus*, gram-negative bacilli, *Candida albicans*
Mouth and esophagus	*C. albicans*, herpes simplex, cytomegalovirus, gram-negative bacilli
Lungs	*P. aeruginosa, E. coli, S. aureus, Aspergillus flavus, A. fumigatus, Pneumocystis carinii*
Urinary tract	*E. coli, K. pneumoniae, P. aeruginosa*
Perianal region	*Bacteroides* spp., *K. pneumoniae, E. coli, P. aeruginosa*

50. Are masks required for healthcare providers and family/significant others when they care for neutropenic patients?

The use of masks varies from center to center. Studies show that masks must be changed every 15 minutes or when they become moist to provide an effective barrier to airborne infections. Most centers have discontinued the use of masks because their limited effectiveness does not justify the cost.

51. Describe the significance of bleeding in leukemia.

Bleeding is another high-risk complication that often occurs with leukemia and its treatment. Patients with acute leukemia are often thrombocytopenic at the time of diagnosis. The aggressive therapy causes thrombocytopenia for an extended period, placing patients at high risk for hemorrhage. Patients with M3 promyelocytic leukemia also have a propensity to develop disseminated intravascular coagulopathy (DIC). Multiple platelet transfusions are required for leukemic patients. Standard thrombocytopenic precautions should be strictly upheld (i.e., no nose blowing, no standard toothbrushes, sexual activity only with platelets > 50,000, sedentary activity, no intramuscular injections, no rectal suppositories or temperature assessments).

52. When can platelet transfusions be given?

Most centers transfuse platelets when the count is ≤ 10,000 μ/L or active bleeding is present. Spontaneous bleeding does not become a significant risk until the platelet count drops below this level. Alloimmunization (antibody production to antigens expressed on red cells or platelets) can occur in patients who have received multiple blood product transfusions. Minimizing transfusions can help to prevent this complication.

53. Define blast crisis. How is it treated?

In blast crisis the leukemia becomes extremely aggressive, and an inordinate number of blasts are circulating in the peripheral blood. The widely accepted definition is > 30% blasts in peripheral blood. Treatment is based on protocols for acute leukemia. If white blood cell counts are > 100,000 μ/L, leukopheresis may be considered.

54. What resources are available for patient support, counseling, education, and information?

National Cancer Institute Cancer Information Service: 1-800-422-6237

American Cancer Society: 1-800-ACS-2345 or www.cancer.org

Leukemia Society of America: 1-800-955-4LSA or www.leukemia.org

REFERENCES

1. Greenlee RT, Hill-Harmon MB, Murray T, Thun M: Cancer statistics, 2001. CA Cancer J Clin 51:15–36, 2001.
2. Hoffman R, Benz EJ, Shattil SJ, et al (eds): Hematology: Basic Principles and Practice, 3rd ed. Philadelphia, Churchill Livingstone, 2000.
3. Lee GR, Foerster J, Lukens J, et al (eds): Wintrobe's Clinical Hematology. Philadelphia, Lippincott Williams & Wilkins, 1999.
4. Sawyers C, Hochhaus A, Feldman E, et al: A phase II study to determine the safety and antileukemic effects of ST1571 in patients with Philadelphia chromosome positive chronic myeloid leukemia in myeloid blast crisis [abstract]. American Society of Hematology, 2000.
5. Sievers EL, Appelbaum FR, Spielberger RT, et al: Selective ablation of acute myeloid leukemia using antibody-targeted chemotherapy: A phase I study of an anti-CD33 calicheamicin immunoconjugate. Blood 93:3678–3684, 1999.
6. Tallman MS, Mocharnuck RS: Hematology–Oncology Clinical Management: Acute Myeloid Leukemia. http://www.medscape.com/Medscape/oncology/Clinicalmgmt/CM.v04/public/index-CM.v04.html, 2000.
7. Wujcik D: Leukemia. In Yarbro CH, Frogge MH, Goodman M, Groenwald SL (eds): Cancer Nursing: Principles and Practice, 5th ed. Boston, Jones & Bartlett, 2000, pp 1244–1268.

19. MULTIPLE MYELOMA

Paul Seligman, MD, and Cathy E. Pickett, RN, BSN

Quick Facts—Multiple Myeloma

Incidence	1% of all malignancies; in 2001, approximately 14,400 new cases will be diagnosed in the United States
Mortality	In 2001, estimated 11,200 deaths
Etiologic factors	No single predisposing factor; suggested factors include chronic exposure to various types of low-level radiation, occupational exposures (agriculture, chemicals, rubber plant, leather tanners), and chemical exposure to benzene formaldehyde, hair dyes, paint sprays.
Risk factors	Increasing age (median age: 50–70 yr); increased risk in men; more common among African-Americans than Caucasians (2:1)
Signs and symptoms	Many patients present with complications because the disease is a slow-growing neoplasm typified by a long prodromal or asymptomatic period. Most patients present with systemic involvement indicated by bony disease (many present with back pain), renal disease, increased calcium, anemia, and/or infections.
Diagnostic studies	Urinary and serum protein electrophoresis (UPEP/SPEP) to assess for presence of monoclonal protein
	Quantitative immunoglobulins to evaluate specific amounts of immunoglobulin
	Skeletal survey to evaluate degree of bone marrow involvement as indicated by percentage of plasma cells
	Complete blood count to evaluate for anemia, neutropenia, and thrombocytopenia
	$\beta 2$ microglobulin (prognostic indicator) increases with advancing disease

Staging*   Stage I < 0.5 myeloma cells $\times 10^{12}/m^2$ plus **all** of the following:
         1. Hemoglobin value > 10 gm/100 ml
         2. Serum calcium value normal (< 12 mg/100 ml)
         3. On radiographs, normal bone structure (scale 0) or solitary bone plasmycytoma only
         4. Low M-component production rates
           a. IgG value < 5 mg/100 ml
           b. IgA value < 3 gm/100 ml
           c. Urine light-chain M-component on electrophoresis: < 4 gm/24 hr

        Stage II > 0.6–1.20 myeloma cells $\times 10^{12}/m^2$ (intermediate)
        Fitting neither stage I nor stage III

        Stage III > 1.20 myeloma cells $\times 10^{12}/m^2$ (high) plus **one or more** of the following:
         1. Hemoglobin < 8.5 gm/100 ml
         2. Serum calcium value > 12 mg/100 ml
         3. Advanced lytic bone lesions (scale 3)
         4. High M-component production rate
           a. IgG value > 7 mg/100 ml
           b. IgA value > 5 gm/100 ml
           c. Urine light-chain M-component on electrophoresis: > 12 gm/24 hr

Subclassification
    A = Relatively normal renal function (serum creatinine value < 2.0 mg/100 ml)
    B = Abnormal renal function (serum creatinine value > 2.0 mg/100 ml)

---

* Criteria vary, and standard definitions are lacking. Some clinicians monitor serum levels of $\beta 2$ microglobulin, which correlate with renal function and myeloma cell tumor burden. Although good indicators of prognosis and survival, current staging systems do not indicate treatment. The staging system presented above was developed by Durie GB, Salmon SE: A clinical staging system for multiple myeloma. Cancer 36:852, 1975. © 1975 by the American Cancer Society. Reprinted by permission of Wiley-Liss, Inc., a subsidiary of John Wiley & Sons, Inc.

1. What is multiple myeloma?

Multiple myeloma is a malignant proliferation of plasma cells that results in an overproduction of a specific immunoglobulin, generally detected in the blood or urine. M-protein is the abnormal immunoglobulin produced by the malignant plasma cell. It is produced excessively and is not able to make effective antibodies. Plasma cells are responsible for production of immunoglobulin (the basic unit of antibodies) and arise from stem cells in the bone marrow. Myeloma cells are present in bone marrow and in the outer part of bones.

2. How is multiple myeloma diagnosed?

A few patients are diagnosed by chance with the identification of abnormal protein in the blood or urine. Most present with a common complication of myeloma and are further evaluated using diagnostic studies (see Quick Facts).

Diagnostic Criteria for Various Forms of Monoclonal Gammopathies

Multiple myeloma
1. Plasmacytoma on tissue biopsy
2. > 30% marrow plasmacytosis
3. Monoclonal spike
   a. IgG > 3.5 gm/dl
   b. IgA > 2.0 gm/dl
   c. Urinary light chain > 1.0 gm/24 hr
4. Additional features
   a. Lytic bone lesions
   b. Low residual immunoglobulins

Diagnosis requires 1, 2, or 3 plus either 4a or 4b if plasmacytosis and monoclonal spike are present but lower than above. Diagnosis can be made if 4a or 4b is present.

Indolent myeloma
Same as for myeloma except
1. 0–3 bone lesions, no fractures
2. Monoclonal spike< 7 gm/dl IgG; < 5 gm/dl IgA
3. No associated features: anemia, hypercalcemia, renal dysfuntion, infection; good performance

Smoldering myeloma
Same as for indolent myeloma except
1. No bone lesions
2. Marrow plasmacytosis < 30%

Monoclonal gammopathy of unknown significance (MGUS)
1. Monoclonal gammopathy
   a. IgG < 3.5 gm/dl
   b. IgA < 2.0 gm/dl
   c. Urinary light chain < 1.0 gm/dl
2. Marrow plasmacytosis < 10%
3. No bone lesions
4. No symptoms

From Gautier M, Cohen H: Multiple myelomas in the elderly. J Am Geriatr Soc 42:653–654, 1994, with permission.

3. What is monoclonal gammopathy of unknown significance (MGUS)?

The diagnosis of MGUS is made when patients have no symptoms, no skeletal involvement, a marrow plasmacytosis of < 10%, and M protein levels lower than described. Because 20–25% of patients eventually develop multiple myeloma, frequent and ongoing evaluation is necessary.

4. What is a plasmacytoma?

A plasmacytoma is a single isolated collection of malignant plasma cells in the bone that can be treated with local therapy such as surgery and/or radiation. Because some of these patients eventually develop multiple myeloma, close monitoring is necessary.

5. What is the significance of Bence-Jones protein in the urine?

Some malignant plasma cells produce only the light-chain part of the immunoglobulin. These low-molecular-weight proteins are excreted in the urine; they allow the diagnosis of light-chain myeloma and may contribute to the development of renal failure (referred to as **myeloma kidney**).

6. Why are patients with multiple myeloma so prone to the development of renal failure?

Renal failure in patients with multiple myeloma is multifactorial. The causes generally include an accumulation of Bence-Jones proteins, hypercalcemia, hyperuricemia, and dehydration. It is important that patients with multiple myeloma receive adequate hydration before receiving diagnostic dyes or contrast media. The degree of hydration depends on the patient's creatinine value and stage of disease, but treatment generally involves the administration of at least 1 liter of normal saline and reevaluation of the patient's renal function and fluid status.

7. What are lytic lesions?

Many patients present with skeletal involvement and bony destruction caused by the accumulation of plasma cells. Plasma cells also increase bone resorption, resulting in further bony destruction that may present as "punched-out" lesions on radiographs. A lytic lesion is a destructive loss of bone in an isolated area secondary to metastatic cancer infiltration. Diffuse osteoporosis also may result. Skeletal involvement may lead to pathologic fractures, increased serum calcium, and severe pain. The administration of intravenous biphosphonates, such as pamidronate, which inhibit osteoclastic activity and decrease bone resorption, is currently recommended every 3–4 weeks to minimize bony destruction.

8. If patients with multiple myeloma have an increase in a specific immunoglobulin, why are they at increased risk for infection?

The elevated monoclonal protein is impaired and does not function normally to provide protection. Because it is produced in large quantities, it also results in a decrease in the levels of other normal and functional immunoglobulins. As the percentage of bone marrow infiltration by plasma cells increases, neutropenia further predisposes patients to infection.

9. What medical emergencies are patients with multiple myeloma prone to develop?

The common oncologic emergencies in patients with multiple myeloma are hypercalcemia, spinal cord compression, and hyperviscosity.

10. Define hyperviscosity. How is it exhibited?

The presence of high concentrations of M protein in the blood may lead to occlusion of blood vessels and circulatory problems. The patient may develop claudication, visual disturbances, and neurologic symptoms such as headache, drowsiness, and confusion.

11. How is multiple myeloma treated?

Systemic treatment begins when symptoms appear. Because multiple myeloma has a long prodromal phase in which patients are asymptomatic, treatment is generally reserved for patients who have developed complications. Radiation may be used effectively to treat a solitary lesion or palliatively to treat bony lesions and control pain.

12. What chemotherapy is used for the treatment of multiple myeloma?

The combination of melphalan and prednisone (MP), which has been a primary treatment modality since the 1960s, induces a temporary (duration of 2 years) remission in 40% of previously untreated patients. There is a low frequency of complete response. (Response is defined as a 75% reduction in the rate of myeloma protein production, a 95% decrease in the rate of Bence-Jones protein excretion, and < 5% marrow plasma cells, as determined by bone marrow biopsy). A continuous infusion of vincristine and doxorubicin combined with oral dexamethasone (VAD) is used primarily as a treatment for relapses or patients who fail MP therapy. VAD has response rates of

55% and quicker remission but no improvement in long-term survival. Patients younger than 60 years usually receive VAD initially or other combinations at higher doses with some evidence of longer remissions.

13. What are the major complications of treatment?

Side effects of all treatments include drug resistance, infection in an already immunocompromised patient, and leukemia as a result of long-term use of alkylating agents.

14. What is the prognosis for patients with multiple myeloma?

Multiple myeloma is normally treated with chemotherapy, and initially patients respond well. It is considered an incurable disease, because most patients relapse and fail to respond to chemotherapy as the disease progresses. Once symptoms develop, the median survival time without treatment is 7 months. Standard treatment can extend survival to 2–3 years. The 5-year survival rate increased from 12% in the 1960s to 27% in the 1980s. Although this increase represents progress, the lack of a cure has led to ongoing investigation of other treatment modalities.

15. What current studies are under way in the management of multiple myeloma?

Studies investigating the use of interferon after chemotherapy have produced conflicting results. Although trials are still in progress, little evidence indicates that interferon improves survival. The use of interferon as maintenance therapy (after chemotherapy), however, may prolong response to initial treatment. Recent research suggests that thalidomide, a drug with antiangiogenesis and immunologic properties, is an active agent in the treatment of patients with relapsed myeloma. Administered orally at a dose of 200 mg/day for 2 weeks and titrated gradually to 800 mg/day maximally, thalidomide has a side-effect profile that includes constipation, weakness or fatigue, somonolence, and rash. Some patients may tolerate a dose of only 50 mg/day. Bone marrow transplantation (generally autologous transplants after high-dose chemotherapy) is also under investigation; results indicate prolonged remission and increased survival but increased morbidity.

16. If bone marrow transplantation can increase survival and achieve a complete response in some patients, why is it not a standard treatment?

Many patients with multiple myeloma are elderly and, thus, more susceptible to the major side effects of the regimen. They may choose to enjoy a period of symptom-free survival with standard chemotherapy. Younger patients in early stages of the disease may be the best candidates for bone marrow transplantation, but they must accept the increased risk of morbidity. Until morbidity is decreased, many patients may be hesitant to accept bone marrow transplantation as a treatment option. Trials are under way to determine the most effective chemotherapy regimen, the best source of stem cells (peripheral or bone marrow), and the best time for transplantation.

17. How can nurses promote safety and improve the quality of life in patients with multiple myeloma?

The nurse's role involves facilitating diagnosis and managing disease-related complications or treatment-induced side effects.

Nurses can help patients with skeletal involvement to achieve optimal pain control while avoiding side effects of medication. Education about positioning and ambulation also may help to prevent further pathologic fractures and continued bone destruction.

Nurses also can educate patients about the importance of hydration and avoidance of renal toxic drugs and hypercalcemia to promote optimal renal function and prevent further damage. Because infection is the leading cause of death, patient education about prevention, recognition, and treatment of infection is critical.

18. What resources are available to provide patients and families with more information?

Patients and families should contact their local American Cancer Society for resources and support group information. The Physician Data Query is a valuable resource for patients and families looking for current information and investigational trials in progress. The Leukemia Society of America (800-955-4LSA) can be accessed by computer and also has pamphlets and resources for patients with multiple myeloma. "Surfing the net" is recommended to explore a variety of resources. The International Myeloma Foundation (800-452-CURE; e-mail: TheIMF@aol.com) offers patient seminars, a newsletter, resources, publications, and a patient-to-patient directory.

REFERENCES

1. Alexanian R, Dimopoulos M: The treatment of multiple myeloma. N Engl J Med 330:484–489, 1994.
2. Bensinger W, Rowley S, Demirer T, et al: High-dose therapy followed by autologous hematopoietic stem-cell infusion for patients with multiple myeloma. J Clin Oncol 14:1447–1456, 1996.
3. Berenson J, Lichtenstein A, Porter L, et al: Efficacy of pamidronate in reducing skeletal events in patients with advanced multiple myeloma. N Engl J Med 334:488–493, 1996.
4. Bubley G, Schnippe L: Multiple myeloma. In Holleb A, Fink D, Murphy G (eds): American Cancer Textbook of Clinical Oncology. Atlanta, American Cancer Society, 1991, pp 397–409.
5. Fishman MN, Dalton WS: Considerations in the treatment of myeloma. Oncology 14:72–81, 2000.
6. Gautier M, Cohen H: Multiple myeloma in the elderly. J Am Geriatr Soc 42:653–664, 1994.
7. Greenlee RT, Hill-Harmon MB, Murray T, Thun M: Cancer statistics, 2001. CA Cancer J Clin 51:15–36, 2001.
8. Hjorth M, Westin J, Dahl I, et al: Interferon-α2b added to melphalan–prednisone for initial and maintenance therapy in multiple myeloma. Ann Intern Med 124:212–222, 1996.
9. Lawrence J: Critical care issues in the patient with hematologic malignancy. Semin Oncol Nurs 10:198–207, 1994.
10. Rajkumar SV, Fonseca R, Dispenzieri A, et al: Thalidomide in the treatment of relapsed multiple myeloma. Mayo Clin Proc 75:897–901, 2000.
11. Sheridan C, Serrano M: Multiple myeloma. In Yarbro CH, Frogge MH, Goodman M, Groenwald SL (eds): Cancer Nursing: Principles and Practice. Boston, Jones & Bartlett, 2000, pp 1354–1370.
12. Whitley P: Multiple myeloma: Thalidomide Nursing Roundtable Report. University of Nebraska Medical Center Continuing Education Monograph. PharmaCom Group, 2000, pp 6–13.

20. NON-HODGKIN'S LYMPHOMA

Scott Kruger, MD, and Lynn Ellis, RN, MEd, OCN

Quick Facts—Non-Hodgkin's Lymphoma	
Incidence	4% of all cancers in the United States, with an estimated 56,200 new cases in 2001 (increase associated with AIDS and elderly). In adults, the median age at diagnosis is over 50 years.
Mortality	Overall survival has improved with newer treatments. It is estimated that in the United States, 26,300 people will die from the disease in 2001.
Cause	The exact causes of non-Hodgkin's lymphoma (NHL) are unknown.
Risk Factors	**Infections** • Human immunodeficiency virus (HIV) • Epstein-Barr virus (African Burkitt's lymphoma) • Human T-cell lymphoma virus (HTLV-1) (T-cell lymphoma) • *Helicobacter pylori* associated with gastric mucosa-associated lymphoid tissue lymphomas (MALT) **Environmental factors:** pesticides and fertilizers, wood and cotton dust, early and prolonged use of hair dyes, and possibly smoking **Therapy-related factors** • Chemotherapy (alkylating agents) and radiation therapy with latency period of about 5–6 years • Immunosuppressants (azathioprine or cyclosporine) **Congenital immune deficiencies:** ataxia telangiectasia, Bloom's and Wiskott-Aldrich syndromes, severe combined immune deficiency, common variable hypo-gammaglobulinemia, and acquired immunodeficiency states (e.g., HIV, organ transplantation) **Autoimmune disorders:** Sjögren's syndrome, systemic lupus erythematosus, rheumatoid arthritis, celiac disease
Signs and symptoms	B symptoms of fevers, weight loss, and drenching sweats may be present. **Low-grade lymphomas** present with painless, slowly progressive lymphadenopathy that at times may spontaneously regress in size and then grow at a later time. Extranodal involvement and B symptoms may be found in advanced disease. Patients with low-grade lymphomas often present with higher-stage disease (stages III and IV) than patients with intermediate and high-grade lymhomas. **Intermediate- and high-grade lymphomas** sometimes present with rapidly growing adenopathy. One-third present with extralymphatic disease in the GI tract, skin, sinuses, and central nervous system (CNS). B symptoms are common. Patients often present with lower-stage disease (I and II). Lymphoblastic lymphoma may present with a large mediastinal mass, superior vena cava syndrome, or cranial nerve involvement due to leptomeningeal disease. American Burkitt's lymphoma often starts with a large abdominal mass and obstructive symptoms.
Staging	NHL is staged according to the Ann Arbor Staging System.
	Stage I Involvement of a single lymph node region or lymphoid structure (spleen, thymus, or Waldeyer's ring)
	Stage II Involvement of 2 or more lymph node regions on same side of diaphragm (the mediastinum is a single site, hilar nodes are lateralized). The number of anatomic sites should be indicated by a suffix (e.g., stage II$_3$).
	Stage III Involvement of lymph node regions or structures on both sides of diaphragm

Table continued on following page

Quick Facts—Non-Hodgkin's Lymphoma (Continued)

Stage III₁   Splenic, celiac, or portal nodes

Stage III₂   Paraaortic, iliac, or mesenteric nodes

Stage IV   Multifocal involvement of extranodal sites with or without associated lymph node involvement or isolated extralymphatic organ involvement with distant nodal involvement.

Each stage is subdivided into **category A** (no symptoms) or **category B** (fever > 101.5° F, drenching sweats, loss of > 10% body weight within past 6 months).

X = bulky disease (>⅓ widening of mediastinum and > 10 cm maximal dimension of nodal mass).

E = extranodal site, contiguous or proximal to known nodal sites. Sites are identified by the following notations: **P** = lung or pleura, **H** = liver, **M** = bone marrow, **S** = spleen, **O** = bone, **D** = skin.

Patients are also assigned a **clinical stage (CS)**, based on node and bone marrow biopsy studies, physical exam, and radiologic evaluation. and a **pathologic stage (PS)** based on results of invasive procedures beyond initial biopsies (e.g., additional biopsies).

---

1. What are the non-Hodgkin's lymphomas (NHLs)? How are they diagnosed?

The NHLs are a diverse group of seemingly unrelated diseases arising from lymphoid tissues. NHL is caused by a malignant clonal expansion of one of the elements of a lymph node. Because lymphatic tissue is present throughout the entire body, the disease may develop anywhere. It may begin in a lymph node, spleen, liver, or bone marrow as well in extralymphatic sites such as skin, gastrointestinal tract, pharynx, and central nervous system. The diagnosis is established by biopsy of abnormal tissue and evaluation with histologic and immunophenotypic examination.

2. What are the most common cytogenetic abnormalities? How do they correlate with histology?

Chromosomal abnormalities are associated with oncogene expressions involved in lymphogenesis, as depicted below:

CYTOGENETIC ABNORMALITY	ONCOGENE EXPRESSION	HISTOLOGY
t(14;18)	bcl-2	Follicular and diffuse large cell
t(11;14)	bcl-1	Mantle zone
t(14;19)	bcl-3	B-cell chronic lymphocytic lymphoma (CLL)
t(8;14), t(2;8), t(8;22)	c-myc	Burkitt's and non-Burkitt's lymphoma
Trisomy 12		B-cell CLL
14q11 abnormalities	tcl-1, tcl-2	T-cell acute lymphocytic lymphoma (ALL)
7q35 abnormalities	tcl-4	T-cell ALL and lymphoblastic lymphoma
t(2;5)	npm;alk	Anaplastic large cell

3. What characteristics of an enlarged node raise the suspicion of lymphoma?

A painless, enlarging lymph node that feels rubbery is suspicious for lymphoma. Infectious nodal enlargement is usually tender. Supraclavicular nodes are always suspicious for malignancy.

4. Why is the classification of NHL so confusing?

The classification is confusing because the NHLs are a heterogeneous group of diseases that seem to have little relationship to each other. They are named according to growth pattern (follicular vs. diffuse) within the lymph node, cell size (large vs. small), and appearance (cleaved or noncleaved). Until the mid 1980s, the Rappaport classification was widely used in the United States, but it has been replaced by the Working Formulation, which attempts to simplify classification into risk categories of low, intermediate, and high grade. However, the Working

Formulation does not include all lymphomas. The REAL (Revised European American Lymphoma) classification was recently proposed by the International Study Group in an effort to accommodate newly described lymphomas not included in the Working Formulation.

Classification of Non-Hodgkin's Lymphomas

WORKING FORMULATION	RAPPAPORT
Low grade	**Low grade**
A Small lymphocytic	Diffuse, well-differentiated lymphocytic
B Follicular, small cleaved cell	Nodular, poorly differentiated lymphocytic
C Follicular, mixed, small cleaved and large cell	Nodular, mixed
Intermediate grade	**Intermediate grade**
D Follicular, large cell	Nodular, histiocytic
E Diffuse, small cleaved cell	Diffuse, poorly differentiated lymphocytic
F Diffuse, mixed, small cleaved and large cell	Diffuse mixed
G Diffuse, large cell	Diffuse, histiocytic
High grade	**High grade**
H Immunoblastic	Diffuse, histiocytic
I Lymphoblastic	Lymphoblastic
J Diffuse, small noncleaved cell	Burkitt's and non-Burkitt's types

5. Which lymphomas are not classified by the Working Formulation?

DISEASE	DESCRIPTION
Mantle zone	Resembles follicular small cleaved cell but is derived from a cell in mantle zone surrounding B-cell follicles. Aggressive disease with high risk for extranodal spread. Low potential for cure.
Monocytoid B-cell lymphoma	Low-grade indolent disease. Predominant lymph node involvement.
Mucosa-associated lymphoid tissue (MALT)	Low-grade indolent disease. Affects GI tract, lung, breast, thyroid, and salivary glands.
Anaplastic large cell Ki-1 lymphoma	Skin is often involved. Cells infiltrate the sinusoids of nodes. Often confused with Hodgkin's disease or carcinoma. Most cases are of T-cell origin. Behaves as an intermediate-grade lymphoma.
Mycosis fungoides	Indolent cutaneous T-cell lymphoma that may later spread to lymph nodes and invade other organs. More advanced forms with peripheral blood involvement and diffuse erythema are called Sezary syndrome. Involvement of organs results in poor prognosis.
Angiocentric lymphoma	T-cell disease that invades and destroys blood vessels.
T-cell–rich B-cell lymphoma	Usually aggressive and behaves like large cell lymphomas.
Angiotropic large cell	Diffuse intravascular proliferation, usually of B-cell lineage.
Angioimmunoblastic lymphadenopathy (AILD)	Diffuse adenopathy, hepatosplenomegaly, skin rash, cytopenias, systemic symptoms, polyclonal hypergammaglobulinemia. Often evolves into T-cell lymphoma.
Divergent or discordant lymphoma	Large cell histology in lymph node but low grade in marrow. The low-grade component usually turns into high-grade disease.
Composite lymphoma	Two histologic subtypes in the same node; sometimes coexists with Hodgkin's disease.
Castleman's disease	Benign lymphoproliferative disorder, sometimes related to HIV. Increased rate of evolving into malignancy.
Adult T-cell leukemia lymphoma	Aggressive malignancy associated with skin infiltration, hypercalcemia, and lytic bone lesions.

Adapted from Molina A, Pezner RD: Non-Hodgkin's lymphoma. In Pazdur R, Coia LR, Hoskins WJ, Wagman LD (eds): Cancer Management: A Multidisciplinary Approach—Medical, Surgical, and Radiation Oncology, 3rd ed. Melville, NY, PRR, 1999, pp 525–558.

6. What are favorable and nonfavorable lymphomas? Are favorable lymphomas more curable?

Favorable lymphomas are low-grade lymphomas. Unfavorable lymphomas are intermediate- and high-grade lymphomas. Low-grade lymphomas are considered "favorable" because of their relatively long natural course without treatment. Unfortunately, they are not considered curable. Most patients with low-grade lymphoma require treatment for a few years, but it is generally for palliation rather than cure. The 5-year survival rate for patients with low-grade lymphomas ranges from 50–70%. In contrast, the unfavorable lymphomas are potentially curable with combination chemotherapy regimens. The higher-grade lymphomas are considered "unfavorable" because without active treatment the natural prognosis is poor. The 5-year survival rate for intermediate-grade lymphoma ranges from 33–45%; for high-grade lymphomas, from 23–32%. Treatment may achieve complete remission in 60–80% of patients with diffuse, aggressive NHL.

7. What is the International Index?

The International Index consists of five factors used by the major cooperative groups to predict overall survival in patients with unfavorable lymphomas. Two or more of the following risk factors signify a less than 50% chance of relapse-free and overall survival at 5 years.

- Age (> 60 years)
- Elevated levels of serum lactate dehydrogenase (LDH)
- Performance status (levels ≥ 2)
- Stage III or IV disease
- Two or more sites of extranodal involvement

8. What other prognostic factors are useful in unfavorable lymphomas?

- Tumor biology: Ki-67 (marker for cellular proliferation), abnormal cytogenetics, T-cell lymphoma
- Presence of B symptoms
- Tumor burden: bulky sites (diameter > 7 cm), elevated B2 microglobulin
- Drug resistance

9. Explain the significance of immunophenotyping in NHLs.

NHLs are typed for T and B cells; however, whether this distinction influences patient outcome is still debated. Some studies indicate a shorter disease-free survival time in patients with T-cell, diffuse large cell lymphoma than in patients with B-cell lymphomas of similar histology.

10. How does Hodgkin's lymphoma differ from non-Hodgkin's lymphomas?

Pathologically the characteristic Reed-Sternberg cell is not found in NHLs. NHLs spread by skipping lymph node areas, whereas Hodgkin's disease is orderly and does not skip lymph node groups. NHLs are usually seen in older adults, whereas Hodgkin's disease has a bimodal incidence with the first peak in young adults.

11. What is the treatment of low-grade lymphomas?

Low-grade lymphomas are characterized by indolent behavior and median survival times of 6–10 years. Most patients are elderly and have advanced disease at presentation. Only 10–20% have stage I or II disease.

Stage I or II disease. Radiation alone is rarely used because NHLs do not spread contiguously and often skip to other lymph node areas. It has been used for localized tumors of the head and neck, orbit, and other single sites of disease. Many oncologists use a combination of radiation and chemotherapy for localized disease with the hope that it will produce long-term disease-free survival and even cure. For patients with comorbid illnesses, a watch-and-wait approach is a reasonable alternative. Chemotherapy is used when patients become symptomatic. Total nodal irradiation is not generally used because of its relapse rate (> 50%).

Stage III and IV. Treatment options include watching and waiting. Various systemic chemotherapy regimens are begun when patients become symptomatic. Chemotherapy is usually started early in patients with unfavorable prognostic features such as marrow involvement, bulky disease, high levels of serum LDH, many extralymphatic sites of disease, and decreased performance status.

12. Describe the treatment of intermediate-grade lymphomas.

Intermediate-grade lymphoma is frequently diagnosed in early stages. High-grade immunoblastic lymphoma is treated like intermediate-grade diseases.

Stage I and II. A combination of chemotherapy and radiation is the treatment of choice. The 5-year disease-free survival rate ranges from 78–95% for stage I disease and from 70–75% for stage II disease. Patients usually receive 3–4 cycles of chemotherapy followed by involved-field radiation therapy. For patients who do not receive radiation, 6–8 cycles of chemotherapy are used.

Stage III and IV. Most patients are treated with 6–8 cycles of systemic chemotherapy. Radiation is sometimes added to sites of bulky disease to decrease the risk of local recurrence. Despite the availability of multiple chemotherapy regimens, the 5-year disease-free survival rate is approximately 40%.

13. What chemotherapy regimens are commonly used for treating NHL?
Palliation of low-grade disease
 Oral chlorambucil with or without prednisone
 Oral cyclophosphamide with or without prednisone
 Fludarabine with or without mitoxantrone
Intermediate and high-grade disease
 CVP (cyclophosphamide, vincristine, prednisone)
 CHOP (cyclophosphamide, doxorubicin, vincristine, prednisone)
 MACOP-B (methotrexate, doxorubicin, cyclophosphamide, vincristine, bleomycin, prednisone
 ProMACE-CytaBOM (cyclophosphamide, etoposide, doxorubicin, cytarabine, bleomycin, vincristine, methotrexate, leucovorin, prednisone)
 m-BACOD (methotrexate, leucovorin, bleomycin, doxorubicin, cyclophosphamide, vincristine, dexamethasone)
Salvage chemotherapy
 DHAP (dexamethasone, cytarabine, cisplatin)
 IMVP (ifosfamide with mesna, methotrexate, etoposide)
 ESHAP (etoposide, methyl prednisone, cisplatin, cytarabine)
 MIME (mesna, ifosfamide, mitoxantrone, etoposide)
 CEPP (cyclophosphamide, etoposide, procarbazine, prednisone)
Note: Some regimens include trimethoprim-sulfamethoxazole (Septra) to prevent *Pneumocystis carinii* pneumonia.

14. Discuss the role of interferon therapy.

Interferon has significant activity in NHL and is useful in follicular, cutaneous T-cell, and diffuse large cell disease. Interferon is safe but toxic. Side effects of flu-like syndrome and myelosuppression can be dose-limiting, particularly in older patients. It is not clear whether interferon improves survival rates compared with other chemotherapy agents. The combination of interferon with an anthracycline-based regimen has produced encouraging results; some studies have demonstrated a survival benefit. Future trials are needed to determine the role of interferon in treating NHL.

15. Which of the above regimens is the best treatment for intermediate- or high-grade NHL?

Many researchers believe that CHOP, one of the first combination regimens to be used, is the gold standard for treatment of intermediate- or high-grade NHL. New clinical trials suggest that it may be beneficial to add Rituxan to the standard chemotherapy regimen. This may result in improved disease-free survival and overall survival compared with CHOP alone. Burkitt's lymphoma requires a more aggressive and dose-intense treatment, including intrathecal chemotherapy.

16. What is tumor lysis syndrome?
While undergoing therapy for leukemia and high-grade lymphomas, patients develop multiple electrolyte abnormalities due to the release of chemicals in the blood from the dying cancer cells. All patients should be adequately hydrated and receive allopurinol to decrease the production of uric acid. Alkalinization of the urine is sometimes performed to increase the solubility of uric acid. Hyperkalemia, hypocalcemia, and hyperphosphatemia may be life-threatening. Despite prevention, in some patients dialysis is needed to treat metabolic abnormalities. Risks for the patient include renal failure, cardiovascular collapse, and death.

17. What is the best treatment for low-grade NHL?
Any of the alkylators (e.g., cyclophosphamide), used alone or in combination, are highly active in low-grade NHL. Fludarabine and pentostatin (adenosine deaminase inhibitors) are also highly active. Traditionally they have been used for relapsed disease, but because of their high efficacy they are under study as first-line therapy in combination with anthracycline.

18. What paraneoplastic syndromes are associated with NHL?
• Non–parathyroid hormone-induced hypercalcemia
• Subacute motor neuropathy
• Polymyositis

19. How is lymphoblastic lymphoma treated?
Lymphoblastic lymphoma is uncommon in adults, but in children it is the most common type of NHL. Treatment is the same as for acute lymphoblastic leukemia: high-dose chemotherapy, including treatment of CNS involvement with chemotherapy and/or radiation therapy. Patients usually require several years of treatment.

20. Which patients should receive CNS prophylaxis with radiation or intrathecal therapy?
All patients with Burkitt's, non-Burkitt's, and lymphoblastic lymphoma receive treatment to the CNS. Other patients with involvement of bone marrow, testes, nasopharynx, or sinuses should be evaluated for CNS disease. Epidural and brain disease is treated with intrathecal therapy using methotrexate or cytarabine (Ara-C) or with radiation therapy.

21. What is the treatment of mycosis fungoides and other cutaneous T-cell lymphomas?
Topical chemotherapy with nitrogen mustard or carmustine (BCNU) and ultraviolet light A activation of skin with psoralen (PUVA) are usually the initial therapies. Bexarotene, a retinoid that is available as a cream and orally as a pill, has significant activity against the disease. Ontak, a new monoclonal antibody, is a diphtheria toxin targeted to cells that express the IL2 receptor (cd 25). It is FDA-approved for treatment of cutaneous T-cell lymphoma. Extracorporeal photopheresis and total skin electron beam therapy are used for more advanced disease. Systemic chemotherapy may be used to palliate symptoms.

22. What is the role of bone marrow transplant and stem cell rescue in NHLs?
The role in initial presentations is unclear. In relapsed disease, high-dose therapy with autologous bone marrow transplant or stem cell support may be used; initial results are encouraging. An unrelated or related allogenic transplant sometimes is considered because of the added graft vs. lymphoma effect on killing the cancer. This type of transplant has a higher risk of rejection and graft vs. host disease than any of the autologous transplants. In a randomized study of patients with relapsed chemotherapy-sensitive diffuse, aggressive NHL, the event-free 5-year survival rate was 46% vs. 12% and the 5-year survival rate was 53% vs. 32% in the autotransplant group. Patients who relapsed within 1 year of diagnosis were less likely to benefit from transplant than patients who had a longer remission. Patients with an International Prognostic Index score of 1–3, including those with poor performance status, did better with transplant than with standard treatment. Poor

results have been obtained in patients with truly chemotherapy-refractory disease. In low-grade disease, transplantation usually is reserved for patients who have relapsed or are in second or later remission. It is suggested that transplantation changes the natural history of the disease by providing durable remissions and delaying relapses. Randomized studies are needed to determine the exact role of transplantation.

23. What is Richter's transformation?

Evolution of a low-grade lymphoma into a diffuse large cell lymphoma is called Richter's transformation. The term was first used in 1928 to describe a case of CLL that developed into aggressive lymphoma.

24. Which lymphomas can be treated with antibiotics?

MALT lymphoma in the stomach has been associated with *H. pylori* infection. Treatment of this infection with antibiotics (bismuth, metronidazole, tetracycline, omeprazole) can lead to complete remission of the lymphoma. Patients with systemic advanced disease require chemotherapy.

25. What is rituximab?

Rituximab (Rituxan) is a monoclonal antibody used in the treatment of relapsed and refractory low-grade and follicular NHL. It is a genetically engineered mouse antibody directed against the CD20 receptor, commonly expressed in NHL. Once bound to B cells, rituximab induces lysis of the abnormal cells. It is used alone and with standard chemotherapy.

26. What is bexxar?

Bexxar is a radioactive iodine conjugate of the same type of antibody used in rituximab, but it also targets B cells. Bexxar carries radiation directly to the tumor cells. Trials have been conducted in patients with low-grade lymphomas and are now being expanded to include other forms of the disease.

27. Describe the treatment for lymphoma of the central nervous system (CNS).

Patients with CNS lymphoma have a poor prognosis. All tumors are high-grade, and some are associated with HIV. The frequency of CNS lymphoma in HIV-infected patients is decreasing because of the effectiveness of antiviral therapy. Treatment with a combination of whole-brain radiation and chemotherapy seems to give the best long-term results. Chemotherapy includes drugs that cross the blood-brain barrier, such as high-dose cytarabine and methotrexate, with intrathecal treatments of the same drugs. High doses of steroids (e.g., dexamethasone) can be helpful in palliation of symptoms. It is important to make the diagnosis before initiating steroids because the tumor can be highly sensitive to this treatment and may shrink before a diagnosis can be made. With treatment the median survival time is 41 months. The treatment is highly toxic, producing long-term leukoencephalopathy and dementia in 25% of patients at 5 years. Age and performance status are important prognostic factors.

28. What public resources are available for patients with lymphoma?

- Cure for Lymphoma Foundation
  Website: www.cfl.org; telephone: 212-319-5857; E-mail: InfoCFL@aol.com
  Raises funds for research and provides patient educational materials. Patient support is available through a patient-to-patient telephone network, library, and newsletter.
- Leukemia and Lymphoma Society of America
  Website: www.leukemia-lymphoma.org; telephone: 800-955-4LSA; 212-573-8484
  National voluntary health agency that offers support groups and financial assistance.
- Lymphoma Research Foundation of America
  Telephone: 310-204-7040; E-mail: Irfa@aol.com
  Nonprofit agency that provides research grants and educational information. It offers a support group (Los Angeles) and a national "buddy system."

• Lymphoma Foundation of America
  Telephone: 202-223-6181
  Nonprofit agency that provides educational materials, patient support groups, treatment up-
  dates, and patient advocacy.
• Lymphoma Information Network
  Website: www.lymphomainfo.net

REFERENCES

1. Abeloff M (ed): Oncology and Hematology 2000: An Internet guide. eMedguides, 2000.
2. Armitage JO: Treatment of non-Hodgkin's lymphoma. N Engl J Med 328:1023–1030, 1993.
3. Beutler E, Lichtman M, Coller B, Kipps T (eds): Williams' Hematology, 6th ed. New York, McGraw-Hill, 2000.
4. DeVita V, Hellman S, Rosenberg S: Cancer: Principles and Practice of Oncology, 6th ed. Philadelphia, J.B. Lippincott, 2001.
5. Engelking C, Hubbard SM: Current Issues and Controversies in the Management of Non-Hodgkin's Lymphoma. New York, Triclinica Communications, 1996.
6. Greenlee RT, Hill-Harmon MB, Murray T, Thun M: Cancer statistics, 2001. CA Cancer J Clin 51:15–36, 2001.
7. Haskell C: Cancer Treatment, 5th ed. Philadelphia, W.B. Saunders, 2000.
8. Hauke RJ, Armitage JO: A new approach to non-Hodgkin's lymphoma. Intern Med 39:197–203, 2000.
9. Hauke RJ, Armitage JO: Treatment of non-Hodgkin's lymphoma. Curr Opin Oncol 12:412–418, 2000.
10. Lessin LT (ed): Medical Knowledge: Self Assessment Program in the Specialty of Hematology, 2nd ed. Philadelphia, American College of Physicians, 1998.
11. Molina A, Pezner RD: Non-Hodgkin's lymphoma. In Pazdur R, Coia LR, Hoskins WJ, Wagman LD (eds): Cancer Management: A Multidisciplinary Approach—Medical, Surgical, and Radiation Oncology, 3rd ed. Melville, NY, PRR, 1999, pp 525–558.
12. Nasir S, DeAngelis L: Update on the management of primary CNS lymphoma. Oncology 14:228–237, 2000.
13. Winter J: High-dose therapy with stem cell transplantation in the malignant lymphomas. Oncology 13:1635–1645, 1999.

IV. Solid Tumors

21. AIDS-RELATED MALIGNANCIES

David C. Faragher, MD

1. What are the AIDS-defining malignancies?

Kaposi's sarcoma (KS), non-Hodgkin's lymphoma (NHL), and invasive cervical cancer. Cumulatively through the end of 1998, 56,615 cases of KS, 18,879 cases of NHL, and 1,166 cases of invasive cervical cancer have been reported among persons with AIDS in the United States. The outbreak of *Pneumocystis carinii* pneumonia (PCP) and KS signaled the onset of the epidemic in 1981.

2. Does KS occur with equal frequency in all groups of patients with AIDS?

KS is much more frequent in homosexual and bisexual men with human immunodeficiency virus (HIV) than in other risk groups. Studies from the early 1980s revealed that up to 50% of homosexual/bisexual men presented with KS as the initial manifestation of AIDS. In 1991 this percentage had decreased to 11%. Over 90% of all AIDS-related KS occurs in homosexual/bisexual men. KS also has been described in non-HIV infected homosexual men. It is quite uncommon in intravenous drug users, heterosexual men, and women. However, KS is more common in women who have bisexual male sexual partners than in women who are intravenous drug users. Compared with the general population, KS risk is increased approximately 100,000-fold for homosexual men with AIDS and approximately 13,000-fold for others with AIDS.

3. Does KS occur only in patients with AIDS?

KS initially was described by Moricz Kaposi in 1872 in elderly men of eastern European or Mediterranean descent. It was limited primarily to skin involvement of the legs and was rarely life-threatening (classic type). Cases of lymph node involvement or visceral disease were rare. An endemic form also has been described in younger men and women of sub-Saharan Africa. The endemic form is more aggressive with visceral and lymph node involvement as well as cutaneous disease. A third category of non–HIV-related KS involves patients who are immunocompromised from organ transplantation or autoimmune diseases. The incidence of KS is 200–400 times greater in patients with organ transplants than in the general population. KS in patients with AIDS is the epidemic form of the disease.

4. Why are malignancies included in the Centers for Disease Control and Prevention (CDC) list of AIDS-defining conditions?

Malignancies are a relatively common complication of a broad range of immunodeficiency states. There have been many reports of malignancies in patients with organ transplants as well as various congenital immunodeficiency conditions. Immunosuppression predisposes to malignancies for several possible reasons: (1) absence of protective immune surveillance to eliminate abnormal clones; (2) dysregulation of cell proliferation and differentiation; and (3) chronic antigenic bombardment of the immune system by various infections. The marked rise in incidence of lymphoma and KS in HIV-infected people has been noted since 1982. KS was one of the first recognized conditions in AIDS. Epidemiologic studies subsequently showed that non-Hodgkin's lymphoma and, most recently, invasive cervical cancer in women are much more common in patients with AIDS than in age-matched controls. The greater-than-expected frequency of these malignancies led to their inclusion as AIDS-defining conditions.

5. Have other malignancies been associated with AIDS?

Several non–AIDS-defining malignancies have been described in patients with AIDS, including Hodgkin's disease (HD; relative risk = 8-fold), squamous cell carcinomas (SCC) of the head and neck, SCC of the anus (relative risk = 31.7-fold), germ cell cancer (relative risk = 2.9-fold), lung cancer (relative risk = 2.5-fold), melanoma, basal cell carcinomas of the skin, colon cancer, and plasmacytoma/multiple myeloma (relative risk = 4.5-fold). There are also several reports of myelodysplastic syndrome (preleukemia) and acute myeloid leukemia (relative risk = 3-fold) in patients with AIDS. Some of these malignancies, such as HD and germ cell cancers, are more common in 30–45-year-old people, which is the age group most often afflicted with AIDS. The results of epidemiologic studies to determine whether these cancers have a higher incidence in patients with AIDS than in age-matched controls are conflicting. There is also some controversy about different biologic behavior of malignancies in patients with AIDS compared with immunocompetent patients. Many malignancies are significantly more aggressive and more advanced in patients with AIDS.

6. Is HTLV-1 associated with AIDS-related malignancies?

The human T-cell leukemia/lymphoma virus (HTLV-1) is not the AIDS virus. It is a retrovirus endemic to southwest Japan, the Caribbean basin, Melanesia, and parts of Africa. There have been some reports of HTLV-1 in urban areas of the United States, such as New York City and Miami. Transmission routes are the same as for HIV: transplacental transmission, blood transfusions, sexual contact, and sharing of contaminated intravenous needles. In 1988, the Food and Drug Adminstration (FDA) formally recommended screening all whole blood and blood component donations for HTLV-1. In the United States, seroprevalence rates are approximately 0.016%. HTLV-1 is associated with adult T-cell leukemia/lymphoma as well as HTLV-1–associated myelopathy and tropical spastic paresis, a neurologic disease.

7. What causes KS?

There have been multiple theories about the cause of KS in AIDS. Because KS was seen primarily in homosexual and bisexual men, it was hypothesized that KS was caused by an infectious agent such as cytomegalovirus (CMV), Epstein-Barr virus (EBV), or human papillomavirus (HPV). These viral DNA sequences were reported in some, but not all, samples of KS tumors. It is known that various soluble factors (cytokines) stimulate growth of KS in tissue culture systems as well as in the human body. These cytokines include interleukin-1 (IL-1), IL-6, tumor necrosis factor-beta (TNF-β), platelet-derived growth factor (PDGF), and oncostatin-M. Cytokine production is also stimulated by opportunistic infections and some medications (e.g., steroids). In addition to cytokines, KS production and growth are stimulated by a protein product of the HIV virus. The HIV-*tat* protein induces and stimulate KS in animal systems. In the search for a sexually transmissible KS agent, Chang, Moore, and colleagues discovered a previously unknown herpes virus—KS-associated herpes virus (KSHV), also known as human herpes virus-8 (HHV-8). HHV-8 has been isolated from virutally 100% of AIDS-KS tumor cells by polymerase chain reaction, but it is not found in normal cells from the same patients. HHV-8 has numerous genes capable of deregulating mitosis, interrupting apoptosis (programmed cell death), increasing angiogenesis, and blocking presentation of antigenic epitopes. It is thought that HHV-8 may be the agent that transforms normal mesenchymal cells into pre-KS cells. Further activation by cytokines (e.g., IL-1, HIV-*tat*, TNF) may trigger a true monoclonal malignant condition.

8. What types of NHL occur in AIDS?

The predominant types of NHL in AIDS are high-grade B-cell NHLs, such as immunoblastic, Burkitt's lymphoma, non-Burkitt's small noncleaved lymphoma (70%), intermediate-grade large cell lymphomas (30%), and primary NHLs of the CNS. Epidemiologic studies have shown a sharp rise in the incidence of NHL since 1983, predominantly in men aged 20–54 years. In a study of 100,000 patients with AIDS from 1981 to 1989, 3% had NHL—a 150–250-fold increase in incidence compared with the general population. NHL also may be clinically undetected before death. In an autopsy study of 101 patients with AIDS, 20 were found to have NHL. Herpes virus infections play a distinct role in AIDS NHL. HHV-8 was discovered in essentially every case of the newly defined clinicopathologic condition currently termed *primary effusion lymphoma.* EBV can be detected in virtually 100% of primary CNS lymphomas in patients with AIDS.

9. Does HIV-related NHL follow the same natural history as NHL in immunocompetent patients?

AIDS-associated NHL is significantly more aggressive than NHL in immunocompetent patients. Typically it is more extensive and frequently involves extranodal sites (central nervous system, bone marrow, gastrointestinal tract); it is, therefore, diagnosed as stage IV disease. Patients also frequently have B symptoms (fevers, night sweats, and weight loss). Lymphomas of the central nervous system may occur as mass lesions or with leptomeningeal involvement only. The risk for NHL rises significantly as immunosuppression worsens. The incidence of NHL is much greater in patients with CD4 lymphocyte counts < 50. (A healthy person normally has a CD4 count of 500–1000). Opportunistic infections are likely in people with CD4 counts < 200. Another unique finding in AIDS-associated NHL is the presence of polyclonal malignant cells. Monoclonality generally is considered a hallmark of malignancy. However, the patient with AIDS is exposed to repeated infections and subsequent polyclonal B-lymphocyte activation and transformation to a polyclonal malignancy.

10. How is KS staged?

Most malignancies are staged by parameters developed and standardized by the American Joint Committee on Cancer (AJCC). This system uses the tumor-node-metastasis (TNM) classification. However, KS has a unique presentation, prognosis, and natural history. Many staging systems modeled after the TNM classification have been proposed, but none accurately predicts the prognosis of AIDS-associated KS. Recently, the Oncology Subcommittee of the NIH-sponsored AIDS Clinical Treatment Group (ACTG) proposed a new staging scheme based on factors that more accurately predict the natural history and prognosis of KS.

Good risk (all of the following)	Poor risk (any of the following)
Tumor confined to skin and/or lymph nodes	Extensive oral, GI, or other visceral disease, tumor associated with edema or ulceration
CD4 ≥ 200	CD4 < 200
No opportunistic infection, thrush, or B symptoms	History of opportunistic infection or B symptoms
Karnofsky performance status ≥ 70%	Karnofsky performance status < 70

11. Describe the treatment for HIV-associated NHL.

Because AIDS-associated NHL is an aggressive disease that usually presents with multiorgan involvement, chemotherapy is generally the standard of care. However, patients most likely to develop AIDS-associated NHL are severely immunocompromised and frequently have active opportunistic infections. A complete evaluation must be done to determine whether any treatment is appropriate. If treatment is chosen, multiagent chemotherapy is necessary. In immunocompetent patients, multiagent chemotherapy yields response rates as high as 80% and long-term survival rates of approximately 40%. However, in AIDS-associated NHL, response rates are 50% and median survival is approximately 5–6 months. Survival is significantly better in subgroups of patients, including those with CD4 count > 100, Karnofsky performance status > 70%, no opportunistic infections, and no extranodal disease. Because of the higher toxicity associated with standard NHL regimens in patients with AIDS, numerous studies have compared the response, relapse rate, and overall survival of AIDS NHL patients with standard dose vs. low-dose combination chemotherapy regimens. Randomized studies have revealed no significantly improved survival rates with standard dose regimens compared with low-dose regimens. Furthermore, randomized studies have confirmed the safety of concurrent use of highly active antiretroviral therapy (HAART) with combination chemotherapy in patients with NHL. The overall rates of response and survival may be favorably affected by the use of HAART along with chemotherapy.

12. What special precautions are needed in giving chemotherapy for AIDS-associated NHL?

Completing full courses of chemotherapy may be more difficult because of frequent dose reductions and delays due to prolonged bone marrow suppression and opportunistic infections. Recent studies confirm improved outcomes with modified chemotherapy regimens and generous use of hematopoetic growth factors (granulocyte colony-stimulating factor [G-CSF], granulocyte-macrophage colony-stimulating factor [GM-CSF]). Original studies, using full-dose chemotherapy, revealed excessive morbidity and mortality as a result of infections. The likelihood of morbidity increases as the degree of immunosuppression increases. Current recommendations include use of attenuated doses and/or use of hematopoetic growth factors if CD4 < 100 and standard chemotherapy doses (with or without G-CSF or GM-CSF) if CD4 > 200. Because the risk of leptomeningeal relapse is extremely high, use of meningeal prophylaxis is encouraged for all patients with AIDS-associated NHL. Such patients also should be treated with aggressive antiviral therapy and prophylaxis against PCP.

13. What are the indications for treatment of AIDS-associated KS?

The first factor to consider in the treatment of KS is the indications for treatment. KS often presents with limited skin involvement, which may not require immediate treatment. Some patients request immediate treatment for body image and cosmetic reasons. But if KS is asymptomatic, treatment may be postponed until there is further indication. The primary indications for treatment include (1) cosmetic control; (2) painful, bulky lesions; (3) oral lesions interfering with eating or swallowing; (4) lymphedema from lymph node or lymph vessel infiltration; (5) pulmonary involvement; (6) extensive GI involvement, causing GI obstruction; and (7) rapidly progressive disease.

14. Which treatment modalities are used for AIDS-associated KS?

The many options for treatment of KS include local or systemic therapy. Local treatments include radiation therapy, intralesional therapy, and cryotherapy (liquid nitrogen). Intralesional therapy usually involves dilute solutions of vincristine, but other agents have been used. Systemic treatment includes single-agent chemotherapy, multiagent chemotherapy, and alpha-interferon (with or without concomitant antiretroviral therapy). Life-threatening disease, usually pulmonary disease, requires aggressive treatment with multiagent chemotherapy. Response rates have ranged from 70–100%. Alpha-interferon has response rates up to 65% in a select subset of patients with good prognosis (CD4 > 200, no opportunistic infection or B symptoms). HAART has had a dramatic impact on KS, with regression of some lesions when HAART is used alone. All patients with AIDS and KS should be given a trial of HAART. The combination of antiretroviral therapy with alpha-interferon has allowed continued high response rates with lower doses of interferon. Although many older chemotherapy agents have had response rates of 15–30% with KS, the current systemic chemotherapy treatments for KS revolve around liposomal formulations of anthracyclines and paclitaxel. The liposomal coating allows long circulation time, higher intralesion drug levels, and high response rates (up to 70%) with lower toxicity. A side effect common to nearly all of these treatments is neutropenia. Paclitaxel, a relatively new microtubule toxin, has response rates up to 70%. Hematopoetic growth factors have helped to minimize cytopenia and infections while maximizing tolerated doses of therapy. All treatment for KS is palliative; therefore, risks and benefits must be weighed before initiating therapy. Future research in the treatment of KS will target HHV-8 as the etiologic agent.

15. Can treatment of HIV with antiretroviral therapy increase the risk of NHL?

This question is controversial. Several reports have investigated the possibility. An autopsy study in 1992 found an association of increasing incidence of NHL with cumulative doses of zidovudine (AZT). An animal study also found a higher incidence of NHL in mice treated with didanosine. However, a study in 1991 revealed no increase in the incidence of NHL with increased cumulative doses of AZT. The authors reported a risk of approximately 0.8% for each 6 months of AZT treatment, with an incidence up to 3.2% after 24 months of AZT treatment. This study suggests that an increased incidence of NHL correlates with increased survival due to antiretroviral therapy. If patients treated with antiretrovirals live longer, they have more time to become immunosuppressed, leading to increased exposure to lymphomagenic stimuli (e.g., viruses, oncogenes).

16. Why has invasive cervical SCCA been included as a AIDS-defining malignancy?

The percentage of women infected with HIV has risen significantly. HIV infection in women now accounts for 40% of all infections worldwide and for up to 12% in the United States. In selected regions in the U.S., such as New York City, up to 25% of HIV patients are female. Most HIV infections in American women result from heterosexual transmission. It is also known that the incidence of cervical neoplasia is significantly higher in congenital immunodeficiencies, autoimmune diseases, and acquired immunodeficiency states (e.g., organ transplantation). Reported rates of cervical neoplasia in such patients reach as high as 40%; the risk of anogenital neoplasia is 9–14-fold compared with matched controls. Immunosuppressed women with HIV have a much higher incidence of monilial vaginitis, sexually transmitted diseases, genital ulcers, and pelvic inflammatory disease. Vaginal candidal infection may occur much earlier than oral thrush and be more resistant to conventional therapies. The association of HPV and cervical neoplasia is well known. The oncogenic HPVs have been identified in 80–90% of invasive cervical cancers as well as high-grade cervical intraepithelial neoplasia (CIN). Several studies have reported a high incidence of HIV in women under 50 years of age with invasive cervical cancer. Furthermore, cervical cancer in the setting of HIV appears to be much more biologically aggressive, less responsive to conventional therapies, and associated with a poorer prognosis. Because of these findings, CDC revised the AIDS-defining criteria in 1993 to include invasive cervical cancer.

17. Is preinvasive neoplasia of the cervix included in the revised AIDS-defining CDC list?

CIN generally refers to cervical dysplasia, carcinoma in situ, and preinvasive neoplasia. The incidence of HIV infection in women with CIN varies by risk group and geographic region. In high-risk areas, such as New York City, up to 13% of women in screening clinics were found to be HIV-positive. The risk of abnormal cervical cytology is increased by as much as 10-fold in HIV-positive women; some studies report abnormal cervical cytology in 30–60%. However, a high degree of discordance between cytology and biopsy has been found in HIV-positive women with negative cytology and abnormal cervical biopsies. Although preinvasive cervical neoplasia is not included in the AIDS definition, cervical dysplasia and CIS are considered AIDS-related conditions. The degree of cervical neoplasia is correlated with the degree of immune suppression. Women with CIN tend to have lower CD4 counts than HIV-positive women without CIN.

18. Describe the proper screening for cervical neoplasia in HIV-positive women.

Papanicolaou smears should be done every 6 months as well as baseline colposcopy or cervicography. There is also an extremely high association between HPV and anal neoplasia. All HIV-positive women with HPV or cervical dysplasia should have a thorough anal examination, including visual and digital exam, anal cytology smear, and anoscopy.

19. Describe the appropriate treatment for invasive malignancy of the cervix in women with AIDS.

Patients with AIDS-associated cervical cancer present with more advanced disease than age-matched controls. Incidence of high-grade tumors, lymph node involvement, and aggressive biologic behavior is more common in women with AIDS. In addition, risk of recurrence is higher and survival times are shorter for patients with AIDS. Therapy for invasive disease should be based on the patient's condition and stage of malignancy. Patients with relatively good immune function tolerate surgery quite well. Patients with advanced inoperable disease should be considered for chemotherapy or radiation therapy. Patients with poor immune function do not tolerate pelvic radiation treatment or chemotherapy because of depressed hematologic reserve.

20. Are any nursing considerations different in patients with AIDS-related malignancies and other patients with cancer?

Nursing care and symptom control are similar in patients with AIDS-related malignancies and other patients with cancer, except that even more vigilance may be required for early identification of life-threatening infectious complications and assessment of neurologic abnormalities. Patients need to be well educated about prevention of infection and signs and symptoms of opportunistic infections, particularly PCP. Symptoms of PCP include shortness of breath with or without exertion and dry, nonproductive cough. In addition to other neutropenic precautions, HIV-infected patients should be instructed not to handle or eat raw meat, to avoid eating raw shellfish due to risk of *Vibrio* spp. infection, and to wear gloves when handling litter boxes because of the potential for contacting toxoplasmosis. Assessment of neurologic abnormalites can be complicated because mental status changes may be associated with HIV-related dementia, central nervous system involvement, drug side effects, viral or opportunistic infections, or depression.

21. What problems are associated with medications for people with AIDS and cancer?

A particularly difficult nursing challenge in patients with AIDS-related malignancies is keeping track of various drug interactions and incompatibilities in patients who are on multiple drug regimens to treat malignancy, underlying HIV disease, and opportunistic infections. Patients need to be encouraged to inform health care providers if they are taking any other drugs, remedies, or alternative substances that may interact with prescribed therapies. The large potential for drug interactions may be synergistic or antagonistic and result in increased effect, decreased effect, or enhanced toxicity.

22. Are there any "red flags" to alert health care providers about potential drug interactions in HIV-infected patients?

Red flags that should alert nurses to potential drug interactions include the following: treatment or prophylaxis for mycobacterial infections with rifamycins (e.g., rifampin, rifabutin) or macrolides (e.g., erythromycin); therapy with azole antifungal drugs (e.g., ketoconazole) or protease inhibitors (e.g., ritonavir); and any multidrug regimen. Although most interactions do not require changes in drug selection, nurses should be aware of clinically significant interactions. For example, patients with advanced HIV disease and cancer frequently receive palliative care drugs such as opioids, antidepressants, sedatives, and/or hypnotics. Serious clinical consequences may result from increased concentrations due to altered clearances when these drugs are taken with ritonavir (an antiretroviral protease inhibitor).

23. What psychosocial issues are involved?

Psychosocial issues and stresses may be more complicated than in oncology patients without AIDS. Even in communities that are accepting of AIDS, the patient with AIDS and cancer may experience more social isolation, particularly as the illness progresses.

REFERENCES

1. Emmanoulides C, Miles SA, Mitsuyasu RT: Pathogenesis of AIDS-related KS. Oncology 10:335–341, 1996.
2. Goedert JJ: The epidemiology of acquired immunodeficiency syndrome malignancies. Semin Oncol 27:390–401, 2000.
3. Kaplan LD, Northfelt DS: Malignancies associated with AIDS. In Sande MA, Volberding PA (eds): The Medical Management of AIDS, 5th ed. Philadelphia, W.B. Saunders, 1997, pp 413–439.
4. Levine AM: Acquired immunodeficiency syndrome-related lymphoma. Blood 80:8–20, 1992.
5. Levine AM, Bernstein L, Sullivan-Halley J, et al: Role of zidovudine antiretroviral therapy in the pathogenesis of AIDS-related lymphoma. Blood 86:4612–4616, 1995.
6. Moore PS, Chang Y: Detection of herpesvirus-like DNA sequences in KS in patients with and those without HIV infection. N Engl J Med 332:1181–1185, 1995.
7. Northfelt DW: Cervical and anal neoplasia and HPV infections in persons with HIV infection. Oncology 8:33–37, 1994.
8. Piscitelli SC, Flexner C, Minor JR, et al: AIDS commentary: Drug interactions in patients infected with human immunodeficiency virus. Clin Infect Dis 23:685–693, 1996.

22. BLADDER CANCER

Carmel Sauerland, RN, Tauseef Ahmed, MD, and Muhammad Choudhry, MD

Quick Facts—Bladder Cancer

Incidence	54,300 estimated new cases in 2001. Bladder cancer is the fourth leading cancer in men.
Mortality	The estimated number of deaths in 2001 is 12,400.
Risk factors	Cigarette smoking Exposure to chemical compounds—aromatic amines and aniline dyes Exposure to *Schistosoma haematobium*, a parasite common in Egypt and developing countries Previous radiation to the pelvic area Previous treatment with the antineoplastic agent, cyclophosphamide
Histology	Transitional cell carcinoma: most common (90%); 75% are invasive at presentation Squamous cell carcinoma (8%) Adenocarcinoma (1%)
Signs and symptoms	Painless hematuria (80–90%), which may be persistent, microscopic, or gross at presentation Irritative symptoms (20%) such as urgency, frequency, and dysuria (burning on urination)
Diagnosis and staging studies	• History and physical examination (including bimanual examination at the time of transurethral resection) • Complete blood count, chemistry profile, urinalysis, chest radiograph, urine cytology • Intravenous pyelography (IVP) • Cystoscopy and transurethral resection of bladder tumor (TURBT) + bladder mapping and sampling of the floor of the prostatic urethra in men with high-grade bladder cancer • Abdominal computed tomography (CT) scan and bone scan should be considered in patients with muscle invasion • CT scan of the chest should be considered in patients with high-grade, muscle-invading tumors
Staging	**Tumor, node, metastasis (TNM) staging system for bladder cancer*** **Tumor**

TX	Primary tumor cannot be assessed
T0	No evidence of primary tumor
Ta	Noninvasive papillary tumor
Tis	Carcinoma in situ: "flat tumor"
T1	Tumor invades subepithelial connective tissue
T2	Tumor invades muscle
T2a	Tumor invades superficial muscle (inner half)
T2b	Tumor invades deep muscle (outer half)
T3	Tumor invades perivesical tissue
T3a	Microscopically
T3b	Macroscopically (extravesical mass)
T4	Tumor invades any of the following: prostate, uterus, vagina, pervic wall, abdominal wall
T4a	Tumor invades prostate, uterus, vagina
T4b	Tumor invades pelvic wall, abdominal wall

Table continued on following page

Quick Facts—Bladder Cancer (Continued)

Nodes

NX	Regional lymph nodes cannot be assessed
N0	No regional lymph node metastases
N1	Metastasis in a single lymph node, ≤ 2 cm in greatest dimension
N2	Metastases in a single lymph node > 2 or ≤ 5 cm, or multiple lymph nodes, none > 5 cm in greatest dimension
N3	Metastasis in a lymph node > 5 cm in greatest dimension

Metastasis

MX	Distant metastasis cannot be assessed
M0	No distant metastases
Ml	Distant metastases

Stage groupings

Stage 0a	Ta	N0	M0
Stage 0is	Tis	N0	M0
Stage I	T1	N0	M0
Stage II	T2a	N0	M0
	T2b	N0	M0
Stage III	T3a	N0	M0
	T3b	N0	M0
	T4a	N0	M0
Stage IV	T4b	N0	M0
	Any T	N1-3	M0
	Any T	Any N	M1

* The TNM staging system is preferred over the Jewett-Strong staging system.

1. What epidmiologic characteristics are known about bladder cancer?

Bladder cancer is a disease of the elderly. The average age at diagnosis is 65 years. In the United States, it is a disease primarily of Caucasian men, who are twice as likely to develop bladdder cancer as African-American men. There is also a significant gender difference with a four times higher incidence in men than in women.

2. What is the greatest risk factor for bladder cancer?

Cigarette smoking. Smokers are twice as likely to develop bladder cancer. In men, 50% of bladder cancers are attributed to smoking.

3. Who is at risk for bladder cancer related to chemical exposure?

People who are exposed to aromatic amines (contained in cigarettes) and aniline dyes are at risk for developing bladder cancer. These chemicals are used in various industrial trades, including dry cleaning, printing, and painting. Other exposed workers are hair dressers (hair dyes), janitors, and leather, rubber, aluminum, and textile workers. Although exposure to these chemicals is probably small, new evidence suggests that host factors may play a significant role in determining the effect of the exposure. Specifically, people of the slow acetylator phenotype are more likely to have difficulty with ridding the body of these harmful chemicals.

4. What type of bladder cancer is related to chronic irritation and infection?

Squamous cell carcinoma, the second most common type, is usually seen in the bladder after chronic irritation secondary to infection, stones, and chronic indwelling Foley catheters. Infections with the *Schistosoma haemotobium* parasite often lead to the development of bladder cancer due to chronic irritation. Transitional cell carcinoma, the most common (90%) type of bladder cancer in the United States, arises from the transitional epithelial lining of the bladder. Seventy-five percent of the transitional cell carcinomas are invasive (through the muscle wall of the bladder) at presentation.

5. What are the important prognostic features?

In general, bladder cancer can be divided into two groups: noninvasive (stages Ta, Tis, and T1) or invasive (stages T2–T4). Noninvasive cancers tend to recur throughout the patient's life but remain superficial; they require continued monitoring and local treatment. The most important prognostic factor in superficial or noninvasive bladder cancers is the tumor grade (level of cell differentiation). Tumors are typically graded as low (G1), moderate (G2), or high (G3). For invasive cancers (almost all are G3), the stage, not the grade, is the most important prognostic factor. Such patients usually require radical surgery and have a higher probability of developing metastatic disease.

6. What are the most common sites of metastases?

Invasive bladder cancer tends to invade *directly* the sigmoid colon, rectum, prostate (in men), ureters, and vagina (in women). The most common metastatic sites are lymph nodes, bones, liver, and lungs. Of interest, in patients who have been successfully treated with combination chemotherapy, the central nervous system is a common site of metastasis.

7. Describe the treatment of superficial tumors after cystoscopy.

Stage Tis tumors should be treated with intravesical agents, such as bacillus Calmette-Guérin (BCG; an attenuated strain of *Mycobacterium bovis*), doxorubicin, mitomycin, and thiotepa. The agent with the best response rate is BCG. In controlled trials, BCG has been shown to be superior to most available intravesical agents. BCG decreases both the risk of recurrence and the rate of progression. Low grade Ta and T1 lesions can be managed with surveillance, cystoscopy, and cytology every 3 months. Recurrent and high-grade superficial tumors may be treated with intravesical agents after tumor resection. Current clinical trials are examining biologic agents (e.g., interferon, interleukin 2) to determine whether they enhance the effect of BCG.

8. How often is intravesical BCG administered?

The standard treatment regimen is weekly intravesical BCG for 6 weeks with repeat cystoscopy approximately 6 weeks after the last treatment. Some evidence suggests that maintenance BCG improves results.

9. What are the local effects of intravesical instillation of BCG?

Three to four hours after instillation, patients may experience dysuria, frequency of urination, and urgency.

10. What systemic reactions occur in some patients treated with BCG?

Approximately 3% of patients receiving BCG develop fever > 103° F. They require immediate attention and may be hospitalized and treated with cycloserine, isoniazid (INH), and rifampin, especially if the high fever occurs within the first 2 hours of BCG therapy. BCG therapy should not be reinstituted. Some patients experience low-grade fevers, usually 4–8 hours after BCG treatment. They usually resolve in response to antipyretics and do not last longer than 24 hours. No INH or rifampin is necessary, and BCG may be continued with close monitoring. Patients with low-grade fevers lasting longer than 24 hours can be pretreated with INH. BCG therapy may be safely continued.

BCG sepsis occurs in 0.4% of patients. Traumatic catheterization with bleeding is the most common cause of intravascular absorption of BCG and development of sepsis syndrome. Treatment includes INH, rifampin, and cycloserine; prednisone use is controversial. Patients definitely should not receive BCG again.

11. Which patients should never be treated with BCG?

BCG should be avoided in patients who are immunosuppressed, who have active urinary tract infections, or who have exhibited previous sensitivity to BCG.

12. How is muscle-invading transitional cell carcinoma (TCC) treated?

In the United States, radical cystectomy is the treatment of choice for muscle-invading TCC. This procedure involves removal of the local pelvic lymph nodes and radical cystoprostatectomy in men and anterior exenteration in women. Patients have urinary diversions (e.g., ileal-conduit with external bag or continent urinary diversions that do not involve external drainage). For patients with T2–T3a disease without ureter obstruction, the benefit of multmodality therapy (partial cystectomy, radiation therapy, and chemotherapy) vs. radical cystectomy is debated. Unfortunately, only a small number of patients are in clinical trials examining the multimodality approach, thus, making it difficult to determine whether this approach improves survival.

13. What factors determine eligibility for a neobladder (continent urinary diversion) vs. an ileal-conduit?

The absence of impaired renal function, dilated ureters, and bowel disease, no contraindications to prolonged surgery, and performance status.

14. What morbidities are associated with cystectomy? How can they be decreased?

- Impotence. Potency can be maintained by surgical techniques that spare the nerves traveling posteriorly to the prostate gland. However, most patients become impotent if classic surgical techniques are used.
- Need for urinary stoma. Neobladders, such as Indiana, Studer, and Koch pouches, prevent continuous loss of urine. A neobladder is formed from the bowel and may enable a patient to achieve urinary continence.

15. What is an ileal conduit?

An incontinent type of diversion that requires an external drainage bag. The ureters are not brought to the skin directly after removal of the bladder because of the high rate of stoma stenosis, which may lead to renal obstruction and failure. By interspersing a segment of ileum between the ureters and skin, this complication is virtually eliminated. The ileal conduit maintains its blood and nerve supply and continues to peristalse and eliminate urine. An ileal conduit may have less morbidity compared with continent diversions.

16. Describe the Indiana pouch. How is it formed?

An Indiana pouch is a continent, catherizable neobladder made from the terminal ileum and proximal colon. The colon portion is opened, then folded back on itself to decrease the pressure and increase the volume within the pouch. The terminal ileum is left attached to the colon and brought to the skin. The ileal-cecal valve keeps the urine from leaking out of the colon and can be catheterized through the stoma to drain the pouch. No bag is required over the stoma because it should not leak. The pouch should be catheterized every 4–6 hours, using clean technique. Only a 4 × 4 gauze pad is necessary to cover the stoma.

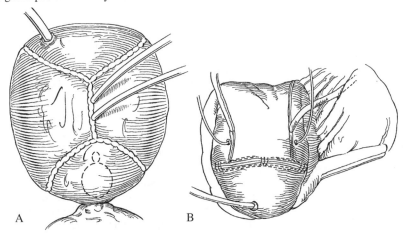

The illeoneobladder (A) and the Indiana reservoir *(B)*. (From Herr HW, Shipley WH, Bajorin DF: Cancer of the gladder. In DeVita VT, Hellman S, Rosenberg S (eds): Cancer: Principles and Practice of Oncology, 6th ed. Philadelphia, Lippincott Williams & Wilkins, 2001, p 1402, with permission.)

17. What is a Studer pouch? How is it formed?

A Studer pouch is a neobladder made entirely from ileum. In men, it can be connected to the urethra so that they can void through the urethra and maintain continence. In the future, more of these pouches will be seen in men with bladder cancer.

18. What types of bladder alterations should nurses expect after cystectomy?

- Because the bowels normally make mucus, neobladders and ileal conduits continue to do so. Mucous passes freely from ileal conduits but may need to be irrigated from continent neobladders.
- Urine cultures are always positive because of intestinal colonization by bacteria. True infections, manifested by fever and possible flank pain, are managed with antibiotics.
- Reflux of urine to the kidneys may contribute to pyelonephritis and late renal deterioration.
- Stones may develop in the kidney or pouch if urinary stasis is present.

19. What metabolic alterations may patients experience after surgery for bladder cancer?

Patients may develop metabolic disturbances depending on the type of urinary diversion and segment of intestine used. The intestine is responsible for absorption; therefore, if urine is in prolonged contact with the intestine, metabolic disturbances may result. Ileal conduits probably have the least amount of metabolic abnormalities because of the short time of urine contact. Continent diversions using ileum and colon may cause hyperchloremic metabolic acidosis, which in turn may cause osteoporosis over the long term. Patients may have frequent loose bowel movements after an intestinal urinary diversion. This symptom may resolve over a 3-month period. A few patients have persistent change in bowel habits, especially if the ileal-cecal valve is removed.

Patients with presurgical renal dysfunction (creatinine > 2.0) may have a problem compensating for this metabolic alteration and probably are candidates for ileal conduits only. Patients with neobladders and patients with resection of large amounts of terminal ileum are at risk for vitamin B12 deficiency, possibly leading to megaloblastic anemia. Blood levels should be monitored.

20. Does neoadjuvant or adjuvant therapy have a role in bladder cancer?

Evidence suggests that in high-risk patients combination cisplatin-based therapy before or after surgery decreases the risk of recurrence and increases cure rates. Specifically, extravesical tumor extension, evidence of vascular invasion in the resected specimen, and evidence of nodal involvement are justifications for offering adjuvant chemotherapy.

21. What role does radiation therapy play in the treatment of bladder cancer?

Radiation therapy is a treatment option for bladder cancer in several settings. If a patient is not a candidate for surgery or chemotherapy, radiation therapy becomes the primary treatment. It also can be used as a part of multimodality treatment plan, in combination with surgery and chemotherapy, to achieve bladder preservation. When metastatic disease to the bones is present, radiation may be used as a palliative treatment to obtain pain relief. The potential acute reactions to radiation therapy to the bladder are cystitis, stress incontinence, diarrhea, local skin inflammation, and fatigue. The late reactions consist of decreased bladder capacity and chronic cystitis. Radiation therapy also may affect sexual function.

22. Is there an effective treatment for metastatic TCC?

Cisplatin-based chemotherapy is effective in metastatic TCC. Methotrexate, vinblastine, doxorubicin (Adriamycin), and cisplatin (M-VAC) is a commonly used regimen. The patient should have good performance status, adequate myocardial reserve, and adequate renal function. Growth factors may be useful in conjunction with M-VAC. An alternative regimen is paclitaxel and cisplatin. Adequate hydration and vigorous use of antiemetics are necessary. Carboplatin may be substituted for cisplatin. Ifosfamide has been added to this regimen as well. Gemcitabine has also shown significant activity in TCC.

23. What is the nurse's role in caring for a patient diagnosed with bladder cancer?

The nurse plays a critcal role in assisting the patient with bladder cancer. The nurse should focus on several key areas: patient education, quality of life assessment, and supportive services.

24. What areas should be covered when educating the patient and family about bladder cancer treatment?

Basic anatomy of the genitourinary tract. The use of diagrams can help the patient and family to understand the normal anatomy of the urinary tract and how it changes with surgery.

Treatment options with rationale. Review the treatment with the patient and family. Is standard treatment being offered, or is the patient being asked to participate in a clinical trial? Do patient and family understand the difference?

- **Surgery.** Review the patient/family's understanding of the surgical procedure(s). Do they understand the changes that will result from surgery, such as creation of an ileoconduit/ neobladder? Are they aware of the self-care measures that will be required as a result of these changes?
- **Intravesical treatment.** Review the process of intravesical instillation treatment. The patient and family should understand that this treatment requires weekly visits to the doctor's office for 6 weeks. At each visit a bladder catheter is placed, followed by BCG instillation and cathether removal.
- **Chemotherapy.** Explain the chemotherapy agents, the route of administration, and the frequency and length of the treatment.
- **Radiation therapy.** Explain to the patient and family how radiation therapy is administered, the frequency and length of treatments, and the overall course.

25. What potential complictions or side effects should the nurse address?

After surgery: pneumonia, clots, fistula formation, infection, and electrolyte changes.

After intravesical treatment: cystitis, fever.

After chemotherapy: myelosuppression, mucositis, bleeding, change in bowel patteren (constipation and/or diarrhea), and increased risk of infection.

After radiation therapy: see question 21.

Instruct the patient to call the nurse or physician if a problem or question arises, especially if the patient receives multimodality therapy. It should be clear to patient and familiy whom they should call for what problems.

26. Which self-care measures should the nurse address?

After surgery. Teach ostomy care or self-catheterization, monitoring for signs and symptoms of urinary infection, and (for patients at increased risk) ways to decrease the risk of osteoporosis (change in diet, exercise).

After intravesicular treatment. Avoid an excessive amount of fluids and caffeine-containing beverages 6–8 hours before and for approximately 12 hours after treatment. Try to hold the BCG for approximately 2 hours. Good hygiene (hand washing after voiding, cleansing of toilet seat with bleach) should be practiced at home to avoid BCG exposure to household members. Men receiving BCG therapy should be instructed to use a condom, and women should be instructed to avoid vaginal contact for 1 week after treatment.

After chemotherapy. Review infection and bleeding precautions and mucositis care. Hygiene measures should be reinforced to reduce the risk of infection during myelosuppression.

After radiation therapy. Symptoms of cystitis can be controlled with increased fluid intake (2–3 L/day), avoiding caffeine-containing beverages, and use of analgesic agents (e.g., phenazopyridine hydrochloride). Stress incontinence can be controlled with alpha-adrenergic agonists (e.g., pseudoephedrine, tricyclic antidepressants) or nonpharmacologic measures such as biofeedback.

27. How does bladder cancer affect quality of life?

Each patient defines the components that provide him or her with a good quality of life. In addition to the frequent issues raised during diagnosis and treatment of cancer (e.g., the threat of death, the ability to work, carry on activities of significance, and maintain family responsibilities), patients with bladder cancer may have to contend with body image and sexual function changes. For patients who are not candidates for neobladder or bladder conservation surgery, the creation of a stoma for the ileal conduit and the use of a permanent drainage bag will alter body image and lifestyle. The patient and family need assistance to learn to cope with such changes.

28. How does bladder cancer diagnosis and treatment affect sexuality?

Alterations in body image affect sexuality in most patients. For men undergoing a radical cystectomy, there is a possibility of impotence even with the nerve-sparing technique. Most women experience discomfort during intercourse due to vaginal shrinkage. Intravesicular instillation therapy, chemotherapy, and radiation therapy may further affect sexual function. Education about these potential side effects and interventions available to assist the patient should take place throughout the continuum of care. The nurse may need to initiate discussion about sexuality concerns because the patient may be too uncomfortable to ask questions.

29. How do fatigue and pain due to bladder cancer or its treatment affect quality of life?

Fatigue can interfere with activities of daily living as well as roles and responsibilities within the family and on the job. A thorough assessment of the patient's nutritional status, blood work (to determine whether anemia is present), activity level, and degree of fatigue should be done so that information can be used to create an intervention plan specific to the patient's needs. Pain, associated with acute and chronic cystitis or bone metastasis, can negatively affect quality of life and should be treated immediately. Frequent assessments and patient/family education can help to achieve an acceptable pain management program.

30. What's new in bladder cancer diagnosis and treatment?

Hyaluronic acid (HA) and hyaluronidase (Haase) are currently under investigation as tumor markers. If found to be sensitive enough, they may eliminate more invasive diagnostic procedures. The potential value of the tumor suppressor gene (p53) in the diagnosis of bladder cancer, determination of treatment outcome, prediction of the risk of tumor development, and assessment of the benefit of adjuvant chemotherapy is also under investigation. Gene therapy is in the early phases of investigation for the treatment of bladder cancer. Easy access to the bladder makes it an ideal target for this type of therapy.

ACKNOWLEDGMENT

The authors acknowledge the contributions of Pat Judson, MD, and Mark Nishiya, MD, to the Bladder Cancer chapter in the first edition of Oncology Nursing Secrets.

REFERENCES

1. Basselli E, Greenberg R: Intravesical therapy for superficial bladder cancer. Oncology, 14:719–725, 2000.
2. Beltran A: Bladder treatment. Urol Clin North Am 26:535–554, 1999.
3. Carlson R: Bladder cancer: Sorting out the treatment options. Oncol Times 21:50–54, 1999.
4. Droller M: Bladder cancer: State of the art care. CA Cancer J Clin 48:269–284, 1998.
5. Duque J L, Loughlin K: An overview of the treatment of superficial bladder cancer. Urol Clin North Am 27:125–135, 2000.
6. Engelking C, Sauerland C: Maintenance of normal elimination. In Watkins-Bruner D., Moore-Higgs G,. Haas M (eds): Outcomes in Radiation Therapy (Multidisciplinnary Management). Sudbury, MA, Jones & Bartlett, 2001, pp 530–562.
7. Fleming ID, Cooper JS, Henson DE, et al: AJCC Cancer Staging Handbook, 5th ed. Philadelphia, Lippincott-Raven, 1998.
8. Greenlee RT, Hill-Harmon MB, Murray T, Thun M: Cancer statistics, 2001. CA Cancer J Clin 51:15–36, 2001.

9. Hsieh J, Dinney C, Chung L: The potential role of gene therapy in the treatment of bladder cancer. Urol Clin North Am 27:103–113, 2000.
10. Kantoff P, Zietman A, Wishnow K: Bladder cancer. In Holland J, Frei E (eds): Cancer Medicine, 5th ed. Philadelphia, B.C. Decker, 2000, pp 1543–1558.
11. Kelly LP, Miaskowski C: An overview of bladder cancer: Treatment and nursing implications. Oncol Nurs Forum 23:460–468, 1996.
12. Kim HL, Steinberg GD: The current status of bladder preservation in the treatment of muscle invasive bladder cancer. J Urol 164(3 Pt 1):627–632, 2000.
13. Vogelzang N, Scardino P, Shipley W, Coffey D: Comprehensive Textbook of Genitourinary Oncology, 2nd ed. Philadelphia, Lippincott Williams & Wilkins, 2000.
14. Watkins-Bruner D, Hurwitz M: Bladder cancer. In Watkins-Bruner D, Moore-Higgs G, Haas M. (eds): Outcomes in Radiation Therapy (Multidisciplinary Management). Sudbury, MA: Jones & Bartlett, 2001, pp 331–350.

23. BONE AND SOFT TISSUE SARCOMAS

Kyle M. Fink, MD, and Ioana Hinshaw, MD

Quick Facts—Sarcomas

Incidence	**Rare tumors**, < 1% of all cancers; 8,700 estimated new cases of soft tissue sarcomas and 2,900 estimated new cases of bone sarcomas in 2001
Mortality	< 1% of all cancer deaths; 4,400 estimated deaths from soft tissue sarcomas and 1,400 estimated deaths from bone sarcomas in 2001
Risk factors	Most patients have no known risk factors; rarely, genetically inherited diseases (von Recklinghausen's disease), prior radiation therapy, Paget's disease (osteosarcoma)
Histology	**Soft tissue sarcomas** have at least 70 histologic subtypes (liposarcoma, rhabdomyosarcoma, leiomyosarcoma, malignant fibrous histiocytoma) **Bone sarcomas** (osteosarcoma, Ewing's sarcoma, chondrosarcoma, malignant fibrous histiocytoma of bone)
Symptoms	Local pain, soft tissue swelling, palpable mass
Staging	**Soft tissue sarcomas** (tumor, node, metastasis [TNM]) Stage I Well differentiated, no nodes, no metastases Stage II Moderately differentiated, no nodes, no metastases Stage III Poorly differentiated, no nodes, no metastases Stage IV Any differentiation, with nodes and/or metastases Stages I, II, and III are subclassified into A (< 5 cm) and B (> 5 cm) **Bone sarcomas** (surgical staging more often used) Stage I Low grade Stage II High grade Stage III Any grade, with regional and/or distant metastasis Stages I and II are subclassified into A (intracompartmental) and B (extracompartmental)
Treatment	**Soft tissue sarcomas**

Small, well differentiated tumors	Surgery alone
Large, poorly differentiated tumors	Multimodality treatment, including chemotherapy, surgery, and radiation therapy
Osteosarcoma, Ewing's sarcoma	Chemotherapy followed by surgery followed by chemotherapy with or without radiation therapy

1. What are sarcomas?

Sarcoma is derived from the Greek *sarkoma*, meaning fleshy growth; it refers to a group of malignant tumors that originate from a common embryologic ancestry, the primitive mesoderm. The mesoderm gives rise during embryogenesis to soft tissues (e.g., muscles, tendons, fibrous tissue) as well as bone and cartilage. Sarcomas are tumors derived from any of these structures.

2. Are any risk factors associated with the development of sarcomas?

Most sarcomas appear in patients with no known predisposing factors. Some genetically transmitted diseases, however, are associated with an increased incidence of sarcomas. For example, von Recklinghausen's disease (neurofibromatosis) carries a 7–10% risk of developing neurofibrosarcoma, an otherwise rare sarcoma. Patients with chronic lymphedema secondary to mastectomy and lymph node dissection are at increased risk for angiosarcoma. A few cases of sarcomas arising in damaged tissues after radiation therapy have been reported. Radiation therapy-related sarcomas, more common after high doses of radiation, tend to be high grade and occur after a latency of more than 10 years. Their distribution involves the sternum, sternoclavicular joint, cervical/thoracic spine, and soft tissue areas in the radiation fields used for treatment of lymphomas, seminomas, and Hodgkin's disease. Paget's disease carries an increased risk for developing osteosarcoma in the affected bones (estimated to be 1000 times higher than that of the normal population).

3. How are sarcomas classified?

Sarcomas are divided into soft tissue sarcomas and bone sarcomas. There are at least 70 different histologic subtypes of soft tissue sarcomas, which are classified according to the appearance of the tissue that the sarcoma has formed (e.g., fibrosarcoma, liposarcoma). Bone sarcomas include osteosarcoma, Ewing's sarcoma, and malignant fibrous histiocytoma (MFH) of bone.

4. What are the most common sarcomas in adults? In children?

In adults the most common sarcomas are malignant fibrous histiosarcoma, liposarcoma, leiomyosarcoma, and osteosarcoma. Children most often have rhabdomyosarcoma, osteosarcoma, or Ewing's sarcoma.

5. Describe the importance of histologic grade in sarcomas.

Histologic grade is of paramount importance in evaluating the aggressiveness of sarcomas and is included in the pathology report along with the exact histopathologic type. The grade may be low, intermediate, or high; high-grade sarcomas are the most aggressive. High-grade tumors more often have distant metastasis and are associated with a lower survival rate. Low-grade tumors, in general, have a better prognosis. The histopathologic grade is based on the degree of differentiation, cellularity, number of mitoses, pleomorphism, and amount of necrosis.

6. Describe the clinical presentation of patients with sarcomas.

The early symptoms of sarcomas are nonspecific and include mild pain and mild soft tissue swelling; they are often attributed to local trauma, which leads to frequent delay in diagnosis. Eventually they grow to form palpable masses. Of interest, in osteosarcoma the pain precedes the soft tissue swelling and is caused by stretching of the periosteum by the tumor.

7. What steps are necessary in the diagnosis and staging of sarcomas?

The steps needed in diagnosing sarcomas include computed tomography (CT) and magnetic resonance imaging (MRI) of the affected area and open biopsy. MRI is the most sensitive imaging modality because of high resolution and accurate distinctions between normal and abnormal tissues. After MRI confirmation an open incisional biopsy is done. Although fine-needle aspiration (FNA) and core biopsy can give a diagnosis of malignancy, they rarely provide the exact histopathologic type and grade of the tumor. The incision should be made in a direction that allows incorporation into the subsequent excision, which prevents local recurrence. Therefore, it is recommended that the biopsy be done by the surgeon who will excise the tumor. Once the diagnosis is made, the next step is complete staging to define the extent of disease. This step includes CT of the chest and bone scan to exclude metastasis in these two most frequent sites of distant spread.

8. How does staging differ between soft-tissue and bone sarcomas?

Bone sarcomas are staged using the TNM system with the additional factor of tumor confined within or beyond the cortex and including pathologic grade. The staging of soft tissue sarcoma depends on tumor size, pathologic grade, location (superficial vs. deep), and presence or absence of lymph node involvement and distant metastasis. The grade and size of the malignancy have greater bearing on treatment planning and prognosis than anything else.

9. What are the most important prognostic factors in sarcomas?

The TNM stage has direct influence on survival: stage I is associated with a 5-year survival rate of 90%; stage II, 70%; stage III, 20–50%; and stage IV, < 20%. High-grade tumors > 5 cm have a more than 50% chance of recurrence, whereas tumors < 2 cm have an excellent prognosis with a cure rate of approximately 90%. It is important to emphasize the poor prognosis of local recurrence, which almost always correlates with the presence of systemic disease.

10. Describe the prognosis and management of pulmonary metastasis from sarcomas.

The lung represents the most common site of distant spread of sarcomas. It is important to recognize a subset of patients who benefit from surgical resection of pulmonary metastasis. This subset includes patients whose primary tumors have been controlled, who lack extrapulmonary disease, and who have adequate cardiac and pulmonary function. Important prognostic factors are number of pulmonary nodules (preferably < 5), disease-free interval (> 1 year), and completeness of resection. Resection of up to 5 nodules or aggressive repeated metastectomies result in a long-term disease-free survival rate of 20–35%. The prognosis of patients who present with pulmonary metastases at diagnosis is uniformly fatal.

11. Where do soft tissue sarcomas most commonly arise?

Soft tissue sarcomas most often arise in the extremities with more frequent involvement of the lower (38%) than upper extremities (11%); rarely they are seen in other parts of the body, such as the retroperitoneal area (15%), trunk (13%), viscera (5%), and head and neck region (5%).

12. To what sites do soft tissue sarcomas metastasize?

The lungs are the most frequent site (33%), followed by bones (23%) and liver (15%).

13. Describe the current therapy for soft tissue sarcomas of the extremities.

For low-grade sarcomas the treatment is complete surgical excision with negative margins, a prerequisite for local control and cure. Low-grade sarcomas are relatively chemo- and radioresistant; therefore, chemotherapy and radiation therapy play no role in their management. High-grade sarcomas show higher response rates to chemotherapy and radiation. For small high-grade tumors the preferred modality is still surgery; however, for larger tumors (> 5 cm) a multimodality approach that involves both chemotherapy and surgery is preferred. In this setting, some centers have used intra-arterial neoadjuvant chemotherapy followed by limb-sparing surgery.

14. Which chemotherapy agents are most effective against soft tissue sarcomas?

The most effective drugs are doxorubicin and ifosfamide, which have response rates of 15–25% when used as single agents. The preferred approach is a combination regimen that includes both agents and shows response rates as high as 40–50%.

15. Define osteosarcoma.

Osteosarcomas are malignant tumors, usually arising in the bone, that are characterized by bone or osteoid production.

16. Which age group and gender are most often affected by osteosarcoma?

Osteosarcoma usually affects young patients, 10–20 years of age, with a peak incidence around the adolescent growth spurt. The second peak occurs during the sixth decade of life. Osteosarcoma affects men more than women (male-to-female ratio = 1.5:1).

17. Which sites does osteosarcoma most often involve?

The knee is most often affected, and the distal femur is the most frequent primary site. The proximal tibia is second in frequency, followed by the proximal humerus.

18. What is the recommended management of osteosarcomas?

In the past osteosarcomas were treated by amputations one joint above the location of the primary tumor. Despite this mutilating surgery, survival was poor (in the range of 20%), with patients succumbing to metastatic disease. The modern approach involves preoperative (neoadjuvant) chemotherapy followed by limb-sparing surgery and more adjuvant chemotherapy. Preoperative chemotherapy decreases the size of the tumor and permits limb-sparing surgery; most importantly, however, response to chemotherapy is a significant prognostic factor and correlates with survival. Limb salvage surgery is now possible in close to 90% of cases. Some institutions use preoperative intra-arterial cisplatin with great success.

19. What is considered a good histologic response to chemotherapy in osteosarcoma? What are the clinical implications?

The response to preoperative chemotherapy as assessed by the pathologist through examination of the surgical specimen is an important piece of information and correlates with long-term survival. A good pathologic response is defined by more than 90% necrosis of the specimen. In general, patients with good response to chemotherapy have a 10-year survival rate approaching 90%, whereas the rate is much lower in patients without such a response.

20. What are the most effective drugs for treatment of osteosarcoma?

The most active drugs are high-dose methotrexate, cisplatin, doxorubicin, cyclophosphamide, and ifosfamide. Unfortunately, the newer chemotherapeutic agents have not shown beneficial response rates in sarcoma.

21. What is the long-term prognosis for osteosarcomas?

With modern therapy the long-term survival rate is approximately 60–80%. Almost 80–90% of patients are able to undergo limb-sparing surgeries. The local recurrence rate is approximately 5–10%.

22. What is Ewing's sarcoma? How does it differ from osteosarcoma?

Ewing's sarcoma is a rare tumor of the bone that affects mainly adolescents. It differs from osteosarcoma morphologically because of the presence of small, round, blue cells as opposed to the typical spindle cells of osteosarcomas. It also has a preference for the midshaft of the bone rather than the diaphysis and tends to involve the pelvic bones, scapula, and spine in addition to the femurs. Bone metastases are more common than in osteosarcoma.

23. Describe the usual plan of therapy and prognosis in Ewing's sarcoma.

Therapy should involve a multimodality approach; the initial step is preoperative chemotherapy followed by limb-sparing surgery and adjuvant chemotherapy. The usual treatment program involves extended periods of chemotherapy (9–12 months). With this approach the long-term disease-free survival rate is approximately 70-80%.

24. How do you choose between limb-sparing surgery and amputation in the surgical treatment of sarcomas?

In experienced hands, limb-sparing surgery is considered safe and routine for a large number of carefully selected patients. Use of neoadjuvant chemotherapy increases the number of patients who undergo this procedure. Because limb-sparing surgery offers local control rates similar to amputation and provides better quality of life, it is the procedure of choice. However, in large and poorly differentiated tumors, the risks and benefits must be carefully weighed by the surgeon, keeping in mind that local recurrence is almost a death warrant.

25. What are contraindications for limb-salvage surgery?

Bone tumors with major neurovascular involvement	Pathologic fracture with hematoma at tumor site
Infection	Muscle involvement (extensive)
Inappropriate biopsy site	Immature skeletal age (< 10 years; rare)

26. What are the major nursing issues in patients with osteosarcoma?

Patients facing limb surgery with or without amputation have reduced mobility, which may affect self care (e.g., dressing, personal hygiene) and activities of daily living. Some restrictions affect employment status, relationships, house adaptation, and body image.

REFERENCES

1. Bacci G, Ferrari S, Bertoni F, et al: Long-term outcome for patients with nonmetastatic osteosarcoma of the extremity treated at the Istituto Ortopedico Rizzoli according to the Istituto Ortopedico Rizzoli/osteosarcoma-2 protocol: An updated report. J Clin Oncol 18:4016–4027, 2000.
2. Daliani D, Patel SR: Soft-tissue and bone sarcomas. In Padzur R (ed): Medical Oncology: A Comprehensive Review. Huntington, NY, PRR, 1995, pp 511–529.
3. De Vita VT Jr, Hellman S, Rosenberg SA: Cancer: Principles and Practice of Oncology, 6th ed. Philadelphia, Lippincott-Raven, 2001.
4. Fink K, Wilkins R: Intra-arterial chemotherapy and limb preservation in osteosarcoma in children. ASCO 1001:1126, 1991 [abstract].
5. Greenlee RT, Hill-Harmon MB, Murray T, Thun M: Cancer statistics, 2001. CA Cancer J Clin 50:15–36 2001.
6. Lenhard RE Jr, Lawrence W Jr, McKenna RJ: General approach to the patient. In Murphy GP, Lawrence W Jr, Lenhard RE Jr (eds): American Cancer Society Textbook of Clinical Oncology, 2nd ed. Atlanta, American Cancer Society, 1995, pp 64–74.
7. Lewis IJ, Weeden S, Machin D, et al: Received dose and dose-intensity of chemotherapy and outcome in nonmetastatic extremity osteosarcoma. J Clin Oncol 18:4028–4037, 2000.
8. Pisters PWT, Leung DHY, Woodruff J, et al.: Analysis of prognostic factors in 1,041 patients with localized soft tissue sarcomas of the extremities. J Clin Oncol 14:1679–1689, 1996.
9. Roth JA: Resection of pulmonary metastases from osteogenic sarcoma. Cancer Bull 42:344–346, 1990.
10. Rougraff B: The diagnosis and management of soft tissue sarcomas of the extremities in the adult. Curr Probl Cancer 23:1–52, 1999.
11. Sim FH, Bowman WE, Wilkins RM, Choa EYS: Limb salvage in primary malignant bone tumors. Orthopedics 8:574–581, 1985.
12. Tierney JF, Stewart LA, Parmar MKB, et al: Adjuvant chemotherapy for localised resectable soft-tissue sarcoma of adults: Meta-analysis of individual data. Lancet 350:1647–1654, 1997.
13. Wilkins RM, Sim FH: Evaluation of bone and soft tissue tumors. In D'Ambrosia (ed): Musculoskeletal Disorders: Regional Examination and Differential Diagnosis, 2nd ed. Philadelphia, J.B. Lippincott, 1986.

24. BRAIN TUMORS

Kim Pollmiller, RN, MS, CNRN, and Kevin O. Lillehei, MD

1. Why do people develop brain tumors?

With a few exceptions, the cause is unknown. Exposure to certain chemicals is loosely associated with a higher incidence of brain tumors, but the only clear association is with radiation therapy. The most common tumor, astrocytoma, has not been associated with a causal factor. Although familial clustering is rare, some families have a predisposition to develop brain tumors; they are under study.

2. Do cellular phones really cause brain tumors?

No. In addition, no evidence suggests that electromagnetic fields or power lines contribute to brain tumor development.

3. Who gets brain tumors?

- Brain tumors develop in persons of all ages, but the two peak age ranges are 3–8 and 40–60 years.
- The overall incidence is slightly higher in males than females. The incidence of brain tumors is thought to be increasing, but only time will prove this hypothesis true or false.
- Patients with von Hippel-Lindau disease develop multiple benign vascular tumors called hemangioblastomas.
- Patients with neurofibromatosis develop multiple benign tumors called neurofibromas and have a higher risk of developing meningiomas, astrocytomas, and schwannomas.

4. Give the incidence and mortality rates for brain tumors.

In 2001, the estimated number of new cases of primary brain and central nervous system tumors in the United States was 17,200. By gender this incidence includes 13.55 new cases per 100,000 males and 12.25 per 100,000 females. Over 13,100 estimated deaths in 2001 will be attributed to brain tumors.

5. What is the difference between benign and malignant brain tumors?

The major difference between benign and malignant brain tumors is the aggressiveness of histology. For example, meningioma usually is considered a benign tumor because it grows very slowly, does not invade normal brain, and has distinct borders. Thus, tumor removal can be accomplished with minimal risk of damage to surrounding brain. The most aggressive and malignant primary brain tumors, gliomas, start within the brain itself—not within the neurons but within the glial cells that carry nourishment to and waste from the neurons. Gliomas infiltrate normal brain and do not have distinct borders. This infiltrating border makes total surgical resection virtually impossible. Most gliomas have a relatively high growth rate. Even those that are initially low grade have the potential to degenerate into a more aggressive lesion.

6. Why is the location of the tumor important?

In determining whether a tumor is benign or malignant, its location in the brain must be considered. Histologically benign tumors may be located near critical structures and, therefore, cannot be surgically removed. Such tumors eventually cause neurologic deficits and possibly death. Thus a tumor may be benign by histology but cause severe problems because of its location within the brain. The term *benign* should be used cautiously in describing brain tumors. Perhaps the best approach is to describe the nature of the tumor as it is now and what it may become, leaving the patient with hope but indicating that no one knows when and if the tumor will recur.

7. Which type of brain tumor is considered the most aggressive? Why?

Grade IV astrocytoma (glioblastoma multiforme) strikes the greatest fear in health professionals and eventually in patients and family members as they learn the prognosis. These tumors grow at a phenomenal rate, quickly leading to significant neurologic problems. Prognosis without treatment is death within a few weeks. With surgery, radiation, and chemotherapy, survival can be extended to 12–18 months. Even within this classification, the growth rate of individual tumors varies. Glioblastoma behaves just as aggressively in children.

8. Describe the common problems experienced by patients with brain tumor.

All symptoms of a brain tumor are caused by tumor infiltration, pressure on normal brain, or treatment of the tumor. Headaches are common but usually can be managed by adjusting the doses of corticosteroids. Seizures occur frequently and, if not controlled, can be quite disturbing for patient and family. Focal deficits involving motor or sensory loss, vision, or speech are common and relate to the location of the tumor within the brain. Fatigue is often a complaint and is managed by frequent rest periods. With conventional radiotherapy, hair loss is usually temporary but may be permanent, depending on the skin surface dose. Weight gain is caused by steroids, fluid retention, and ravenous appetite. Nausea and vomiting may be late signs of increased intracranial pressure from tumor growth or result from radiation and/or chemotherapy. Diarrhea, stomatitis, anorexia, and dyspnea are rarely experienced.

9. What is the most difficult problem to manage?

Cognitive impairment. For short periods, living with a brain tumor is tolerable, but long illness becomes trying for patient and family. Family members may find it difficult to believe that the patient cannot control his or her behavior and need repeated explanations and support.

10. Which impairments are most common?

1. **Reasoning and judgment** may decline before patients are diagnosed. For example, a business owner may make poor decisions, not follow through with plans, or fail to meet deadlines. If there are no other overt symptoms of the brain tumor, the business may become bankrupt before someone challenges the owner's judgment or recognizes the problem.

2. **Lack of initiative** is particularly common in patients with frontal lobe tumors. For example, the patient is aware that he or she needs to do something but cannot get started. The family may think that the patient is lazy or obstinate, and the supervisor at work knows only that the job is not getting done. Often relationships at work and home suffer, and the patient may be fired or divorced before the brain tumor is diagnosed.

3. **Lack of awareness of neurologic deficits** is also common. If a family member tries to point out such deficits, the patient may refuse to believe that anything is wrong. Athough the patient does not intend to be obstinate, this situation becomes exasperating for both patient and family member.

4. **Short-term memory deficit** may complicate the lack of awareness. The patient asks the same question over and over again and cannot follow through on tasks because he or she does not remember. Many of these symptoms are similar to those of Alzheimer's disease.

5. **Personality change** is particularly difficult for the family. Roles usually change because the patient cannot perform normal physical tasks or offer the usual emotional support and companionship.

11. When is surgery indicated?

After a brain tumor is diagnosed by computed tomography (CT) or magnetic resonance imaging (MRI), the physician, patient, and family determine which treatment approach is best. If at all possible, a tissue diagnosis is made. Tissue may be obtained from an open or needle biopsy; the method is determined by the location of the tumor, its proximity to critical structures, and the damage that may result from an open craniotomy or needle biopsy. Another factor in this decision is the predicted diagnosis——whether the tumor is thought to be benign or malignant by histology.

In most situations, the goal is to remove as much of the tumor as safely possible. If neurologic risk is minimal, gross total resection may be attempted. If neurologic risk is great, partial resection or biopsy may be the procedure of choice. For example, a brain scan may demonstrate that a meningioma is attached to a dural surface and has clear, distinct borders. If totally removed, a meningioma may not recur; even if only partially removed, it will probably grow back very slowly. The surgeon may choose to perform an open craniotomy and to remove as much tumor as is safe. On the other hand, if the tumor is thought to be an astrocytoma and is in a critical area, biopsy alone may be performed, followed by radiotherapy. Total or partial removal of an aggressive tumor may not be warranted if deficits result; in most cases, even with gross total removal, microscopic cells remain. The goal of surgery is to extend survival without sacrificing quality of life.

12. What is the role of PET scanning in the diagnosis and treatment of brain tumors?

Positron emission tomography (PET) scanning is a relatively new imaging modality that allows visualization of the metabolic rate of different areas of the brain. The scan is performed by injecting the patient with a radioactively labeled marker (either fluoro-deoxyglucose [FDG] or an amino acid), which is taken up by the brain cells during active metabolism. The picture that is generated is similar to a CT or MRI scan but with less detail. By comparing the CT or MRI with the PET scan, you can determine areas of abnormal metabolism.

13. When is knowledge of metabolic rates particularly helpful?

Low-grade gliomas are generally hypometabolic, showing very little uptake of the metabolic marker on PET scanning. If the clinician is concerned about areas of higher-grade tumor within a low-grade glioma, a PET scan may help to pin-point such regions. A second application is in patients with high-grade glioma after radiation therapy. Occasionally the clinician needs to determine whether recurrent contrast enhancement seen on MRI or CT is recurrent tumor or radiation necrosis. Recurrent high-grade tumor usually is hypermetabolic, showing increased uptake of the marker, whereas radiation necrosis is hypometabolic.

14. When is radiation therapy given?

After optimal tumor removal, radiotherapy is the treatment of choice for malignant lesions. Conventional fractionated radiotherapy is generally preferred, but in certain situations other modalities (e.g., hyperfractionated radiotherapy, stereotactic radiosurgery, brachytherapy) are indicated.

15. Define stereotaxis.

Stereotaxis is based on the concept that the location of a lesion can be determined more precisely by a fixed frame of reference in relation to the brain. Stereotactic technology has greatly improved the quality and safety of neurosurgical procedures for patients with brain tumors.

16. How are stereotactic biopsy and stereotactically guided craniotomy accomplished?

A spherical open frame (similar to a halo) is pinned to the skull, and the patient is taken for a CT or MRI scan. The subsequent films show not only the tumor but also points of reference on the frame. With the aid of a computer program, the surgeon can determine the x, y, and z coordinates of the lesion. During surgery, a special frame with degree markings is placed over the head and attached to the stereotactic halo. A needle is attached to the frame at a precise degree and trajectory and then passed to the target. If a biopsy is indicated, the target is usually the center of the lesion. Multiple samples are taken to ensure that representative tissue is obtained. If a craniotomy is indicated, the periphery of the lesion is targeted. During the craniotomy, the needle points to the edges of the lesion. A stereotactically guided craniotomy is indicated when the tumor is close to critical areas and its consistency makes it difficult for the surgeon to differentiate between tumor and normal brain.

17. What other technique may be used to target the tumor more precisely?

A computerized robotic microscope. Instead of a stereotactic frame, small markers are glued to the skin of the head. An MRI is obtained immediately before surgery. The markers (rather than a frame) are the fixed reference points. In the operating room, the MRI images are inserted into a special computer, using magnetic datatape attached to the robotic microscope. The MRI images are displayed on the computer screen, and the surgeon outlines the tumor on each image. Critical structures, such as a major artery or the central sulcus, also can be outlined. With these data, the computer can create a three-dimensional image of the tumor, showing the tumor's proximity to critical structures. Looking through the microscope, the surgeon registers the location of the fixed reference markers on the patient's head into the computer. With this information, the computer superimposes an image of the tumor through the microscope lens onto the operative surface. As the surgeon is operating, he or she can see where the edges of the lesion should be. As the microscope is moved during surgery, laterally or by depth, the computer adjusts the outline to accommodate the move. Such technology allows better resection with less risk to nearby critical areas, particularly when it is difficult to differentiate visually between normal brain and tumor.

18. What is stereotactic radiosurgery?

Stereotactic radiosurgery is effective treatment for small, well-defined lesions of the brain. The same stereotactic principle is used: a frame provides fixed reference points when an MRI or CT scan is obtained. The location of the lesion is determined, and a treatment plan is developed. Radiosurgery can be delivered by the linear accelerator with adaptive equipment for the stereotactic frame or gamma knife. In both cases, treatment is delivered by narrow beams of radiation so that all beams come together at an isocenter, delivering a high dose to the isocenter with little radiation to surrounding tissues. The goal of radiosurgery is to deliver a dose of radiation that destroys everything in the target area. A full day is required to plan and prepare for the treatment, which takes approximately 30 minutes.

19. Is chemotherapy effective for brain tumors?

The answer depends on whom you ask. Optimists reply, "Yes, definitely," whereas pessimists ask, "Why bother?" The truth probably lies somewhere between the two responses. After radiotherapy, chemotherapy may be given immediately or when the tumor recurs. Chemotherapy is potentially effective only for aggressive tumors. Statistically, chemotherapy extends survival in patients with high-grade lesions by a few weeks to several months. On the other hand, a few patients may benefit significantly.

20. What are the most commonly used chemotherapy regimens?

Intravenous 1,3-bis-(2-chloroethyl)-1-nitrosourea (BCNU) alone, PCV (procarbazine, lomustine, and vincristine), temozolomide (Temodar), or a biodegradable wafer impregnated with BCNU (Gliadel), which can be implanted directly into the tumor resection site at the time of surgery. Because high doses of radiation therapy are toxic to the developing brain, more extensive chemotherapy regimens with multiple drugs are used in children. New drugs and new combinations of drugs are under investigation.

21. What long-term problems do children with a brain tumor face?

The long-term toxicity caused by multimodal therapy is a major concern in children because of the critical stage of brain development. Radiotherapy is delayed until after 2 years of age to decrease the risk and severity of long-term problems. Long-term toxicities are related to cognition (intelligence), growth, and development. Degrees of cognitive deficits range from mild to severe. Throughout the school life of the child it is imperative to assess cognitive function periodically and to adjust classroom work to fit specific deficits. Annual evaluation of the child should include input from teachers and other appropriate school personnel. Growth and development need to be assessed at least annually. Radiotherapy to the pituitary area may impair production of growth hormone. Sexual development, which is controlled by the pituitary, should be assessed, with appropriate hormone replacement as the child nears puberty.

Such physical and cognitive changes affect social development. Problems continue as the young adult pursues an independent life away from parents and considers marriage and fertility issues. Evaluations and interventions may be required throughout life.

22. Why are corticosteroids given to patients with brain tumors?

Patients with brain tumors most commonly present with neurologic deficits or symptoms of increased intracranial pressure (headache, nausea, vomiting) caused by mass effect of the tumor plus surrounding edema. The edema is caused by abnormal blood vessels within the tumor, which allow fluid to leak from the intravascular space into surrounding brain tissue. Corticosteroids (most commonly dexamethasone) decrease the area of edema and improve symptoms, often dramatically. Corticosteroids are believed to improve the cell-to-cell adherence of endothelial cells within the tumor blood vessels, thereby lessening leakage of fluid into the surrounding brain. This in turn decreases the abnormal mass effect responsible for symptoms.

23. What regimen is appropriate for administration of corticosteroids?

Because of their significant toxicity, the smallest effective dose of corticosteroids should be prescribed for the least amount of time. A patient should not discontinue treatment abruptly without instructions from a physician, because the body adjusts to the artificial steroids and stops producing natural steroids. Steroids taken for longer than 7–14 days must be gradually tapered. The longer a patient has taken steroids and the higher the dose, the longer and slower the taper must be.

24. List the major side effects of corticosteroids.

- Alterations in body image caused by fluid retention and weight gain in varying degrees. Patients often complain about a ravenous appetite. The patient should be reassured that the weight can be lost after stopping the steroids. Other effects on body image include flushed face, abdominal striae, and growth of facial or body hair.
- Increased susceptibility to infection
- Stomach irritation, which can be relieved with an antacid
- Mood changes and irritability
- Muscle weakness in the proximal extremities, degenerative bone disease, and cataracts (caused by long-term use)

25. Which corticosteroid is used? How is it dosed?

Dexamethasone is commonly prescribed in oral doses of 0.25–40 mg/day. Patients often are given an average dose of 2–4 mg every 6 hours. The maximal effective dose is considered to be 40 mg/day. The patient should be cautioned not to discard unused medication because it may be prescribed intermittently throughout the course of the illness.

26. Are anticonvulsants prescribed for most patients?

Anticonvulsants are often prescribed, depending on the physician's judgment and whether the patient has had a seizure. Seizures are caused by irritation to the brain. The brain tumor functions as an irritant, as can normal scar formation after a craniotomy. Even if anticonvulsants are not prescribed for long-term use, most patients receive a bolus before surgery, which is continued for 3–4 weeks postoperatively. Patients who experience a seizure are likely to remain on anticonvulsants for a longer period.

27. Do patients have to remain on anticonvulsants for life?

If a patient remains seizure-free, anticonvulsants may be stopped after 6 months or 1 year. Although anticonvulsants may be stopped abruptly, often they are tapered to reduce the risk of severe seizure. In patients with brain tumors, attention should be paid to all minor complaints, which in fact may represent unrecognized seizure activity. Seizures occur in various forms and degrees and often are not identified as seizures by the patient or family.

28. What should patients be told about taking anticonvulsants?

The most commonly used anticonvulsant is phenytoin (Dilantin), followed by carbamazepine (Tegretol). Both drugs must be taken for 7–10 days to reach a therapeutic blood level. The patient should take a missed dose if it is remembered on the same day. If a day has passed, the patient should not try to make up the dose. Do *not* take a double dose!

29. What are the side effects of anticonvulsants?

If a patient is allergic to phenytoin and develops a skin rash, the drug should be stopped immediately. Because the rash may become severe, even life-threatening, it is imperative to instruct the patient to call the physician if a rash develops. Many patients feel sleepy and drowsy after taking anticonvulsants. Major toxicities include nystagmus, slurred speech, dysarthria, hypotension, and coma (rare). Because anticonvulsants are metabolized by the liver, liver function should be evaluated at least annually. Often combinations of drugs are used if a single agent is not effective. Many new drugs are also available, including clonazepam (Klonopin), gabapentin (Neurontin), valproic acid (Depakote), lamotrigine (Lamictal), and levetiracetam (Keppra).

30. Should patients with brain tumors be allowed to drive?

Patients and families often ask when it is safe for the patient to drive. Reasons for restriction of driving privileges include seizures and cognitive deficits that affect processing of information and judgment. If a patient has had a seizure, many states have laws that restrict driving for 6–12 months. Although each state differs, most require a physician's approval. Rehabilitation programs often offer a safe driving evaluation. The patient who is not fit to drive but lacks awareness of deficits may resist the judgment of family and physician.

31. How does a patient or family know that the tumor is recurring?

In 90% of cases, the tumor recurs in the same general location, and the symptoms are similar to those at initial presentation. As the tumor continues to grow, intracranial pressure increases, neurologic problems worsen, and the patient tends to sleep more hours each day. Eventually the patient can be awakened only with difficulty, usually for meals, and then quickly falls asleep again.

32. How does a patient with a brain tumor die?

As the patient spends more and more time in bed and ingests less fluid and nutrition, he or she is more prone to infections, thrombophlebitis, and other problems related to extended bedrest. In fact, an infection such as pneumonia may be the cause of death. Headaches are rarely a problem for patients with brain tumors. As the patient becomes more lethargic, he or she becomes less aware of deficits. Although watching neurologic deterioration is extremely difficult, families find comfort in the fact that the patient does not experience pain and is usually not aware of changes in mental status. Sudden death is possible but rare. Death usually occurs over days to weeks, depending on the growth rate of the tumor.

33. What factors influence survival? How do they affect treatment decisions?

Age, neurologic status at diagnosis, histology of the tumor, and extent of surgical resection are the primary factors that influence survival in adults. Younger patients with a good neurologic status at diagnosis statistically have a better chance of survival. If corticosteroids improve the neurologic deficit, it is likely that surgery will help as well. Tumor histology is a major factor influencing survival. The more aggressive the lesion, the poorer the prognosis. Complete (as opposed to partial) resection favors longer survival. Patients with multiple aggressive tumors have a poor prognosis and often are biopsied only and then treated with radiation. During craniotomy, as much tumor as possible is removed to relieve pressure and to reduce the tumor burden for subsequent therapies. Location is also a factor; the extent of tumor resection is often limited by its location. Tumors near or in the brainstem or adjacent to areas of motor or speech function are more difficult to treat.

34. What factors affect treatment decisions?

Age alone does not usually affect treatment decisions; however, an aggressive surgical approach may not be recommended for elderly patients with an aggressive lesion, poor neurologic status, and other health problems that increase surgical risk. For such patients, diagnostic biopsy and radiotherapy may be the best treatment options. Intrinsic brainstem lesions often cannot be biopsied because the operative risks of neurologic deficit and death are too great.

35. What is the prognosis for common tumor types?

Survival is poorest for high-grade gliomas. The most common primary brain tumor is astrocytoma. Survival for glioblastoma (grade IV astrocytoma) treated with surgery, radiation, and chemotherapy is 12–18 months; for anaplastic (grade III) astrocytoma, 18–24 months; and for grade II astrocytoma, 6–7 years.

36. Describe new treatment options.

Progress in the treatment of brain tumors has been slow; in the past decade, however, neuro-oncology has gained the attention of the healthcare community. New efforts focus on basic science as well as clinical research. Both local and systemic approaches are under evaluation:

- Localized approaches for high-grade gliomas, including radiosurgery, radiosensitizers, brachytherapy, hyperthermia, and hyperfractionization.
- Localized chemotherapy approaches, including direct delivery to the tumor via drug-impregnated, biodegradable wafers placed in the operative cavity and intra-arterial delivery of chemotherapeutic agents.
- Tumor vaccines that augment or manipulate the immune system. Because gliomas infiltrate normal brain, systemic treatment must include a way to search out the infiltrated abnormal tumor cells.
- Temporary interruption of the blood-brain barrier, which allows passage of chemotherapy agents to the tumor.
- High-dose chemotherapy with bone marrow rescue
- Gene therapy

37. What resources are available to patients and families for education and support?

The foundations listed below provide free information about brain tumors and treatment to the public and health professionals. Related associations, often affiliated with rehabilitation medicine, provide education and support for patients with physical and mental disabilities related to traumatic brain injury. Such information also may be helpful to patients with brain tumor. A brain tumor support group is located on the Internet; however, patients should be cautioned to validate information with a trusted nurse or physician.

American Brain Tumor Association (ABTA)

2720 River Road, Suite 146

Des Plaines, IL 60018

(800) 886-2282, (847) 827-9910)

E-mail: ABTA@aol.com

Services include a listing of support groups, pen-pal program, newsletter, and information about treatment facilities and research funding.

National Brain Tumor Foundation (NBTF)

785 Market Street, Suite 1600

San Francisco, CA 94103

(800) 934-CURE, (415) 284-0208

E-mail:sstf39f@prodigy.com

NBTF provides free information and counseling and support services to patients with brain tumor, survivors, and families. It also provides a newsletter, patient-to-patient telephone support line, free resource guide, and list of support groups.

ACKNOWLEDGMENT

The authors thank Betty Owens, RN, MS, for her contribution to this chapter in the first edition of *Oncology Nursing Secrets*.

REFERENCES

1. Broderson JM: Surgical options for brain tumor treatment. Crit Care Nurs Clin North Am 7:91–102, 1995.
2. Bronstein KS: Epidemiology and classification of brain tumors. Crit Care Nurs Clin North Am 7:79–89, 1995.
3. Central Brain Tumor Registry of the United States: Year 2000 Standard Statistical Report. Chicago, Central Brain Tumor Registry of the United States, 1999.
4. Greenlee RT, Hill-Harmon MB, Murray T, Thun M: Cancer statistics, 2001. CA Cancer J Clin 51:15–36, 2001.
5. Lamb SA: Radiation therapy options for management of the brain tumor patient. Crit Care Nurs Clin North Am 7:103–114, 1995.
6. Laperriere NL, Bernstein M: Radiotherapy for brain tumors. Cancer J Clin 44(2):96–108, 1994.
7. Moore IM: Central nervous system toxicity of cancer therapy in children. J Pediatr Oncol Nurs 12(4):203–210, 1995.
8. Perry GF Jr: What occupations have been associated with brain cancer, and, more specifically, what is the connection between brain cancer and electric utility work? J Occup Environ Med 37:1067–1069, 1995.
9. Roman DD, Sperdoto PW: Neuropsychological effects of cranial radiation: Current knowledge and future directions. Int J Radiat Oncol, Biol Physics 31:983–998, 1995.
10. Shiminski-Maher T, Wisoff JH: Pediatric brain tumors. Crit Care Nurs Clin North Am 7:143–149, 1995.

25. BREAST CANCER

Patrice Y. Neese, MSN, RN, CS, ANP, and Dev Paul, DO, PhD

Quick Facts—Breast Cancer

Incidence	30% of new cancers in women annually. In 2001, approximately 193,700 new cases will be diagnosed.
Mortality	40,600 estimated deaths in 2001.
Risk factors	Increased age
	History of breast cancer
	Early menarche, nulliparity, late menopause
	Increased age at birth of first child
	Use of exogenous hormones
	History of atypical hyperplasia, lobular carcinoma in situ (LCIS)
	Family history
	Radiation exposure
Histology	Adenocarcinoma most common, followed by lobular carcinoma
Symptoms	Painless mass more common than painful mass
	Nipple discharge, nipple erosion
	Diffuse erythema of the breast
	Axillary adenopathy
Staging	**Tumor, node, metastasis (TNM) system**

Primary tumor (T)

TX	Primary tumor cannot be assessed
T0	No evidence of primary tumor
Tis	Carcinoma in situ: intraductal carcinoma, lobular carcinoma in situ, or Paget's disease of the nipple with no tumor
T1	≤ 2 cm in greatest dimension
T2	2–5 cm in greatest dimension
T3	> 5 cm in greatest dimension
T4	Tumors of any size with direct extension to chest wall or skin (e.g., peau d'orange, skin ulceration, satellite nodes, inflammatory carcinoma)

Regional lymph nodes (N)

NX	Regional lymph nodes cannot be assessed
N0	No regional lymph node metastasis
N1	Metastasis to movable ipsilateral axillary lymph node(s)
N2	Metastasis to ipsilateral axillary lymph node(s) fixed to one another or other structures
N3	Metastasis to ipsilateral internal mammary lymph node(s)

Distant metastasis (M)

MX	Distant metastasis cannot be assessed
M0	No distant metastasis
M1	Distant metastasis, including metastasis to ipsilateral supraclavicular lymph node(s)

Stage grouping			
Stage 0	Tis	N0	M0
Stage I	T1	N0	M0
Stage IIA	T0	N1	M0
	T1	N1	M0
	T2	N0	M0
Stage IIB	T2	N1	M0
	T3	N0	M0

Table continued on following page

Quick Facts—Breast Cancer (Continued)

Stage grouping (continued)	Stage IIIA	T0	N2	M0
		T1	N2	M0
		T2	N2	M0
		T3	N1, N2	M0
	Stage IIIB	T4	Any N	M0
		Any T	N3	M0
	Stage IV	Any T	Any N	M1

Surgical treatment Mastectomy or lumpectomy plus radiation (for any tumor > 5 cm or > 4 positive lymph nodes, offer radiation after mastectomy)

Summary of adjuvant treatment options (individualize for each patient)

Any stage with positive estrogen or progesterone receptors: tamoxifen

Tumor > 1 cm (lymph node positive or negative): offer chemotherapy with or without tamoxifen, depending on estrogen and progesterone receptor status

Positive lymph nodes: offer chemotherapy with or without tamoxifen, depending on estrogen and progesterone receptor status

1. What is the incidence of breast cancer among American women?

An estimated 193,700 new cases of breast cancer will be reported in the United States during 2001. With a life expectancy of 85 years, about 1 in 9 women will develop breast cancer at some time during their lives. Although the incidence has increased over the years, the mortality rate has been fairly stable for the past 60 years at about 27 per 100,000 patients. Breast cancer is the most common cancer diagnosis in women and the second major cause of cancer-related death. In addition, an estimated 1,500 cases of breast cancer in men will be diagnosed during 2001.

2. What are the signs and symptoms of breast cancer?

Breast masses that are firm, nontender, irregular without distinct borders, nonmovable, and fixed to skin or deep fascia are often suspicious for cancer. Skin dimpling and nipple retraction are sometimes present. Erythema and peau d'orange (orange peel) skin are worrisome signs. Unilateral nipple discharge, especially serous or bloody, is suspicious in older women. Enlarged axillary or supraclavicular lymph nodes are less common.

3. In which area of the breast are more cancers found?

The primary site of breast cancer is described by the quadrant of the breast in which it is detected. The most common area is the upper outer quadrant, where approximately 50% of tumors are found. The upper inner quadrant is associated with a 15% incidence, the lower outer quadrant with 11%, the lower inner quadrant with 6%, and the central region (near the areola) with approximately 17%.

4. Which imaging modalities are used before biopsy is performed? Why?

Before biopsy of a dominant mass, a patient should have a mammogram to define the extent of the lesion and to identify other suspicious areas. Because mammograms are not sensitive to approximately 15% of cancers, a negative test should not dissuade a physician from performing a biopsy on a dominant, palpable mass. Breast ultrasound often is used for highly dense breast tissue because it can distinguish between fluid-filled and solid masses. Digital mammography, magnetic resonance imaging (MRI), and positive emission tomography (PET) scanning are under study for screening, diagnosis, and staging of breast cancer.

5. What are the various biopsy methods for diagnosing breast cancer?

Fine-needle aspiration (FNA) is often performed on palpable nodules because it is quick, relatively painless, and inexpensive. FNA cannot distinguish between ductal carcinoma in situ (DCIS) and invasive cancers, however, and its use is somewhat limited. **Core-cutting needle biopsy** has advantages similar to those of FNA, and a larger sample is usually obtained, giving a higher degree of accuracy.

Stereotactic core biopsy is performed with the patient lying face down with the breast suspended through an opening in the table. The breast is compressed, and multiple core samples can be obtained. **Mammotome** uses a vacuum-assisted system that yields a larger tissue sample with less discomfort for the patient. A sterile probe is placed into the breast and rotated to obtain multiple samples. Both techniques require experience in performing the test and interpreting cytopathologic results.

If a suspicious, nonpalpable nodule is seen on mammogram, it may be localized with needles guided by mammography. The needle-localized lesion is excised. **Excisional biopsies** are performed on any palpable nodule to provide the greatest diagnostic information, including size, receptor status, and margins. Most are performed in outpatient settings under local anesthesia.

6. What are the most common histologic types of breast cancer?

Approximately 80% of invasive or infiltrating cancers originate in the ductal system and are called **ductal cancer**. About 5–10% of infiltrating (invasive) cancers arise from the lobules and are called **lobular cancers**.

7. What histologic types account for the remaining invasive breast cancers?

Medullary, tubular, mucinous, papillary, micropapillary, and invasive cribriform carcinoma.

8. How is noninvasive breast cancer classified?

Cancer that is confined within the lumen of the ducts is classified as ductal carcinoma in situ (DCIS).

9. Define lobular carcinoma in situ (LCIS) and inflammatory cancer.

LCIS is not considered a true cancer; it is a marker for increased risk of future cancer in either breast. **Inflammatory cancer** (an aggressive form of breast cancer) is not a histologic sub-type but a clinical diagnosis based on the presence of erythema and edema (peau d'orange) of the skin of the breast.

10. Do all breast cancers grow at a steady rate?

No. Most breast cancers have a doubling time of approximately 60–90 days. On average, it takes 5–8 years for an invasive breast cancer to be detected by mammogram or physical examination. However, a small percentage double in size as quickly as every 15 days or as slowly as every 600 days. The latter are associated with late recurrences (> 10 years and sometimes 20 years after the original diagnosis).

11. Discuss the significance and incidence of lymph node metastasis.

Axillary lymph node metastases are associated most closely with tumor size. Prognosis is related to the number of axillary lymph nodes involved; the greater the number, the poorer the overall survival rate. Medial tumors are more likely to metastasize to internal mammary and mediastinal lymph nodes. A complete axillary lymph node dissection is the standard procedure for breast cancer staging and, based on studies from the 1990s, is associated with a 10–20% chance of lymphedema. The true incidence of lymphedema is difficult to ascertain because of the many years needed for follow-up, differences in reporting how lymphedema is measured, and the year in which the surgery was performed.

12. What is a sentinel lymph node biopsy?

The sentinel node is the first lymph node that drains a cancer. The principle of sentinel lymph node biopsy (SLNBx) rests on the theory that if metastatic spread has occurred, it involves the sentinel node first. Biopsy of this node should be an accurate determinant of stage.

13. How is SLNBx performed?

A blue dye and technetium-99m–labeled sulfur colloid are injected around the tumor. Nodes that appear blue and are found to be be "hot" by a hand-held gamma probe are sampled as the sentinel lymph nodes. Once the sentinel lymph node is identified, it can be removed through a small incision, with little disruption to the lymphatics and low complication rates. The incidence of lymphedema with this procedure is about 3%.

14. List the contraindications to SLNBx, according to the American College of Surgeons.
- Tumor size > 5 cm
- Locally advanced disease
- Palpable axillary lymph nodes
- Multicentric disease
- Use of preoperative chemotherapy
- Prior radiation to the breast or axilla
- Large biopsy cavity
- Prior axillary surgery
- Pregnancy or lactation

15. What are the credentialing requirements for performance of SLNBx?
Because of the learning curve associated with performance of SLNBx, the American College of Surgeons recommends credentialing be granted after completion of 20 cases that include SLNBx and axillary node dissection, with an average false-negative rate ≤ 5%. Currently several national clinical trials are under way to evaluate the appropriate use of SLNBx in breast cancer surgery. Most likely SLNBx will become the standard of care in a few years because it has been shown to be more sensitive in detecting axillary lymph node metastasis than standard axillary dissection.

16. What should be done if the SLNBx is positive?
Complete axillary dissection.

17. What are the cardinal prognostic factors in breast cancer staging?
The tumor-nodes-metastasis (TNM) staging system is used to predict the outcome of disease by analysis of prognostic factors and survival rates. Tumor size, extent of lymph node involvement, and presence of metastasis are graded and grouped according to the extent of disease. Approximately 96% of patients with stage I disease are alive at 5 years after diagnosis. The survival rates at 5 years for patients with stages II and III cancers are approximately 55% and 35%, respectively. Less than 15% of patients with metastatic disease or stage IV breast cancer are alive 5 years after diagnosis. Also important for prognosis, although not part of the staging system, are estrogen (ER) and progesterone receptor (PR) status, Her-2/*neu*, and S-phase status.

18. Define ER and PR status.
Receptor levels are measured in the primary tumor and provide valuable information for determining treatment. In general, tumors that are estrogen and/or progesterone receptor positive have a better prognosis than tumors that are negative. Approximately 60% of breast cancers are ER positive. Postmenopausal women are more likely to be positive than premenopausal women. Receptor-positive tumors are generally responsive to endocrine therapies such as selective estrogen receptor modulators (SERMs) and aromatase inhibitors (see question 33).

19. What other prognostic criteria are helpful?
1. **Elevated S-phase status** indicates a tumor that divides more rapidly and correlates with a more aggressive tumor.
2. **Angiogenesis** (increased blood vessel/capillary development in primary tumors) is currently under study and has been linked to more aggressive tumors.
3. **HER-2/*neu*** (erbB2) oncogene, one of several epidermal growth factor receptors (EGFrs), is overexpressed in 20–30% of breast tumors. Overexpression is associated with increased tumor growth, increased rate of metastases, ER negativity, and decreased overall survival.

20. What is trastuzumab?
Identification of HER/*neu* has led to the development of the monoclonal antibody trastuzumab (Herceptin), which in combination with chemotherapy has greater efficacy in patients with metastatic breast cancer. Clinical trials combining trastuzumab with chemotherapy as adjuvant therapy in lymph node-positive patients are under way.

21. What are the surgical options for treatment of breast cancer?

The most common surgical interventions for breast cancer are **lumpectomy** (breast conservation) with axillary node dissection and **modified radical mastectomy** (removal of breast and lymph nodes). Multiple randomized trials have demonstrated that the 10–20-year survival rate of patients with stage I or II breast cancer treated with lumpectomy and radiation therapy is equivalent to that of patients treated with mastectomy alone. Lumpectomy must be combined with radiation therapy for equivalent local control. Immediate or delayed reconstructive surgery is also an option for women who choose mastectomy. The decision is often difficult for women to make; it is based on personal preference, values, feelings about the body, priorities, and perceptions of risk.

22. The preoperative plan for patient education should include what basic points?

Because short-stay and outpatient procedures are becoming more common for both lumpectomy and mastectomy, preoperative patient education from the nurse is imperative. The nurse should remind patients to stop taking aspirin and nonsteroidal anti-inflammatory agents, which may decrease platelet function. Hormonal therapy (birth control or replacement) should be stopped as soon as a diagnosis of breast cancer is made. The nurse also should teach the signs and symptoms of infection, wound care, Jackson-Pratt drain management, prevention and management of lymphedema, pain control, and comfort measures at home; recommend purchase of a postoperative bra (see question 25); and initiate referral to the Reach to Recovery Program of the American Cancer Society.

23. Explain the Reach to Recovery Program.

It is a one-on-one visitation program designed to help women meet the physical, emotional, and cosmetic needs related to breast cancer. Trained volunteers who have had breast cancer are available to visit women postoperatively. Information about exercises, temporary prosthetic devices, bras, and available support services is part of the program.

24. What additional information should be covered in the postoperative phase of patient education?

In addition to reinforcement of preoperative teaching, the postoperative phase of patient education should remind patients that individual coping is affected by exhaustion, anesthesia, change in body image, and emotional aspects of dealing with a new diagnosis. The nurse should recommend moderation of habits related to eating, drinking, resting, socializing, and exercise. The patient should avoid lifting weights above 5 pounds for a few weeks. If the patient is a candidate for adjuvant chemotherapy, there is usually a period of several weeks between surgery and start of chemotherapy. This is an ideal time to have a dental examination and cleaning, which should be avoided during chemotherapy treatments when blood counts are low. In addition, it may be necessary to discuss appropriate birth control methods.

25. What kind of bra, if any, should be worn in the postoperative period?

Women are most comfortable after biopsy or lumpectomy if the breast is well supported. A sports bra is ideal, especially one with frontal closure, which is easier to put on than the overhead type. Wearing a bra to bed for the first few nights helps some women, as does lying on the opposite side with a towel rolled under the breast for support. Women should avoid underwire support postoperatively and during radiation therapy when the breast is tender and edematous.

26. What techniques are used for delivery of radiation therapy to the breast?

In general, 4500–5000 cGy are administered 5 days/week for 5–6 weeks after lumpectomy. Several other techniques are currently under investigation, including brachytherapy (short-term radiation seed implants) and more rapid fractionalization (more radiation in less time).

27. Discuss the side effects of radiation therapy to the breast.

Because the majority of radiation exposure is via tangential beam (through the breast instead of the body to avoid the heart and lungs), most women can expect few systemic effects. The most common side effect is local skin irritation similar to a bad sunburn. This symptom varies among women and may cause pruritus, edema, and occasionally moist desquamation in severe cases. Women should be encouraged to avoid ointments or oil-based products on the skin as well as all deodorant soaps and deodorants, most of which which have a high aluminum content that may interact with the radiation. A dusting of cornstarch may be used as a deodorant. Radiation to the axilla may increase the incidence of lymphedema (see Chapter 41). Fatigue is another often reported side effect of therapy (see Chapter 40). Rare side effects include radiation pneumonitis and development of skin cancers and even rarer sarcomas years later in the irradiated field.

28. Why do some women with a modified radical mastectomy receive radiation therapy?

Postmastectomy radiation therapy is recommended for women with a tumor > 5 cm, skin or chest wall involvement, positive surgical margin, or > 4 positive lymph nodes. Depending on institutional protocols, radiation therapy is administered at different times during treatment. Most commonly it is administered after completion of chemotherapy. Patients tend to have more severe side effects with concomitant therapy (especially doxorubicin) and radiation therapy. Radiation therapy also is used to treat some spot bone or brain metastases.

29. Explain the role of neoadjuvant chemotherapy in breast cancer.

Neoadjuvant chemotherapy is administered before surgery in an effort to decrease the size of the primary tumor so that breast conservation is possible. Patients who present with locally advanced or inflammatory breast cancers (stage IIIB) may benefit from neoadjuvant chemotherapy. Response rates appear to be 80% with a combination of doxorubicin and cyclophosphamide. The same patients also may receive adjuvant chemotherapy. Results of the recently closed National Surgical Adjuvant Breast and Bowel Project (NSABP) B237 trial are pending.

30. Why do some women receive adjuvant chemotherapy whereas others do not?

The potential increase in long-term survival weighed against the potential side effects determines whether a patient should be offered adjuvant chemotherapy. The general health of the patient is important in making this decision. According to the National Institutes of Health (NIH) Consensus Development Conference Statement on Adjuvant Therapy for Breast Cancer (2000), most women with primary invasive breast tumors > 1 cm in diameter (both node-negative and node-positive) should be offered cytotoxic chemotherapy. The decision to consider chemotherapy should be individualized for women with node-negative tumors < 1 cm. For women with positive lymph nodes and any size tumor, adjuvant chemotherapy should be offered.

31. What are the most common chemotherapy drug combinations?

Several hundred chemotherapy trials for breast cancer have provided data for the efficacious use of the following regimens:

1. Combination of cyclophosphamide, methotrexate, and 5-fluorouracil (CMF), administered on days 1 and 8 every 28 days for 6 cycles.

2. Combination of 5-fluorouracil (5-FU), doxorubicin (Adriamycin), and cyclophosphamide (FAC), administered on day 1 every 21 days. Alternatively, 5-FU may be administered on days 1 and 8 of a 28-day cycle for 6 courses. A variation is oral cyclophosphamide for 14 days with administration of doxorubicin and 5-FU on days 1 and 8 (CAF).

3. Doxorubicin with cyclophosphamide (AC), administered in slightly higher doses every 21 days for 4 cycles.

4. In Europe, regimens containing epirubicin instead of doxorubicin are commonly used.

5. The NIH Consensus Development Statement states that inclusion of anthracyclines in adjuvant chemotherapy regimens produces a small but significant improvement in survival.

6. The Food and Drug Administration (FDA) recently approved 4 cycles of doxorubicin and cyclophosphamide, followed by 4 cycles of paclitaxel, for use in node-positive patients.

7. The exact role of taxanes is still investigational.

32. When is bone marrow transplant recommended for women with breast cancer?

Autologous bone marrow transplant is still investigational for patients ≥ 4 positive lymph nodes and no evidence of metastatic disease.

33. How does tamoxifen work? How long does treatment last?

Tamoxifen is considered a standard adjuvant therapy for women with estrogen receptor and/or progesterone receptor positive breast cancer. The overall response rate is 60%. Formerly known as an anti-estrogen, it is now classified as a SERM. Tamoxifen essentially blocks the binding of estrogen to breast cancer cells. It does not stop estrogen production in the body. Women taking tamoxifen generally are less likely to develop osteoporosis and usually have lower serum cholesterol levels.

34. Describe the currently recommended regimen for tamoxifen therapy.

In the adjuvant setting, the current recommendation is 20 mg/day orally for 5 years.

35. What are the side effects of tamoxifen?

The more common side effects are hot flashes and vaginal discharge. However, tamoxifen also may lead to a 2.5-fold increase in the incidence of endometrial cancer, a 2–4-fold increase in strokes and blood clots, and a slight increase in the incidence of posterior subcapsular cataracts.

36. Describe the role of aromatase inhibitors in management of breast cancer.

Because aromatase is important for the conversion of androgens into estrogens in post-menopausal women, drugs have been developed to inhibit this enzyme. Aminoglutethimide was the first aromatase inhibitor used with some effectiveness. Newer agents (anastrozole and letrozole) have been studied with promising results.

37. How are hot flashes treated?

Hot flashes induced by treatment with SERMs or early menopause as a side effect of chemotherapy have been reported by 65% of women with breast cancer. Several treatments have been tried, with little supporting research: vitamin E (800 IU/day orally), transdermal clonidine, Bellargal (1 tablet orally twice daily), and Megace (20 mg/day orally). All of these therapies have side effects with minimal or no improvement compared with placebo. Recently the antidepressant venlafaxine hydrochloride (12.5 mg orally twice daily) was reported to be well tolerated with significant reduction of hot flash severity and duration. Additional research is needed.

Nonmedical interventions include dressings in layers, relaxation, exercise, herbs, and avoidance of caffeine, alcohol, and spicy foods.

38. How often does breast cancer spread from one breast to the other?

It is rare for cancer to metastasize from one breast to the other. A woman who has had cancer in one breast, however, is at a higher risk of developing a new primary contralateral breast cancer. The risk in the opposite breast is 0.5–1.0% during each year of follow-up. Therefore, most malignancies of the other breast are new cancers. It is also possible for one person to have one estrogen/progesterone receptor positive tumor and a second tumor that is receptor-negative.

39. What are the most common sites of metastases?

Metastatic spread from breast cancer may involve various organs. Bone, liver, lung, brain, and skin are reported most frequently. Breast cancer in the ovaries, spleen, peritoneum, adrenal glands, stomach, leptomeninges, and retina of the eye is rare.

40. Discuss the prognosis of metastatic disease.

Although metastatic disease is considered incurable, it does not always mean that death is imminent. In fact, one-half of patients live more than 2 years, and 10% live a decade or more. Women with only bone metastases may live for a considerable time with the use of radiation, hormonal therapy, and chemotherapy.

41. What is the role of bisphosphonates in the treatment of metastatic bone disease?

Recently bisphosphonates have become a standard part of the treatment regimen. They interfere with tumor-mediated osteolysis by modulating the function and maturation of osteoclasts and can reduce significantly the risk of nonvertebral pathologic fractures as well as decrease the need for radiation therapy and surgery to treat bone complications, the incidence of hypercalcemia, and the degree of bone pain. Bisphosphonates also prevent or reduce the incidence of bone metastasis. The standard dose of pamidronate is 90 mg given intravenously over 2 hours every 3–4 weeks.

42. Should multiple regular screening tests be performed to monitor for metastatic disease or recurrence in women diagnosed with breast cancer?

The American Society of Clinical Oncology issued guidelines for the follow-up of patients with breast cancer. Routine screening for distant recurrences with laboratory tests, radiographs, computerized tomography, or bone scans in asymptomatic patients offers no survival advantage over performing the same tests when patients become symptomatic. Women with a history of breast cancer have several unique health issues. Long-lasting effects of treatment may include early menopause, osteoporosis, and lymphedema. Survivors may have questions about childbearing, lactation, and hormone replacement. Long-term follow-up needs to address these issues as well as assessment of psychosocial well-being.

43. What is the ideal interval between mastectomy and breast reconstruction?

No interval can be considered ideal for all patients. Most mastectomy patients are candidates for reconstruction, which often may be performed at the same time that the breast is removed. For some women, delayed reconstruction may be best.

44. List the goals of breast reconstruction.

To enhance body image and to provide symmetry of the breasts when the woman is wearing a bra.

45. Discuss the options for breast reconstruction.

The options, which should be discussed with a plastic surgeon, depend on body type and breast size. Breast reconstruction may be accomplished as a prosthetic implant, tissue expansion, or flap procedure. After mastectomy, a balloon expander is inserted beneath the skin and chest muscle. Through a port mechanism, saline is injected periodically, stretching the skin until a more permanent saline implant may be inserted. Some patients do not require expansion before receiving an implant. An alternative approach involves creation of a skin flap using tissue from other parts of the body, such as the transverse rectus abdominis myocutaneous (TRAM) or the latissimus dorsi (LD). Although these alternatives do not require the use of implants and generally result in a more natural contour, they involve more extensive surgical procedures and scarring. Additional surgical procedures are available to reconstruct the areola and nipple.

46. What critical psychological issues may confront families of patients with breast cancer?

Breast cancer is a crisis for the entire family. It may result in depression among family members, impaired marital relationships, lowered self-esteem, developmental delays in children, and behavioral problems with adolescents. Functional patterns of families are influenced by their structure and organization in both traditional and nontraditional modes; history of coping styles; and cultural, ethnic, and religious or spiritual influences. The oncology nurse is often the first observer of family dynamics in response to cancer. Identification of problems, provision of clear information, and referral to appropriate resources may help the family to develop a successful coping style. This approach hopefully enables family members to use the experience as an opportunity for growth and to avoid destructive outcomes as well as assists the patient with her emotional response.

47. How can the oncology nurse support a couple coping with cancer?
Changes in the quality of a couple's intimate relationship, communication problems, and fear of recurrence have been documented in the literature. The oncology nurse can support the partner by being available to answer questions about procedures and treatments. Anticipatory guidance and education about possible challenges can facilitate the couple's sense of control and reduce feelings of uncertainty. Active listening is a valuable intervention, as is validation of concerns.

48. What care interventions should guide nurses working with women who have a family history of breast cancer?
Mutations in *BRCA1* and *BRCA2* genes account for approximately 5–10% of breast cancers, 45% of hereditary breast cancer, and the majority of heritable breast/ovarian cancer. The implications of a family history of breast cancer affect people differently, depending on various psychosocial issues (e.g., confidentiality, insurance coverage) and family dynamics. Some women consider prophylactic surgery as means of risk reduction. Patients and family members should be referred to centers that offer genetic screening and counseling for women at risk. Nurses should recognize and discuss why some women exhibit high-risk behaviors or seem reluctant to comply with screening; they also should provide information about the benefits of early detection. By emphasizing and facilitating breast cancer screening and detection through monthly breast self-examination, periodic clinical examination, and screening mammography, the oncology nurse may reduce the fear of breast cancer.

49. Discuss the relationship between dietary fat intake and incidence of breast cancer.
Epidemiologists have long pondered whether a low-fat diet can prevent breast cancer. The incidence of breast cancer is clearly lower in countries where intake of animal fat is lower, but reproductive habits are also different in these countries. It is difficult to design a study of the relationship between low-fat diets and rates of breast cancer. The ongoing Nurses' Health Study has not demonstrated an association between the two, but compliance has been a problem with many studies to date. Diets high in raw fruits and vegetables are also under study. Although current data do not support specific dietary guidelines for reducing the risk of breast cancer, the American Cancer Society still recommends that women maintain a healthy weight and limit intake of high-fat foods, particularly those from animal sources, as part of a healthy lifestyle.

50. What is the modified Gail Model?
The modified Gail Model is a computerized method of predicting a woman's 5-year and lifetime risk of developing invasive breast cancer. Risk factors include race, patient age, age at first mensis and first live birth, number of first-degree relatives with breast cancer, number of previous breast biopsies, and biopsies showing atypical hyperplasia.

51. Does tamoxifen lower the risk of developing breast cancer?
The Breast Cancer Prevention Trial (BCPT) included 13,388 women at high risk for the development of breast cancer, based on the modified Gail Model. Patients were randomized to take either tamoxifen or placebo for 5 years. After a median follow-up of 54.6 months, the risk of invasive breast cancer was reduced by 49% in women receiving tamoxifen. Based on these results, tamoxifen has been approved in the U.S. for breast cancer prevention in high-risk women who meet criteria established by the National Cancer Institute.

52. What other preventive agents are under study?
Several trials are under way to evaluate the efficacy of newer agents with fewer side effects than tamoxifen. The Multiple Outcomes of Raloxifene Evaluation (MORE) trial, designed to assess the value of raloxifene in prevention of osteoporosis, also evaluated as a secondary end point the incidence of newly diagnosed breast cancer. Although preliminary results show a reduction in new diagnoses, raloxifene currently is approved only for the treatment of osteoporosis. The Study of Tamoxifen and Raloxifene (STAR) trial is recruiting patients to compare the efficacy and side effects of both drugs.

53. What issues related to breast cancer should we expect to hear about in the coming years?

In addition to chemoprevention, the chemical actions of flax seed and isoflavones in soy are under investigation. Identification of additional oncogenes and genetic predisposition has scientific interest as well as ethical and legal implications. New screening and diagnostic tools currently under study include ductal lavage and ductoscopy. Advances in surgical management of breast cancer also are under study. The use of lymphoscintigraphy or lymph node mapping (sentinel node procedure) will reduce the morbidity of lymph node dissections. New and improved treatments with less systemic toxicity are always of interest. Data about taxanes and other agents in the adjuvant setting are pending. Survivorship (e.g., quality of life, fatigue, exercise, diet, hormone use, pregnancy, financial impact, body image) is an area of increased interest. Complementary and alternative therapies are of interest to many practitioners and women with breast cancer. The oncology nurse must keep up to date and encourage patients to seek information from randomized trials rather than anecdotal recommendations.

54. What resources offer support, counseling, education, and information for patients with breast cancer?
- American Cancer Society
  800-ACS-2345
  www.cancer.org
  Reach to Recovery Program
- Susan G. Komen Breast Cancer Foundation
  800-IM-AWARE (800-462-9273)
  Services include research and program grants, helpline.
  www.komen.org
- ENCORE–YWCA of USA
  hn2202@handsnet.org
  Exercise program for women with breast cancer available through most local YWCA branches
- Mothers Supporting Daughters with Breast Cancer (MSDBC)
  (410) 778-1982
  lillie@ix.netcom.com
  MSDBC helps women whose daughters have breast cancer so that they can better help their daughters cope with the disease and treatment.
- National Alliance of Breast Cancer Organization (NABCO)
  9 East 37th Street, 10th Floor
  New York, NY 10016
  (212) 709-0154 or 800-719-9154
  www.nabco.org
  Nonprofit agency representing over 300 organizations concerned about breast cancer; services range from physician referrals to job discrimination and professional education.
- Women's Healthcare Network
  800-991-8877
  Organization made up of independent businesses that specialize in serving women who have had breast surgery.
- Y-ME National Breast Cancer Organization
  800-221-2141
- National Institutes of Health clinical trials site
  www.clinicaltrials.gov
- National Surgical Adjuvant Breast and Bowel Project (NSABP)
  www.nsabp.pitt.edu

REFERENCES

1. Barse PM: Issues in the treatment of metastatic breast cancer. Semin Oncol Nurs 16:197–205, 2000.
2. Burstein HJ, Winer EP: Primary care for survivors of breast cancer. N Engl J Med 343:1086–1093, 2000.
3. Carpenter JS: Hot flashes and their management in breast cancer. Semin Oncol Nurs 16:214–225, 2000.
4. Dietz JR, Kim JA, Malycky BA, et al: Feasibility and technical considerations of mammary ductoscopy in human mastectomy specimens. Breast J 6:161–165, 2000.
5. Early Breast Trialists' Collaborative Group: Polychemotherapy for early breast cancer: An overview of the randomized trials. Lancet 352:930–942, 1998.
6. Fisher B, Costantino JP, Wickerham DL, et al: Tamoxifen for prevention of breast cancer: Report of the National Surgical Adjuvant Breast and Bowel Project P-1 study. J Natl Cancer Instit 90:1371–1388, 1998.
7. Fleming ID, Cooper JS, Henson DE, et al: AJCC Cancer Stating Handbook, 5th ed. Philadelphia, Lippincott-Raven, 1998.
8. Goodman H: HER-2, Herceptin, and breast cancer. Oncol Nurs Updates 7:1–11, 2000.
9. Greenlee RT, Hill-Harmon MB, Murray T, Thun M: Cancer statistics, 2001. CA Cancer J Clin 51:15–36, 2001.
10. Gross R: Breast cancer: Risk factors, screening, and prevention. Semin Oncol Nurs 16:176–184, 2000.
11. Haber J, Noll Hoskins C: Meeting the challenges of adjuvant therapy: Strategies for partners and significant others. Innov Br Cancer Care 5:49–50, 2000.
12. Hilton BA: Issues, problems, and challenges for families coping with breast cancer. Semin Oncol Nurs 9:88–100, 1993.
13. Hsueln EC, Hansen N, Giuliano AE: Intraoperative lymphatic mapping and sentinel lymph node dissection in breast cancer. CA Cancer J Clin 50:279–291, 2000.
14. Maunter BD, Schmidt KV, Brennan MB: New diagnostic techniques and treatments for early breast cancer. Semin Oncol Nurs 16:176–184, 2000.
15. McMasters KM, Tuttle TM, Carlson DJ, et al: Sentinel lymph node biopsy for breast cancer: A suitable alternative to routine axillary dissection in multi-institutional practice when optimal technique is used. J Clin Oncol 18:2560–2566, 2000.
16. O'Rourke Clothier A: Advanced breast cancer: Recent developments in hormonal therapy. Semin Oncol Nurs 16:206–213, 2000.
17. Vogel VG: Breast cancer prevention: A review of current evidence. CA Cancer J Clin 50:156–170, 2000.

26. COLORECTAL CANCER

Diane K. Nakagaki, RN, BSN, ET, Brenda M. Hiromoto, RN, MS, CETN, OCN, Kelly Mack, RN, MSN, AOCN, NP-C, and Allen Cohn, MD

Quick Facts—Colorectal Cancer

Incidence	15% of all new cancer cases in the United States. Steady decline during 1992–1996 (~2.1% per year) due to increased screening and removal of polyps that might progress to invasive cancer. In 2001, 135,400 estimated new cases (98,200 colon and 37,200 rectal cancers). Colon cancer affects 1 in 20 people. Incidence = < 1 per 100,000 in persons under age 30 years and 500 per 100,000 in people over age 80 years.
Mortality	In 2001, an estimated 56,700 deaths will be due to colorectal cancer; 48,100 related to colon cancer and 8,600 to rectal cancer; 11% of total cancer deaths annually. Mortality unchanged for three decades.
Cause	Unknown; diet may be an influencing factor.
Risk factors	Adenomatous polyps are the most common risk factor. The larger the polyps, the greater the likelihood of malignancy (up to 40% in polyps > 2 cm) Family history and genetic syndromes: familial adenomatous polyposis (FAP), Gardner syndrome, Oldfield syndrome, Turcot syndrome, Peutz-Jeghers syndrome, hereditary nonpolyposis colorectal carcinoma (HNPCC) (originally named cancer family syndrome) Inflammatory bowel disease; ulcerative colitis, especially > 10 years' duration; Crohn's disease History of pelvic irradiation for gynecologic cancers Diets rich in fat and cholesterol (high in red meat) Alcohol consumption, especially beer Sedentary employment Increased risk begins at 40 years and increases with age
Histology	**Adenocarcinomas** account for 98% of colon cancers and 95% of rectal cancers **Anal carcinomas:** 65% squamous cell carcinomas, 25% transitional (cloacogenic or basaloid), < 10% adenocarcinoma, and < 5% miscellaneous
Symptoms	Early: no symptoms; vague abdominal pain or flatulence Vary according to location of tumor, but usually change in bowel movements is first symptom Other signs and symptoms include weakness due to anemia, pain, blood in stool, and bowel obstruction
Diagnosis and staging tests	Digital rectal exam and fecal occult blood test (FOBT) Colonoscopy with biopsy of any lesions and/or air contrast barium enema Endoscopic ultrasound Chest radiograph, computed tomography (CT) scan of abdomen and pelvis Complete blood count, liver and renal function tests, urinalysis, preoperative tests for carcinoembryonic antigen (CEA) Immunoscintigraphy (antibody scan) to detect extrahepatic disease and radiolabeled monoclonal antibodies are under investigation to improve detection rates
Staging	**Astler-Coller modification of Dukes' classification** Stage A Tumor confined to mucosa (2% of cases) Stage B1 Tumor penetrates into muscularis layers (11%) Stage B2 Tumor penetrates through muscularis into serosa or perirectal fat (30%) Stage C1 B1 tumor with positive regional lymph nodes (2%)

Table continued on following page

218

Quick Facts—Colorectal Cancer (Continued)

Staging	**Astler-Coller modification of Dukes' classification** *(cont.)*
	Stage C2 B2 tumor with positive regional lymph nodes (22%)
	Stage D Distant metastases to other organs (33%)
Staging	**Tumor, nodes, metastasis (TNM) system**
	Tumor stage
	TX Primary tumor cannot be assessed
	T0 No evidence of tumor
	Tis Carcinoma in situ
	T1 Tumor invades submucosa
	T2 Tumor invades muscularis propria
	T3 Tumor invades through muscularis propria into submucosa
	T4 Tumor perforates visceral peritoneum or invades other organs or structures
	Lymph node stage
	NX Regional lymph nodes cannot be assessed
	N0 No regional lymph nodes involved
	N1 One to three pericolic lymph nodes involved
	N2 Four or more pericolic lymph nodes involved
	N3 Regional nodes along major named vascular trunk
	Metastatic stage
	MX Distant metastases cannot be assessed
	M0 No distant metastasis
	M1 Distant metastasis
	Stage grouping
	Stage 0 Tis N0 M0
	Stage I T1 or T2 N0 M0 (Dukes' stage A)
	Stage II T3 or T4 N0 M0 (Dukes' stage B)
	Stage III Any T N1, N2, or N3 M0 (Dukes' stage C)
	Stage IV Any T Any N M1 (Dukes' stage D)

1. What are the epidemiologic differences between colon cancer and rectal cancer?

The prevalence of colon cancer is nearly equal in men and women. Rectal cancer has a slight male predominance. Colorectal cancer is the third most common cancer for both genders and the second leading cause of death.

2. What other factors are related to the incidence of colorectal cancers?

The incidence of colorectal cancers is higher after the age of 40. The mean age of patients at presentation is 60–65 years. The incidence of colon cancer is higher in African Americans; the incidence for Native Americans is less than half the incidence for white Americans. The risk of colorectal cancer is much lower among Mormons and Seventh Day Adventists, who avoid alcohol and tobacco and eat mainly vegetables, fruits, and whole-grain cereals.

Other predisposing factors include history of colorectal or other cancer (e.g., breast, endometrial, or ovarian cancer); sedentary employment; and women with no or low parity or history of pelvic irradiation for gynecologic cancer. Alcohol consumption, especially beer, has been associated with a higher incidence of colorectal cancer. Charcoal or smoked meats and irradiated foods have no conclusive correlation to the risk of colorectal cancer. Irritation of the anal canal related to condylomata, rectal intercourse, fistulas, fissures, abscesses, and hemorrhoids may increase the risk for colorectal cancer. HIV-positive patients have a higher incidence of anal canal carcinomas.

3. Is the incidence of colorectal cancer similar in the United States and other countries?

The incidence varies widely among cultures and countries. Countries in which people consume large amounts of fruits and vegetables and low amounts of fat have a lower incidence of colorectal cancer. For example, the incidence is 3 per 100,000 in Nigeria and 7 per 100,000 in Japan vs. 40 per 100,000 people in the United States.

4. What is the survival rate for colorectal cancer?

The 1-year survival rate is 83%, and the 5-year survival rate is 61%. In general, the 5-year survival rate is based on the stage of disease (Astler-Coller modified Dukes' classification):

Stage A	75–100%	Stage C1	40%
Stage B1	65%	Stage C2	15%
Stage B2	50%	Stage D	< 5%

For anal cancer the 5-year survival rate is 48–66%.

5. What are the most common signs and symptoms of colorectal cancer?

Right colon: vague, achy abdominal pain; bleeding (dark or mahogany red); weakness due to anemia (common); obstruction (infrequent); palpable abdominal mass.

Transverse colon: blood in stool; change in bowel pattern; potential bowel obstruction.

Left colon: colicky pain; bleeding (red, mixed with stool); obstruction (common); weakness due to anemia (infrequent); nausea, vomiting; constipation alternating with diarrhea; decreased caliber of stool (pencil stools).

Rectum: steady gnawing pain; bleeding (bright red, coating stool); change in bowel movements (constipation or diarrhea); pencil stools; rectal urgency or fecal incontinence; spasmodic contractions with pain; perineal and buttock pain.

Anal: bleeding; pain; sensation of a mass; severe anal itching.

6. What percentage of cancer is accounted for by the different segments of the colon?

Descending and sigmoid colon: 52%
Ascending colon: 32%
Transverse colon: 16%

7. What is the value of carcinoembryonic antigen in monitoring patients with colorectal cancer?

Carcinoembryonic antigen (CEA) is a glycoprotein present in gastrointestinal mucosa. It is useful as a tumor marker for patients who have CEA-producing adenocarcinomas. CEA is most useful as a marker for tumor recurrence and in monitoring response to chemotherapy. An elevated, sustained postoperative CEA is related to tumor recurrence in most patients. Rising CEA levels (serial changes > 35% of baseline) may indicate progressive disease. Elevations in CEA are found in gastrointestinal, breast, and lung cancers and in smokers and patients with liver disease or cirrhosis, pancreatitis, inflammatory bowel disease, or rectal polyps.

8. What are common sites of colon and rectal metastases?

Common sites of metastasis for colon cancer are the liver, lungs, and peritoneum (with carcinomatosis). Colon cancer has a tendency to metastasize to the liver because most of the colon's venous drainage is through the portal system. Uncommon sites are brain, bone, ovaries, and adrenal glands. Rectal cancer has a tendency to metastasize to the lungs because its venous drainage is via the hemorrhoidal veins. Anal cancer may metastasize to the lung, liver, and inguinal nodes.

9. How is colorectal cancer detected if no symptoms are present?

Screening guidelines are controversial; however, the American Cancer Society recommends the following tests to screen for colorectal cancer in asymptomatic patients with no risk factors:

Digital rectal examination + fecal occult blood test (FOBT) for 3 specimens annually after age 50, in addition to one of the following screening tests:

- Flexible sigmoidoscopy starting at age 50; repeat every 5 years if the initial flexible sigmoidoscopy is normal, or
- Double–contrast barium enema (if normal, repeat every 5–10 years), or
- Colonoscopy after age 50; repeat every 10 years if normal.

Screening examinations are recommended at more frequent intervals and should be started earlier in high-risk patients and in patients with history of colorectal cancer.

10. What may cause false-positive or false-negative occult blood results?

False positives: red meat, poultry, fish, turnips, horseradish, iron, aspirin, skin of cherries and tomatoes. Avoid for 72 hours before and during test.

False negatives: vitamin C and low-fiber diet 72 hours before test

11. What foods are thought to reduce the risk of colorectal cancer?

A diet low in fat and animal protein may reduce the formation of carcinogenic metabolites produced from the enzymatic activity of bacterial flora. The consumption of a diet high in vegetables, fruits, whole grains, and beans is associated with a decreased incidence of colorectal cancer. Additional studies have shown that cruciferous vegetables (e.g., cabbage, broccoli, cauliflower, brussels sprouts) reduce the risk for colorectal cancer. The recommendation is to eat 5 or more servings of fruits and vegetables (30–35 gm of dietary fiber) daily and to keep dietary fat intake to less than 25–30% of daily caloric intake.

More recent studies have questioned the effect of dietary fiber on the risk of colorectal cancer. In a comprehensive review of published colorectal prevention studies, the American Gastroenterological Association found most of the retrospective case-controlled studies showed a benefit to increasing dietary fiber. But the prospective studies failed to show a clear benefit or have shown only a modest improvement in risk reduction with increasing dietary fiber. The issue is complex: several different types/sources of dietary fiber have been described, other dietary factors were not controlled (e.g., fat intake), and different endpoints were used to evaluate efficacy (measurement of levels of intermediate chemical precursors vs. polyp formation vs. development of cancer). The effect is likely to be dose-dependent and of modest-to-moderate impact.

12. How does a high-fiber diet protect against colon cancer?

Fiber in the diet may act as a protective agent against colon cancer by reducing the contact of possible carcinogens with bowel mucosa in five ways:
- Decreasing transit time within intestine
- Diluting carcinogens in stool
- Altering pH in colon
- Binding of possible carcinogens
- Decreasing ammonia concentration in intestine

13. Have any studies proved that the consumption of vitamins or other nutrients prevents colorectal cancer?

The following products have not been shown to reduce the risk of colon cancer: vitamins, beta carotene, antioxidants, calcium, coffee, fish oils, fluorides, folic acid, food additives, garlic, olestra, olive oil, soybeans, salt, selenium, and tea.

14. Can nonsteroidal anti-inflammatory drugs (NSAIDs) prevent colorectal cancer?

Clinical studies showed that sulindac (Clinoril) decreased the formation of colonic polyps and regression of rectal polyps in familial adenomatous polyposis (FAP). In 1999, Celebrex (cyclooxygenase-2 inhibitor) was approved for the regression and reduction of adenomatous polyps in patients with FAP. Indomethacin and aspirin have demonstrated a protective effect against bladder and colon cancer. Tumors may produce large amounts of prostaglandins, which can promote carcinogenesis. The role of prostaglandins in cancer initiation or promotion may be related to their activation of procarcinogens. Several studies have shown that after reaction with cyclooxygenase, certain substances in food may become mutagenic. By inhibiting cyclooxygenase, anti-inflammatory agents may be able to block this activation. In addition to the inhibition of prostaglandin H synthetase (cyclooxygenase) and other enzymes important in carcinogenesis, NSAIDs may have important anticancer effects through modulation of the immune system, antiangiogenic effects, induction of apoptosis, and reduction of certain growth factor synthesis. In general, the degree of benefit is positively correlated with dose and duration of NSAID therapy. There is estimated to be a 10-year delay before positive benefits of NSAID prophylaxis can be seen.

15. What is the treatment of choice for colorectal cancer?

Surgical resection is the primary treatment of choice in colorectal cancer. More than one-half of all patients can be cured by surgical resection of the involved intestinal segment and reanastomosis. Even if distant metastases are present, surgery is often performed to avoid problems related to bleeding or obstruction. Abdominal-perineal resections may be indicated for low rectal lesions, and newer sphincter-sparing procedures are under study. Clinical trials are ongoing to compare laparoscopic surgery with traditional open surgery. For anal canal carcinomas, a combination of radiation and chemotherapy is the treatment of choice. Surgery is reserved for patients who fail this combination.

Treatments for Colorectal Cancer

SITE	PROCEDURE	PHYSICAL ALTERATIONS
Appendix, cecum, ascending colon, hepatic flexure	Right hemicolectomy	Possible temporary or permanent cecostomy or ascending colostomy
Transverse colon	Transverse colectomy	Possible temporary or permanent transverse colostomy
Distal transverse colon	Left hemicolectomy	Possible temporary or permanent colostomy
Splenic flexure, descending colon	Left partial colectomy	Possible temporary or permanent descending colostomy
Sigmoid colon	Sigmoid colectomy	Possible temporary or permanent sigmoid colostomy
Rectum	Low anterior resection for tumors > 10 cm from anal verge (upper third of rectum)	Possible temporary or permanent sigmoid colostomy
	Abdominal perineal resection (APR)	Permanent sigmoid colostomy (APR) in distal 6 cm of rectum
	Low anterior resection or APR controversial (cancer in mid-rectum 7–11 cm from anal verge)	Permanent sigmoid colostomy with APR

16. When is radiation therapy indicated?

- Preoperatively to reduce bulky rectal cancers, improve the rate of surgical resectability, and eradicate microscopic disease.
- Postoperatively in stage B or C rectal cancers to prevent local recurrence. Postoperative radiation is given to eliminate remaining disease if surgical margins are positive or for Dukes' stage B or C cancer of the rectum.
- Postoperatively in colon cancer if disease invades other organs (i.e., bladder, abdominal wall)
- Palliatively to decrease painful metastases or control bleeding for inoperable patients.

Note: Adjuvant postoperative radiation therapy combined with a chemotherapy regimen containing 5-FU may have a detrimental effect on long-term bowel function with patients experiencing liquid stools, frequent defecation, increased use of antidiarrheal medications, perineal skin irritation, and inability to differentiate stool from flatulence.

17. What is the role of chemotherapy in colorectal cancer?

- Adjuvant treatment after surgery
- Radiation sensitizer
- Palliation of advanced disease

18. Why is chemotherapy important for patients with cancer of the colon, rectum, or anus?

Chemotherapy often is used for patients with colorectal cancer, either as an adjuvant or for advanced disease. Adjuvant therapy is important because almost 50% of patients with colorectal cancer die of metastases primarily due to residual disease at surgery.

19. Which chemotherapeutic agents are used for cancer of the colon and rectum?

Fluorouracil (5-FU) is the most widely used chemotherapy agent, with an overall response rate of 17–30%. Gastrointestinal effects (diarrhea and mucositis) or myelosuppression related to 5-FU vary according to total dose, timing, combinations of drugs used, and method of administration. For example, continuous infusions commonly cause more gastrointestinal toxicity or hand-foot syndrome, whereas bolus dosing causes more myelosuppression.

Leucovorin (a vitamin that enhances the effectiveness of 5-FU) is given with 5-FU postoperatively as adjuvant therapy in patients with Dukes' stage B and C colon cancer.

Irinotecan (Camptosar) is used in patients with advanced disease refractory to 5-FU; it has a response rate of 23%. Irinotecan in combination with 5-FU and leucovorin has been shown to be superior to 5-FU and leucovorin alone in the metastatic setting. Studies are currently under way to explore the role of irinotecan in the adjuvant setting.

20. How is anal canal cancer treated?

5-FU and mitomycin C frequently are given concurrently with radiation therapy. 5-FU has radiosensitizing effects that improve the efficacy of radiation therapy. Other radiation sensitizers include paclitaxel, gemcitabine, and cisplatin.

21. What newer agents show promise?

Newer agents with impending approval include oxaliplatin (SAR96669) for previously treated colorectal cancer and capecitabine (Xeloda), an oral 5-FU prodrug, for metastatic colorectal cancer. Other experimental approaches include signal transduction inhibition (for example, inhibiting an epidermal growth factor receptor, causing downregulation of malignant cellular behavior), monoclonal antibody therapy against the colon carcinoma-associated antigen CO17-1A, and vaccination against the tumor-associated antigen, CEA. Folate-based specific inhibitors of thymidylate synthases (D1694) and inhibitors of tyrosine kinase vascular endothelial growth factor (VEGF) receptors are also under study. The second group of agents inhibits microvessel formation (anti-angiogenesis) and promotes endothelial cell apoptosis. UFT, another oral 5-FU prodrug, is also in clinical trial.

22. What novel administration technique may be used for hepatic metastases?

Hepatic arterial infusion of chemotherapy (5-FU or FUDR).

23. What rare adverse effects can occur from 5 FU therapy?

Severe reactions to standard doses of 5 FU are seen in 3% of patients with a rare genetic enzyme deficiency called dihydropyrimidine dehydrogenase deficiency (DPD). This enzyme is responsible for 5 FU catabolism. Adverse effects include diarrhea, stomatitis, mucositis, myelosuppression, neurotoxicity, hand and foot syndrome, nausea and vomiting, and mental status changes.

24. Are other treatments available for metastatic disease?

Treatment depends on the symptoms and extent of metastatic disease. Metastatic disease in the liver can be treated with radiation, hepatic artery chemoinfusion, or surgical resection if disease is limited to one area of the liver.

25. How is a colostomy managed?

Approximately 15% of all patients diagnosed with colorectal cancer require a permanent colostomy. The care of a colostomy is ideally taught by a nurse trained in enterostomal therapy (ET). Patients should be taught the following tasks:
- Clean the peristomal skin with soap and water.
- Apply the disposable pouch over the stoma.
- Empty the pouch when it is one-third full of stool and/or flatus.

• Change the pouch every 4–7 days if there is no leakage. Because pouches are now odor-proof and water-proof, they should not be punctured with holes, as recommended in the past.

26. What instructions about lifestyle changes should be given to patients with a colostomy?

Diet. No restrictions. Continue to eat well-balanced meals with fluid intake of 6–8 glasses/day. Avoid or eat in moderation foods that may cause odor or gas.

Activity. Avoid heavy lifting, pushing, and pulling during the first three postoperative months. Continue participation in sports, including swimming, but avoid contact sports.

Traveling. No restrictions. Always hand-carry supplies and take along extras.

Social issues. Be aware of initial reactions, including feelings of despair, invalidism, fear of accidents, feeling mutilated, loss of control, and fear of death and dying. Body image disturbance is greatest during the first year after surgery. As recovery from ostomy surgery progresses, patients become increasingly comfortable with their bodies, the ability to care for their pouch, and the desire to return to a normal lifestyle, including sexual activity. Ask to see an enterostomal therapist and/or trained ostomy visitor from the local ostomy association.

Hygiene. Bathe with or without pouch; be aware that stool can pass while bathing. Hot tubs should be avoided or used with caution.

27. What suggestions may help to lower anxiety about sexual activity?

• Empty the pouch before sexual activity.
• Deodorize the pouch 6–12 hours before sexual activity, and avoid foods that can cause gas, urinary odor, or loose stools.
• Wear opaque pouch covers to conceal fecal material, or use lingerie or underwear made with pockets on the inside to hold the pouch.
• Experiment with sexual positions other than the missionary position.
• For women, consider vaginal lubricants for dyspareunia.
• For men, consider prostheses or reconstructive surgery (high incidence of impotence in men after abdominal perineal resection).

28. Should colostomies be irrigated?

Irrigations generally are taught for bowel regularity and may be necessary to cleanse the bowel for procedures. Colostomy irrigations can be done to regulate bowel activity in descending or sigmoid colostomies with formed stool. Irrigations are not recommended for the ascending or transverse colon because of the loose consistency of stool.

29. What resources are available to patients with colorectal cancer?

The American Cancer Society (800-ACS-2345) offers many educational and support services to all patients with cancer. The United Ostomy Association (800-826-0826) has local chapters that offer complete rehabilitative services and support groups to patients with ostomies. The Johns Hopkins Colorectal Cancer Registry (410-955-3875) and Myriad Genetics laboratories (1-800-469-7423) provide information about genetic screening and counseling. The Wound, Ostomy, Continence Nurses Society provides educational and support services for patients with ostomies, incontinence, and wounds.

REFERENCES

1. American Cancer Society 1996 Advisory Committee: Guidelines on diet, nutrition, and cancer prevention: Reducing the risk of cancer with healthy food choices and physical activity. Cancer J Clin 46(6):325–341,1996.
2. American Gastroenterological Association Clinical Practice and Practice Economics Committee: AGA technical review: Impact of dietary fiber on colon cancer occurrence. Gastroenterology 118:1235–1257, 2000.
3. Bryant RA, Buls JG: Pathophysiology and diagnostic studies of gastrointestinal tract disorders. In Hampton BG, Bryant RA (eds): Ostomies and Continent Diversions: Nursing Management. St. Louis, Mosby, 1992, pp 299–348.

 4. Diaz-Canton EA, Padzur R: Colorectal cancer: Diagnosis and management. In Padzur R (ed): Medical Oncology: A Comprehensive Review, 2nd ed. New York, PRR, 1995, pp 263–284.
 5. Diaz-Rubio E, Sastre J, Zaniboni A, et al: Oxaliplatin as single agent in previously untreated colorectal carcinoma patients: A phase II multicentric study. Ann Oncol 9:105–108, 1998.
 6. Ellis C, Saddler DAH: Colorectal cancer. In Yarbro CH, Frogge MH, Goodman M, Groenwald SL (eds): Cancer Nursing: Principles and Practice, 5th ed. Boston, Jones & Bartlett, 2000, pp 1117–1137.
 7. Fleming ID, Cooper JS, Henson DE, Hutler R: AJCC Cancer Staging Handbook, 5th ed. Philadelphia, Lippincott-Raven, 1998.
 8. Fuchs CS, Giovannucci EL, Colditz GA, et al: Dietary Fiber and the risk of colorectal cancer and adenoma in women. N Engl J Med 340:169–176, 1999.
 9. Giardiello FM: Clinical trials of non-aspirin NSAIDs to prevent colorectal neoplasia. In American Society of Clinical Oncology: Educational Book, 32nd Annual Meeting (May 18–21). Philadelphia, American Society of Clinical Oncology, 1996, p 425.
10. Greenlee RT, Hill-Harmon MB, Murray T, Thun M: Cancer statistics, 2001. CA Cancer J Clin 51:15–36, 2001.
11. Kollmorgen CF, Meagher AP, Wolff BG, et al: The long-term effect of adjuvant postoperative chemoradiotherapy for rectal carcinoma on bowel function. Ann Surg 220:676–682, 1994.
12. Lorenz M, Muller HH: Randomized multicenter trial of fluorouracil plus leucovorin administered either via hepatic arterial or intravenous infusion versus flurordeoxyuridine administered via hepatic arterial infusion in patients with nonresectable liver metastases from colorectal carcinoma. J Clin Oncol 18:239, 2000.
13. Morrison GB, Bastian A, Rosa TD, et al: Dihydropyrimidine dehydrogenase deficiency: A pharmacogenetic defect causing severe adverse reactions to 5-fluorouracil-based chemotherapy. Oncol Nurs Forum 24:83–88, 1997.
14. Rosen N: Cancers of the gastrointestinal tract. In DeVita VT, Hellman S, Rosenberg SA (eds): Cancer Principles and Practice of Oncology, 5th ed. Philadelphia, Lippincott-Raven, 1997, pp 971–980.
15. Rothenberg ML, et al: Phase II trial of irinotecan in patients with progressive or rapidly recurrent colorectal cancer. J Clin Oncol 14:1128–1135, 1996.
16. Salz LB, Cox JV, Blanke C, et al: Irinotecan plus fluorouracil and leucovorin for metastatic colorectal cancer. N Engl J Med 343:905–914, 2000.
17. Shell JA: The psychosexual impact of ostomy surgery. Progr Develop Ostomy Wound Care 4:3–15, 1992.
18. Smalley W, Ray WA, Daugherty J, Griffin MR: Use of nonsteroidal anti-inflammatory drugs and incidence of colorectal cancer. Arch Intern Med 159:161–166, 1999.
19. Steele GD Jr: Colorectal cancer. In Murphy GP, Lawrence W Jr, Lenhard RE Jr (eds): American Cancer Society Textbook of Clinical Oncology. Atlanta, American Cancer Society, 1995, pp 236–250.
20. Steele GD Jr: The national cancer data base report on colorectal cancer. Cancer 74:1979–1989, 1994.
21. Steinbach G, Lynch PM, Phillips RKS, et al: The effect of celecoxib, acyclooxygenase-2 inhibitor, in familial adenomatous polyposis. N Engl J Med 342:1946–1952, 2000.
22. UKCCCR Mal Cancer Trial Working Party: Epidermoid anal cancer results from the UKCCCR randomized trial of radiotherapy alone versus radiotherapy, 5-fluorouracil, and mitomycin. Lancet 348:1049–1054, 1996.
23. Wolmark N, Rockette H, Mamounas E, et al: Clinical trial to assess the relative efficacy of fluorouracil and leucovorin, fluorouracil and levamisole, and fluorouracil, leucovorin, and levamisole in patients with Dukes' B and C carcinoma of the colon: Results from National Surgical Adjuvant Breast and Bowel Project C-04. J Clin Oncol 17:3553–3559, 1999.

27. ENDOCRINE CANCERS

Michael T. McDermott, MD

1. What are endocrine neoplasms?

The endocrine glands secrete hormones directly into the bloodstream for transport throughout the body. Benign or malignant tumors may develop in these glands and cause clinical disease by secreting excessive amounts of hormones, by compressing or invading surrounding structures, or by metastasizing to distant sites. An estimated 21,400 new cases of endocrine neoplasms will occur in 2001; 19,500 of these cases will be due to thyroid cancer. Only 2,300 deaths are estimated for 2001, of which 1,300 deaths will be related to thyroid cancer.

Location of endocrine neoplasms. Endocrine neoplasms arise from the hormone-secreting glands. The most common are tumors of the pituitary, thyroid, parathyroid, and adrenal glands and pancreatic islet cells. Carcinoid tumors, which may secrete large amounts of physiologic substances, are also often classified with the endocrine tumors, although they do not arise from an endocrine gland.

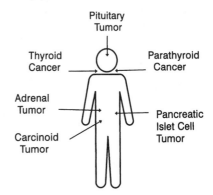

2. Name the different types of pituitary tumors.

The pituitary gland is the master gland that controls most of the other endocrine glands. It consists of five distinct cell types, each having a specific function. Any cell type may become neoplastic and produce excessive amounts of its specific hormone. Thus, pituitary tumors may secrete growth hormone (GH), prolactin (PRL), adrenocorticotropic hormone (ACTH), thyrotropin (TSH), or gonadotropins (luteinizing hormone [LH] and follicle-stimulating hormone [FSH]). Some tumors produce combinations of hormones, and others are nonsecretors.

Regulation and Function of the Pituitary Gland

CELL TYPE	HORMONE	TARGET	ACTION
Somatotroph	Growth hormone (GH)	All tissues	Tissue growth
Lactrotroph	Prolactin (PRL)	Breast	Milk production
Corticotroph	Corticotropin (ACTH)	Adrenal	Cortisol production
Thyrotroph	Thyrotropin (TSH)	Thyroid	Thyroxine production
Gonadotroph	Follicle-stimulating hormone (FSH)	Ovary	Ovum development
		Testes	Sperm development
	Luteinizing hormone (LH)	Ovary	Ovulation induction
		Testes	Androgen production

3. What syndromes are associated with pituitary tumors?

GH-secreting tumors produce gigantism in children and acromegaly in adults. Prolactinomas cause galactorrhea (abnormal milk discharge from the breast) and amenorrhea (cessation of menstruation) in women and impotence in men. ACTH-producing tumors cause the many manifestations of Cushing's disease. TSH-producing tumors result in hyperthyroidism, whereas gonadotropin-producing tumors paradoxically cause hypogonadism because of loss of pulsatile hormone secretion.

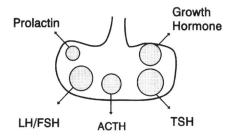

Functioning pituitary tumors. Pituitary tumors often secrete excessive amounts of one or more of the pituitary hormones: growth hormone, prolactin, thyrotropin, corticotropin, or gonadotropins (LH and FSH). Although the tumors are usually histologically benign, significant morbidity and mortality may result from the syndromes of hormone oversecretion or tumor mass compression of surrounding vascular or neural structures.

Clinical Features of Acromegaly

Enlargement of acral parts and multiple organs		Other features
Hands	Ears	Skin tags
Feet	Nose	Sleep apnea
Skull	Tongue	Osteoarthritis
Jaws	Heart	Hypertension
Sinuses	Liver	Diabetes mellitus

Clinical Features of Cushing's Syndrome

Central obesity	Purple striae	Emotional lability
Facial plethora	Easy bruising	Hypertension
Moon face	Muscle weakness	Diabetes mellitus
Buffalo hump		

4. Are pituitary tumors usually benign or malignant?

Pituitary tumors are almost always benign histologically and rarely metastasize to distant sites. However, they often undergo progressive growth and frequently compress or invade local structures such as the optic nerves and cavernous sinuses. Invasion may result in severe headaches, significant visual defects, vascular thrombosis, and, occasionally, hydrocephalus.

5. How are pituitary tumors treated?

Prolactinomas are most often treated with medications such as bromocriptine and cabergoline, which produce significant reductions in tumor size and prolactin secretion. The treatment of choice for other pituitary tumors is surgical resection; the tumor is usually removed through an incision inside the nose or under the lip (transsphenoidal hypophysectomy). Because many large and invasive tumors cannot be completely removed, radiation therapy is often given postoperatively.

6. Name the most common types of thyroid cancer.

The thyroid gland is composed of follicular cells, which synthesize thyroid hormones, and parafollicular c-cells, which produce calcitonin. Three main histologic types of cancer arise from the follicular cells: papillary, follicular, and anaplastic carcinomas. Medullary carcinoma, on the other hand, develops from the parafollicular c-cells.

7. How do thyroid cancers present clinically?

Thyroid cancer usually presents as a painless thyroid mass, much like a benign thyroid nodule. Features suggesting that such a mass is malignant include size greater than 3 cm, rock-hard consistency, lymphadenopathy, and hoarseness due to vocal cord paralysis. The diagnosis is most reliably made by fine-needle aspiration biopsy.

8. What is the prognosis for patients with thyroid cancers?

The prognosis for papillary carcinoma is excellent. The cure rate exceeds 90%, and the 10-year mortality rate is only 5%. Similarly, follicular carcinoma has a cure rate of over 80% and a 10-year mortality rate of 10%. Medullary carcinoma, however, results in a 10-year mortality rate of approximately 30%, and most patients with anaplastic carcinoma die within 8 months of diagnosis.

9. How are thyroid cancers treated?

Papillary and follicular carcinomas are best treated with surgery, radioiodine (I-131) ablation and chronic levothyroxine (LT4) suppression therapy. The surgical procedure of choice for most patients is a near-total thyroidectomy, in which only a small amount of thyroid tissue around the parathyroid glands and the recurrent laryngeal nerves is preserved. I-131 will then destroy the remaining thyroid tissue and, hopefully, any residual or metastatic thyroid cancer tissue. Prior to receiving I-131 therapy, the patient must not take LT4 for 4–6 weeks to allow the serum TSH level to become elevated. Once this is done, suppressive doses of LT4 are instituted to inhibit pituitary TSH secretion since TSH can stimulate the growth of both normal and malignant thyroid tissue. The goal of LT4 suppression is to maintain the serum TSH level below or at the lower end of the normal range. Medullary carcinoma requires a total thyroidectomy and LT4 replacement therapy, which maintains the serum TSH level within the normal range. The treatment of anaplastic carcinoma is total thyroidectomy, LT4 suppression and, in some cases, external beam irradiation. A variety of adjunctive but largely unproven medications that can also be used in these patients include doxorubicin, paclitaxel, alpha interferon and retinoic acid.

10. What are the features of parathyroid carcinoma?

Parathyroid carcinoma may present as a neck mass with associated lymphadenopathy or as hypercalcemia discovered on serum testing. The most strongly suggestive finding is moderate to marked hypercalcemia in association with extremely elevated serum levels of parathyroid hormone (PTH). The diagnosis of parathyroid cancer, however, ultimately depends on tissue examination.

11. Is there an effective treatment for parathyroid carcinoma?

The treatment of choice is aggressive neck dissection by an experienced surgeon. Chemotherapy and radiation therapies are rarely beneficial. The 5-year survival rate is less than 50%.

12. What are the most common tumors of the adrenal glands?

The adrenal glands consist of an outer cortex, in which steroid hormones are produced, and an inner medulla, in which catecholamines are made. Benign and malignant tumors may arise in either site. Adrenal cortical tumors may produce excessive cortisol, aldosterone, or androgens. Adrenal medullary tumors, called pheochromocytomas, often secrete norepinephrine and epinephrine.

Functioning adrenal tumors. Adrenal tumors may arise from the outer zone (cortex) or the inner zone (medulla) of the adrenal glands. Tumors of the cortex often secrete excessive amounts of cortisol, aldosterone, or testosterone. Tumors of the medulla, known as pheochromocytomas, secrete catecholamines (epinephrine and norepinephrine). Symptoms result from hormone overproduction or, when tumors are malignant, from local invasion and distant metastases.

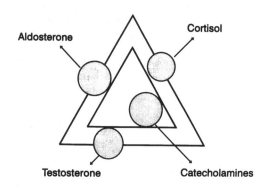

13. Describe the clinical manifestations of adrenal tumors.

Cushing's syndrome results when tumors secrete cortisol. An excess of aldosterone causes hypertension and hypokalemia. Androgen-producing tumors bring about virilization in women but may be asymptomatic in men. Pheochromocytomas often produce severe hypertension, headaches, sweating, and palpitations. Nonsecreting tumors, when large or malignant, present with abdominal or flank pain, and weight loss.

14. How are adrenal tumors treated?

Surgery is the treatment of choice for nearly all hormone-secreting adrenal tumors and for any nonsecreting tumors over 6 cm in diameter. When tumors prove to be malignant on pathologic examination, mitotane treatment has produced partial or complete tumor regression, reduced production of adrenal hormones, and improved survival in nonrandomized, noncontrolled trials. The combination of mitotane with etoposide, cisplatin and doxorubicin has shown some promise but responses to chemotherapy have, in general, been disappointing. Radiation therapy has not been shown to be effective.

15. What is the prognosis for patients with adrenal tumors?

The prognosis for patients with benign adrenal tumors is usually excellent. For those with adrenal carcinoma, however, the mean survival is about 15 months and the 5-year survival rate is approximately 20–35%. Prognosis is improved by younger patient age, smaller tumor size, localized disease (in nonfunctioning tumors), and complete tumor resection.

16. Name the most common types of pancreatic islet cell tumors.

The pancreatic islets normally secrete three major hormones: insulin, glucagon, and somatostatin. Nonetheless, the most common islet cell tumor is gastrinoma, a neoplasm that secretes gastrin, which is normally made only in the stomach. Insulinoma is the second most common islet cell tumor; glucagonomas and somatostatinomas are rare. Occasionally islet cell tumors will also secrete pancreatic polypeptide.

17. What syndromes do pancreatic islet cell tumors produce?

Gastrinomas hypersecrete gastrin, which stimulates prolific acid overproduction by the stomach, resulting in the development of multiple, recurrent peptic ulcers, and chronic watery diarrhea. This complex is also known as the Zollinger-Ellison syndrome. Excessive insulin secretion by insulinomas causes episodes of severe hypoglycemia, manifested by confusion, convulsions, and coma.

18. Are most islet cell tumors benign or malignant?

Insulinomas are usually benign (80%), whereas all other pancreatic islet cell tumors are most often (80% of cases) malignant.

19. Is there an effective treatment for islet cell tumors?

The treatment of choice for islet cell tumors, whenever possible, is surgical resection. For gastrinomas that are unresectable, symptomatic relief can be achieved by reducing gastric acid secretion with medications such as omeprazole or octreotide. Hypoglycemia from a persistent insulinoma may be prevented by frequent ingestion of small meals and administration of diazoxide, propranolol, or verapamil.

Since most islet cell tumors are malignant, chemotherapy is often necessary. The most effective chemotherapy combinations include the following: streptozotocin, 5-fluorouracil and leucovorin; lomustine and 5-fluorouracil; etoposide, doxorubicin, and 5-fluorouracil; cisplatin, dacarbazine, and alpha interferon. Finally, tumor embolization in conjunction with direct intra-arterial infusions of chemotherapy agents has shown additional promise as a palliative procedure.

20. What is the difference between carcinoid tumors and carcinoid syndrome?

Carcinoid tumors are neoplasms that arise from cells called enterochromaffin cells because of their peculiar histologic staining characteristics. They may occur in the lungs or gonads and throughout the digestive tract; the most common site is the appendix. Carcinoid syndrome is a symptom complex consisting of cutaneous flushing, diarrhea, and wheezing; it is associated with a tendency to develop progressive fibrosis of the right heart valves, endocardium, pleura, peritoneum, and retroperitoneum.

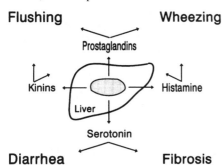

Carcinoid syndrome consists of a constellation of symptoms and signs that include flushing, wheezing, diarrhea, and growth of scar tissue in internal organs and body cavities. This syndrome most often occurs when an intestinal carcinoid tumor metastasizes to the liver and secretes into the systemic circulation active substances such as serotonin, prostaglandins, kinins, and histamine.

21. Describe the pathophysiology of carcinoid syndrome.

Many carcinoid tumors produce substances such as serotonin, bradykinin, tachykinin, histamine, prostaglandins, neurotensin, and substance P, all of which are readily metabolized by the liver. When carcinoid tumors metastasize to the liver, these humoral mediators gain access to the systemic circulation and cause the manifestations of carcinoid syndrome. The diagnosis is usually made by finding elevated serum levels of serotonin or increased urinary excretion of 5-hydroxyindoleacetic acid (5-HIAA), a breakdown product of serotonin.

22. Can carcinoid syndrome be treated or controlled?

Almost all patients who develop carcinoid syndrome have metastatic disease and cannot be cured; chemotherapy and radiation therapy are usually ineffective. However, because of the relatively slow growth rate of most carcinoid tumors, prolonged survival is common and control of the symptoms becomes necessary. Flushing may be most effectively alleviated with antihistamines (H_1 and H_2 antagonists), steroids or octreotide injections, whereas diarrhea most commonly responds to codeine, diphenoxylate (Lomotil), loperamide (Immodium), clonidine or octreotide.

Although not generally curative, chemotherapy may reduce the total tumor burden sufficiently to reduce carcinoid symptoms. The following chemotherapy regimens have thus far shown the greatest efficacy in these patients: streptozotocin, 5-fluorouracil and leucovorin; lomustine and 5-fluorouracil; etoposide, doxorubicin and 5-fluorouracil; cisplatin, dacarbazine, and alpha interferon. Another promising approach to hepatic tumor debulking has been hepatic artery embolization along with direct intra-arterial chemotherapy infusions.

23. What are the endocrine paraneoplastic syndromes?

Endocrine paraneoplastic syndromes occur in association with some tumors but are not due to tissue invasion or metastases. They result from secretion by the tumor of hormones into the circulation. The three best known examples are the syndrome of inappropriate antidiuretic hormone (SIADH), hypercalcemia of malignancy, and ectopic ACTH syndrome.

24. Explain the pathophysiology of SIADH.

Antidiuretic hormone (ADH) is normally secreted by the posterior pituitary gland and acts on the kidney to promote water retention. In doing so, it protects the body against dehydration. Tumors, particularly those of the lung and brain, sometimes secrete large amounts of ADH that result in excessive water retention and dilutional hyponatremia. Dilutional hyponatremia may result in confusion, convulsions, and coma due to edema of the brain. For more information on SIADH, please refer to chapter 56.

25. What are the mediators of the hypercalcemia of malignancy?

Most cases of hypercalcemia of malignancy result from tumor elaboration of a hormone known as parathyroid hormone-related peptide (PTHrp). Refer to chapter 52 for more information on hypercalcemia. Similar in some ways to PTH, this hormone normally functions to concentrate calcium in breast milk. When secreted in excessive quantities by tumors, such as those of the lung, it stimulates bone resorption and renal calcium retention, which combine to raise the serum calcium level.

26. Describe the pathophysiology of ectopic ACTH syndrome.

ACTH is normally secreted by the anterior pituitary gland and stimulates the adrenal glands to produce cortisol. Tumors of various organs, especially the lungs, occasionally produce ACTH in quantities sufficient to stimulate excessive secretion of adrenal cortisol. This results in development of Cushing's syndrome, the manifestations of which are partly masked by tumor cachexia.

REFERENCES

1. Feldman JM: The carcinoid syndrome. Endocrinologist 3:129–135, 1993.
2. Friesen SR: Tumors of the endocrine pancreas. N Engl J Med 306:580–590, 1982.
3. Gagel RF, Robinson MF, Donovan DT, Alford BR: Medullary thyroid carcinoma: Recent progress. J Clin Endocrinol Metab 76:809–814, 1993.
4. Galanis E, Kvols LK, Rubin J: Carcinoid syndrome. J Clin Oncol 16:796–798, 1998.
5. Greenlee RT, Hill-Harmon MB, Murray T, Thun M: Cancer statistics, 2001. CA Cancer J Clin 51:15–36, 2001.
6. Hirshberg B, Livi A, Bartlett DL, et al: Forty-eight hour fast: The diagnostic test for insulinoma. J Clin Endocrinol Metab 85:3222–3226, 2000.
7. Jaffe BM: Current issues in the management of Zollinger-Ellison syndrome. Surgery 111:241–243, 1992.
8. Janmohamed S, Bloom SR: Review. Carcinoid tumours. Postgrad Med J 73:207–214, 1997.
9. Jensen RT: Pancreatic endocrine tumors: Recent advances. Ann Oncol 10 Suppl 4:170–180, 1999.
10. Klibanski A, Zervas NT: Diagnosis and management of hormone-secreting pituitary adenomas. N Engl J Med 324:822–831, 1991.
11. Kulke MH, Mayer RJ: Review. Carcinoid tumors. N Engl J Med 340:858–868, 1999.
12. Luton J-P, Cerdas S, Billaud L, et al: Clinical features of adrenocortical carcinoma, prognostic factors, and the effect of mitotane therapy. N Engl J Med 322:1195–1201, 1990.
13. Mazzaferri EL, Samaan NA (eds): Endocrine Tumors. Boston, Blackwell Scientific Publications, 1993.
14. Robbins J (moderator): Thyroid cancer: A lethal endocrine neoplasm. Ann Intern Med 115:133–147, 1991.
15. Wajchenberg BL, Albergaria Pereira MA, Medonca BB, et al: Adrenocortical carcinoma: Clinical and laboratory observations. Cancer 88:711–736, 2000.
16. Williamson SK, Lew D, Miller GJ, et al: Phase II evaluation of cisplatin and etoposide followed by mitotane at disease progression in patients with locally advanced or metastatic adrenocortical carcinoma: A Southwest Oncology Group study. Cancer 88:1159–1165, 2000.
17. Wynne AG, Heerden JV, Carney JA, et al: Parathyoid carcinoma: Clinical and pathologic features in 43 patients. Medicine 71:197–205, 1992.

28. GASTRIC, PANCREATIC, HEPATOCELLULAR, AND GALLBLADDER CANCERS

Susan Morgan, MD

Quick Facts—Gastric Cancer

Incidence	In the United States the incidence is 10/100,000 persons compared with 78/100,000 persons in Japan. The number of new cases in the United States in 2001 is estimated at 21,700. Emigrants from high-incidence to low-incidence countries often have a decreased risk of developing gastric cancer. For unknown reasons, both incidence and mortality rates have decreased in all regions of the world.
Mortality	Highest in East Asia (Hong Kong, Japan, Singapore) and lowest in the United States. In 2001, an estimated 12,800 deaths in the United States will be due to gastric cancer.
Risk factors	Environment: lower socioeconomic status, diets low in fruits and vegetables, ingestion of salt-preserved or smoked foods, and cigarette smoking. Precursor conditions: previous partial gastrectomy for benign disease, chronic atrophic gastritis, pernicious anemia, achlorhydria, mucosal dysplasia, history of Barrett's esophagus, *Helicobacter pylori* infection, gastric adenomatous polyps. Heredity: type A blood, hereditary nonpolyposis colorectal cancer (Lynch syndrome 2), Li-Fraumeni syndrome.
Histology	Approximately 95% of gastric cancers are adenocarcinomas. The remainder are predominantly lymphomas or leiomyosarcomas. Other rare histologies include carcinoid tumors and squamous cell carcinomas.
Symptoms	Gastric cancer often progresses to an advanced stage before symptoms develop. Symptoms and signs of advanced disease include anorexia, early satiety, weight loss, palpable abdominal mass, dysphagia, severe anemia, and weakness.
Staging	**Tumor, node, metastasis (TNM) system** based on postgastrectomy pathologic specimen:

Primary tumor (T)

TX	Primary tumor cannot be assessed
T0	No evidence of primary tumor
Tis	Carcinoma in situ
T1	Tumor invades lamina propria or submucosa
T2	Tumor invades muscularis propria or submucosa (classified as T3 with perforation of visceral peritoneum over gastric ligaments or omenta)
T3	Tumor penetrates serosa without invasion of adjacent structures
T4	Tumor invades adjacent structures

Regional lymph nodes (N)

NX	Regional lymph node(s) cannot be assessed
N0	No regional lymph node metastasis
N1	Metastasis in 1 to 6 regional lymph node(s) within 3 cm of edge of primary tumor
N2	Metastasis in 7 to 15 regional lymph node(s) more than 3 cm from edge of primary tumor or in lymph nodes along left gastric, common hepatic, splenic, or celiac arteries
N3	Metastasis in > 15 regional nodes

Table continued on following page

Quick Facts—Gastric Cancer (Continued)

Distant metastasis (M)

MX   Presence of distant metastasis cannot be assessed

M0   No distant metastasis

M1   Distant metastasis

Stage grouping

Stage 0	Tis, N0, M0	Stage IIIA	T2, N2, M0
Stage IA	T1, N0, M0		T3, N1, M0
Stage IB	T1, N1, M0		T4, N0, M0
	T2, N0, M0	Stage IIIB	T3, N2, M0
Stage II	T1, N2 M0	Stage IV	T4, N1–2, M0
	T2, N1, M0		Any T, N3, M0
	T3, N0, M0		Any T, Any N, M1

Treatment
- Complete surgical resection of the tumor and adjacent lymph nodes is the only chance for cure. Survival rates are best improved in patients with stage I disease. Patients with T3, T4, or any nodal involvement have a significant risk for relapse after surgical resection.
- Postoperative adjuvant chemotherapy combined with radiation therapy is under clinical evaluation.
- Preliminary results of the Intergroup Study INT-0116 show improved disease-free and overall survival rates for curative-intent resection of stage IB–stage IV (M0) adenocarcinoma of the stomach or gastroesophageal junction. A combined approach with external-beam radiation therapy and chemotherapy was used and may become the new standard of care. More time is needed for the study results to mature.
- When chemotherapy is combined with radiation therapy in patients with locally advanced gastric carcinoma, survival is prolonged compared with either radiation therapy or chemotherapy alone.
- For patients with locally advanced tumors that are unresectable, external beam radiation therapy may be palliative in reducing pain, relieving obstruction, and controlling bleeding.
- For patients with metastatic gastric carcinoma, chemotherapy is the treatment of choice vs. supportive care.

1. Is there an association between *Helicobacter pylori* infection and gastric cancer?

Yes. Patients infected with *H. pylori* may have a 2–8-fold increased risk for the development of gastric cancer. Infection with *H. pylori* causes a sequence of events that leads to a chronic inflammatory process in the gastric mucosa, which can proceed in some patients to atrophic gastritis (loss of gastric glands) and in a minority of patients to gastric cancer. Because only a minority of infected patients develop gastric cancer, gastric carcinogenesis cannot be explained by *H. pylori* infection alone.

2. Does treatment for gastric *H. pylori* infection reduce the risk of developing gastric cancer?

Unknown. Data are insufficient to recommend mass screening programs of asymptomatic people for *H. pylori* infection for prevention of gastric cancer.

3. List the names associated with specific metastatic deposits in gastric cancer.

Virchow's node: left supraclavicular lymph node enlargement

Irish's node: left axillary lymph node enlargement

Sister Mary Joseph nodule: periumbilical nodule

Krukenberg's tumor: metastatic disease to ovaries

Blumer's shelf: mass in the cul-de-sac or rectal shelf

4. What paraneoplastic syndromes occasionally are seen in gastric cancer?

The following paraneoplastic syndromes are systemic manisfestations of gastric cancer, but they are rarely seen at initial presentation:

Acanthosis nigricans: a black or brownish wart-like eruption in intertriginous areas (axilla, groin, under breast); also may appear on palms of hands and soles of feet.

Trousseau's syndrome (hypercoagulable state): recurrent, idiopathic deep vein thrombosis.

Polymyositis/dermatomyositis: symmetrical proximal muscle weakness with or without skin rash.

Diffuse seborrheic keratosis

5. Describe the clinical manifestations of the "dumping syndrome." What is its probable cause?

The dumping syndrome is a postoperative complication of gastric resection. Clinical manifestations include nausea, vomiting, diarrhea, epigastric fullness, tachycardia, diaphoresis, and weakness. Dumping syndrome most likely is due to removal of the reservoir function (antrum) of the stomach. Hypertonic foodstuffs empty directly into the small bowel, resulting in a major fluid shift out of the intravascular space and into the bowel. To improve symptoms, the patient needs to decrease the osmotic load presented to the small bowel by eating small, frequent meals that are low in carbohydrate and high in protein.

6. Monthly injections of which vitamin are necessary after subtotal or total gastrectomy? Why?

After gastric resection, vitamin B12 deficiency occurs within 6–10 years. The several-year delay in clinical evidence of vitamin B12 deficiency is due to adequate liver stores. Once these stores are exhausted, the deficiency becomes evident because the parietal cells of the stomach are responsible for producing intrinsic factor, which is necessary for absorption of vitamin B12 (distal ileum). Monthly administration of vitamin B12 prevents deficiency.

7. Is there a role for adjuvant (postoperative) chemotherapy or radiation therapy after curative resection for gastric cancer?

Now under clinical investigation. The recent Intergroup Study showed improved disease-free and overall survival rates. Investigators are waiting for results to mature. However, the best approach for cure is subtotal gastrectomy with resection of adjacent lymph nodes. Patients with stage I disease are the best candidates for surgical resection for cure.

8. How often does cancer recur after curative resection?

Cancer recurs in most patients within the first 2 years. The 5-year survival rate for stage I disease is 50–60%; for stage II disease, 29%; and for stage III disease, 13%. Continued research is needed to improve these dismal outcomes.

9. Does radiation therapy in conjunction with chemotherapy confer a survival benefit for patients with locally advanced (nonmetastatic) gastric cancer?

Yes. Patients with locally advanced disease are unable to undergo resection for cure. Radiation alone may be palliative in reducing pain or relieving obstruction but does not improve survival. Nor does chemotherapy alone appear to improve survival. However, when radiation therapy (4000–5000 cGy) is combined with chemotherapy (5-fluorouracil [5FU]-based), survival appears to be prolonged. In one study comparing 5FU plus radiation therapy with radiation therapy alone, the median survival was 12 months vs. 5.9 months, respectively.

10. What treatment options are available for patients with advanced (metastatic) gastric cancer?

Advanced gastric cancer is incurable. Most patients die within a few months of diagnosis. Treatment options include investigational protocols; single-agent chemotherapy with 5FU; multi-agent chemotherapy such as 5FU, Adriamycin, high-dose methotrexate, and leucovorin rescue (FAMTX); etoposide, leucovorin, and 5FU (ELF); and palliative radiation therapy for symptoms (bleeding, pain, obstruction) or comfort-directed supportive care. Depending on the patient's performance status (debilitated vs. good activity level), any one of the previous options is acceptable. No single appraoch is considered standard of care.

Single-agent 5FU has a response rate of about 20%. Complete responses are rare, and partial responses are of brief duration. FAMTX has a higher response rate (40–50%) and is associated with survival times of 6–10 months. Palliative resection should be reserved for patients with continued bleeding or obstruction.

Quick Facts—Pancreatic Cancer

Incidence	In the United States, the incidence of pancreatic cancer is 9/100,000 people; the estimated number of new cases for 2001 is 29,200. Incidence has been stable for the past 20 years. Men are 1.5–2.0 times more likely to develop pancreatic cancer than women. African-Americans are more frequently affected, with an incidence of 15/100,000 people.
Mortality	The median survival of patients with pancreatic cancer is 3–4 months, and the 5-year survival rate is only 3%. In the U.S., the number of estimated deaths in 2001 is 28,900. The prognosis is so dismal because most patients have advanced disease at the time of diagnosis.
Risk factors	Cause remains unknown but several factors are associated with its occurrence: • Cigarette smoking: most prominent risk factor for pancreatic cancer • Diet: high fat, low intake of fruits and vegetables, excessive alcohol • Previous partial gastrectomy for benign conditions • Diabetes mellitus • Occupational exposure: solvents, petroleum compounds, beta-naphthylamine, and benzidine • Lower socioeconomic status • Hereditary pancreatitis
Histology	Pancreatic cancer arises from both exocrine parenchyma and endocrine islet cells. Approximately 95% of pancreatic cancers occur within the exocrine portion of the pancreas. Of exocrine malignancies, 80–90% are adenocarcinomas. The majority arise in the proximal portion of the pancreas, which includes the head, neck, and uncinate process. Other less common malignant tumors of the pancreas include pancreatic islet cell tumors, lymphomas, and cystadenocarcinomas.
Symptoms	Most patients are symptomatic at the time of diagnosis. Symptoms include abdominal pain, anorexia, weight loss, early satiety, jaundice, nausea, vomiting, and diarrhea.
Staging	**Tumor, node, metastasis (TNM) system** **Primary tumor (T)** TX Primary tumor cannot be assessed T0 No evidence of primary tumor Tis In situ carcinoma T1 Tumor limited to the pancreas 2 cm or less in greatest dimension T2 Tumor limited to the pancreas more than 2 cm in greatest dimension T3 Tumor extends directly into duodenum, bile duct, or peripancreatic tissues T4 Tumor extends directly into stomach, spleen, colon, or adjacent large vessels **Regional lymph nodes (N)** NX Regional lymph nodes cannot be assessed N0 No regional lymph node metastasis N1 Regional lymph node metastasis **Distant metastasis (M)** MX Distant metastasis cannot be assessed M0 No distant metastasis M1 Distant metastasis

Table continued on following page

Quick Facts—Pancreatic Cancer (Continued)

Stage grouping			
Stage 0	Tis, N0, M0	Stage III	Any T, N1, M0
Stage I	T1-2, N0, M0	Stage IVA	T4, Any N, M0
Stage II	T3, N0, M0	Stage IVB	Any T, Any N, M1

Treatment

- The approach to therapy differs according to stage of disease at presentation. Complete surgical resection remains the only effective treatment (possible in only 5–15% of patients). Procedures include pancreatoduodenectomy (Whipple procedure) for tumors in the head of the pancreas, distal pancreatectomy for lesions in the tail, and total pancreatectomy for large or diffuse lesions. Despite complete resection, locoregional recurrence still occurs in > 70% of patients.
- Survival is improved with adjuvant chemotherapy (5FU) plus radiation therapy after curative resection and no evidence of lymph node metastases. Clinical trials are evaluating pre- and postoperative radiation therapy with 5FU vs. gemcitabine.
- For patients with a good performance status and unresectable locally advanced disease, chemoradiation (5FU/XRT) has been shown to improve survival compared with radiation therapy alone or chemotherapy alone.
- Gemcitabine alone, as first-line therapy in locally advanced or metastatic pancreatic cancer not amenable to curative surgical resection, improves survival. Clinical benefits include decreased pain, increased appetite, weight gain, and improved functional status.
- For patients with metastatic disease, clinical trials, chemotherapy, and supportive care are the treatment options. The newest agent under evaluation in clinical trials is 9-nitro-camptothecin (oral agent).

11. What is the name of the standard operation for pancreatic tumors located in the head of the pancreas? What is removed?

The Whipple procedure (pancreatoduodenectomy) is the only potentially curative approach to cancer in the head of the pancreas. This procedure includes removal of the distal stomach, common bile duct, gallbladder, duodenum, pancreatic head to the midbody en bloc, and vagotomy. Unfortunately, resection is feasible in only 5–15% of cases because most patients have advanced disease (liver metastases, tumor extension into spleen, colon, or stomach, vascular invasion, or nerve invasion) at presentation. Resection also is typically limited to patients with cancer in the head of the pancreas because patients with tumors in the body or tail invariably have advanced disease (asymptomatic until well advanced). Patients with stage I tumors (T1–T2, N0, M0) are the best candidates for curative resection. However, even with resection, 90% of patients die from tumor recurrence within 1–2 years. The expected median survival is only 12–18 months.

12. Is there a role for adjuvant therapy after curative resection for pancreatic cancer?

Yes. Adjuvant therapy appears to be a reasonable approach for the few patients who are able to undergo curative resection and have no lymph node metastases identified on pathologic review. Only one prospective randomized trial (Gastrointestinal Tumor Study Group trial) has shown a survival benefit with the addition of postoperative 5FU and radiation therapy. Patients who received this combination showed significant improvement in median survival (20 months vs. 11 months), 2-year survival (43% vs. 18%), and 5-year survival (14% vs. 5%).

13. What is the newest chemotherapeutic agent for unresectable (locally advanced or metastatic) pancreatic cancer?

Gemcitabine. A randomized study demonstrated an advantage with gemcitabine over 5FU in survival time and symptom control (pain, weight, performance status). Gemcitabine was given at 1000 mg/m^2 weekly for 7 doses, followed by a week of rest, and then weekly for 3 doses every 4 weeks thereafter. Approximately 24% of gemcitabine-treated patients experienced improved symptom control compared with only 4.8% of 5FU-treated patients. The median survival for gemcitabine-treated patients was 5.65 months compared with 4.41 months for 5FU-treated patients. Common side effects included nausea, vomiting, diarrhea, and neutropenia. At present, gemcitabine should be considered as first-line management of symptomatic patients with advanced pancreatic adenocarcinoma.

14. Which ganglion plexus is commonly involved in pancreatic cancer?

Pancreatic cancers may invade the celiac plexus, causing significant neuropathic pain. This pain is one of the worst symptoms experienced by patients with advanced pancreatic cancer. Treatment to control pain includes opioid analgesics, surgical neurotomy, chemical neurolysis (celiac block), and radiation therapy. Medical management alone often is not enough. Chemical neurolysis involves the injection of 50% alcohol directly into the region of the celiac plexus either intraoperatively or percutaneously and is associated with pain relief in 90% of cases. External-beam radiation therapy is effective in relieving neuropathic pain in approximately 50–70% of patients with advanced pancreatic cancer.

15. When Courvoisier's sign is present, what organ of the body can be palpated?

Gallbladder. Carcinoma of the head of the pancreas may cause biliary obstruction, resulting in a distended gallbladder. The distended gallbladder is typically nontender.

16. Are there any new treatments for pancreatic cancer?

Yes. A phase 3 randomized study is under way to compare the efficacy of 9-nitro-camptothecin and gemcitabine in chemo-naive patients with pancreatic cancer. Gemcitabine recently demonstrated a survival advantage and disease-related symptom improvement compared with 5FU.

Quick Facts—Hepatocellular Cancer

Incidence	The incidence of hepatocellular carcinoma is greatest in Southeast Asia, sub-Saharan Africa, and the Orient. The incidence in the United States, Canada, Britain, Australia, and South America is low. In 2001 in the United States, 16,200 new cases of liver and biliary passage cancers are estimated.
Mortality	High fatality rate. The 5-year survival rate is approximately 3–5%. In 2001 in the U.S., an estimated 14,100 deaths will be due to liver and biliary passage cancers.
Risk factors	Chronic infection with either hepatitis B or hepatitis C, with or without underlying cirrhosis. Preexisting cirrhosis: approximately 10% of patients with cirrhosis develop hepatocellular carcinoma. Aflatoxin: proved to be a potent hepatocarcinogen; appears to cause a specific mutation in the p53 tumor suppressor gene, leading to hepatocellular carcinoma. Hormones: the risk of liver cell adenomas and hepatocellular carcinoma is increased in women who use oral contraceptives for 8 or more years; hepatocellular carcinoma also has been observed in patients with long histories of androgen use.
Histology	80–90% of primary liver cancers are hepatocellular; other less common tumors include hepatoblastomas, sarcomas, and primary lymphomas.
Symptoms	Usual presenting symptoms are right upper quadrant pain, fatigue, abdominal swelling, and weight loss.
Staging	**Tumor, node, metastasis (TNM) system** **Primary tumor (T)** TX Primary tumor cannot be assessed T0 No evidence of primary tumor T1 Solitary tumor ≤ 2 cm in greatest dimension without vascular invasion

Table continued on following page

Quick Facts—Hepatocellular Cancer (Continued)

T2	Solitary tumor ≤ 2 cm in greatest dimension with vascular invasion, or multiple tumors limited to one lobe, none > 2 cm in greatest dimension without vascular invasion, or a solitary tumor > 2 cm in greatest dimension without vascular invasion
T3	Solitary tumor > 2 cm in greatest dimension with vascular invasion, or multiple tumors limited to one lobe, none > 2 cm in greatest dimension, with vascular invasion, or multiple tumors limited to one lobe, any > 2 cm in greatest dimension, with or without vascular invasion
T4	Multiple tumors in more than one lobe or tumor(s) involving a major branch of portal or hepatic vein(s) or invasion of adjacent organs other than gallbladder

Regional lymph nodes (N)
NX   Regional lymph nodes cannot be assessed
N0   No regional lymph node metastasis
N1   Regional lymph node metastasis
Distant metastasis (M)
MX   Distant metastasis cannot be assessed
M0   No distant metastasis
M1   Distant metastasis
Stage grouping

Stage 1	T1, N0, M0	Stage IIIB	T1–3, N1, M0
Stage II	T2, N0, M0	Stage IVA	T4, Any N, M0
Stage IIIA	T3, N0, M0	Stage IVB	Any T, Any N, M1

Treatment   Surgery is the only potential curative modality for hepatocellular carcinoma, but its use depends on tumor size, location, and condition of the uninvolved liver. Only 10% of patients with hepatocellular carcinoma are resectable at the time of diagnosis (solitary or unilobar hepatic lesions). There is no role for adjuvant chemotherapy or radiotherapy after curative resection. Other treatment options include hepatic intraarterial infusion of chemotherapy, chemoembolization, radiofrequency ablation, cryosurgery, ethanol injections, liver transplantation, radiation therapy, and single-agent chemotherapy (doxorubicin).

17. What tumor marker is commonly ordered for evaluating hepatocellular carcinoma?

Alpha-fetoprotein (AFP) is elevated in approximately 70% of patients diagnosed with hepatocellular carcinoma. Unfortunately, AFP is not specific for hepatocellular carcinoma and may be elevated in benign liver disease, germ cell tumor, gastric cancer, and pancreatic cancer. A normal level of AFP does not exclude the diagnosis of hepatocellular carcinoma.

18. List several paraneoplastic syndromes associated with hepatocellular carcinoma.

Fever	Gynecomastia
Hypercalcemia	Erythrocytosis
Hypoglycemia	Dysfibrinogenemia

19. What is transarterial chemoembolization?

Transarterial chemoembolization is a treatment used in some patients with hepatocellular carcinoma. It takes advantage of the fact that the majority of the blood supply to the cancer is via the hepatic artery, whereas the rest of the liver relies on the portal system. The goal is to eliminate the blood supply to the cancer by occluding the hepatic artery with gelfoam while at the same time administering cytotoxic chemotherapy directly to the tumor to cause necrosis (cell death). Transarterial chemoembolization is frequently complicated by abdominal pain and fever (postembolization syndrome) and is usually self-limiting. It has been used in patients with large unresectable hepatocellular carcinoma, prior to resection, and prior to transplant. Careful patient selection is important and depends on several patient characteristics (e.g., AFP, tumor volume).

20. What is the survival rate for patients with hepatocellular carcinoma?

The 5-year survival rate is approximately 40–45% for patients with small tumors (2–5 cm) and 10% for patients with tumors > 5 cm. Disease recurs in most patients undergoing resection. Unfortunately, curative resection is appropriate for only 10% or fewer cases because of advanced disease (bilobar involvement), underlying cirrhosis (poor hepatic reserve), portal/vena caval thrombus, or other comorbid diseases. Survival for patients with unresectable disease is about 2–6 months.

GALLBLADDER CANCER

21. What risk factors are possibly associated with the development of gallbladder cancer?

The cause of gallbladder cancer is unknown. Chronic cholecystitis and cholelithiasis have been associated with the development of gallbladder cancer in 50% and 75% of cases, respectively. A calcified gallbladder ("porcelain gallbladder") has about a 15–20% chance of harboring cancer. Ulcerative colitis increases the risk for development of gallbladder cancer. The incidence of gallbladder cancer increases with age and peaks in the 6th–7th decades of life; it is rare before the age of 40. In 2001, 6,900 new cases and 3,300 deaths are estimated. Women are affected more commonly than men (female-to-male ratio of 3:1–4:1). The incidence of gallbladder cancer is considerably higher in Mexicans, American Indians, and Alaskan natives. Employees of rubber industries have a higher incidence and earlier onset of gallbladder cancer.

22. Why is the prognosis for gallbladder cancer so dismal?

Gallbladder cancer is typically asymptomatic in its early resectable stages; by the time symptoms occur, the disease is advanced and unresectable. The cancer usually grows into the liver, stomach, and duodenum by direct extension, making resection impossible. The median survival period is approximately 6 months, and the 5-year survival rate is < 5%. Patients who are incidentally found to have stage I or II tumors at cholecystectomy for presumed symptomatic benign disease have an improved survival rate and are potentially cured.

23. Klatskin tumor refers to a cancer in what location?

A Klatskin tumor is a primary extrahepatic bile duct cancer (cholangiocarcinoma) located near the bifurcation of the left and right hepatic bile ducts.

The views contained in this manuscript are solely those of the author and do not reflect the views or policies of Tripler Army Medical Command, the Department of Defense, or the U.S. Government.

REFERENCES

1. Barber FD, Nelson J: Liver cancer: Looking to the future for better detection and treatment. Am J Nurs (Suppl):41–46, 2000.
2. Brain MC, Carbone PP (eds): Current Therapy in Hematology-Oncology, 5th ed. St. Louis, Mosby, 1995.
3. Casciato DA, Lowitz BB (eds): Manual of Clinical Oncology, 3rd ed. Boston, Little, Brown, 1995.
4. DeVita VT, Hellman S, Rosenberg SA (eds): Cancer: Principles and Practice of Oncology, 6th ed. Philadelphia, Lippincott Williams & Wilkins, 2001.
5. Fleming ID, Cooper JS, Henson DE, Huttler R: AJCC Cancer Staging Manual, 5th ed. Philadelphia, Lippincott-Raven, 1998.
6. Greenlee RT, Hill-Harmon MB, Murray T, Thun M: Cancer statistics, 2001. CA Cancer J Clin 51:15–36, 2001.
7. Huang, JQ: Meta-analysis of the relationship between helicobacter pylori seropositivity and gastric cancer. Gastroenterology 114:1169, 1998.
8. Macdonald JS, Haller DG, Mayer RJ (eds): Manual of Oncologic Therapeutics, 3rd ed. Philadelphia, J.B. Lippincott, 1995.
9. Macdonald JS, Proceedings of the American Society of Clinical Oncology, Abstract 1, 2000.
10. Padzur R (ed): Medical Oncology: A Comprehensive Review, 2nd ed. New York, PRR, 1995.
11. Sung, JY, Lin, SR, Ching, JY, et al: Effects of curing helicobacter pylori infection on precancerous gastric lesions: One year follow-up of a prospective randomized study in China [abstract]. Gastroenterology 114:A296, 1998.

29. GYNECOLOGIC CANCERS

Patricia Novak-Smith, RN, MS, AOCN, Susan Adnan-Koch, RN, MS, OCN, and Susan A. Davidson, MD

1. What are the primary sites of gynecologic cancer?

Gynecologic cancers are associated with the female reproductive organs. The principal sites include the ovaries, fallopian tubes, uterus, cervix, vagina, and vulva. Additional rare cancers that are classified as gynecologic include gestational trophoblastic neoplasias (GTN), a group of pregnancy-related tumors that may persist and metastasize (e.g, hydatidiform mole, choriocarcinoma), and primary peritoneal carcinoma, a tumor that originates on the peritoneal surfaces but demonstrates behavior similar to epithelial ovarian cancers. The three most commonly diagnosed gynecologic cancers are the focus of this chapter: endometrial (epithelial surface of the uterus), ovarian, and cervical.

2. How are gynecologic cancers staged?

Gynecologic cancers are staged according to guidelines established by the International Federation of Gynaecology and Obstetrics (FIGO). FIGO adapted the traditional primary tumor-regional lymph nodes-distant metastasis (TNM) system to ensure consistency on the international level. The primary features that distinguish this system from other staging systems are (1) reliance on clinical staging for cervical and vaginal cancer, which includes but is not limited to physical examination, chest radiograph, and intravenous pyelogram; (2) use of specific surgical staging for all other gynecologic cancers; and (3) adherence to the original staging designation for all disease sites despite later findings of persistence, metastasis, or recurrence.

Quick Facts—Cervical Cancer

Incidence	< 2% of new cancer cases in women annually. In 2001, 12,900 estimated new cases.
Mortality	< 2% of cancer deaths in women annually. In 2001, 4,400 estimated deaths.
Risk factors	Early coitus Human papillomavirus (HPV), especially types 16 and 18 Human immunodeficiency virus (HIV) Low socioeconomic status—decreased access to routine Pap smear screening Smoking (nicotine byproducts, measured in cervical secretions, are thought to favor development of precancerous changes of the cervix)
Histology	Squamous carcinomas are most common; other cell types include adenocarcinoma, adenosquamous carcinoma, small cell, and glassy cell.
Symptoms	Thin, watery vaginal discharge, heavier menses, and postcoital spotting are most common; other symptoms include spontaneous, intermittent, painless uterine bleeding (menometrorrhagia); back, flank, or leg pain; lower extremity edema; dysuria; hematuria or rectal bleeding; and cough.

Staging	Stage I Confined to cervix
	     IA_1 Invasion of stroma ≤ 3 mm deep and ≤ 7 mm wide
	     IA_2 Invasion of stroma > 3 mm to ≤ 5 mm deep and ≤ 7 mm wide
	     IB_1 Invasion of stroma > 5 mm deep or > 7 mm wide, and clinical lesions ≤ 4 cm in size
	     IB_2 Clinical lesions > 4 cm in size
	Stage II Extension beyond cervix and/or upper two-thirds of vagina
	     IIA No parametrial involvement
	     IIB Parametrial involvement

Table continued on following page

Quick Facts—Cervical Cancer (Continued)

	Stage III	Extension to lower third of vagina
	IIIA	No extension to pelvic side wall
	IIIB	Extension to pelvic side wall and/or hydronephrosis
	Stage IV	Extension beyond true pelvis
	IVA	Involvement of adjacent organs (bladder, rectum)
	IVB	Distant metastasis
Treatment	Stage I	Cone biopsy up to radical hysterectomy
	Stages IB, IIA	Radical hysterectomy with lymph node dissection or radiation has equivalent prognosis. For some IB tumors, combination therapy (radiation and surgery) is sometimes used.
	Stages IIB, III, IVA	Radiation therapy with chemotherapy used as radiation sensitizer
	Stage IVB	Palliative radiation and/or chemotherapy

3. Why is cervical cancer considered preventable?

It is characterized by a lengthy premalignant, preinvasive state that is amenable to early detection through routine Papanicolaou (Pap) smear sampling. These premalignant conditions may be eradicated completely with currently available treatment. Abnormalities of the cervix may be invisible to the naked eye. Exfoliative cytologic sampling of the cervix permits microscopic examination to detect the presence of cells with either atypical appearance or abnormal development. All premalignant lesions have the potential to regress, persist, or become invasive. It may take as long as 7 years for early changes to progress to an invasive cancer. Cervical cancer is thus prevented when premalignant lesions are detected and treated before they undergo malignant transformation.

4. What terms are used to explain an abnormal Pap smear?

Atypia refers to cells with abnormal features that are not diagnostic and are considered to be of undetermined significance.

Dysplasia indicates a distinct abnormality of cellular development and is associated with premalignant disease of the cervix. It is reported as mild, moderate, or severe, depending on the degree of deviation from the normal cells found on the cervix.

Cervical intraepithelial neoplasia (CIN) correlates with three dysplastic categories: (1) mild dysplasia/CIN 1; (2) moderate dysplasia/CIN 2; and (3) severe dysplasia/carcinoma in situ (CIS)/CIN 3.

Squamous intraepithelial lesions (SIL) were introduced in the current Bethesda classification system to include the emergence of human papillomavirus (HPV) as a deviation from normal cervical cytology and its association as a risk factor in the development of cervical cancer. Low-grade SIL (LSIL) encompasses changes due to HPV as well as CIN 1 or mild dysplasia. High-grade SIL (HSIL) includes CIN 2 or moderate dysplasia, CIN 3 or severe dysplasia, and CIS.

5. How should the nurse explain abnormal Pap smear findings to the patient?

Stress that the classification is used to identify degrees of abnormality that are universally understood and to direct appropriate treatment and follow-up. Patients should be reminded that the Pap smear is only a screening test; the actual cervical abnormality may be better or worse than the screening test indicates. To determine the extent of any abnormal Pap smear, the cervix must be examined with a colposcope, and diagnostic biopsies may be required.

6. How should the nurse explain treatment for abnormal Pap smear findings?

The treatment recommendations for an abnormal Pap smear depend on the colposcopy findings and, if necessary, the biopsy results. Colposcopy allows the clinician to examine thoroughly the surface of the cervix using a colposcope for magnification. The colposcope, like a pair of binoculars or a microscope, enhances visual inspection. Patients should be informed that the procedure is comparable to the process of obtaining a Pap smear, although it takes longer to complete. After insertion of the speculum, the cervix is thoroughly examined through the magnification of the colposcope. A

3–5% acetic acid (household vinegar) or other staining solution, such as Lugol's (strong iodine), may be used to demarcate cervical abnormalities. These solutions may cause a stinging or burning sensation, but they are not harmful to cervical mucosa. Biopsies of abnormal areas, as well as curettage (scraping) of the endocervical canal above the external opening of the cervix, are then performed. These procedures are associated with mild discomfort, such as pinching or cramping sensations, and light vaginal bleeding or spotting. If precancerous changes are detected, further treatment is necessary. Treatment options that may be discussed with the patient include laser ablation, cryotherapy (freezing of abnormal tissue), loop excision, cold knife cone biopsy, and hysterectomy.

7. What should the nurse tell a patient who asks about the use of Pap smear screening for gynecologic cancers?

Patients often believe that Pap smears are used as screening tests for all gynecologic cancers. In reality, the Pap smear is specifically intended to detect abnormalities in the cells on the surface of the cervix, particularly preinvasive CIN (see question 4). On occasion, cellular abnormality of vaginal, endometrial, or ovarian origin may be detected. In these situations, additional work-up is required to determine the exact origin and significance of the abnormality. Overall, patients should be informed that the Pap smear is not intended to screen for either invasive cervical cancer or other gynecologic malignancies. Despite this limited application, the process of obtaining the Pap smear provides valuable information to the practitioner. Before insertion of the speculum, inspection of the external genitalia under bright light facilitates identification of abnormal or suspicious lesions on the vulva. Direct visualization of the cervix and vaginal tissue may reveal the presence of a gross lesion in an asymptomatic woman. After the speculum examination, palpation during bimanual examination assesses the ovaries for enlargement, a possible symptom of ovarian pathology.

8. When should women begin annual Pap smear screening?

Women should be encouraged to begin annual Pap smear screening and pelvic examination with the initiation of sexual activity or by age 18. After three or more consecutive normal annual screening tests and examinations, the Pap smear may be done less frequently as suggested by the clinician. Establishing a life-long habit of annual testing as part of a well-woman examination offers the most consistent method of detecting abnormalities early. Both the American Cancer Society and the American College of Obstetricians and Gynecologists recommend annual examinations. After hysterectomy, Pap smear recommendations vary according to patient history.

9. Why is a pelvic examination often performed under anesthesia in patients with cervical cancer?

Cervical cancer spreads primarily by direct extension to surrounding tissues and organs and involvement of regional lymph node chains. In the presence of visible, measurable tumor, it is important to assess the surrounding parametrial tissue for evidence of tumor infiltration. Although a pelvic examination is performed in the office, full assessment is not possible because of patient discomfort during the examination, presence of stool in the bowel, and anxiety about the findings. Patients, therefore, are frequently examined under anesthesia so that a thorough pelvic examination may be performed with the benefit of complete relaxation. This promotes a more accurate assessment of the clinical stage of disease. In addition, cystoscopic and sigmoidoscopic examinations may be carried out at the same time to rule out bladder and bowel involvement. Although computerized axial tomographic (CAT) examination helps to determine lymph node involvement, it may be inconclusive in the determination of tissue invasion.

10. What is meant by parametrial spread in cervical cancer?

The parametrium is the space between the lateral portion of the cervix and the bony structure of the pelvic sidewall. It contains the supporting structures, such as the uterosacral and transverse cervical ligaments, that maintain the cervix in its relatively immobile position. The ureters pass through this area in rather close proximity to the uterus before insertion into the urinary bladder. Invasion of this space is common when a cervical tumor expands laterally. It may extend and become adherent to the bony structure of the pelvic side wall. Patients with parametrial spread have an increased incidence of hydronephrosis, which requires ureteral stent placement because of compression by tumor growth. In addition, such patients commonly complain of radiating hip or back pain secondary to mass effect, nerve infiltration, and possible bony metastasis. Spread of tumor to this location is an indication for primary treatment with radiation therapy. Chemotherapy is used as a radiation sensitizer. Surgical excision after radiation therapy is generally not undertaken because of the poor healing properties of radiated tissue and the subsequent propensity for fistula formation. Nurses should understand that when parametrial spread is documented on bimanual pelvic examination, the patient has a more advanced stage of disease, which, as described above, affects treatment recommendations.

11. When is hysterectomy indicated in patients with cervical cancer?

The use of hysterectomy for treatment of cervical cancer varies. The decision is based on the stage of the cancer, age and health status of the patient, treatment plan, and preference of the patient. Proper treatment of cervical cancer and potential sites of spread with surgery alone requires a radical hysterectomy with lymph node dissection. Patients with early cancers, characterized by tumors confined to the cervix that are smaller than 4 cm, may be the most appropriate candidates for this procedure if surgery does not expose them to increased morbidity. Patients with tumors that are larger than 4 cm but still confined to the cervix usually receive radiation therapy and weekly sensitizing chemotherapy first. This may be followed by a simple hysterectomy to remove any residual cervical tumor.

When the cancer extends beyond the cervix to the parametrium and other surrounding tissue, radiation therapy without hysterectomy is the most effective treatment. It should be emphasized that cervical cancer may be effectively treated with radiation therapy. In the event that the patient has an early cervical cancer in the presence of comorbid factors that significantly increase operative risks, treatment with definitive radiation therapy offers survival rates comparable to those of the surgical procedure.

12. Distinguish among an extrafascial, modified radical, and radical hysterectomy.

The nurse caring for a patient with gynecologic cancer should be aware that several classes of hysterectomies are routinely used. The differences have significance for recovery and potential postoperative complications.

An **extrafascial hysterectomy** is essentially synonymous with a simple hysterectomy, in which the entire uterus and cervix are removed vaginally or abdominally. The adjacent supporting ligaments and vagina remain intact. This procedure may be used for benign conditions, such as fibroids. It is also the procedure of choice after administration of pelvic radiation because it allows removal of the uterus and cervix with minimal cutting damage to radiated tissue. The associated complications are low and include common surgical risks such as bleeding and infection.

In a **modified radical hysterectomy**, a small portion of the upper vagina and the inner third of the parametrium (the space containing the uterosacral and cardinal ligaments) are removed along with the entire uterus and cervix. The ureters are partially dissected out of the uterosacral ligaments, along with the bladder and rectum. The higher complication rate is due to the increased potential for blood loss, ureteral injury, and postoperative bladder dysfunction. Patients commonly experience a more lengthy postoperative recovery period characterized by the need for either an indwelling Foley or suprapubic catheter until normal voiding patterns are reestablished. Some patients may be required to perform self-catheterization as a result of continued bladder dysfunction.

In a **radical hysterectomy**, the upper 3 cm of the vagina and most of the parametrium are removed along with the entire uterus and cervix. The ureters are completely dissected out of the uterosacral ligaments. The bladder and rectum must be dissected further from the supporting tissue than for the modified radical hysterectomy. The complication rate is approximately 5%. Possible complications include infection, blood loss, ureteral injury, chronic bladder or rectal dysfunction, fistula formation (from ureter, bladder, or rectum), small bowel obstruction, and nerve injury. As with the modified radical hysterectomy, patients should expect the need for an indwelling Foley or suprapubic catheter for 1–4 weeks after surgery. In addition, chronic problems such as urinary frequency or incontinence, change in bowel elimination patterns, and pain or hypersensation associated with femoral-genital nerve disruption may be encountered.

13. Why is lymph node dissection often performed during hysterectomy?

Regional pelvic lymph nodes are removed in patients with a diagnosis of cancer to check for cancer spread. Lymph node dissection is frequently combined with the more radical hysterectomy procedures. Increased complications may be seen because the procedure lengthens operative time. Examples include lymphocyst formation and lower extremity edema.

14. What is salpingo-oophorectomy? Why is it performed?

Salpingo-oophorectomy (removal of the Fallopian tubes and ovaries) at the time of hysterectomy depends on the age of the patient and prior treatments. Women over the age of 45, who are approaching menopause, may choose to have the ovaries removed at the time of hysterectomy. For women with nonfunctioning ovaries, such as those who are postmenopausal or have received prior pelvic radiation therapy, removal of the ovaries is often recommended to reduce future risk of ovarian cancer. Surgical induction of menopause in pre- or perimenopausal patients results in an abrupt reduction in circulating estrogen and thus causes an acute vasomotor response. Depending on the diagnosis, estrogen replacement may be recommended for such patients.

15. What is a pelvic exenteration?

Pelvic exenteration is a radical surgical procedure that involves the removal of the uterus (if it is still present), vagina, parametrium, bladder (in a total or anterior exenteration), and rectum (in a total or posterior exenteration). The type of exenterative procedure—anterior, posterior, or total—is determined by the location of the cancer in the pelvis. The exenteration is followed by reconstructive procedures that include formation of a neovagina (with skin grafts or flaps), a urinary drainage system (either a conduit or continent pouch) fashioned from bowel, and either a colostomy or reanastomosis of the lower rectum to the sigmoid colon.

16. When is pelvic exenteration used?

Pelvic exenteration is used most commonly for cervical cancer that recurs in the central pelvis after radiation therapy. It also may be used for recurrent vaginal or endometrial cancer as well as for primary treatment of some extensive pelvic cancers. The rationale for complete and radical removal of tissues and organs in the pelvis after radiation therapy, as opposed to simple local excision, is based on the circulatory compromise and poor healing properties of radiated tissue and the need to achieve free margins around the tumor. Once tissue has been radiated, it is less likely to heal normally. This compromise further increases the risk of infection, abscess, and fistula formation, requiring ongoing intervention and corrective procedures. The intent of an exenterative procedure is curative. It should not be performed for palliation because of the high morbidity rate. For this reason, evidence of disease outside the central pelvis is a contraindication for exenteration.

17. What nursing skills are required to care for patients with pelvic exenteration?

Patients undergoing pelvic exenteration require intensive nursing care in the postoperative period. Patients may be hemodynamically unstable because of the length of the surgical procedure, blood loss, and fluid shifts. Infection and possible sepsis are concurrent concerns, along with early signs of failure of reconstructive procedures. Once the patient has stabilized, the process of patient teaching and adjustment to variations in elimination becomes the focus of nursing intervention.

18. Why are radiation implants used in the treatment of cervical cancer?

The successful use of radiation therapy depends, in part, on the ability to deliver an adequate dose of radiation to the source of the cancer. Tissue tolerance of the effects of radiation varies throughout the body. Continued administration of radiation beyond the known level of tolerance may result in permanent tissue damage. The vagina and cervix are relatively radiation-resistant compared with the surrounding bowel and bladder. Higher doses of radiation therapy, therefore, may be used to deliver a curative dose to the cervix. The usual radiation treatment plan for cervical cancer is biphasic. Approximately 5 weeks of external beam radiation therapy along with weekly sensitizing chemotherapy is administered to the pelvis to shrink the tumor and treat regional lymph nodes. This is followed by brachytherapy, which is the placement of an intracavitary radiation source kept in place by a holder, such as a tandem and ovoid device, vaginal cylinder, or interstitial template. When loaded with the radioactive source, these devices deliver additional high doses of radiation to the vagina, cervix, and adjacent parametrial tissue. While the implanted radiation source is in place, the uterus insulates the small bowel from higher doses of radiation. In addition, packing placed into the vagina pushes the bladder and rectum further away from the implanted radiation source. Thus, the cervix and vagina receive at least twice the dose of radiation that could be delivered by external radiation alone.

19. What nursing care should be provided to patients receiving a radiation implant?

Nursing care should focus on safe delivery of the treatment and recognition and prevention of complications. The most common devices used to deliver intracavitary radiation in gynecologic cancer are tandem and ovoid devices, vaginal cylinders, and interstitial afterload needles. After placement in the operating room of one of these hardware devices, adequate recovery from anesthesia, and final planning in the radiation oncology department, the patient returns to her room. Before the radioactive sources are loaded in the hardware, the nurse should have adequate time to perform a thorough postoperative assessment of the patient, review the postoperative orders, inform the patient of restrictions on activity, and prepare the patient for the loading procedure. The nurse should expect the patient to be on strict bed rest with minimal side-to-side turning to prevent dislodging the hardware. The head of the bed may be elevated no more than 30° to prevent perforation from the tandem or interstitial afterload needles. A Foley catheter to gravity drainage is used to eliminate use of the bedpan for urination. Complete bowel rest is desired to prevent hardware dislodgement. Patients are given a low-residue diet along with Lomotil and/or opioid pain medications around the clock to promote constipation and discourage defecation. Intravenous fluids may be administered until the patient has recovered from nausea due to anesthesia.

20. What preventive measures are used?

Deep vein thrombosis (DVT) is prevented through the use of antiembolism or intermittent inflation stockings. Subcutaneous heparin also may be used. Patients should be encouraged to use an incentive spirometer hourly during the day to promote adequate lung expansion and to prevent atelectasis. A patient-controlled analgesia (PCA) pump or epidural analgesia catheter may be used to prevent discomfort from the hardware placement.

21. Describe the nurse's assessment duties.

Vital signs and pain should be assessed every 4 hours, and intake and output should be measured during every shift to monitor subtle changes in the patient's status. Assessment of the patient every shift is a key nursing function. Specific attention should be given to signs and symptoms of: (1) embolic episodes secondary to a diagnosis of pelvic malignancy, bed rest, and postoperative state; (2) perforation of the uterus by the tandem or bowel by the interstitial needles; (3) sepsis from the introduction of a foreign object (tandem or interstitial needle) through the necrotic tumor mass; and (4) dislodgement of the hardware through activity, bowel function, or inadvertent shifting of the device.

22. How are staff members protected from radiation exposure?

In performing required activities, the nurse must be organized and efficient so that minimal time is spent at the bedside after the radiation source has been placed. As a result, routine care activities, such as bathing, oral hygiene, and changing linens, are severely restricted. Whenever possible, the nurse should increase the distance from the source of radiation to decrease the amount or concentration of radiation that reaches a specific area. Lead shields may be placed around the patient's bed and/or just inside the entrance to the room as a protective device intended to absorb emitted radiation. Staff members are expected to position themselves behind a shield when inside the room to minimize their exposure to radiation. Shields may be impractical, however, when the patient requires direct care. Lead aprons do not afford additional protection from the gamma rays of this type of radiation; therefore, their use is not advocated. The nursing care of patients with radiation implants represents a challenge to all staff members. A coordinated team effort is required to ensure that the principles of time, distance, and shielding are followed without compromising the patient's physical and emotional care needs.

23. What is high-dose-rate brachytherapy?
In some institutions, high-dose-rate brachytherapy is used to deliver radiation directly to the tumor source. This method follows the principles of conventional implant devices through the insertion of an applicator or holder into the tumor (cervix) or cavity (vagina, uterus). The radiation source emits a much higher rate of radiation on an hourly basis. As a result, the time that the implant needs to stay in place is reduced dramatically. In addition, the procedure can be done on an outpatient basis. The major disadvantages are the requirements for specialized equipment and a highly trained staff.

Quick Facts—Ovarian Cancer

Incidence	4% of new cancers in women annually. In 2001, 23,400 estimated new cases.
Mortality	5% of cancer deaths in women annually. In 2001, 13,900 estimated deaths.
Risk factors	Age—risk increases with age until age 70
	Family history of ovarian cancer, breast-ovarian cancer, or breast-ovarian-endometrial-colon cancer
	Incessant ovulation—conditions such as nulliparity or infertility
	Northern European ancestry
	Industrialization/higher socioeconomic class
	Association with perineal talc use, high dietary fat, and excessive coffee and alcohol consumption have been suggested but are considered weak
Histology	Adenocarcinoma of mucinous or serous papillary origin is most common; other types include endometrial, clear cell, Brenner, undifferentiated, and sarcomas.
Symptoms	Abdominal distention and bloating are most common; others include increased abdominal girth, nonspecific changes in GI function, increased flatus, weight gain, and pain.
Staging	Stage I — Limited to ovaries
	IA — One ovary; capsule intact; no tumor on ovarian surface
	IB — Two ovaries; capsules intact; no tumor on ovarian surface
	IC — Tumor limited to one or both ovaries with any of the following: ruptured capsule, surface tumor, positive cytology
	Stage II — Pelvic extension
	IIA — Uterus or tubes
	IIB — Other tissues
	IIC — Ruptured capsule, surface tumor, positive cytology
	Stage III — Abdominal or nodal metastasis
	IIIA — Microscopic seeding of abdominal-peritoneal surfaces
	IIIB — Abdominal-peritoneal implants $\leq$ 2 cm, negative nodes
	IIIC — Abdominal peritoneal implants > 2 cm and/or positive nodes
	Stage IV — Distant metastasis; includes pleural effusion with positive cytology, parenchymal liver metastases
Treatment	Staging laparotomy with tumor debulking (< 1 cm residual disease is optimal)
	Chemotherapy (six cycles of paclitaxel/platinum-based preferred) for all stages except stage IA and IB with well- or moderately well-differentiated cancer

24. Are any screening studies useful in detecting ovarian cancer?
Unfortunately, no reliable tests are available for screening asymptomatic women for ovarian cancer. Although a combination of bimanual pelvic examination, transvaginal ultrasound, and CA-125 assay has been suggested, little evidence supports the effectiveness of this triad in an asymptomatic population. Bimanual pelvic examination may not alert the practitioner to the presence of an abnormality, particularly if the cancer is in an early stage or if the body habitus of the patient

prevents optimal examination. Transvaginal ultrasound is helpful in defining the characteristics of an enlarged ovary but, like many radiographic studies, has limited diagnostic value. Although serum tumor marker CA-125 is useful for monitoring treatment response, it lacks specificity for distinguishing ovarian cancer from various benign and malignant conditions. CA-125 tumor marker is elevated in approximately 80% of patients with ovarian cancer. The degree of elevation varies, and the actual CA-125 level may not be a direct reflection of the amount of tumor present.

25. When is the CA-125 assay useful?

If CA-125 is elevated when ovarian cancer is diagnosed, the assay is useful to monitor response to treatment and to detect cancer recurrence. The CA-125 level may be obtained monthly during treatment and every few months during follow-up after remission is achieved. Although the return of the CA-125 to normal levels early in the course of chemotherapy treatment may be considered a favorable prognostic indicator, it is not an indication of cure. Approximately one-half of women with ovarian cancer who have a normal CA-125 after initial debulking surgery and chemotherapy have residual cancer if a second-look operation is performed. Residual cancer is frequently microscopic or of small volume; it may not be visible on radiographic studies or palpable on bimanual pelvic examination.

26. How does heredity contribute to increased risk for the development of ovarian cancer?

Several familial cancer syndromes contribute to increased risk for the development of ovarian cancer. All are autosomal dominant conditions and account for 5–10% of all ovarian cancers. Ovarian cancer in two first-degree relatives (mother, sister) may increase the risk to as much as 50%. In addition, women with family histories of both breast-ovarian cancers and breast-ovarian-endometrial-colon cancers have a higher incidence of ovarian cancer.

27. Can anything protect women from developing ovarian cancer?

Oral contraceptive pills (OCPs) significantly reduce the risk of ovarian cancer by as much as 50% in women who use them consistently for 5 years. This reduction is attributed to the ovulatory suppression of OCPs. Protection is also obtained from breastfeeding and one or more full-term pregnancies because both situations suppress ovulation. Tubal ligation also gives some protection, although the reasons are unclear. A prophylactic oophorectomy should be considered in women with a gene mutation associated with breast-ovarian syndrome or a strong family history suggestive of hereditary syndrome.

28. A patient with ovarian cancer is told by her gynecologic oncologist that all visible cancer was removed at the time of debulking surgery, but she still needs chemotherapy. Why?

Although the removal of all visible tumor markedly improves prognosis, microscopic tumor is still present because of the spread patterns of ovarian cancer. Epithelial ovarian cancer, the most common type, arises from the surface of the ovary. The cancer cells can exfoliate and spread throughout the abdominal cavity early in the course of disease. This often results in peritoneal seeding of tumor, which may form microscopic implants of tumor on the peritoneal surfaces. Without chemotherapy, these implants have the potential to grow and reform bulky tumor. The patient should be informed by her physician that chemotherapy is needed to treat the microscopic tumor.

29. What is a second-look laparotomy? When should a nurse expect a patient to undergo this procedure?

A second-look laparotomy is an exploratory procedure performed after completion of the initial chemotherapy regimen for ovarian cancer. It is initiated when there is no evidence of cancer on physical examination or radiographic evaluation, such as CAT scan. The purpose is to determine whether residual cancer is present. Residual cancer is possible in 50% of women who have undergone debulking surgery and chemotherapy despite the lack of physical evidence of disease. During the procedure, the abdominal and pelvic cavities are thoroughly explored. Visible tumor is removed when possible, and multiple biopsies of the peritoneal surfaces are obtained.

Although it was considered standard practice for many years, second-look laparotomy has limited value. Gynecologic oncologists moved to abandon the procedure when it became apparent that as many as 50% of women with negative second-look surgeries developed recurrent disease at a future time. Thus, survival was not positively affected, and patients were exposed to the increased morbidity and mortality of additional surgery. The procedure may be used on an individual basis or when a patient is enrolled in a study protocol examining the efficacy of existing or new treatment regimens.

30. How should the nurse explain borderline ovarian cancer to patients?

Borderline ovarian cancer is also known as ovarian adenocarcinoma of low malignant potential. These terms can be confusing to both patients and nurses. Pathologically, the cells resemble those of an ovarian carcinoma, but they are not invasive. Patients generally present with symptoms similar to ovarian carcinoma, such as increased abdominal girth, ascites, and enlarged ovaries. Tumors usually occur in the fourth and fifth decades of life, are more commonly confined to the ovary at diagnosis, and are associated with a good prognosis. When they have spread beyond the ovary, which is uncommon, the primary treatment is surgical debulking. In the event that they recur, surgical debulking may be repeated. Chemotherapy is rarely used because few data indicate that it improves survival. Patients should be informed that borderline ovarian cancer can be extensive and recurrent, but it is treated primarily with surgical excision and has a much more favorable prognosis than epithelial ovarian cancers.

Quick Facts—Endometrial Cancer

Incidence	6% of new cancer cases in women annually. In 2001, 38,300 estimated new cases.
Mortality	2% of cancer deaths in women annually. In 2001, 6,600 estimated deaths.
Risk factors	Unopposed exogenous estrogen (progesterone is protective) Nulliparity, infertility, anovulation Late menopause (after age 52) Obesity (increased levels of endogenous estrogen) Diabetes mellitus, hypertension Family history (breast-ovarian-endometrial-colon cancer) Complex atypical hyperplasia (thickened endometrium with cytologic atypia of glands)
Histology	Endometrial adenocarcinoma most common; other types include adenosquamous, squamous, mucinous, serous papillary, clear cell, and undifferentiated.
Symptoms	Abnormal uterine bleeding in postmenopausal women (80% of patients) Pap smear abnormality, presence of endometrial cells suspicious; symptoms of uterine enlargement or pelvic pressure may be signs of advanced disease.
Staging	Stage I　　Confined to corpus 　IA　Tumor limited to endometrium 　IB　Tumor invades < half of myometrium 　IC　Tumor invades > half of myometrium Stage II　Extends to cervix 　IIA　Involves endocervical glands 　IIB　Invades cervical stroma Stage III　Involves adjacent structures 　IIIA　Invades uterine serosa, adnexae, or peritoneal cytology positive 　IIIB　Vaginal extension 　IIIC　Positive pelvic or paraaortic lymph nodes Stage IV　Distant metastasis, including intraabdominal or inguinal lymph nodes, lungs
Treatment	Total abdominal hysterectomy with bilateral salpingo-oophorectomy and lymph node dissection considered gold standard; adjuvant radiation therapy and/or chemotherapy generally recommended for stage IC and above, poorly differentiated tumor, or aggressive histology (e.g., clear cell, serous papillary)

31. How are estrogen and estrogen replacement therapy related to endometrial cancer?

The association of estrogen and endometrial cancer should be known by all nurses caring for women, regardless of practice setting. Endometrial cancer depends on the unopposed supply of estrogen from endogenous (within the body) and exogenous (outside the body) sources. During the reproductive years, neuroendocrine changes occur each month to promote regularity of the menstrual cycle. Cyclical estrogen production in the form of estradiol from the ovary promotes proliferation of the lining of the uterus in anticipation of implantation of a fertilized ovum. After ovulation, secretion of estradiol continues, and progesterone is initiated to maintain the endometrial lining. In the absence of pregnancy and the associated appearance of human chorionic gonadotropin (HCG) from the developing placenta, the level of progesterone falls dramatically. The drop in progesterone causes the organized shedding of the endometrial lining within 1–2 days.

Estrogen production that is not challenged or opposed by progesterone causes ongoing proliferation of the endometrial lining. Continued growth of the endometrial lining favors the development of atypical cells and cancer. When a woman has either increased endogenous sources of estrogen (e.g., with anovulation and obesity) or increased exogenous sources of estrogen (e.g., estrogen replacement without progesterone), the risk of developing endometrial cancer is greater. Any woman with an intact uterus who takes estrogen replacement also should receive progesterone either cyclically or daily to counteract the proliferative effects of estrogen on the lining of the uterus. Women who have had the uterus removed do not require progesterone therapy when estrogen replacement is initiated.

32. How should the nurse respond to the woman who asks if obesity increases the risk for endometrial cancer?

Associations among obesity, excessive estrogen levels, and endometrial cancer have been documented. Obese women typically have higher levels of endogenous estrogen because of two mechanisms. First, the adrenal cortex produces androstenedione, which is converted to estrogen by adipose tissue. Consequently, excessive fat tissue leads to excessive production of estrogen. Second, obesity depresses the level of sex hormone-binding globulin (SHBG) and thus leads to higher free (unbound) levels of estrogen. Unbound estrogen is the hormonally active form. The nurse should explain that obese women face a higher risk for the development of endometrial cancer because increased levels of endogenous estrogen promote proliferation of the uterine lining.

33. After hysterectomy for endometrial cancer, a patient is told by her physician that the final surgical pathology report will determine the need for additional radiation or chemotherapy. How may the nurse clarify this statement?

Several pathologic determinations are required to ascertain the need for adjunctive treatment, including histology, tumor grade, myometrial invasion, cytologic washings, and lymph node status. Adenocarcinomas are the most common histologic types of endometrial cancer. Additional cell types, such as clear cell or papillary serous carcinomas, are considered more aggressive and require adjuvant treatment. Tumor grade is applied to all histologic types and is stated in degree of differentiation—well, moderately, or poorly differentiated cells. A less favorable prognosis is associated with moderately to poorly differentiated tumors; thus, adjuvant treatment is desirable.

The extent of myometrial invasion is another important predictor of the need for additional treatment after surgery. Myometrial invasion refers to the depth of cancer cell penetration into the wall of the uterus. The pathologist provides this information in the form of a measurement on the final pathology report. Myometrial invasion that is less than one-half the thickness of the uterine wall is less likely to have spread beyond the uterus than tumors that invade the outer half. Such patients require treatment with radiation or chemotherapy. Cytologic washings from the abdominal-peritoneal cavity collected at the beginning of the surgery are checked for malignant cells that may have disseminated through either the fallopian tubes or the uterine wall before removal of the uterus. Lymph nodes sampled at the time of the surgery are also examined microscopically for evidence of disease. Positive findings in either sample require additional treatment, usually chemotherapy or radiation, due to disease spread outside the uterus. Despite the appearance of "normal" tissue at the time of gross visual inspection, any of these pathologic findings may alter the treatment recommendations. The nurse needs to be aware that the treatment plan cannot be determined until the final pathology report has been received so that he or she can offer emotional support to the patient during this time of uncertainty.

34. What resources offer support, counseling, education, and information for women with gynecologic cancer?
- National Ovarian Cancer Coalition
  888-OVA-RIAN
- Gilda Radner Familial Ovarian Cancer Registry
  800-OVA-RIAN

Services include general counseling, data collection registry on the link between heredity and ovarian cancer, support groups, and assistance with genetic screening.
- Gynecologic Cancer Foundation
  800-444-4441
  www.wcn.org/gcf

Services include information about gynecologic cancer, counseling, and support resources.

REFERENCES

1. Berek JS, Hacker NF (eds): Practical Gynecologic Oncology, 3rd ed. Philadelphia, Lippincott Williams & Wilkins, 2000.
2. Dow KH, Hilderley LJ (eds): Nursing Care in Radiation Oncology, 2nd ed. Philadelphia, W.B. Saunders, 1997.
3. Fleming ID, Cooper JS, Henson DE, et al: AJCC Cancer Staging Handbook, 5th ed. Philadelphia, Lippincott-Raven, 1998.
4. Greenlee RT, Hill-Harmon MB, Murray T, Thun M: Cancer statistics, 2001. CA Cancer J Clin 51:15–36, 2001
5. Moore-Higgs GJ, Almadrones LA, Colvin-Huff B, et al (eds): Women and Cancer: A Gynecologic Oncology Nusing Perspective, 2nd ed. Boston, Jones & Bartlett, 2000.
6. Thomas GM: Improved treatment for cervical cancer: Concurrent chemotherapy and radiotherapy. N Engl J Med 340:1198–1200, 2000.

30. CANCERS OF THE HEAD AND NECK

R. Lee Jennings, MD, and Lenore L. Harris, RN, MSN, AOCN

Quick Facts—Head and Neck Cancer

Incidence	3% of new cancer cases annually; 30,100 estimated new cases in United States in 2001
Mortality	2% of all cancer deaths; one-third of patients die from this disease; 7,800 estimated deaths in 2001; 5-year survival rate: 53%; 10-year survival rate: 43%
Risk factors	Any type of habitual tobacco use (greatest risk factor): cigarette, cigar, pipe, smokeless tobacco, or marijuana
	Advancing age (more common after age 50)
	Male gender (male-to-female ratio = 3:1)
	Excessive use of alcohol (synergistic with tobacco)
	Epstein-Barr virus (EBV; associated with nasopharyngeal cancer)
	Industrial exposure to wood dust, leather, metal (nickel), asbestos, chemical inhalants (woodworking)
	Daily exposure of skin to sun
Histology	Squamous cell carcinomas (approximately 95% of all head and neck cancers)
	Salivary gland primaries
	Sarcomas (rare)
Symptoms	Pain, tenderness — Unilateral sinusitis
	Nonhealing ulceration — Unilateral nasal obstruction
	Neck mass — Persistent hoarseness or change in voice
	Submucosal mass — Unilateral ear pain, not explained by infection
	Chronic dysphagia
Staging	**Tumor, node, metastasis (TNM) system**
	Primary tumor (T) for lip and oral cavity

	T1	Greatest diameter of primary tumor ≤ 2 cm
	T2	Greatest diameter of primary tumor > 2–4 cm
	T3	Greatest diameter of primary tumor > 4 cm
	T4	Lip: invades adjacent structure such as bone, tongue, skin
		Oral cavity: invades adjacent structures such as deep muscles of tongue, bone (deep invasion), maxillary sinus, skin

Primary tumor (T) for salivary glands

	T1	Greatest dimension of tumor ≤ 2 cm (no local extension)
	T2	Greatest dimension of tumor > 2–4 cm (no local extension)
	T3	Greatest dimension of tumor > 4–6 cm (with local extension but no CN VII involvement)
	T4	Invades base of skull, CN VII, and/or greatest dimension of tumor > 6 cm; local extension is defined as clinical or macroscopic evidence of spread to skin, nerve, or bone

Cervical node involvement (N), oral cavity and salivary glands

	NX	Regional nodes cannot be assessed
	N0	No nodal involvement
	N1	Single clinically positive ipsilateral node ≤ 3 cm
	N2a	Single clinically positive ipsilateral node > 3–6 cm
	N2b	Multiple clinically positive ipsilateral nodes, none > 6 cm
	N2c	Bilateral or contralateral positive nodes, none > 6 cm
	N3	One clinically positive lymph node > 6 cm

Table continued on following page

251

Quick Facts—Head and Neck Cancer (Continued)

Staging (cont'd)	**Distant metastasis (M)**			
	MX	Distant metastasis cannot be assessed		
	M0	No known distant metastasis		
	M1	Distant metastasis present		
Stage grouping	**For cancer of lip, oral cavity, and pharynx**			
	Stage I	T1 N0 M0	Stage IVA	T4 N0 M0
	Stage II	T2 N0 M0		T4 N1 M0
	Stage III	T3 N0 M0		Any T N2 M0
		T1 N1 M0	Stage IVB	Any T N3 M0
		T2 N1 M0	Stage IVC	Any T Any N M1
		T3 N1 M0		
	For salivary glands			
	Stage I	T1 N0 M0	Stage IV	T4 N0 M0
	Stage II	T2 N0 M0		T3 N1 M0
	Stage III	T3 N0 M0		T4 N1 M0
		T1 N1 M0		Any T N2 M0
		T2 N1 M0		Any T N3 M0
				Any T Any N M1

1. Describe the types and sites of head and neck cancer.

All cancers arising in the upper food and airway passages (upper aerodigestive tract) are included for reporting purposes: lips, oral cavity, pharynx (oropharynx, nasopharynx, hypopharynx), nasal cavity, and paranasal sinuses. Also included are the major and minor salivary glands and the thyroid gland (see chapter on endocrine tumors). Subdivisions of the major sites include buccal mucosa, gingiva, palate, tongue, tonsil, pyriform sinus, and larynx. Each subsite is important because prognosis, treatment, and morbidity of treatment may change dramatically from subsite to subsite. Cancers arising in the skin (melanoma, basal cell and squamous cell carcinoma, skin adnexal tumors) and lymphomas are excluded for reporting purposes but are important in any discussion of malignancies of the head and neck (see chapter on melanoma).

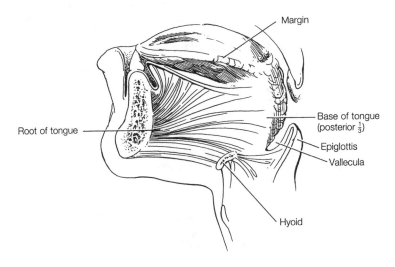

Posterior oral anatomy. (From Jennings RL: Tumors of the head and neck. In Ritchie WP Jr, Steele G Jr, Dean RH (eds): General Surgery. Philadelphia, Lippincott-Raven, 1995, p 35, with permission.)

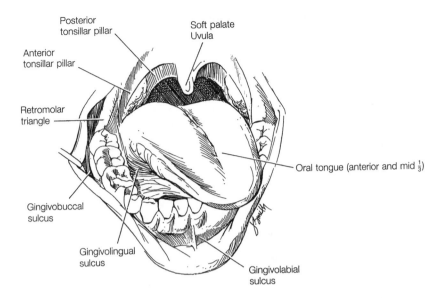

Anterior oral anatomy. (From Jennings RL: Tumors of the head and neck. In Ritchie WP Jr, Steele G Jr, Dean RH (eds): General Surgery. Philadelphia, Lippincott-Raven, 1995, p 35, with permission.)

2. How do patients with head and neck cancer differ from patients with other types of cancer?

The head and neck region is unique among the sites requiring care for cancer. The complex interaction of the face, oral cavity, voice, and air passages in personal presentation, food intake, and comfort makes treatment planning highly demanding. Even the smallest cosmetic or functional defect is viewed with concern by the patient and caregivers as well as the surgeon. The importance of maintaining acceptable cosmetic and functional results must be balanced with the necessity of adequately treating the primary cancer. Primary tumors of the head and neck create functional and cosmetic problems if the cancer is not adequately treated and controlled. Good palliation is seldom achieved without cure of the primary cancer.

3. Describe the role of chemoprevention.

Chemoprevention using retinoids, including natural vitamin A and synthetic analogs, beta carotene, and vitamin E, has shown some promise in reversing premalignant lesions and preventing second primary tumors.

4. What are the risk factors for skin and lip malignancies?

Malignancies arising on the skin, including the lips, are usually caused by prolonged, excessive exposure to the sun. Lip cancer is more common in outdoor workers, including farmers, construction workers, oil field workers, and those in recreation occupations (e.g., ski instructors, lifeguards). Light skin and red or blonde hair are also predisposing factors for skin cancer.

5. Discuss the risk factors for cancers of the oral cavity, pharynx, and larynx.

Habitual tobacco use is the most significant risk factor. Ninety percent of patients with primary tumors in the oral cavity, pharynx, or larynx have a smoking history. Smokeless tobacco plays a less significant role. Alcohol consumption is also linked with these cancers. Heavy alcohol use is common in this population, and a high percentage of patients present with cirrhosis of the liver or consumption levels high enough to place them in danger of delirium tremens on sudden withdrawal. Such patients have a lower survival rate and a higher rate of second primary tumors than nonusers.

6. What are the risk factors for nasopharyngeal cancers?

Nasopharyngeal cancers have a more complicated etiology. They are common among Cantonese Chinese and rare among Caucasians. There are weak links to history of chronic sinusitis and exposure to smoke from cooking fires but a strong link to infection with Epstein-Barr virus. Cancer of the turbinates and paranasal sinuses also has a complex etiology. Industrial exposures are significant. However, most patients present without a history of exposure to known environmental carcinogens.

7. Discuss the risk factors for salivary and thyroid cancers.

No cause has been found for salivary cancers. The cause of thyroid cancer is mostly unknown. Convincing evidence suggests that radiation exposure, especially in children and adolescents, increases the risk of thyroid cancer. In addition, about one-third of medullary carcinomas of the thyroid (carcinomas arising in the calcitonin-secreting cells) are familial.

8. What are the presenting symptoms of head and neck cancer?

Presenting complaints are quite varied because of the complex anatomy of the region and the variety of functions represented in the head and neck. Significant changes in facial appearance, sight, smell, swallowing, and/or speech may be early symptoms of cancer. Nonhealing ulceration, pain at the primary site, and referred pain also may be early symptoms. Often the patient consults the dentist first because of one of these symptoms, loosening teeth, or ill-fitting dentures. Pharyngeal primary tumors are the most subtle and varied in presentation. They are much harder for the patient to detect because these areas are not easily visible; hoarseness and throat irritation commonly occur with the habitual use of tobacco.

Symptoms According to Site of Primary Tumor

SITE	PRESENTING SYMPTOMS	LATE SYMPTOMS
Lip	Sore that does not heal	Large ulceration, mass
Oral cavity		Pain, ulceration, foul breath, loss of function
Buccal mucosa	Ulceration or mass; acidic drinks may cause burning	Pain, mass in cheek
Gingiva	Ulceration, dentures do not fit	Pain, loose teeth, trismus (lock jaw)
Oral tongue	Ulceration, mild pain, mass	Decreased range of motion, pain, dysphagia, malnutrition, ear pain
Hard palate	Ulcer or mass	Ulceration, loose teeth
Floor of mouth	Ulceration	Pain, ear pain, mass, invasion of tongue with same symptoms
Pharynx		
Nasopharynx	Nasal stuffiness, nosebleeds	Bleeding, nasal obstruction, cranial nerve paralysis, pain, vision changes
Oropharynx	Sore throat, usually unilateral and persistent	Dysphagia, pain, malnutrition, muffled voice
Base of tongue (posterior one-third)	Same	Same
Tonsil, soft palate	Ulceration or mass	Mass or large ulceration, dysphagia
Pharyngoesophageal junction	Possible dysphagia	Same
Hypopharynx (pyriform sinus)	Same	Dysphagia, pain, aspiration, voice change
Larynx	Hoarseness	Severe hoarseness, airway obstruction, aspiration

Table continued on following page

Symptoms According to Site of Primary Tumor (Continued)

SITE	PRESENTING SYMPTOMS	LATE SYMPTOMS
Salivary gland, major and minor	Preauricular or submandibular mass, mucosa-covered mass in oral cavity (no ulceration)	Enlarged mass, ulceration in oral cavity, (minor salivary gland), neck masses, facial nerve paralysis with parotid, mandibular invasion with submandibular gland cancers
Thyroid gland	Thyroid mass	Neck masses, vocal cord paralysis, dysphagia, enlarged mass

9. How is head and neck cancer diagnosed?

The initial examination should start with a complete history and physical examination. Pay attention to the time that suspicious symptoms have been present. Document tobacco and alcohol use. The combination of heavy tobacco and alcohol use may make it impossible for the patient to tolerate radiation therapy to the oral mucous membranes. Obtain nutritional assessment, baseline complete blood count, and chemistry profile (including albumin and magnesium). Plan to monitor nutritional status to prevent weight loss so that nutritional repair can start as the work-up continues. Documenting and understanding the patient's psychosocial history may determine whether the patient accepts treatment, complies with stopping smoking/alcohol use, and whether rehabilitation will be successful.

10. When does treatment planning begin?

Planning for rehabilitation starts with the initial history.

11. What does the practitioner need to perform a head and neck examination?

Instruments required for clinical head and neck examination are simple, fairly inexpensive, and easily available in the head and neck surgeon's office but often absent from the hospital unit or outpatient clinic. They include a high-backed chair for the patient and a stool for the examiner. A flashlight is inadequate. Examiners (and caregivers) need a headlight to free both hands. Also needed are laryngeal mirrors, a heat source to warm the mirror to prevent fogging, tongue blades, finger cots, local and topical anesthetic, and forceps for biopsy. A fiberoptic laryngoscope may be needed to examine the nasopharynx of patients with a severe gag reflex. Extensive, complex cancers require several visual examinations and direct palpation to evaluate their extent.

Physical examination of the oral cavity, pharynx, and larynx requires visualization of all surfaces. The oral cavity, base of tongue, and tonsils are palpated with a gloved finger. The nasopharynx, hypopharynx, and larynx are visualized with a mirror or fiberoptic laryngoscope. All findings are described and documented on a diagram for staging and treatment planning.

12. How is the histologic diagnosis of head and neck cancer obtained?

Diagnosis and staging of any primary site require biopsy. Lip, skin, and oral carcinomas are usually biopsied with forceps under local anesthesia at the time of the initial examination. Fine-needle aspiration cytology is helpful in evaluating thyroid, salivary gland, and neck masses. Cancers of the pharynx and larynx are examined for staging and biopsy with direct laryngoscopy under general anesthesia. Sinus cancers require general anesthesia for biopsy and staging examination through the nostril or through the anterior wall of the sinus.

13. What diagnostic studies may be necessary to confirm head and neck cancer?

Direct laryngoscopy (panendoscopy with esophagoscopy) under anesthesia may be necessary to visualize the tumor and obtain biopsies. Selected imaging and laboratory studies are necessary to complete the initial examination, including biochemical survey, complete blood count, urinalysis, and chest radiographs for all patients. Selected patients require computerized tomography or magnetic resonance imaging for oral, pharyngeal, laryngeal, and sinus primaries. Patients with thyroid primaries need radioactive thyroid scans and thyroid ultrasound. Other studies depend on the findings from the history and physical examination (e.g., evaluation for cirrhosis, emphysema, diabetes). More extensive imaging and/or laboratory evaluation is necessary if any evidence of distant metastasis is found.

14. What histologic types of cancer occur on skin surfaces of the head and neck, including the lip?

Malignant tumors of the skin are the most common cancers requiring surgical care. Over 800,000 skin malignancies are reported each year, along with 2,300 deaths. Basal cell and squamous cell carcinomas are by far the most numerous, with 85% occurring in the head and neck region. Ninety-four percent of recurrent basal cell cancers occur in the head and neck region, with 75% occurring in the central face.

15. How are skin cancers of the head and neck treated?

Most basal cell malignancies are small and can be treated adequately by dermatologists and primary care physicians with desiccation and curettage. Biopsy for pathology examination is mandatory. Larger skin cancers, multicentric basal cell cancers, or recurrent skin cancers should be treated with wide excision and pathology confirmation that margins are free of cancer. Wide elliptical excision is usually adequate, but flap reconstruction should be considered if the pathologist reports close or positive margins. Lymph node metastasis is unusual except with large squamous cell skin cancers. Merkel cell cancer and skin appendage cancers are rare but important because nodal metastasis and distant spread are more likely. Sentinel lymph node biopsy should be considered for melanoma and Merkel cell carcinoma. Wide surgical removal with flap or skin graft reconstruction is necessary, and lymph node dissection may be required, depending on the location of the primary tumor. Melanoma may occur on any skin surface in the head and neck and on mucosal surfaces such as the oral cavity and nasal cavity (see the chapter on melanoma).

16. What are salivary gland malignancies? How are they treated?

Malignancies may occur in the major (parotid, submandibular, sublingual) and minor salivary glands. Minor salivary glands are present in all mucosal surfaces in the upper food and airway passages. A mass in one of the major salivary glands has a 20–50% chance of being malignant. A mass covered by intact mucosa in the oral cavity may be a minor salivary tumor, and the risk of malignancy is as high as 50%.

17. How are salivary gland malignancies treated?

Complete surgical excision is the treatment of choice, even at the time of the biopsy. Most benign tumors of the salivary glands are pleomorphic adenomas (mixed tumors); incomplete excision results in a recurrence rate of 70%.

Treatment of Major Salivary Neoplasms

BENIGN MIXED OR WARTHIN'S TUMOR NONNEOPLASTIC BENIGN MASSES	TI OR T2 LOW-GRADE TUMOR MUCOEPIDERMOID OR ACINIC CELL CARCINOMA	TI OR T2 HIGH-GRADE TUMOR*	T3, N0, OR N+ RECURRENT SALIVARY CANCERS	T4
Parotid				
Superficial parotidectomy	Total parotidectomy	Total parotidectomy	Radical parotidectomy	Radiacal parotidectomy
Preservation of facial nerve	Preservation of facial nerve	Preservation of facial nerve unless involved	Resection of facial nerve	Resection of ear canal, muscle, etc.
	No radiation therapy	No postoperative radiation therapy	Neck dissection if N+	Sacrifice of facial nerve
			Postoperative radiation therapy	Postoperative radiation therapy

Table continued on following page

Treatment of Major Salivary Neoplasms (Continued)

BENIGN MIXED OR WARTHIN'S TUMOR NONNEOPLASTIC BENIGN MASSES	TI OR T2 LOW-GRADE TUMOR MUCOEPIDERMOID OR ACINIC CELL CARCINOMA	TI OR T2 HIGH-GRADE TUMOR*	T3, N0, OR N+ RECURRENT SALIVARY CANCERS	T4
Submandibular				
Digastric triangle dissection	Digastric triangle dissection	Digastric triangle dissection	Radical neck dissection	Resection of involved structures
Preserve marginal branch of facial nerve	Preserve marginal branch of facial nerve	Preserve marginal branch of facial nerve unless involved	Removal of marginal branch of facial nerve and lingual nerve as necessary	Radical neck dissection
	No radiation therapy	Neck dissection if N+	Postoperative radiation therapy	Postoperative radiation therapy
		Postoperative radiation therapy		

* Includes malignant mixed, squamous, and poorly differentiated adenocarcinomas and anaplastic and adenoid cysts.

From Jennings RL: Tumors of the head and neck. In Ritchie WP Jr, Steele G Jr, Dean RH (eds): General Surgery. Philadelphia, Lippincott-Raven, 1995, p 35, with permission.

18. Should all patients with thyroid masses have surgery?

Definitely not. Benign nodular goiter has been calculated to be 500 times more common than thyroid cancer, which makes up only 1% of all malignancies. History and physical examination provide clues that suggest malignancy in a thyroid nodule:

- History of low-dose radiation exposure to thyroid gland
- Risk of malignancy for a new nodule increases with patient age (especially > 40 years)
- Nodule fixation if thyroiditis is excluded
- Rapid growth of a nodule
- Onset of hoarseness
- Palpable cervical lymph nodes
- Solitary thyroid nodule in a male of any age
- Surgery is indicated in a patient < 20 years old with a thyroid nodule

19. When the patient has a thyroid nodule and cancer is suspected, what type of thyroidectomy operation is advised?

It is unusual to have a definitive diagnosis of cancer before thyroidectomy. Total thyroid lobectomy on the side of the nodule is the preferred procedure. An attempt to excise the nodule for biopsy is not advised because of (1) the risk of contaminating the surgical field if cancer is found, (2) the greater risk of injury to the recurrent nerve, and (3) the greater difficulty of making a definitive diagnosis from frozen section. A later diagnosis of cancer requires return to surgery for completion of the thyroidectomy, again placing the recurrent nerve and parathyroid glands at greater risk for injury. When cancer is identified on frozen section, many surgeons favor total thyroidectomy to allow total thyroid ablation with I-131 and later radioactive iodine scanning for metastasis. Small (< 2 cm), well-differentiated cancers contained within the thyroid capsule require only total lobectomy. Lymph node dissection for well-differentiated thyroid cancer is necessary only if nodes are clinically involved.

20. How are special situations managed?

Special situations, such as medullary cancer, require total thyroidectomy and node dissection because of a 70% risk of bilateral gland involvement and nodal metastasis. Undifferentiated carcinoma of the thyroid is one of the most malignant of human cancers, but it is rare. Treatment consists of a combination of radical surgery, chemotherapy, and radiation therapy, but it is rarely successful.

21. What are the types of lip cancer?

Most lip malignancies involve the lower lip and are squamous in type. Basal cell carcinoma usually involves the upper lip. Other lip malignancies are minor salivary gland cancers.

22. How are the various types of lip cancer treated?

Minor salivary gland cancers are treated with wide excision, including the mucosal surface. Postoperative radiation therapy is used for advanced or high-grade malignancies. Basal cell and squamous cell cancers are best treated with surgery, but radiation therapy may be used with equal cure rates. Radiation therapy has the disadvantage of requiring 5 weeks of daily (Monday through Friday) treatment, further damaging surrounding skin already injured from sun exposure and making surgical care quite difficult if the primary tumor recurs or new skin cancers occur in the same area. Locally advanced cancers or node-positive cancers may require a combination of radiation and surgery. Surgical procedures are usually done in one stage. Tumors requiring removal of up to one-third of the lip width are treated with a V excision and primary repair. Cosmetic and functional results are excellent. Upper neck dissection is necessary for the node-positive neck cancers and advanced cancers directly invading skin and bone. Basal cell cancers of the upper lip require special attention. They are more likely to recur locally, perhaps because wide excision and cosmetic repair are more difficult.

23. What are other types of oral and pharyngeal cancers?

Well over 90% of malignancies involving the mucosal surfaces are squamous cell. The remainder are minor salivary gland tumors (see question 16).

24. How are T1 squamous cell cancers treated?

Small (T1) squamous cancers located in the anterior oral cavity may be treated with radiation therapy or surgery with equal cure rates. Many believe that early cancers with minimal risk of nodal spread are better treated with surgery because it is quickly accomplished, morbidity is usually minimal, and the risk of xerostomia (dryness) is avoided, along with the risk of dental caries and bone loss (osteoradionecrosis).

25. How are T2 and more advanced squamous carcinomas best treated?

Many are best treated with a combination of surgery and radiation therapy. It is important for both radiation therapist and surgeon to see the patient for treatment planning before treatment begins. When combined treatment is chosen, most surgeons prefer that the surgical procedure be done first if the primary tumor is sufficiently well defined to allow complete excision with free margins. Surgery also may be scheduled between 3 and 7 weeks after completion of radiation therapy. Surgery sooner than 3 weeks usually results in excessive bleeding because of inflammation and, after 7–8 weeks, excessive fibrosis increases the risk of poor wound healing.

Nasopharyngeal primary tumors are usually treated with radiation therapy; skull base surgical techniques are reserved for radiation failures and primary tumors with local extension that are not treatable with radiation therapy for cure. Hypopharyngeal and laryngeal cancers are usually treated with primary radiation therapy for malignancies that are diagnosed early. A combination of surgery and radiation is reserved for advanced-stage primary tumors. Surgical salvage is necessary for radiation failures and usually results in partial or total laryngectomy.

26. What repair techniques are used for advanced cancer?

Advanced cancers of the posterior oral cavity and oropharynx treated with surgery require repair techniques, usually involving flaps, to replace the large amount of functional tissue removed. Repair techniques improve functional and cosmetic results. Microvascular free-flap procedures allow use of bone and soft tissue from distant sites to repair mandible, tonsil, and tongue defects.

27. What is a carotid rupture? How common is it?

Carotid rupture is rare because of improved techniques for both radiation therapy and surgery. The carotid artery may become exposed as a result of flap necrosis, fistula formation and associated infection, or recurrent cancer around the artery. The first hint of this complication may be a trickle of blood hours or even days before rupture.

28. How is carotid rupture managed?

Preparations are made at the first signs of rupture. The patient must be moved to a bed near the nurse's station. Blood should be typed and cross-matched, intravenous access ensured, tracheotomy established, and a hemostat placed in the room. If rupture occurs, the nurse should apply firm pressure over the artery with a towel, immediately call for help, initiate oxygen and intravenous fluids, and call for blood. When rupture occurs in a palliative setting, surgery is usually not done, but comfort measures, reassurance, and support are appropriate. The process is not painful but may be terrifying.

29. What is important in the postoperative nursing care of patients with head and neck cancer?

Many patients are treated on an outpatient basis, making it difficult for inpatient nurses to gain adequate experience. Inpatient and ambulatory care nursing draws from a comprehensive knowledge base of preoperative, intraoperative, and postoperative requirements as well as patient care needs during radiation therapy, chemotherapy, and combination therapy (involving 2–3 modalities, given in sequence or concomitantly). Major areas of nursing care include the following:

1. **Assurance of an adequate airway.** Many hospitalized patients have a tracheotomy, which should be sutured in place or securely tied at all times. A dislodged tracheotomy may result in hypoxia or death. Attention to secretion clearance is mandatory for airway maintenance, patient comfort, and wound healing.

2. **Self-care.** Patients should be taught self-care techniques for airway clearance and wound care as soon as possible after surgery. The confidence that results from airway assurance, secretion clearance, and wound care allows the patient to gain control of a terrifying situation.

3. **Speech and swallowing rehabilitation.** Techniques taught by a speech pathologist should be reinforced by nursing staff. This reinforcement supports the patient's ability to control basic functions, gives a sense of control, and allows recovery to begin.

4. **Repair of nutritional defects.** Total parenteral nutrition provides excellent short-term support, but it is not the optimal method of feeding for patients with head and neck cancer. Enteral feeding should start as soon as possible. Oral feedings usually start as soon as suture lines allow. Nasogastric or transcutaneous gastric feeding (PEG) tubes allow patients with long-term swallowing problems to be discharged while outpatient rehabilitation continues. A transcutaneous gastric feeding tube can be placed preoperatively so that nutritional repair may begin preoperatively and continue immediately after surgery.

The postoperative role of the nurse, speech pathologist, and surgeon changes from caregiver to coach and cheerleader as discharge approaches.

30. Outline patient education needs according to tumor site.

Patient Education Guidelines

ORGAN SITE	TREATMENT	PATIENT TEACHING
Nasal fossa/paranasal sinus	Surgery alone or combination therapy	Elevate head of bed Wound care/irrigating graft Oral hygiene Technique for removing, cleaning, and replacing oral obturator Care of prosthesis
Nasopharynx	Radiation therapy Chemoradiation with or without surgery	Wound care Management of xerostomia, pain, otitis media

Table continued on following page

Patient Education Guidelines (Continued)

ORGAN SITE	TREATMENT	PATIENT TEACHING
Oral cavity/oropharynx	Stage I–II: surgery or radiation therapy Stage III–IV: surgery + radiation therapy	Wound care Oral hygiene Speech and swallowing therapy as appropriate Management of pain, xerostomia Tracheostomy care and suctioning Gastric tube care
Salivary gland	Stage I–II: surgery, possibly with radiation therapy Stage III–IV: surgery + chemoradiatin	Wound care Oral hygiene If CN VIII is involved: protection and moisture to affected cornea (eye drops/ointment), taping of eyelids Protect skin from elements (due to facial numbness)
Larynx/hypopharynx/neck	Stage I–II: surgery or radiation therapy Stage III–IV: surgery + chemoradiation or chemoradiation + neck dissection (to preserve larynx)	Prevent aspiration Provide humidification Wound care Management of fistula drainage Oral hygiene Tracheostomy care and suctioning Gastric tube care Swallowing therapy as appropriate With insufficient tissue coverage of carotid artery: carotid artery blow-out precautions

31. What are the choices for speech production after total laryngectomy?

Vocalization requires the movement of air through the larynx and vocal tract and is not possible when the larynx has been removed. Referral to the speech pathologist should include the surgeon's description of the patient's postoperative physiologic status. The speech pathologist provides teaching and supervision for at least one of the following alternatives:

1. **Artificial larynx**
   - Handheld, electronic, battery-powered device with robot-like sound
   - Either neck-type (diaphragm causes vibration of neck tissue with resonance into oral cavity) or mouth-type (directs sound into oral cavity through small tube placed in mouth)
   - Easy to use; minimal training is required
2. **Esophageal speech**
   - Air swallowed into and momentarily held in the esophagus and released as words are articulated (called "burping speech")
   - May require up to 6 months of speech therapy to become proficient
3. **Tracheoesophageal puncture (TEP) speech**
   - Surgical procedure to create a tracheoesophageal fistula and placement of a one-way valve (silicone tube) prosthesis
   - Speech produced by inhaling air and covering the tracheostoma with the thumb; valve may be fitted in place to allow hands-free speech (husky voice results)
   - Cleaning and maintenance of the prosthesis required by the patient (as often as necessary) or practitioner (usually every 6 months)
   - Requires awareness and reporting of possible symptoms of fungal colonization on valve

32. When may radiation therapy alone be the treatment of choice?

Patients with small (T1 or T2) tumors may receive radiation therapy only to achieve better function and cosmesis than can be obtained with surgery alone. If the patient has a stage III or IV unresectable malignancy, radiation therapy may be used temporarily to maintain or improve swallowing and/or speech.

33. What assessments are needed for the patient receiving radiation therapy?
If radiation therapy precedes surgery, the patient's nutritional status should be monitored to prevent malnutrition. Prophylactic dental care is necessary before treatment begins because of the risk of radionecrosis and mandibular bone loss. With preoperative radiation therapy, treatment is usually stopped at around 5500 cGy because most patients develop mucositis at this level. Redness and dysphagia usually disappear by 3 weeks. When radiation therapy is the only method of treatment, additional dosage to the primary site is necessary. This boost may be given with external beam or implant techniques. Implants usually are performed under general anesthesia and require hospitalization and often tracheotomy until the implants are removed.

34. When is chemotherapy used to treat patients with head and neck cancer?
Chemotherapy usually is reserved for patients with metastatic or recurrent disease. Its role in this setting is palliative with the goal of improving quality of life. Chemotherapy also may be given to shrink an inoperable tumor (neoadjuvant therapy) so that resection is possible or given concomitantly with radiation therapy to save function (e.g., laryngeal preservation). The chemotherapy agents showing some responses are methotrexate, carboplatin, cisplatin, 5-fluorouracil with leucovorin, and the taxanes (docetaxel or paclitaxel).

35. Does completion of neoadjuvant chemotherapy reduce the extent of surgery?
Preoperative chemotherapy reduces the extent of surgery in selected cases of advanced laryngeal cancer. This finding has not held true in other primary sites, and neoadjuvant treatment in head and neck cancer remains investigational. Evidence suggests that chemotherapy reduces the rate of distant metastasis, but this advantage affects only a small percentage of patients with head and neck cancer.

36. What are the expected side effects of adjuvant therapy?
- Mucositis
- Infection
- Tube feeding problems
- Xerostomia
- Skin problems

37. How is mucositis managed?
Mouth care: rinse every 3–4 hours; soft-bristle toothbrush; careful, gentle flossing (see chapter on mucositis).
Pain management: prescribed anti-inflammatory/anesthetic rinse; swishing to coat the mucosa, then spit (or swallowing if allowed)

38. Describe the management of xerostomia.
1. Thin saliva with sodium bicarbonate.
2. Pilocarpine usually is prescribed at the start of radiation therapy to stimulate salivary glands.
3. Promote hydration (carry water bottle).

39. What techniques are used to manage infection?
1. Monitor blood counts and manage immunosuppression and mucositis.
2. Inpatient health care team must use sterile technique (gloves and mask) for wound care.

40. How are skin problems managed?
1. Protect skin from irritation (e.g., from abrasion due to folds of shirt neck or collar or tracheostomy tube).
2. Dry desquamation (flaky/itchy skin) is treated with careful skin care, topical cream as prescribed by radiation therapist, and diphenhydramine as needed.
3. Wet desquamation (wound oozing or dripping) is treated with moist dressings, which promote healing. Hydrogel dressings may not need changing for up to 12 hours.

41. What strategies are appropriate for tube feeding problems?
1. Monitor weight and tolerance.
2. A nasogastric tube should be inserted only by a surgical team member familiar with the patient's altered anatomy.

42. What should the nurse include as part of discharge teaching?
• Encourage patient and home caregiver to participate in prescribed care as soon as possible.
• Provide simple verbal and written instructions for self-care and monitoring needs.
• Arrange for supplies for wound care, tracheostomy care/suctioning, humidification, and enteral therapy.
• Reinforce interdisciplinary team members' discharge instructions.

43. What does the home care nurse look for during the first home visit?
The home care nurse should observe the patient's physical and emotional status, including:
• Home environment for safe care (adequate equipment with appropriate set-up and application)
• Patient/caregiver comfort with care and attention to self-care details and the amount of supervision needed
• Plans in place for follow-up appointments

44. What resources are available to assist patients and family with discharge and coping?
• The Cancer Information Service provides booklets on Head and Neck, Larynx, and Skin Cancer (800-4-CANCER; www.nci.nih.gov).
• The International Association of Laryngectomies and I Can Cope are programs established by the American Cancer Society (800-ACS-2345; www.cancer.org; www.larynxlink.com) to assist people who have lost their voice.
• Support for People with Oral and Head and Neck Cancer (SPOHNC) is a patient-run support group with a nationwide newsletter (800-377-0928; www.spohnc.org; e-mail: info @spohnc.org).
• Let's Face It (LFI) (360-676-7325; www.faceit.org) and the National Foundation for Facial Reconstruction (212-263-6656) are nonprofit organizations that help people cope with facial disfigurement. Services include referrals for patients unable to afford private reconstructive surgical care.
• The local Gilda's Club may offer a networking group for patients and family members dealing with head and neck cancer (212-686-9898; www.gildasclub.org).

REFERENCES

1. American Cancer Society: Statistics 2000: Cancer Facts and Figures: Selected cancers—oral cavity and pharynx. www.cancer.org.
2. Blom ED: Current status of voice restoration following total laryngectomy. Oncology 14(6):915–922, 2000.
3. Forastiere AA: Head and neck cancer: Overview of recent developments and future directions. Semin Oncol 27(Suppl 8):1–4, 2000.
4. Greenlee T, Hill-Harmon MB, Murray T, Thun M: Cancer statistics, 2001. CA Cancer J Clin 51:15–36, 2001.
5. Harris LL: Head and neck malignancies. In Yarbro CH, Frogge MH, Goodman M (eds): Cancer Nursing Principles and Practice, 5th ed. Boston, Jones & Bartlett, 2000, pp 1210–1243.
6. Harris LL, Huntoon, MB (eds): Core Curriculum for Otorhinolaryngology and Head-Neck Nursing. New Smyrna Beach, Society of Otorhinolaryngology and Head-Neck Nurses, 1998.
7. Jennings RL, Nelson WR: Pre-and postoperative care. In Loré JM (ed): An Atlas of Head and Neck Surgery, 4th ed. Philadelphia, W.B. Saunders [in press].
8. Jennings RL, Nelson, William R: Tumors of the head and neck. In Ritchie WP Jr, Steele G Jr, Dean RH (eds): General Surgery. Philadelphia, J.B. Lippincott, 1995.
9. Strong EW, Spiro RH: Cancer of the oral cavity. In Suen JY, Myers EN (eds): Cancer of the Head and Neck. New York, Churchill Livingstone, 1981, p 301.
10. Vokes EE, Haraf DJ, Kies MS: The use of concurrent chemotherapy and radiotherapy for locoregionally advanced head and neck cancer. Semin Oncol 27(Suppl 8):34–38, 2000.

31. LUNG CANCER

Linda U. Krebs, RN, PhD, AOCN, and Tina Russell, RN, OCN

Quick Facts—Lung Cancer

Incidence	169,500 newly diagnosed cases estimated in 2001 (90,700 in men, 78,800 in women)
Mortality	157,400 deaths estimated in 2001

Risk factors

Tobacco use	Radon
Environmental tobacco smoke	Asbestos
Air pollution	Nutritional factors
Genetic predisposition	Occupational respiratory carcinogens and radiation exposure

Histology **Non–small-cell lung cancers: 80%**
    Adenocarcinoma (most common form): 30–50%
    Squamous cell (epidermoid): 30%
    Large cell: 10–15%
    Small-cell (oat cell) lung cancers: 20%

Symptoms Cough, hemoptysis, dyspnea, wheezing, weight loss, fatigue, recurring pneumonia or bronchitis, and chest or shoulder pain

Staging **Tumor, node, metastasis (TNM) system**
Primary tumor (T)

TX	Primary tumor cannot be assessed, or tumor proven by the presence of malignant cells in sputum or bronchial washings but not visualized by imaging or bronchoscopy
T0	No evidence of primary tumor
Tis	Carcinoma in situ
T1	Tumor ≤ 3 cm in greatest dimension, surrounded by lung or visceral pleura, without bronchoscopic evidence of invasion more proximal than the lobar bronchus
T2	Tumor with any of the following features of size or extent: • > 3 cm in greatest dimension • Involves main bronchus, 2 cm or more distal to carina • Invades visceral pleura • Associated with atelectasis or obstructive pneumonitis that extends to the hilar region but does not involve the entire lung
T3	Tumor of any size that directly invades any of the following: chest wall (including superior sulcus tumors), diaphragm, mediastinal pleura, parietal pericardium; tumor in main bronchus < 2 cm distal to the carina but without involvement of carina; associated atelectasis or obstructive pneumonitis of entire lung
T4	Tumor of any size that invades any of the following: mediastinum, heart, great vessels, trachea, esophagus, vertebral body, carina; separate tumor nodules in same lobe; tumor with a malignant pleural effusion

Regional lymph nodes (N)

NX	Regional lymph nodes cannot be assessed
N0	No regional lymph node metastasis
N1	Metastasis to ipsilateral peribronchial and/or ipsilateral hilar lymph nodes, and intrapulmonary nodes, including involvement by direct extension of primary tumor
N2	Metastasis to ipsilateral mediastinal and/or subcarinal lymph node(s)
N3	Metastasis to contralateral mediastinal, contralateral hilar, ipsilateral or contralateralscalene, or supraclavicular lymph node(s)

Table continued on following page

Quick Facts—Lung Cancer (Continued)

	Distant metastasis (M)	
	MX	Distant metastasis cannot be assessed
	M0	No distant metastasis
	M1	Distant metastasis present
Stage grouping	**Non–small-cell lung cancer**	
	Stage IA	T1 N0 M0
	Stage IB	T2 N0 M0
	Stage IIA	T1 N1 M0
	Stage IIB	T2 N1 M0 or T3 N0 M0
	Stage IIIA	T3 N1 M0 or T1–3 N2 M0
	Stage IIIB	Any T4 , Any N3, M0
	Stage IV	Any T, Any N, M1 (distant metastasis present)
Stage grouping	**Small-cell lung cancer**	
	Limited	Tumor confined to one hemithorax and regional lymph nodes with or without pleural effusion
	Extensive	Tumor that has spread beyond the boundaries of limited disease
Treatment	**Non–small-cell lung cancer**	
	Stages IA and IB	Surgery is treatment of choice; radiation therapy for nonsurgical candidates
	Stages IIA and IIB	Surgery is treatment of choice; radiation therapy for nonsurgical candidates
	Stage IIIA	Surgery is treatment of choice for surgical candidates; radiation therapy and/or chemotherapy may be added; radiation therapy with or without chemotherapy for nonsurgical candidates
	Stage IIIB	Radiation therapy and chemotherapy are standard treatment; radiation therapy plus chemotherapy followed by surgical resection is under investigation for selected cases (T4 N0 M0)
	Stage IV	Chemotherapy is treatment of choice for patients with good performance status (including elderly); radiation therapy may provide palliation
	Small-cell lung cancer	
	Limited stage	Combination chemotherapy with local radiation therapy
	Extensive stage	Combination chemotherapy
		Prophylactic cranial irradiation (PCI) is of benefit only in patients in complete remission

1. How common is lung cancer?

Lung cancer is the second most common cancer in men and in women, closely following breast cancer in women and prostate cancer in men. The incidence has increased dramatically since the turn of the century. The marked increase in lung cancer in women began in the late 1960s. Lung cancer is the leading cause of death in both men and women; only 14% of patients with lung cancer live more than 5 years after diagnosis.

2. What role does cigarette smoking play in the development of lung cancer?

Cigarette smoking is believed to be the chief preventable cause of cancer in the United States. If people stopped smoking (or never started), death rates from cancer would decrease by approximately 25%. It is estimated that 30% of all cancer deaths and approximately 85% of all lung cancer deaths are directly attributable to smoking. The rate for developing lung cancer in nonsmokers ranges between 12/100,000 and 15/100,000 population. For people who smoke less than 1 pack/day, the risk is 10 times greater, and for people who smoke more than 1 pack/day, the risk is 21 times greater than for nonsmokers. Tobacco smoke is considered a group A (known human) carcinogen and is both an initiator and promoter of carcinogenesis. A causal link has been established between cigarettes and lung cancer; however, only 10–13% of people who smoke eventually develop lung cancer. The risk for developing lung cancer increases with the number of cigarettes smoked per day and the number of years of smoking.

3. How has the pattern of tobacco use changed over the past 15 years?

Although the percentage of Americans who smoke has decreased (approximately 30% of the adult population smoked in 1985, including 10–15% of all physicians and 20–30% of all nurses), it is estimated that 20% of all men and 22% of all women were smokers in the year 2000. In general, women have a shorter smoking history than men at diagnosis but may be more vulnerable to smoking-related risks than men. However, lung cancer mortality rates remain 23 times higher for men who continue to smoke, whereas for women mortality rates are 13 times higher than lifetime nonsmokers. Of major concern is the marked increase in tobacco use by teenagers because the risk of developing lung cancer is higher for people who begin to smoke before age 15 than for people who begin to smoke after age 25.

4. When do the benefits of smoking cessation become apparent?

The benefits of smoking cessation become apparent by 5 years after quitting and increase over time; the risk of developing lung cancer approaches the risk level for nonsmokers at 15 years. Because of lung damage during smoking, a slightly increased risk of developing lung cancer is always present in former smokers.

5. Does passive smoke play a role in the development of lung cancer?

Passive smoking or environmental tobacco smoke (ETS) is the involuntary exposure of non-smokers to tobacco smoke. ETS is believed to be qualitatively similar to smoke inhaled by smokers and has been labeled by the Environmental Protection Agency as a group A carcinogen (known to cause cancer in humans). Although significantly fewer cases of lung cancer have been directly attributable to ETS than to smoking, 20% of all lung cancers and 3,000 lung cancer deaths are estimated to be related to ETS exposure. This number may well increase when the exact amount of smoke exposure in ETS can be better quantified.

6. Does diet play a role in preventing lung cancer?

Diets high in fruits and vegetables appear to protect against lung cancer, whereas diets deficient in vitamin A appear to be associated with disease. Current chemoprevention trials have shown no benefit in preventing lung cancer by using vitamin A, vitamin E, or beta-carotene. In fact, patients who received vitamin A or beta-carotene had a slightly increased risk for lung cancer.

7. What are the symptoms of lung cancer?

The most common symptoms of lung cancer include cough, hemoptysis, dyspnea, wheezing, and chest or shoulder pain. Systemic symptoms include anorexia, weight loss, fatigue, and paraneo-plastic syndromes such as inappropriate secretion of antidiuretic hormone (SIADH), Cushing's syndrome, and hypercalcemia. Other symptoms include facial swelling (from superior vena cava syndrome), headache or seizures (from brain metastases), pleural effusions, bone pain, clubbing of digits, recurrent bronchitis, and hoarseness. Pneumonia that is unresolved after 2 months of treatment should be investigated as a symptom of lung cancer. Ten percent of patients are asymptomatic.

8. How is lung cancer diagnosed?

A combination of history and physical examination, chest radiographs, sputum cytology, and fiberoptic examination is used to diagnose lung cancer. Asymptomatic people often are diagnosed after a chest radiograph for other purposes. Bronchoscopy with washings, brushings, and biopsies of suspicious areas are most common. Transthoracic fine-needle aspiration may be used to obtain a tissue diagnosis. Additional diagnostic measures include lymph node biopsy, mediastinoscopy, thoracoscopy, and thoracotomy. Chest computed tomography (CT) or a positron-emission tomography (PET) scan also may be used. Fewer than 1% of all lung cancers are diagnosed at an occult stage. One-third to one-half of solitary pulmonary nodules (coin lesions) found on chest radiographs are malignant.

9. What are the differences among the types of lung cancer?

Lung cancer is divided into two histologic classes: non–small-cell lung cancer (NSCLC) and small cell lung cancer (SCLC). NSCLC accounts for approximately 80% of all lung cancers and has three major subtypes: squamous cell, adenocarcinoma (including bronchoalveolar), and large cell. Squamous cell lung cancer usually arises centrally, grows more slowly, and tends to remain localized. Adenocarcinomas are the most common type of lung cancer and are found more frequently in women and younger people. Large-cell lung cancers are associated with a poor prognosis. SCLC or oat cell carcinoma accounts for the remaining 20%. SCLC is generally a systemic disease at diagnosis; more than 50% of patients present with extensive (widespread) disease. Approximately 25% have regional involvement, and less than 10% have only local disease at diagnosis. SCLC metastasizes early and is associated with a poor prognosis.

About 5% of lung cancers can be classified in an "other" category. These types are exceedingly rare and include carcinoid tumors and mucoepidermoid lung cancer.

10. Which lung cancers occur in nonsmokers?

If a nonsmoker develops lung cancer, it more than likely will be adenocarcinoma. Adenocarcinoma also occurs in smokers (particularly women who smoke). Lung cancers most commonly associated with smoking include squamous cell or small cell.

11. Are there any differences in the doubling time for the various types of lung cancer?

The doubling time for SCLC is relatively rapid and averages 45 days, whereas the doubling time for NSCLC averages 90–100 days with a range of 30–150 days. Because of rapid cell division, SCLC tends to be more responsive to both radiation therapy (RT) and chemotherapy.

12. How is NSCLC treated?

The mainstay for NSCLC treatment is surgery; however, only 20–25% of patients have localized disease that is amenable for surgery. Surgery is the only modality that offers a chance for cure and is used to treat patients with stage I, stage II, and stage III disease that is deemed to be surgically resectable. The treatment of choice is lobectomy or pneumonectomy. RT is recommended for stage I and stage II patients who are not surgical candidates or for patients who refuse surgery. RT may offer a potentially curative alternative to surgery in highly selective, nonsurgical candidates; however, its effect tends to be limited when used alone.

Patients with stage III disease pose a treatment challenge. For those with resectable disease, surgery is the treatment of choice, with or without the addition of RT. For those with unresectable disease, chemotherapy with a platinum-based regimen is used. RT is usually added. For patients with marginally resectable disease, treatment recommendations remain unclear but may include neoadjuvant or concomitant chemotherapy and RT followed, when possible, by surgical resection.

Chemotherapy is the treatment of choice for stage IV patients with good performance status. For these patients, chemotherapy has been shown to increase survival, improve quality of life, decrease symptoms, and be more cost-effective than the best supportive care alone. Clinical trials are ongoing for all stages, including many phase I and II trials with novel agents and combination therapies (e.g., radiation and/or chemotherapy and/or surgery).

13. How is SCLC treated?

SCLC is considered to be a systemic disease at time of diagnosis; thus surgical resection alone is not appropriate. The mainstay of treatment is chemotherapy, with or without the addition of RT. Regimens including a variety of agents are most commonly used. The standard of care includes treatment with cisplatin or carboplatin plus etoposide. Approximately 40% of patients with limited stage disease survive 2 years. Smoking cessation may improve quality of life but does not necessarily lengthen survival.

14. What is the role of radiation therapy in the treatment of lung cancer?

RT may be used for cure (in combination with other treatment modalities) in certain nonsurgical candidates with NSCLC and also may be used to sterilize tumors preoperatively and treat regional lymph nodes. RT may provide palliation by shrinking tumors and alleviating symptoms. Various radiotherapy methods are currently under investigation, including altered fractionation (increasing the daily, single-dose fraction), accelerated hyperfractionation (multiple, daily fractions), and three-dimensional conformal radiation therapy (pinpointing the tumor in three dimensions rather than the standard 2 dimensions). These methods allow the radiation dose to the tumor to be increased while minimizing the toxicities to nontumor tissues and may lead to increased rates of survivial and cure.

15. What are the most common sites of metastasis in lung cancer?

The most common metastatic sites for lung cancer include the liver, adrenal glands, bones, and brain. Both hematogenous and lymphatic spread are common. Local spread of disease includes direct invasion through the walls of lung structures and spread along the inside of the bronchial lumens.

16. Which lung cancers are most likely to have brain metastases?

Approximately 10% of all patients diagnosed with SCLC have brain metastases at diagnosis. Of those who survive for more than 2 years, 50–80% have brain metastases.

17. Should a patient with SCLC receive brain irradiation?

The role of prophylactic brain irradiation remains controversial and currently is considered only for those who are in complete remission from lung cancer. The side effects of radiation treatment to the brain must be weighed against long-term survival and quality of life. Currently the rate of brain metastases has been decreased with prophylactic brain irradiation, and a survival benefit has been shown in patients in complete remission.

18. What paraneoplastic syndromes are associated with lung cancer?

Paraneoplastic syndromes are common in lung cancer. SCLC is associated with SIADH, Cushing's syndrome (ectopic production of adrenocorticotropic hormone [ACTH]), peripheral neuropathies, Eaton-Lambert syndrome (myasthenia-like transverse myelitis, polymyositis, and weakness), and carcinoid syndrome. Squamous cell lung cancer is associated with hypercalcemia and peripheral neuropathies, whereas adenocarcinoma of the lung is associated with hypercoagulable states and hypertrophic pulmonary osteoarthropathy. Hypercalcemia (rare), hypertrophic pulmonary osteoarthropathy, and peripheral neuropathies are also seen in patients with large cell lung cancers.

19. What oncologic emergencies most commonly occur in lung cancer?

The most common oncologic emergencies seen in patients with lung cancer are superior vena cava syndrome (SVCS) and airway obstruction. Seventy-five percent of all instances of SVCS are related to obstruction by either squamous cell or small cell lung cancers, whereas partial or complete airway obstruction is seen in 53% of patients with squamous cell, 38% with small cell, and 33% with large cell carcinoma. At thoracotomy, endobronchial lesions are found in approximately 70% of all patients with lung cancer. Pericardial effusions, neoplastic cardiac tamponade (direct extension into the pericardium), and spinal cord compression may occur, and metabolic emergencies, including hypercalcemia and hyponatremia (due to SIADH), are not uncommon.

20. What is Pancoast tumor syndrome?

Named after Henry Pancoast (who described the tumor that bears his name) in 1924, it is a lung tumor usually found after a lengthy investigation associated with severe shoulder and arm pain. Ipsilateral Horner's syndrome, characterized by a small pupil and ptosis of the eyelid, also may be present. The tumor has caused rib destruction and nerve root involvement (C8 or T1). It is located near the brachial plexus, major thoracic vessels, and vertebral bodies. Current treatment of choice includes combined modality therapy with chemotherapy and RT followed by surgery. The brain is the most common site for metastatic spread. Neuropathic pain medications are the mainstay of symptomatic treatment for shoulder and arm pain.

21. What are the most significant prognostic indicators for patients with lung cancer?

For both SCLC and NSCLC, the single most common prognostic indicator for overall survival and response to treatment is weight loss. Other indicators include tumor bulk, presence and site(s) of metastases, gender (women usually fare better than men), and performance status. In addition, an increased level of lactate dehydrogenase (LDH) or alkaline phosphatase and a decreased level of serum sodium are associated with a poorer prognosis in patients with SCLC.

22. Which lung cancers can be cured?

Localized lung cancer has the best chance for cure. Approximately 20–25% of patients with SCLC limited to the hemithorax may be cured by aggressive treatment with chemotherapy and radiation; however, most patients with SCLC present with extensive disease. Up to 90% of all patients with SCLC eventually relapse and die of disease, even if complete remission has been achieved with aggressive therapy.

For patients with NSCLC, the potential for cure exists primarily for stages I and II, totally resectable disease. Any patient with distant metastases is not curable, and fewer than 5% of patients with stage III, mediastinal lymph node involvement are cured. Unfortunately, patients with lung cancer are at risk for developing a second primary lung tumor, especially if they continue to smoke. Chemoprevention trials to minimize second primaries are currently under way.

23. What new treatments are in development for lung cancer?

New chemotherapeutic regimens are currently under investigation for the treatment of NSCLC and SCLC, including protocols using the taxanes, paclitaxel (Taxol), and docetaxel (Taxotere); vinorelbine (Navelbine); the camptothecins, irinotecan (Camptosar) and topotecan (Hycamtin); and gemcitabine (Gemzar), alone or in combination with other agents. Combined or multimodal therapy (chemotherapy and radiation therapy), neoadjuvant or preoperative chemotherapy, and chemoprevention agents continue to be investigated. In addition, new approaches using agents with a biologic basis that target growth factors and various aspects of the cell cycle also are under investigation. Included in these trials are angiogenesis inhibitors, gene therapy, and agents such as Herceptin and Iressa. An exciting addition to current therapies is the development of new oral agents in addition to newer intravenous agents.

24. How does mesothelioma differ from lung cancer?

Mesothelioma, a rare neoplasm commonly involving the pleura or peritoneum, is directly linked to asbestos exposure; people with occupational exposure to asbestos (e.g., ship builders, pipe fitters, brake repairers, insulation installers) have a 6- to 7-fold greater risk of death from cancer than an unexposed population. Short-term exposure (< 1 month) carries a continued risk for the development of cancer 25 years later. More than 8 million people are believed to be at risk for developing mesothelioma. Mesothelioma usually presents with pleural effusion. The three subtypes are epithelial, fibrosarcomatous, and mixed. Disease spreads locally in the mediastinum and chest wall through direct tumor extension. Mesotheliomas rarely metastasize distally.

25. Describe the current treatment for mesothelioma.

Currently, no truly effective treatment exists for mesothelioma. Treatment is tailored to the individual patient and varies by stage of disease. It often includes chemotherapy with a platinum-based regimen. Intrapleural therapy with cisplatin, interferon, or interleukin-2 has been undertaken with mixed results. The role of surgery is controversial, the role of radiation therapy is unclear, and experience with combined modality treatment is limited. Clinical trials continue to provide new insights into the treatment of this rare neoplasm.

26. What methods are available for early detection of lung cancer?

No methods currently are approved for the early detection of lung cancer. In asymptomatic people, lung cancer is often diagnosed when a chest radiograph is done for another purpose. Routine sputum cytology and intermittent bronchoscopy are under investigation in high-risk people. In addition, the use of screening CT (in particular the spiral CT) and various forms of bronchoscopy are under investigation in a systematic fashion that will provide information about routine screening for people at high risk. Patient registries and collection of DNA for genetic marker analysis are also components of clinical trials for people at high risk.

27. Does genetics play a role in the development of lung cancer?
Predisposition to lung cancer may be inherited. Research is ongoing.

28. What is the nurse's role in the care of patients with lung cancer?
Because treatment for lung cancer is primarily palliative, the nurse's role is focused on providing support, promoting comfort, and managing cancer- and treatment-related symptoms. Of particular importance are educational and psychosocial interventions to minimize feelings of guilt (patients' beliefs that they have caused their own disease) and to promote quality of life. Role modeling of healthy behaviors and encouraging patients to quit smoking (to minimize further lung compromise) also should be incorporated into nursing care. Comprehensive symptom management, including nutritional interventions, is essential for providing holistic care.

29. What resources are available to aid the nurse in caring for patients with lung cancer?
Alliance for Lung Cancer, Advocacy, Support, and Education (ALCASE)
P.O. Box 849
Vancouver, WA 98666
Web address: http://www.alcase.org
Hotline: 800-298-2436
Telephone: 360-696-2436; e-mail: info@alcase.org
• National nonprofit organization that provides advocacy, support, education, and rehabilitation programs for people with lung cancer
American Lung Association
1740 Broadway
New York, NY 10019-4374
Web address: http://www.lungusa.org
Telephone: 800-LUNG-USA (800-586-4872) or 212-315-8700; e-mail: info@lungusa.org
• National nonprofit organization that provides information about cancer for patients and professionals as well as stop-smoking programs
Agency for Healthcare Research and Quality (AHRQ)
2101 E. Jefferson St., Suite 501
Rockville, MD 20852
Web address: http://www.ahrq.gov
Telephone: 301-594-1364; e-mail:info@ahrq.gov
• National organization that issues smoking cessation guidelines and other materials for healthcare professionals and the general public

30. Describe the nurse's role in smoking cessation.
Smoking cessation decreases the risk of developing lung cancer and developing a second primary tumor after an initial diagnosis of lung cancer. In addition, smoking cessation has the potential to improve the quality of life in patients undergoing treatment for lung cancer. Of current smokers, 70% want to quit smoking and 34% actually attempt to quit. However, only 2.5% of people who attempt to quit smoking are successful. Methods to enhance smoking cessation include (1) behavior modification strategies, such as relaxation techniques, hypnosis, and monitoring and reducing triggers to smoke; (2) group programs that provide skills training, social support, and structure; (3) nicotine replacement therapy (NRT) with gum, transdermal patches, or nasal spray; (5) use of non–nicotine-containing medications such as bupropion or clonidine; and (6) self-help programs using videotapes, literature, or brief telephone counseling and advice.

Ninety-five percent of all people who attempt to quit smoking do so without outside help. Of these, 20% are successful with their first attempt, and up to 60% are successful with repeated attempts. Multiple modalities (e.g., NRT and counseling) appear to improve smoking cessation efforts. A new Public Health Service guideline, "Treating Tobacco Use and Dependence: A Clinical Practice Guideline," and a new consumer guide, "You Can' Quit Smoking," have been developed and are available online through www.guideline.gov or www.surgeongeneral.gov.

31. What are the four As?

The clinical approach recommended for encouraging smoking cessation includes the four A's: (1) **a**sk about smoking, (2) **a**dvise to stop smoking, (3) **a**ssist to quit, and (4) **a**rrange follow-up. These recommendations are included in a manual of practical smoking cessation techniques available from the National Cancer Institute, Office of Cancer Communications. Encouragement by health care providers to stop smoking or not start smoking has been shown to be of benefit and should be incorporated into routine health care practices.

32. Why should smokers with lung cancer quit smoking?

According to Sarna, reasons for the person with lung cancer to quit smoking include (1) decreasing symptoms such as shortness of breath and cough; (2) decreasing the risk of recurrence or a second lung primary and the risk or worsening of tobacco-related diseases; (3) decreasing the risk of second-hand smoking-related lung cancer or heart disease in household members; (4) increasing feelings of control and overall well-being; and (5) being a role model for friends and family.[13]

ACKNOWLEDGMENT

The authors thank Karen Kelly, MD, Professor of Medicine, Division of Medical Oncology, University of Colorado Health Sciences Center, Denver, Colorado, for her thoughtful review of this manuscript.

REFERENCES

1. Bressler TR: Small cell lung cancer. In Miaskowski C, Buchsel P (eds): Oncology Nursing Assessment and Clinical Care, St. Louis, Mosby, 2000, pp 1301–1329.
2. Engstrom PF: Cancer prevention from concept to practice. CA Cancer J Clin 50:140– 142, 2000.
3. Fleming ID, Cooper JS, Henson DE, et al: AJCC Cancer Staging Handbook. Philadelphia, Lippincott-Raven, 1998.
4. Greco FA, Hainsworth JD: Multidisciplinary approach to potentially curable non-small carcinoma of the lung. Oncology 11:27–36, 1997.
5. Greenlee RT, Hill-Harmon MB, Murray T, Thun M: Cancer statistics, 2001. CA Cancer J Clin 51:15–36, 2001.
6. Hoffman PC, Mauer AM, Vokes EE. Lung cancer. Lancet, 355:479-485, 2000.
7. Hughes JR: New treatments for smoking cessation. CA Cancer J Clin 50:143–151, 2000.
8. Ingle RJ: Lung cancers. In Yarbro CH, Frogge MH, Goodman M, Groenwald SL (eds): Cancer Nursing: Principles and Practice, 5th ed. Boston, Jones & Bartlett, 2000, pp 1298–1328.
9. Iwamoto R: Lung cancer. In Nevidjon BM, Sowers KW (eds): A Nurse's Guide to Cancer Care. Philadelphia, Lippincott, 2000, pp 44–61.
10. Lindsey AM, Sarna L: Lung cancer. In McCorkle R, Grant M, Frank-Stromborg M, Baird SB (eds): Cancer Nursing: A Comprehensive Textbook, 2nd ed. Philadelphia, W.B. Saunders, 1996, pp 611–633.
11. Lindsey LP, Thielvoldt D: Non-small cell lung cancer. In Miaskowski C, Buchsel P (eds): Oncology Nursing Assessment and Clinical Care. St. Louis, Mosby, 2000, pp 1331–1351.
12. Mehta MP, Schiller JH: Diagnosis and management of stage III NSCLC. Clin Oncol Updates 1(3):1–15, 2000.
13. Sarna L: Smoking cessation after the diagnosis of lung cancer. Develop Support Care 2:45–49, 1998.
14. Van Cleave JH: Nursing perspectives on the diagnosis and management of stage III NSCLC. Clin Oncol Updates Oncol Nurse 1(3):1A–6A, 2000.
15. White EJ: Lung cancer. In Varrichio C (ed): A Cancer Source Book for Nurses, 7th ed. Atlanta, American Cancer Society, 1997, pp 284–294.

32. MALIGNANT MELANOMA

Maude Becker, RN, BSN, OCN, and Rene Gonzalez, MD

Incidence	51,400 estimated cases in 2001; 4% of all cancers in United States; 9th most common cancer in United States. Lifetime risk of developing melanoma is increasing: 1991, 1 in 105; 2000, 1 in 75.
Mortality	7,800 estimated deaths in 2001
Risk factors	Large number of moles Family history of melanoma History of severe sunburns in childhood and adolescence Light skin type, blue or green eyes, blond or red hair Clinically atypical moles, dysplastic nevus syndrome History of acute and intermittent exposure to sun or ultraviolet radiation
Histology	Superficial spreading is the most common, followed by nodular melanomas. Other forms: acral lentiginous melanoma, lentigo maligna melanoma, desmoplastic melanoma, and uveal melanoma (rare).
Symptoms	Mole that changes in size, elevation, color, surface, surroundings, and sensation
Diagnosis	Biopsy
Microstaging	

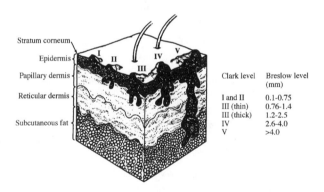

Clark level	Breslow level (mm)
I and II	0.1-0.75
III (thin)	0.76-1.4
III (thick)	1.2-2.5
IV	2.6-4.0
V	>4.0

Both level of invasion and maximal thickness determine the T (primary tumor) classification: **Breslow's thickness** = thickness of tumor tissue; **Clark's level** = anatomic level of invasion. Corresponding thickness of Clark and Breslow levels is shown. (From Gronewald S, Frogge M, Goodman M, Yarbro C: Comprehensive Cancer Nursing Review, 2nd ed. Research Triangle Park, NC, Glaxo Wellcome, 1995, with permission.)

Staging	**Primary tumor (T)**
	T1 ≤ 1.0 mm
	T2 1.01–2.0 mm
	T3 2.01–4.0 mm
	T4 > 4 mm
	    a. without ulceration
	    b. with ulceration

Table continued on following page

Quick Facts—Malignant Melanoma (Continued)

Staging *(cont'd)*	**Lymph nodes (N)**		
	N1	1 lymph node	
	N2	2–3 lymph nodes	
	N3	4 or more nodes, matted lymph nodes, combination of in-transit metastasis/satellite, or ulcerated melanoma and lymph node(s)	
	Distant metastasis (M)		
	M1	Distant skin, subcutaneous, or lymph nodes with normal lactate dehydrogenase (LDH)	
	M2	Lung metastases with normal LDH	
	M3	All other visceral or any distant metastases with elevated LDH	
Stage grouping	Stage 0	Melanoma in situ	
	Stage IA	T1a	N0	M0
	Stage IB	T1b, T2a	N0	M0
	Stage IIA	T2b, T3a	N0	M0
	Stage IIB	T3b, T4a	N0	M0
	Stage IIC	T4b	N0	M0
	Stage IIIA	Any T	N1a	M0
	Stage IIIB	Any T	N1b, N2a	M0
	Stage IIIC	Any T	N2b, N2c, N3	M0
	Stage IV	Any T	Any N	M1–M3
Treatment	Stage IA: Surgical excision of primary tumor		
	Stages IB–II: Consider sentinel lymph node (SLN) biopsy prior to wide excision		
	Stage III: Surgical excision of primary tumor with radical lymphadenectomy and with or without interferon therapy		
	Stage IV: No standard treatment; all patients encouraged to participate in clinical trials		

1. What is melanoma?

Melanoma is a malignant tumor originating from melanocytes, the pigment (melanin)-producing cells in the skin. Melanocytes are found throughout the skin but are most common in the basal layers of the epidermis. Melanoma may arise from a preexisting nevus or occur spontaneously. It is a tumor that strikes fear because of its unpredictable behavior. For example, a melanoma can be completely excised, recur years later in another site, and cause rapid progression and death in less than 1 year.

2. What is dysplastic nevus syndrome (DNS)?

A dysplastic nevus is a distinct melanocytic lesion that may be a precursor to melanoma. It may occur sporadically or be associated with a personal or family history of melanoma (familial DNS). Regardless of family history, persons with DNS have a higher risk of developing melanoma. Clinically, dysplastic nevi tend to be larger than commonly acquired nevi, often measuring > 5 mm. The lesions may have fuzzy or irregular borders, and the pigmentation pattern is often irregular. Another distinctive feature is the "fried-egg" appearance, created when the central nevus component is one color and the peripheral component is another shade. Patients often have dozens or even hundreds of lesions.

3. Where do melanomas commonly occur?

Melanomas can be located anywhere on the body but occur most commonly on the lower extremities in women and on the trunk in men, especially on the back.

4. What type of biopsy should be done if melanoma is suspected?

Because tumor thickness is the most important factor in determining prognosis and treatment, the biopsy should be excisional through the underlying fat, using a punch-type biopsy when possible. After the diagnosis is established, lesions < 1 mm in thickness should be excised with a 1-cm margin, whereas primary lesions of 1–4-mm thickness require a 2-cm margin. Studies have shown that large and disfiguring surgical excisions are unnecessary because they do not improve outcome or decrease local recurrence rates.

5. What are the warning signs of malignant melanoma?
The warning signs of malignant melanoma can be summarized as the **ABCDs**:
Asymmetry in shape, color, or appearance of mole; **a**ppearance of new pigmented lesion
Borders that are notched, irregular in shape, or both; **b**leeding moles
Color of mole is variable or contains blue, gray, white, pink, or red
Diameter > 6 mm in any direction

6. What preventive measures should be taken to reduce the risk of developing melanoma?
1. Avoid peak times of intense ultraviolet (UV) radiation exposure (10 AM–3 PM).
2. Use sunscreen with a sun protection factor (SPF) of at least 15; reapply if swimming, perspiring, or outdoors > 2 hours.
3. Apply 1 ounce of sunscreen evenly over the body at least 30 minutes before sun exposure.
4. Wear protective clothing while outdoors.
5. Do not use artificial suntanning lamps.
6. Do regular self-examinations of skin, and evaluate suspicious lesions using the ABCDs.

7. What is the relationship between melanoma and sunlight?
Sunlight is composed of UV radiation that damages the DNA of skin cells. This damage may result in mutations that lead to the development of all forms of skin cancer, including melanoma. The same process occurs with the use of tanning booths. There is no such thing as a safe tan. The damaging effects of sunlight may occur many years before tumors appear; therefore, sun protection during childhood and youth is particularly important.

8. What does sun protection factor (SPF) mean?
Minimal erythematous dose (MED) is the minimal dose of UV that causes erythema. SPF is the relative protection offered by a sunscreen vs. no sunscreen protection. For example, a person who can be exposed to the sun for only 20 minutes without developing erythema can apply sunscreen with an SPF of 8 and stay outside for 160 (20×8) minutes without burning. More sun protection is offered by sunscreens with higher SPF numbers. A sunscreen with a SPF of 15 offers complete protection in most cases; it is recommended that patients use > 15 SPF for protecting skin after chemotherapy and radiation therapy.

9. What type of sunscreen is recommended?
Newer generations of sunscreens provide UVA and UVB protection. When choosing a sunscreen, check the label to see if it contains both UVA and UVB protection. The SPF refers only to UVB coverage. Research suggests that brief intense exposure to UVA is a risk factor for the development of melanoma.

10. What role do sentinel lymph node mapping and biopsy play in melanoma?
Sentinel lymph node mapping and biopsy have evolved as a means of accurately staging the regional lymph nodes. The draining lymphatic vessels from a high-risk primary melanoma (i.e., T1b or greater) are identified by injecting a vital blue dye and/or radioisotope. The first ("sentinel") lymph node that takes up the dye is surgically removed and subjected to histologic analysis. If this node is not involved with melanoma, there is a < 5% chance that any lymph node in that drainage site is pathologically involved. Preliminary data indicate that this technique is a reliable way of accurately evaluating the lymph node basin(s) at risk and avoiding unnecessary elective lymph node dissections. Likewise, patients at high risk for recurrence (i.e., sentinel lymph node-positive) can be identified and targeted for aggressive systemic therapy.

11. Is there a benefit to prophylactic lymph node dissection?

An elective or prophylactic lymph node dissection is generally performed in patients with deep primary tumors under the assumption that they have a higher risk of regional nodal involvement and that early surgical treatment of the regional nodal basin will improve prognosis. Although this approach seems intuitively reasonable, two large randomized studies failed to demonstrate benefit; thus, its use remains controversial. Most experts do not recommend prophylactic lymph node dissection. In contrast, a therapeutic lymph node dissection is one in which the involved lymph nodes are removed; this technique remains a cornerstone of treatment for patients with stage III melanoma.

12. What are the histologic subtypes of melanoma?

Malignant melanoma has four major subtypes, each with unique clinical features.

Common Melanoma Types

TYPE (%)	INCIDENCE	COLOR AND CHARACTERISTICS	GROWTH	LOCATION
Superficial spread (70–75%)	Male:female ratio of 1:1 5th decade	Tan, brown Flat, crusty, irregular borders	Rapid growth 1–5 years; vertical rapid growth	Women: legs Men: upper back
Nodular (10–15%)	Male:female ratio of 2:1 5th decade	Blue-black, blue-gray, red-blue Raised, bleeding may occur	No radial growth All vertical growth (< 1 year; aggressive)	Head, neck, trunk
Acral lentiginous (5–10%)	African-American Oriental Hispanic	Tan, brown, black	Radial growth: months to years	Palms, soles, subungual
Lentigo maligna (5%)	Male-female ratio of 1:3 7th decade	Tan, brown Mottling, irregular borders	Radial growth: decades; slow-growing; best prognosis of all melanomas	Head, neck, cheek, temple, hands

13. What are the most common sites of metastases?

Malignant melanoma can metastasize to almost any organ in the body. The most frequent sites for metastases are the regional lymph nodes, followed by the lungs. Other sites include skin, subcutaneous tissue, liver, brain, and bone.

14. What is the prognosis of a patient who presents with brain metastases?

Melanoma ranks with small cell lung cancer as the most common tumor that metastasizes to the brain. Headache, seizures, and neurologic deficits are the most common symptoms. The median survival once a patient develops brain metastases is < 6 months.

15. Does melanoma always occur on the skin?

No. Melanoma may originate in any area of the body that contains pigment cells. Unusual variants of melanoma include ocular melanoma (originating in the pigment cells of the retina or iris); conjunctival melanoma; and mucosal melanomas, such as nasopharyngeal, oral, vulvar, and anorectal melanomas. Between 1 and 12% of patients present with metastatic disease originating from an unknown primary site.

16. Where do ocular melanomas commonly spread?

To the liver.

17. What tests are used for diagnosis and staging?

For stages I and II melanomas, a chemistry panel and chest radiograph are recommended. Sentinel lymph node biopsy should be considered before wide excision in patients with tumors >

1 mm. Patients with stage III and IV melanomas may also need a magnetic resonance (MR) brain scan, chest radiograph, computed tomography (CT) scan of the abdomen and pelvis, and chemistry profile because of the higher risk for metastases.

18. What is the role of interferon in the treatment of melanoma?

Alpha interferon is currently indicated for postsurgical adjuvant therapy in patients with tumors > 4 mm in thickness and after therapeutic lymph node dissection. Interferon is also commonly used alone or in combination for treatment of metastatic disease. As a single agent, it produces a 15–20% response rate. The use of interferon is currently under evaluation for the treatment of earlier-stage melanoma.

19. What is the optimal dose of interferon?

The Food and Drug Administration (FDA) has approved a regimen of high-dose interferon for 1 year based on a large randomized study that showed improved disease-free and overall survival in treated patients. However, side effects such as fatigue were substantial. Follow-up studies comparing this regimen with no treatment, low-dose interferon, and a melanoma vaccine have tended to confirm a benefit for the use of high-dose adjuvant alpha interferon.

20. What is the role of chemotherapy in melanoma?

Chemotherapy has generally been considered ineffective in the treatment of melanoma. Studies have shown no benefit in the adjuvant setting in patients at high risk for relapse. In advanced melanoma the only FDA-approved chemotherapy agent is dacarbazine (DTIC), which in many parts of the country remains the standard treatment. The response rate to DTIC is a dismal 15–20%, with a median duration of response of 5–6 months. Complete responses were observed in only 5% of 580 patients entered into phase III trials. Only 3% of patients who achieved a complete response remained disease-free at 6 years. Several multidrug regimens have been evaluated but have shown no benefit over DTIC in randomized trials.

21. What are the latest treatment options for melanoma?

High-dose bolus interleukin-2 (IL-2) was approved by the FDA for stage IV melanoma based on a small but definite proportion of patients who achieve durable complete responses. Newer modalities of diagnosis and treatment are currently under investigation, including sentinel node biopsy with molecular evaluation of lymph nodes, stereotactic radiation with either a gamma knife or linear accelerator for brain metastases, hyperthermic limb perfusion, and chemoembolization for liver metastases. Several new systemic agents and regimens are in various stages of development, including combinations of biologic agents and chemotherapy, gene therapy, agents that inhibit angiogenesis, and various melanoma vaccines.

22. Why should patients with melanoma enroll in clinical trials?

Although substantial progress has been made over the years, all too often patients are confronted with an advanced malignancy, a median survival time of 6–12 months, and no currently available effective treatment. In this circumstance the best option is to enroll in a clinical trial, which provides the hope of more effective treatment and often is the only way to obtain access to experimental drugs. By participating in clinical trials patients also contribute to the rapid progress of science, provide earlier access to new treatment modalities for future patients, and may facilitate the eventual discovery of a cure.

23. Who is at risk for recurrent melanoma?

Patients who have had one melanoma are at greater risk for developing a second melanoma. The lifetime risk of developing a second primary tumor ranges from 3–6%. Patients who have multiple dysplastic nevi or a familial form have an even greater risk of developing multiple primary melanomas. Persons with familial melanoma account for approximately 10% of all patients with melanoma.

24. What is the relationship between pregnancy and melanoma?

The precise influence of pregnancy on melanoma is unknown. During pregnancy, the level of melanocyte-stimulating hormone is higher than normal, and nevi may show an increase in pigmentation. This suggests that hormonal changes secondary to pregnancy may have an abnormal effect on or accelerate melanocyte growth. Other issues to be considered are:

- The effect of the pregnancy on the outcome of the melanoma
- The effects of the melanoma on the fetus and outcome of the pregnancy
- The effects of treatments on the fetus and outcome of the melanoma

In the absence of specific answers to these questions, the decision to become pregnant or to terminate a pregnancy should be left to the patient and her doctor.

25. Does melanoma respond to radiation therapy?

Radiotherapy has a limited role in the management of metastatic disease. It is used mainly for palliation of central nervous system (CNS) or bone metastases. Stereotactic radiation may be beneficial in selected cases with CNS involvement.

26. What follow-up care should a patient have after a diagnosis of melanoma?

All experts agree that lifetime follow-up is indicated because local recurrences and metastases are always possible. Follow-up should include a thorough skin and lymph node examination. The following schedule is recommended: for years 1, 2, and 3, every 3–4 months; for years 4 and 5, every 6 months; and annually thereafter.

27. What are the 10-year survival rates for the various stages of melanoma?

Stage*	10-year Survival Rate
I	85%
II	60%
III	20%
IV	< 5%

* According to the American Joint Committee on Cancer

REFERENCES

1. Atkins MB: Interleukin-2 in metastatic melanoma: What is the current role? Cancer J Sci Am 6 Suppl 1: S8–S10, 2000.
2. Atkins MB, Kunkel L, Sznol M, Rosenberg SA: High-dose recombinant interleukin-2 therapy in patients with metastatic melanoma: Long-term survival update. Cancer J Sci Am 6 Suppl 1:S11–S14, 2000.
3. Balch CM, Buzaid AC, Atkins MB, et al: A new American Joint Committee on Cancer staging system for cutaneous melanoma. Cancer 88:1484–1491, 2000.
4. Balch C, Houghton A, Sober AJ, Soong S-J (eds): Cutaneous Melanoma, 3rd ed. St. Louis, Quality Medical Publishing, 1998.
5. Greenlee RT, Hill-Harmon MB, Murray T, Thun M: Cancer statistics, 2001. CA Cancer J Clin 51:15–36, 2001.
6. Groenwald S, Frogge M, Goodman M, Yarbro C: Comprehensive Cancer Nursing Review, 2nd ed. Research Triangle Park, NC, Glaxo Wellcome, 1995.
7. Hoffman S, Yohn J, Norris D, et al: Cutaneous malignant melanoma. Curr Probl Dermatol 5:7–41, 1993.
8. Kirkwood JM. Adjuvant interferon in the treatment of melanoma. Br J Cancer 82:1755–1756, 2000.
9. Kirkwood JM, Ibrahim JG, Sondak VK, et al: High- and low-dose interferon alfa-2b in high-risk melanoma: First analysis of intergroup trial. J Clin Oncol 18:2444–2458, 2000.
10. Li W, Stall A, Shivers SC, et al: Clinical relevance of molecular staging for melanoma: Comparison of RT-PCR and immunohistochemistry staining in sentinel lymph nodes of patients with melanoma. Ann Surg 231:795–803, 2000.
11. Reintgen D, Albertini J, Berman C: Accurate nodal staging of malignant melanoma. Cancer Control 2:405–413, 1995.
12. Reintgen D, Li W, Stall A, et al: Metastatic melanoma to regional lymph nodes. In Vivo 14:213–220, 2000.
13. Urist M: Surgical management of primary cutaneous melanoma. Cancer J Clin 46: 217–224, 1996.
14. Walsh P, Gibbs P, Gonzalez R: Newer strategies for effective evaluation of primary melanoma and treatment of stage III and IV disease. J Am Acad Dermatol 42:480–490, 2000.

33. PROSTATE CANCER

Susanne K. Cook, RN, BSN, OCN, and Frances Crichton, RN, PhDc

Quick Facts—Prostate Cancer

Incidence	Most common noncutaneous cancer in men; estimated 198,100 new cases in 2001.
Mortality	Second leading cause of cancer deaths in men; 31,500 deaths estimated in 2001.
Cause	Unknown
Risk factors	Increased risk with increasing age African-American Family history
Histology	95% adenocarcinoma

Symptoms	**Early**	**Late**
	May be asymptomatic	Bone pain
	Urinary frequency	Painful defecation
	Nocturia	Obstructive urinary symptoms
	Dysuria	Weight loss
	Slow urine stream	
	Hematuria	
	Urinary retention or hydronephrosis	

Screening	Digital rectal examination Prostate-specific antigen (PSA)
Diagnosis and staging studies	Transrectal ultrasound (TRUS) is controversial Core biopsy Abdominal CT Complete blood count, acid phosphatase, chemistry screen Bone scan

Staging

Tumor, node, metastasis (TNM) and American Urological Association systems

Primary tumor, clinical (T)

TX	Primary tumor cannot be assessed
T0	No evidence of primary tumor
T1	Clinically apparent tumor not palpable or visible by imaging
T2	Tumor confined within prostate
T3	Tumor extends through the prostate capsule
T4	Tumor is fixed or invades adjacent structures other than the seminal vesicles: bladder neck, external sphincter, rectum, levator muscles, and/or pelvic wall

Regional lymph nodes (N)

NX	Regional lymph nodes cannot be assessed
N0	No regional lymph node metastasis
N1	Metastasis in regional lymph node(s)

Distant metastasis (M)

MX	Distant metastasis cannot be assessed
M0	No distant metastasis
M1	Distant metastasis

Histopathologic grade

GX	Grade cannot be assessed
G1	Well differentiated (slight anaplasia)
G2	Moderately differentiated (moderate anaplasia)
G3–4	Poorly differentiated or undifferentiated (marked anaplasia)

Table continued on following page

Quick Facts—Prostate Cancer (Continued)

Stage grouping	Stage I	T1a	N0	M0	G1
	Stage II	T1	N0	M0	Any G
		T2	N0	M0	Any G
	Stage III	T3	N0	M0	Any G
	Stage IV	T4	N0	M0	Any G
		Any T	N1	M0	Any G
		Any T	Any N	M1	Any G
Gleason score	2–4	Well differentiated			
	5–7	Moderately differentiated			
	8–10	Poorly differentiated			

1. How common is prostate cancer?

The incidence of prostate cancer has doubled in the past two decades, partly as a result of early detection as well as aging of the U.S. population. In men, it is currently the number-one cancer and the second leading cause of death due to cancer. A white male born in the United States in the late 1980s has an 8.7% chance of developing prostate cancer and a black male has a 9.4% chance. It is most common in North America and northwestern Europe; it is less common in Asia, Africa, and Central and South America. Although this distinction points to an environmental risk, studies show that Japanese men may have differences in androgen levels that account for the decreased incidence.

2. How much research funding is provided for prostate cancer?

Until recently prostate cancer has received dramatically less publicity and funding than breast cancer and AIDS. Only $60 million was allotted for prostate cancer research in 1996, whereas $550 million was made available for breast cancer and $1.3 billion for AIDS. Disparity between breast cancer research and prostate cancer research has been attributed to the reluctance of men to speak out about healthcare issues. However, increased public awareness has been generated by politicians, actors, musicians, and athletes acknowledging their experiences with prostate cancer. Michael Milken, a prominent financier diagnosed with prostate cancer, founded CaPCURE (Cure for Prostate Cancer). As of 1999, CaPCURE has given $65 million dollars for prostate cancer research. This foundation sponsors more than 80 clinical trials, which are investigating gene and family studies, advanced prostate cancer therapies, and nutritional research into the role of soy protein, selenium, lycopenes, linoleic acids, and the preventive potential of vitamin D and its analogs. The National Cancer Institute has increased annual spending to nearly $90 million. In addition, the government has granted 7.5 million annually for the next 3–5 years for Specialized Programs of Research Excellence (SPORE) in prostate cancer.

3. Can we predict who is at risk for developing prostate cancer?

The strongest predictors for prostate cancer are age, race, and family history. Eighty percent of men are 65 years or older when initially diagnosed. In comparison with Caucasian men, African-American men have a 50% higher chance of being diagnosed with prostate cancer, develop it at an earlier age, have a greater extent of disease at time of diagnosis, and have a mortality rate two times higher. Availability of health care services and beliefs about the health care system may be contributing factors to the disparities.

There seems to be no correlation between prostate cancer and venereal disease, infections, or sexual habits. Exposure to cadmium (a trace mineral found in cigarette smoke and alkaline batteries) has been correlated with prostate cancer. No studies have shown an increased risk of prostate cancer due to vasectomy.

4. How do family history and hereditary risks affect the incidence of prostate cancer?

Family history may genetically predispose men to prostate cancer. This possibility is even greater if the family member was young at the time of diagnosis. A man whose father or brother has been diagnosed with prostate cancer has a three-fold risk of developing the disease. Men with two first-degree relatives are at a 9-fold increased risk. Hereditary risks may result from DNA mutations acquired from parents. For example, *HPC2, HPCX* (found on the X chromosome), and *CAPB* (prostate and brain cancer connection) are two mutations that may contribute to some prostate cancers. The currently much talked about *BRCA1* and *BRCA2* gene mutations, which greatly increase a woman's chance of developing breast and ovarian cancer, contribute minimally to development of prostate cancer.

5. Do hormones play a role in prostate cancer?

High levels of androgens and the more recently discovered insulin-like growth factor-1 (IGF1) hormones may contribute to prostate cancer development. IGF1 is similar to insulin, but its function is to control cell growth, not insulin metabolism.

6. Can dietary habits help to prevent prostate cancer?

Research has shown that high-fat diets, large quantities of vitamin A and C, and diets high in calcium and low in fructose may increase risk. Thus, some research suggests that decreasing dietary fat is probably beneficial. Soybeans (legumes) are considered beneficial because they contain high concentrations of isoflavones. Isoflavones have antiestrogenic effects that were considered potentially beneficial for both breast and prostate cancer. However, studies suggest that the benefit is more promising for prostate cancer than breast cancer. It is currently not known whether dietary intake of retinoids and carotenoids offers any benefit. Synthetic retinoids are under investigation because the therapeutic doses of natural vitamin A necessary to inhibit carcinogenesis are toxic. Vitamin E and selenium studies show strong evidence that they provide protective mechanisms. Selenium supplementation in low doses (200 mg/day) may decrease prostate cancer because of its apoptotic properties. Large quantities of cruciferous vegetables, plus foods that contain a high concentration of lycopenes (e.g., tomatoes, grapefruit, watermelon) are also considered to be risk-reducers.

7. Can pharmacologic intervention help to prevent prostate cancer?

The drug finasteride (Proscar), which inhibits the conversion of testosterone into dihydrotestosterone (DHT), is under evaluation in the NCI-funded Prostate Cancer Prevention Trial (PCPT) to determine whether it can prevent prostate cancer. Men 55–75 years of age, with no evidence of disease, are randomized to receive either 5 mg/day of finasteride for 7 years or a placebo.

8. What are the current recommendations or guidelines for prostate cancer screening?

American Cancer Society Guidelines: men 50 years old with a 10-year life expectancy and high-risk men (African-Americans, men with family history) at 45 years should have both a digital rectal exam (DRE) and prostate-specific antigen (PSA) test annually.

American Urological Association (AUA) Guidelines: All men 50 years and older should be offered an annual DRE and PSA test.

The National Cancer Institute is currently conducting a large prospective, randomized trial to study whether early detection increases survival and decreases disease-related mortality. Results will not be available for 15 years.

9. Discuss the role of PSA in detection of prostate cancer.

Improvements in the ability to diagnose prostate cancer by PSA and transrectal ultrasound (TRUS) have greatly increased the number of men diagnosed with prostate cancer over the past decade. Whether survival rates are increased by early detection remains a controversial issue. PSA is a glycoprotein that acts as an enzyme in liquefying semen. Synthesized in the prostate, PSA is considered to be elevated when it is > 4.0 (normal: 0–4.0 ng/ml). PSA blood screening first became available in 1987 and meets the requirement for sensitivity. Specificity, however, is not as high; 36% of patients with a moderately increased PSA have nonmalignant disease. In addition to detecting prostate cancer cells, PSA may give a false-positive result secondary to benign prostatic hypertrophy, prostatitis, cystoscopy, TURP, and needle biopsy. Manipulating the prostate gland for DRE before drawing the blood sample does not cause significant changes in the PSA level.

10. How is PSA evaluated?

Several approaches—free-to-total PSA ratio, PSA density, PSA velocity, and age-specific PSA—are available to increase the specificity of total PSA. In men with an increased PSA of 4–10 ng/ml, the **free-to-total PSA ratio** is lower in men with prostate cancer than in men with benign disease. The appropriate free-to-total PSA cut-off level remains controversial. Studies suggest that a cut-off level of 25% would enable negative biopsies to be avoided in 20% of patients. **PSA density** adjusts the serum PSA with respect to the prostatic volume, as larger prostates may be associated with a higher PSA level even though the gland is benign. An increase in **PSA velocity** indicates that the change in PSA over time may be greater in men with prostate cancer than in men without cancer.

11. What is meant by age-specific PSA reference ranges?

Because normal PSA levels increase as men become older, many researchers suggest that age-specific reference ranges should be used to increase the sensitivity of the PSA test among younger men and increase the specificity for older men. These ranges have not been approved or accepted by all urologists and clinicians.

Age (yr)	PSA reference range (ng/ml)
40–49	0–2.5
50–59	0–3.5
60–69	0–4.5
70–79	0–6.5

12. Should all patients with prostate cancer be treated aggressively?

Whether all men diagnosed with prostate cancer should be treated is debatable. Most physicians agree that men with moderately differentiated, clinically localized cancers and a life expectancy of more than 10 years should receive treatment. Men who choose watchful waiting for prostate cancer tend to be older and to have a lower serum PSA, and more favorable disease characteristics than men who seek treatment. Watchful waiting defers treatment until the tumor becomes more aggressive (i.e., increasing PSA levels, marked change in DRE, or patient-identified symptoms). Currently the NCI has initiated a research trial called PIVOT (Prostate Cancer Intervention vs. Observation Trial) to determine whether radical prostatectomy leads to a sufficiently significant decrease in mortality to choose surgery over watchful waiting. Patients need information about all treatments and their side effects to make an informed decision about treatment vs. watchful waiting.

13. What are the signs and symptoms of prostate cancer?

Generally, **early-stage prostate cancer** is asymptomatic. However, as the tumor progresses, the patient may complain of symptoms consistent with urinary obstruction: nocturia, hesitancy, straining to void, or irritative symptoms such as urgency, dysuria, feeling of incomplete voiding, or hematuria.

Symptoms of **late-stage prostate cancer** are often associated with bone metastasis; consequently, pain is the most common complaint. Pain often is located in the pelvis and femur areas. The quality of the pain is commonly described as migratory (pain that radiates from one site to another). Complaints of back pain require thorough assessment for possible spinal cord compression. Liver involvement is manifested by elevated liver function tests, tenderness on palpation, anorexia, and nausea. Rarely, coagulopathies, such as thrombophlebitis and disseminated intravascular coagulation, may occur in the late stages. Lung metastasis is rare but may be manifested by shortness of breath.

14. What are the survival rates for prostate cancer?

TNM	AUA Stage	5-Year Survival Rate
T1–T1c	A	90–94%
T2–T2c	B	74–90%
T3-T3c	C	55–72%
T4–M+	D	1–4 years' survival

15. What questions should the patient ask about proposed treatments?

- What is the chance of cure?
- What is the survival rate with each proposed treatment?
- Is the cancer confined to the prostate? How can you tell?
- Are there fewer complications with surgery or radiation?
- What is the risk of impotence?
- What is the chance of incontinence?
- What can I expect from taking hormones?

16. What is a radical prostatectomy?

Radical prostatectomy is an option when the tumor is confined to the prostatic capsule. It involves removal of the entire prostate, including the true prostatic capsule, seminal vesicles, and a portion of the bladder neck. It can be performed by the perineal or retropubic approach.

17. Discuss the complications of radical prostatectomy.

Complications are rare but may include atelectasis, wound infection, pulmonary emboli, and bleeding. Advances in surgical techniques, anesthesia, pain control, and early ambulation have shortened the hospital stay to 2–3 days. Patients are taught catheter care and are sent home with a Foley catheter, which is removed at 2 weeks

18. What are the complications of lymph node dissection?

Edema of the penis or lower extremities and deep vein thrombosis may result.

19. What are the side effects of radical prostatectomy?

The incidence of **incontinence** ranges from 0–57%, depending on the definition and type of incontinence, patient age, and skill of the surgeon. The most frequently reported incidence for stress incontinence (leakage of urine when coughing, straining, or lifting) is approximately 10% for all procedures; the incidence of total incontinence (no control over urine) is 5%.

Loss of potency after radical prostatectomy depends on patient age, potency prior to surgery, and nerve-sparing techniques. In potent patients who have bilateral nerve-sparing techniques, the incidence of reported postsurgical potency is approximately 68%. Men who have unilateral nerve-sparing techniques have an incidence of reported potency of 47%. The use of cavernous nerve mapping and stimulation to identify the nerve may improve nerve sparing.

20. How is incontinence managed?

Surgical techniques to preserve the urethral sphincter and muscle help to improve urinary continence. Treatments such as urethral collagen injections and artificial urinary sphincter are used to correct incontinence when it persists after other methods, such as pelvic floor (Kegel) exercises and biofeedback, do not work.

21. What treatments are available for erectile dysfunction?

The most common treatments, in order of patient ease, are oral medication, vacuum devices, urethral suppository, injectable drugs, and implants. Sildenafil (Viagra), an oral medication, is effective in some patients undergoing nerve-sparing surgery but is rarely effective until at least 6 months after surgery. Vacuum devices are the least invasive and assist the penis to become erect by suction. The vacuum device may be used daily. Its use is encouraged after radical prostatectomy to maintain normal erectile function. Urethral suppositories are easy to use but have poor efficacy (< 20%). A combination of drugs can be injected subcutaneously by the patient or significant other into the corpus cavernosum. Patients must be counseled about potential priapism. Penile implants require surgical intervention. Patients need to know that infection is a potential complication. Hollow tubes are placed in the corpus cavernosum and erection results from pumping a reservoir that inflates the tubes with normal saline. In addition, rods may be surgically placed into the corpus cavernosum to maintain a permanent erection.

22. What forms of radiation therapy are used in the treatment of prostate cancer?

After radical prostatectomy, external-beam radiation therapy may be used in stage A–C tumors as salvage therapy or in advanced disease for palliation. Long-term results of studies comparing external-beam radiation therapy with radical prostatectomy in localized disease suggest that disease-free survival is comparable. Recent evidence also suggests that use of neoadjuvant hormonal suppression in combination with radiation therapy improves disease-free survival.

23. Discuss the role of brachytherapy in prostate cancer.

Recent advances in ultrasound equipment and computer planning techniques have brought a resurgence in the popularity of brachytherapy, the insertion of radionuclides (iodine-125 or palladium 103). Radionuclides are indicated in patients with a PSA < 10 ng/dl, Gleason score < 7, and prostate volume < 40 gm.

24. What are the advantages of brachytherapy?

Radioactive seeds have the advantages of minimal side effects and outpatient administration. The 10-year survival rates of patients receiving brachytherapy are comparable to those in patients who undergo radical prostatectomy.

25. What is high-dose combination radiotherapy? When is it indicated?

High-dose combination radiotherapy is the use of three-dimensional (3-D) conformal therapy with brachytherapy. A fractional dose of 5–7 Gy is followed by 3-D conformal therapy up to 39.6 or 45.0 Gy. Computer planning has greatly increased the efficacy and reduced the toxicity of radiation therapy, thus allowing higher doses of photons directed to the tumor but away from the surrounding tissue. High-dose combination radiotherapy is indicated for patients with a T2a lesion or greater, PSA > 15 ng/dl, Gleason scores of 7 or higher, and prostate volume < 60 ml.

26. Discuss the advantages of high-dose combination radiotherapy.

It allows a shorter course of external-beam radiotherapy, provides treatment of capsular and extracapsular extension of prostate cancer, and provides a higher dose of radiotherapy to the prostate. Ten-year data reveal survival rates comparable to other treatments for high-risk patients.

27. What is the role of particle beam proton therapy in prostate cancer?

Particle beam proton therapy is currently under study in patients with prostate cancer. Protons have different physical and biologic properties than conventional x-ray beams, thus requiring a special building for safe delivery of particle beam therapy. Because the operating costs of particle beam units are much greater than the operating costs of standard x-ray facilities, there is only one such facility in the United States. It is located at Loma Linda Medical Center, where research is currently under way.

28. What are the side effects of radiation therapy for prostate cancer?

Three-dimensional conformal radiation therapy is well tolerated. Minimal fatigue, mild dysuria, and urinary frequency have been reported during therapy. The long-term incidence of impotence is similar to that associated with radical prostatectomy. Brachytherapy has a higher incidence of urinary irritation and obstructive symptoms. Although these side effects resolve over weeks to several months, they may be uncomfortable and require self-catheterization. The incidence of side effects is greater for patients receiving high-dose combination radiation therapy. Approximately 17% of patients experience proctitis, and 5% report irritative urinary symptoms lasting > 1 year. Only 0.5% experience urinary retention. The incidence of proctitis is similar for proton beam therapy.

29. What is the significance of the PSA level after primary treatment?

Patients in whom PSA returns to an undetectable level (< 0.1 ng/ml) after radical prostatectomy are less likely to have a subsequent relapse than patients with levels > 1.0 ng/ml. PSA should decrease rapidly after prostate removal in patients with organ-confined disease. After radiation therapy, however, the PSA may not go to undetectable levels but should reach a nadir of 0.5 ng/ml by 18 months after the end of treatment.

30. What is cryosurgery? When is it used?

Cryosurgery is controlled freezing of the prostate with liquid nitrogen or other agents used for rapid freezing. This procedure consists of implanting percutaneous perineal wire trocars in the prostate. Cryoprobes are placed through cannulas or dilators and positioned over each wire. Urethral freezing is prevented by perfusing a urethral catheter with warm saline. The freezing process begins anteriorly and stops before the freezing agent reaches the rectal serosa. Cryosurgery was popular in the late 1980s and early 1990s but lost its popularity because of poor treatment outcomes and side effects. Currently clinical trials are available for early-stage disease and radiation therapy failures. Five-year follow-up from cryosurgical ablation shows a PSA < 1 ng/ml in 60% of patients with early-stage prostate cancer.

31. What are the side effects of cryosurgery?

Patient-reported side effects compare favorably with the side effects reported after radical prostatectomy. Immediate side effects include urinary leakage (4.3%), erectile dysfunction (85%), urethrorectal fistula (0.4%), bladder outlet obstruction (10%), scrotal swelling (18%), penile tingling (15%), and pelvic pain (12%). These side effects usually resolve over 1 year except for erectile dysfunction, which may take longer. Some men, however, do not regain potency.

32. What hormonal therapy is available for prostate cancer?

Luteinizing hormone-releasing hormone (LHRH) and/or antiandrogens are used in patients with rising PSA levels after initial therapy when salvage therapy is not an option and in patients with advanced disease at diagnosis.

33. What are the side effects of hormonal therapy?

Men who are potent at the time of initiating therapy need to know that the risk of losing potency and libido is almost 100%. In addition, hot flashes, weight gain, loss of bone density, and gynecomastia may occur.

34. How does hormonal therapy work?

Approximately 95% of testosterone comes from the testicles; the other 5% is produced by the adrenal glands. The goal of endocrine manipulation is to inhibit the formation of testosterone. This goal can be achieved surgically by orchiectomy or pharmacologically with oral hormones or injections that inhibit testosterone formation. Response rates are equal. Therapy can be aimed at one or both testosterone-producing systems. Single-agent androgen blockade can be achieved by surgical orchiectomy or by injections of analogs of LHRH agonist, such as a leuprolide (Lupron) or goserelin acetate (Zoladex) implant that interferes with the pituitary feedback system. Analogs can be given as a depot injection monthly or every 3 or 4 months. The hormone injections "trick" the pituitary into thinking that testosterone production does not need to be initiated.

35. What is total hormonal blockade?

Total hormone blockade, or combined therapy, consists of treatment aimed at both the pituitary and adrenal glands. Flutamide and Casodex are oral antiandrogens that inhibit testosterone effects at the target tissue level. In combination with surgical or pharmacologic orchiectomy, both drugs achieve total hormone blockade. Combination hormonal therapy may delay time to relapse in comparison with single-agent therapy; however, it has no advantage over orchiectomy alone. Some patients have a short interval of PSA decline and symptomatic relief of symptoms after antiandrogen withdrawal.

36. Can prostate cancer cells become hormone-refractory over time?

Yes. Relapse occurs 18–36 months after treatment. Studies are under way to determine whether an androgen-independent state can be delayed by the intermittent administration of an LHRH agonist. This therapy may decrease the likelihood that prostate cancer will become hormone refractory by returning cells to their normal pathways of differentiation and apoptosis.

37. How are hot flashes controlled?

Hot flashes are the most frequently reported side effect of hormonal ablative therapy for prostate cancer. Controlling hot flashes is a challenge. Severity may be diminished, but total eradication is rare. A combination of medications and complementary therapies should be offered. Commonly prescribed medications are vitamin E, clonidine, megestrol acetate (Megace), transdermal estrogen patches, and venlafaxine (Effexor). Vitamin E may be obtained over the counter and is recommended in doses of 400 IU twice daily. Clonidine patches (100–400 µg/day) may be prescribed if the patient has no history of hypotension or syncope. Blood pressure is monitored, and, if tolerated, an increase in dosage is prescribed. The most effective drug is Megace at doses of 20 mg/day orally. Transdermal estrogen patches are convenient and effective at a dose of 0.10 mg. Effexor, 12.5–25 mg/day, is a new medication used mostly in women with chemo-induced menopause, but it has been used in men with some success. Acupuncture is reported to reduce hot flashes in 70% of men treated weekly for 10 weeks.

38. When is chemotherapy indicated?

Historically, the efficacy of chemotherapy in prostate cancer has been limited. Only one chemotherapy agent, novantrone, is approved by the Food and Drug Administration (FDA) for painful hormone-refractory disease. Recently, however, efficacy has been reported with the taxanes, particularly taxotere. A > 50% reduction in PSA is found among patients treated with taxotere either weekly or every 3 weeks. This treatment regimen may be enhanced by the addition of estramustine. Paclitaxel also has been used successfully with estramustine. Other treatment protocols include doxorubicin and ketoconazole, cyclophosphamide and dexamethasone, and platinum-based chemotherapy. Side effects are minimal with most therapies. A new drug under study is exisulind, which appears to work through a mechanism of selective apoptosis. The goals of treatment are improved quality of life, palliation of symptoms, and ease of administration.

39. Discuss the role of radionuclides in the treatment of bone metastases.

Strontium-89 and samarium-153 are radioisotopes that are administered intravenously to patients with far-advanced prostate cancer who have failed all other therapy and have a life expectancy > 2 months. These isotopes travel to areas of bone that have become infiltrated by the metastatic process, follow the biochemical pathways of calcium in the body, and are taken into the mineral structure of the bone. Initially they may cause flare pain and myelosuppression. They also have been noted to cause prolonged anemia and thrombocytopenia. Patients should be instructed to continue taking prescribed pain medication for approximately 2–3 weeks after receiving either radionuclide because of the delayed response before pain relief occurs. Pain relief can be maintained for 4–15 months. Response rates have been shown to be 40–80%. Patients also may benefit from a second injection; however, caution must be used because of the prolonged side effects. Use of radionuclides may compromise further chemotherapy.

40. What resources are available to support men with prostate cancer and their families?

The American Cancer Society (800-ACS-2345) offers a group program (Man-to-Man) to men and their partners in a supportive atmosphere with the assistance of qualified health care professionals. US TOO is an international network of chapters providing support and service to survivors of prostate cancer and professional education for health care workers (1-800-808-7866). The American Foundation for Urological Diseases (AFUD) provides public education materials (410-727-2908). Using the Internet to research the latest information can pose a dilemma because not all of the information on the Internet is accurate. Websites that provide accurate sources of information are the American Society of Clinical Oncology (ASCO online, www.asco.org), Prostate Cancer Education Council (PCAW.com), and National Cancer Institute (NCI.gov).

Acknowledgment

The authors thank Michael Glode, MD, Professor of Medicine, Division of Hematology/ Oncology, University of Colorado Health Sciences Center, for his thoughtful review of this manuscript.

REFERENCES

1. Abeloff MD, Armitage JO, Lichter AS, Niederhuber JE (eds): Clinical Oncology. New York, Churchill Livingstone, 1995.
2. American Cancer Society: Prostate Cancer Resource Center. http://www.cancer.org.
3. Avant OL, Jones JA, Beck H, et al: New methods to improve treatment outcomes for radical prostatectomy. Urology 56: 658–662, 2000.
4. Badalament RA, Bahn DK, Kim H et al: Patient-reported complications after cryoablation therapy for prostate cancer. Urology 54:295–300, 1999.
5. Beer T, Raghavan D: Chemotherapy for hormone-refractory prostate cancer: Beauty is in the eye of the beholder. Prostate 45:184–193, 2000.
6. Blander DS, Sanchez-Ortiz RF, Wein AJ, Broderick GA: Efficacy of sildenafil in erectile dysfunction after radical prostatectomy. Int J Impot Res 12:165–168, 2000.
7. Brawley OW, Parnes H: Prostate cancer prevention trials in the USA. Eur J Cancer 36:1312–1315, 2000.
8. Brawer MK, Kirby R: Prostate Specific Antigen. Oxford, Health Press Limited, 1998.
9. Butler WM, Merrick GS, Dorsey AT, et al: Modern prostate brachytherapy. Med Dosim 25:149–153, 2000.
10. Catalona WJ, Carvalhal GF, Mager DE, Smith DS: Potency, continence and complication rates in 870 consecutive radical retropubic prostatectomies. J Urol 162:433–438, 1999.
11. Denis IJ: The role of active treatment in early prostate cancer. Radiother Oncol 57:251–258, 2000.
12. Cohen JH, Kristal AR, Stanford JL: Fruit and vegetable intakes and prostate cancer risk. J Natl Cancer Inst 92:61–68, 2000.
13. Dickie GJ, Macfarlane D: Strontium and samarium therapy for bone metastases from prostate carcinoma. Australas Radiol 43:476–479, 1999.
14. Dreicer R: The evolving role of hormone therapy in advanced prostate cancer. Cleve Clin J Med 67:720–722, 725–726, 2000.
15. Eyre HJ: The American Cancer Society's prostate cancer position. CA Cancer J Clin 47:259–260, 1997.
16. Fitzpatrick JR, Kirby RS, Krane RJ, et al: Sexual dysfunction and prostate cancer therapy. In Carson C, Kirby R, Goldstein I (eds): Textbook of Erectile Dysfunction. Oxford, Books International, 1998, pp 639–644.
17. Fleming I, Cooper JS, Henson DE, et al: AJCC Cancer Staging Handbook. Philadelphia, Lippincott-Raven, 1998.
18. Fowler FJ Jr, McNaughton CM, Albertsen PC, et al: Comparison of recommendations by urologists and radiation oncologists for treatment of clinically localized prostate cancer. JAMA 283:3217–3222, 2000.
19. Gerber GS, Zagaja GP, Ray PS, Rukstalis DB: Transdermal estrogen in the treatment of hot flashes in men with prostate cancer. Urology 55:97–101, 2000.
20. Glode LM, Crawford ED, Gleave ME: Prostatic carcinoma. In Schrier RW, Gottschalk CW (eds): Diseases of the Kidney, 7th ed. Lippincott Williams & Wilkins [in press].
21. Goluboff ET: The role of Exisulind in the treatment of patients with advanced prostate cancer. 10th International Prostate Cancer Update, 2000.
22. Greenlee RT, Hill-Harmon MB, Murray T, Thun M: Cancer statistics, 2001. CA Cancer J Clin 51:15–36, 2001.
23. Hammar M, Frisk J, Grimas O, et al: Acupuncture treatment of vasomotor symptoms in men with prostatic carcinoma: A pilot study. J Urol 16:853–856, 1999.
24. Kamat AM, Lamm DL: Chemoprevention of urological cancer. J Urol 161:1748–1760, 1999.
25. Klotz L, Heaton J, Jewett M, et al: A randomized phase 3 study of intraoperative cavernous nerve stimulation with penile tumescence monitoring to improve nerve sparing during radical prostatectomy. J Urol 164:1573–1578, 2000.
26. Kopple TM, Grossfeld GD, Miller D, et al: Patterns of treatment of patients with prostate cancer initially managed with surveillance: Results from the CaPSURE database, cancer of the prostate strategic urological research endeavor. J Urol 164:81–88, 2000.
27. Laufer M, Sinibaldi V, Eisenberger MA: Treatment of advancd prostate cancer. Clin Oncol 3:1–11, 2000.
28. McEwan AJ: Use of radionuclides for the palliation of bone metastases. Semin Radiat Oncol 10:103–114, 2000.
29. Messina MJ: Legumes and soybeans: Overview of their nutritional profiles and health effects. Am J Clin Nutr 70(3 Suppl):439S–450S, 1999.
30. Nelson MA, Porterfield BW, Jacobs ET, Clark LC: Selenium and prostate cancer prevention. Semin Urol Oncol 17(2):91–96, 1999.
31. Oesterling J, Fuks, Z, Lee C, Scher H: Cancer of the prostate. In DeVita VT., Hellman S, Rosenberg SA: Cancer: Principles and Practice of Oncology, 5th ed. Philadelphia, Lippincott-Raven, 1997, p 1322–1375.
32. Ragde H, Elgamal P, Snow J, et al: Ten year disease free survival brachytherapy with or without 45 Gray external beam irradiation in the treatment of patients with clinically localized, low to high gleason grade prostatic carcinoma. Cancer 83:989, 1998.
33. Sharp J: The internet: Changing the way cancer survivors receive support. Cancer Pract 8:145–147, 2000.
33. Weil M: Protons, neutrons and come-ons. 10th International Prostate Cancer Update, 2000.
34. Wymenga LF, Duisterwinkel FJ, Groenier K, et al: Clinical implications of free-to-total immunoreactive prostate-specific ratios. Scand J Urol Nephrol 34:181–187, 2000.

34. RENAL CELL CARCINOMA

Patrick Judson, MD

1. Discuss the incidence and mortality rate of kidney or renal cell carcinoma.

Estimates for the year 2001 are more than 30,800 new cases of renal cell carcinoma (also called hypernephroma or renal adenocarcinoma) and 12,100 deaths. Men are affected twice as often as women. The median age at diagnosis is 57 years.

2. What risk factors are associated with renal cell carcinoma?
- Cigarette smoking
- Exposure to asbestos
- Von Hippel-Lindau (VHL) syndrome
- Development of renal cystic disease on hemodialysis

3. Is renal cell carcinoma associated with genetic predispositions?

Some families have an inherited autosomal dominant predisposition to renal cell carcinoma. Affected family members have a balanced translocation involving chromosome 3p, whereas members without the disease do not have this translocation. Another form of hereditary renal cell carcinoma is seen with VHL disease, which is characterized by multiple, bilateral renal cysts and carcinomas, pheochromocytomas, retinal hemangiomas, hemangioblastomas of the central nervous system, pancreatic cysts and tumors, and epididymal cystadenomas. Affected families have a germ-line mutation of the VHL gene on chromosome 3p.

4. Summarize the histopathologic findings in renal cell carcinoma.
- 2–4% are bilateral.
- 4–10% have extension into the renal vein or the inferior vena cava.
- The histological types are clear cell, granular cell, papillary, or sarcomatoid. Approximately 85% are adenocarcinomas.

5. List two unusual biologic characteristics of renal cell carcinoma.
- De novo drug resistance
- Complete or partial regression (which has led to research on biologic therapy)

6. What are the signs and symptoms of renal cell carcinoma?

The most common symptom is hematuria. About 25–30% of renal cell carcinomas are found serendipitously on imaging studies obtained for unrelated reasons. The classic triad of flank pain, flank mass, and hematuria is unusual today (10–15% of cases) and indicates advanced disease.

7. Describe the distant effects of renal cell carcinoma.

Paraneoplastic syndromes are relatively common. Examples include an increased erythrocyte sedimentation rate, hypertension, anemia, cachexia and weight loss, fever, abnormal liver functions (e.g., Stauffer's syndrome), hypercalcemia, erythrocytosis, neuromyopathies, and amyloidosis.

8. Where are the usual sites of metastases?

About one-third of patients present with metastatic disease. The usual sites of metastases are the lungs, liver, bones, lymph nodes, and central nervous system (CNS).

9. Summarize the evaluation of patients with renal cell carcinoma.
- History and physical examination
- Complete blood count and chemistry profile
- Ultrasound

- Computed tomography (CT) of chest and abdomen
- Consider venogram of inferior vena cava (IVC) or magnetic resonance imaging (MRI) to evaluate IVC involvement

10. Describe the staging system for renal cell carcinoma.

The TNM system is unwieldy for everyday use in renal cell carcinoma. A staging system modified by Robson is in general use:

Stage I	Tumor is confined within the renal capsule.
Stage II	Tumor invades through the renal capsule but is confined by Gerota's fascia.
Stage III	Tumor has invaded the renal vein (A), regional nodes (B), or both (C).
Stage IV	Distant metastases or involvement of local organs other than the ipsilateral adrenal gland.

11. What determines prognosis and treatment?

Prognosis depends on the size, stage, and grade of the tumor. Sarcomatoid variants are more aggressive and have a poorer prognosis. Resectable, early-stage disease is curable only with surgery. Patients with stage I or II disease have a 5-year survival of 50–80%. Selected patients with stage I disease may have a radical, simple, or partial nephrectomy. Radical resection involves removal of the kidney, adrenal gland, perirenal fat, and Gerota's fascia with or without dissection of regional lymph nodes. Surgical excision of solitary or multiple metastatic lesions also may have a beneficial role.

12. What is the role for adjuvant therapy outside of clinical trials?

There is no proven benefit for adjuvant systemic therapy or radiation therapy.

13. Summarize the prognosis for metastatic disease.

Five-year survival rates of 35–50% have been reported for tumors extending beyond the renal capsule. Patients with stage IV or metastatic disease have a median survival of only 18 months, and approximately 2% survive 5 years.

14. How is metastastic disease treated?

No chemotherapy regimen has a significant benefit (< 10% response rate) for renal cell carcinoma. Patients should be encouraged to participate in clinical trials. Immunotherapy with agents such as interleukin-2 (IL-2) or interferon hold promise. IL-2 has a response rate of approximately 15%. Some complete responders have been disease-free for 5 years. So far long-lasting remissions have been seen only with high doses of IL-2. This therapy can be quite toxic and should be given only to patients with adequate cardiac function and good performance status. Interferon-alpha has a response rate of 15–20% with durations of response of 6–10 months. External-beam radiation can be used to palliate metastatic renal cell carcinoma (bone and CNS lesions).

15. What resources are available for patients with renal cell cancer?

- American Kidney Fund (800-638-8299) provides assistance with finances and medical referrals for people with renal cancer and other kidney diseases.
- Kidney Cancer Association (800-850-9132; website: www.kidneycancerassociation.org; E-mail: office@kidneycancerassociation.org) is a national association that advocates for patients with kidney cancer and provides research funds and professional or patient information.

REFERENCES

1. Clark J, Gaymore E: Renal cell carcinoma. In Foley J, Vose J, Armitage J (eds): Current Therapy in Cancer, 2nd ed. Philadelphia, W. B. Saunders, 1999, pp 199–204.
2. Greenlee RT, Hill-Harmon MB, Murray T, Thun M: Cancer statistics, 2001. CA Cancer J Clin 51:15–36, 2001.
3. Simmons J, Marshall F: Kidney and ureter. In Abeloff M, Armitage J, Lichter A, Niederhuber J (eds): Clinical Oncology, 2nd ed. New York, Churchill Livingstone, 2000, pp 1784–1794.
4. Vogelzang N, Scardino P, Shipley W, Coffey D (eds): Comprehensive Textbook of Genitourinary Oncology, 2nd ed. Philadelphia, Lippincott Williams & Wilkins, 2000, pp 101–278.

35. TESTICULAR CANCER

Jeffrey L. Berenberg, MD, COL, MC

Quick Facts—Testicular Cancer	
Incidence	7,200 new cases are estimated in 2001 (accounts for 1% of all cancers in men). Most common tumor in men between the ages of 20–34 years. Patients with seminoma present one decade later. Incidence is rising in Europe and the United States (doubled in past 40 years); less common in Asia and Africa. One to two percent of all germ cell tumors are bilateral. Both tumors may occur synchronously, or the second tumor may occur years later.
Mortality	400 deaths estimated in 2001. The mortality rate in white U.S. men has decreased from 37% in 1960–1963 to 5% in 1986–1991.
Etiology	Unknown; testicular germinal cell tumors probably start in utero.
Risk factors	History of cryptorchid testis (several-fold increased risk). Successful orchiopexy performed before 6 years of age reduces the risk. Klinefelter's syndrome (mediastinal germ cell tumors) History of previous testis tumor
Genetics	Isochrome of short arm of chromosome 12, i(12p) (80% of germ cell cases), increased copy number in 100%.
Histology	Germ cell neoplasms make up more than 95% of tumors; the remaining 5% are non-germ cell types (e.g., Sertoli and Leydig cells). **Two categories** **Seminoma** (40%) **Nonseminoma** (60%) • Embryonal • Teratoma • Yolk sac (endodermal sinus; most common in children) • Choriocarcinoma (rare; 1%) 40% of tumors are mixed (seminoma ± nonseminoma)
Symptoms	Patients usually present with mass, with or without pain. Often swelling has been present for > 3 months. Gynecomastia and low back pain (secondary to retroperitoneal lymph node involvement) are less common at presentation. Advanced disease: cough, dyspnea, headache, seizures.
Differential diagnoses	Varicocele Spermatocele Epididymitis Hydrocele Torsion
Diagnosis and evaluation	Testicular examination: tumor is unlikely if the mass clearly separates from the body of the testis. Ultrasound examination Radical inguinal orchiectomy (removal of testis, epididymis, part of vas deferens, and parts of gonadal lymphatics and blood vessels) Tumor markers: beta human chorionic gonadotropin (βHCG), alpha-fetoprotein (AFP), and lactate dehydrogenase (LDH) Chest radiograph, CT scan of chest, abdomen, and pelvis MRI for identification of brain metastases

Table continued on following page

Quick Facts—Testicular Cancer (Continued)

Staging	**Tumor, node, metastasis (TNM)**

Primary tumor (pT)

The extent of primary tumor is classified after radical orchiectomy.

pT   Primary tumor cannot be assessed (if no radical orchiectomy has been performed, TX is used)

pT0   No evidence of primary tumor (e.g., histologic scar in testis)

pTis   Intratubular germ cell tumor (carcinoma in situ)

pT1   Tumor limited to testis and epididymis without vascular/lymphatic invasion; tumor may invade tunica albuginea but not tunica vaginalis

pT2   Tumor limited to testis and epididymis with vascular/lymphatic invasion, or tumor extends through tunica albuginea with involvement of tunica vaginalis

pT3   Tumor invades spermatic cord with or without vascular/lymphatic invasion

pT4   Tumor invades scrotum with or without vascular/lymphatic invasion

Regional lymph nodes (N)

NX   Regional lymph nodes cannot be assessed

N0   No regional lymph node metastasis

N1   Metastasis with lymph node mass ≤ 2 cm in greatest dimension or multiple lymph nodes, none > 2 cm in greatest dimension

N2   Metastasis with a lymph node mass > 2 cm but not > 5 cm in greatest dimension or multiple lymph nodes, none > 5 cm in greatest dimension

N3   Metastasis with a lymph node mass > 5 cm in greatest dimension

Distant metastasis (M)

MX   Distant metastasis cannot be assessed

M0   No distant metastasis

M1   Distant metastasis

M1a   Nonregional nodal or pulmonary metastasis

M1b   Nonpulmonary visceral metastasis

Serum tumor markers (S)

SX   Marker studies not available or not performed

SO   Marker study levels within normal limits

S1   LDH < $1.5 \times N$ and HCG (mIU/ml) < 5000 and AFP (ng/ml) < 1000

S2   LDH 1.5-$10 \times N$ or HCG (mIU/ml) = 5000–50,000 or AFP (ng/ml) = 1000–10,000

S3   LDH > $10 \times N$ or HCG (mIU/ml) < 50,000 or AFP (ng/ml) > 10,000

N = upper limit of normal for LDH assay

Stage grouping					
Stage 0	Tis	N0	M0		
Stage I (40%)	Any T	N0	M0		Tumor limited to testis and adjacent structures
Stage IS	Any T	N0	M0	S1–3	Tumor limited to testis and adjacent structures with marker positive
Stage II (40%)	Any T	N1	M0	S0–1	Tumor beyond testis but not beyond
	Any T	N2	M0	S0–1	regional retroperitoneal lymph
	Any T	N3	M0	S0–1	nodes
Stage III (20%)	Any T	Any N	M0	S2–3	Disseminated metastasis beyond
	Any T	Any N	M1	Any S	lymphatic drainage or above diaphragm or regional nodes with S3

In addition to clinical stage definitions, surgical stage may be designated based on results of surgical removal and microscopic examination of tissue.

1. What is unique about testicular cancer?

Testicular carcinoma is the most curable solid tumor in adults (> 90% cure rate in patients with stage I or II disease). It is unique because even in late stages testicular carcinoma can be cured.

2. How often are patients with testicular cancer diagnosed correctly on presentation?

Only 33% in one series. Delay in diagnosis from 1–3 months is not unusual because signs or symptoms are mistaken for benign abnormalities and patients delay seeking medical attention.

3. Is screening for testicular cancer of proven value?

The American Cancer Society recommends monthly testicular self-examination (TSE) starting at puberty; this approach has not been validated and continues to be controversial. Some researchers believe that the potential yield from TSE is outweighed by increased anxiety in an already body-conscious age group. Others believe that testicular examination provides an opportunity to initiate education and discussion about male sexuality and sexually transmitted diseases.

4. What raises the suspicion of cancer when a patient presents with a testicular mass?

The combination of gynecomastia, a swollen left supraclavicular lymph node, and testicular mass almost always means testicular cancer.

5. How is an intrascrotal mass evaluated?

Trauma and infection should be ruled out as a cause of intrascrotal pain or swelling.
1. Examine the patient for the following:
   • Varicocele (vein engorgement within scrotum)
   • Spermatocele (irregular grapelike sac)
   • Hydrocele (accumulation of scrotal fluid)
   • Torsion (swelling)
2. Transilluminate the scrotum with a flashlight. Cysts such as hydroceles often appear transparent, whereas tumors appear dense.

6. Why are needle biopsy and transscrotal orchiectomy contraindicated?

Because of the dual risk of scrotal recurrence from implantation and inguinal spread from change in lymphatic drainage.

7. Where does testicular cancer spread?

Retroperitoneal nodes are usually the first area of spread. With the exception of choriocarcinoma, hematogenous metastases occur later to lung, liver, and brain.

8. Discuss the value of tumor markers.

Tumor markers, such as AFP and βHCG, help to identify nonseminomatous elements, predict prognosis (very high levels), determine residual disease after orchiectomy or retroperitoneal lymph node dissection (RPLND), confirm response to treatment, and detect recurrence. Almost 90% of nonseminomatous tumors have at least one abnormal marker. Patients with pure seminoma do not usually have elevated tumor markers. Occasionally βHCG is mildly elevated in seminoma (< 10% of patients). AFP elevations in seminoma indicate other nonseminomatous elements, whether or not the pathologist can confirm their presence. False-positive results are extremely rare except in hypogonadal patients, in whom βHCG may be falsely elevated when LDH levels are high. AFP may be elevated in hepatoma or liver inflammation due to cirrhosis or hepatitis. Increased LDH levels may correlate with widespread disease.

9. How reliable is the CT scan in staging retroperitoneal disease in patients with nonseminomatous tumors?

About 20–25% of patients with clinical stage I disease are downstaged after RPLND. A similar percentage of patients with clinical stage II disease are upstaged.

10. What prognostic factors are useful in patients with stage I nonseminoma?

Vascular or lymphatic invasion, embryonal histology, and absence of yolk sac tumor/AFP negativity predict a higher relapse rate when patients are observed without RPLND after orchiectomy.

11. When is observation after orchiectomy a reasonable treatment choice?

Orchiectomy followed by RPLND yields an anticipated cure rate of 80–90% in patients with nonseminomatous disease. However, the morbidity associated with RPLND includes injury to nerves supplying the prostate, seminal vesicles, vasa, and bladder neck. Even if erectile potency is preserved, there may be reduction or loss of ejaculate. A nerve-sparing lymphadenectomy may be done to preserve ejaculation.

Observation with assessment of tumor markers every month and chest radiographs and CT scans every 2 months for 2 years yields a relapse rate of 27% and a salvage rate of > 90% with 3 or 4 cycles of platinum-based chemotherapy. However, this approach requires patient commitment and personal involvement of both nurses and physicians in follow-up.

12. What prognostic classifications are commonly used for advanced testis cancer?

An International Germ Cell Cancer Collaborative Group (IGCC-CG) used tumor extent and marker levels to classify prognosis. This system, which has been incorporated into AJCC staging, is based on a combination of primary site (testis/retroperitoneal vs. mediastinal), tumor marker elevation, histology, and metastatic sites (pulmonary or nonpulmonary). Patients with good risk (low serum marker elevations and pulmonary metastases) may need only three courses of chemotherapy. High-risk patients have disseminated visceral metastases, mediastinal primary, or very high marker levels. All patients with seminoma have good prognoses.

13. What is the standard treatment for seminoma?

The tumor is usually localized and especially radiosensitive. All stages of seminoma require removal of the testicle by radical inguinal orchiectomy. After surgery, stage I and II patients have radiation therapy, and stage III patients receive combination cisplatin-based chemotherapy or radiation to the abdominal and pelvic lymph nodes.

14. Does radiation therapy still have a role in primary treatment of testicular cancer?

Yes—in seminoma. Stage I patients typically receive radiation to the ipsilateral iliac and retroperitoneal lymph nodes. This treatment is curative in > 95% of patients. Stage II nonbulky tumors (< 5 cm) are cured in > 90% of patients by irradiation.

15. What is the impact of testicular cancer and its treatment on fertility?

Sterility due to chemotherapy, radiation therapy, and surgery are of major concern to young men diagnosed with testicular cancer. For unknown reasons, oligospermia, azoospermia, and Leydig cell dysfunction often are seen before treatment is initiated. At the time of diagnosis, approximately 80–90 % of men are oligo- or azoospermic. Sperm banking may not be an option because of the urgency of chemotherapy and rapid tumor growth. Chemotherapy may affect spermatogenesis. Patients remain azoospermic for almost 1 year after therapy. Approximately 50% of patients regain both spermatogenesis and Leydig cell function within 2 years. About 33% of patients are able to father children. Oligospermia after radiation is usually reversible. Congenital malformations are not increased.

The size and location of the tumor may preclude the use of nerve-sparing RPLND. Fertility may be affected by retrograde "dry" ejaculation (ejaculate enters the bladder upon orgasm) due to the severing of the sympathetic plexus, which occurs in many patients undergoing RPLND.

16. When should chemotherapy be the initial treatment?

Patients with bulky seminoma and patients with stage III or bulky stage II (> 5 cm or palpable mass) nonseminomatous disease should receive treatment with 3–4 cycles of bleomycin, etoposide, and cisplatin (BEP). Three cycles should result in a long-term disease-free survival rate of > 85% if minimal metastatic disease is present. A recent trial comparing etoposide and cisplatin with either bleomycin or ifosfamide showed that high-risk patients need to receive four cycles and have a disease-free survival rate of > 50%. Modern radiotherapy may be curative for bulky stage II seminoma, but many oncologists prefer cisplatin-based chemotherapy.

17. What is the role of RPLND in nonseminomatous patients after orchiectomy?

RPLND as part of the initial therapy is controversial because of its morbidity and lack of survival benefit in comparison with chemotherapy. Many oncologists believe that it is adequate simply to follow the tumor markers after orchiectomy. If weekly tumor marker values return to normal after orchiectomy, monthly follow-up (e.g., tumor markers, frequent radiologic exams) for 2–3 years should be sufficient. However, if the marker does not return to normal after orchiectomy or rises after an initial decrease, chemotherapy may be instituted immediately even if no discernible disease can be found. RPLND is indicated after chemotherapy when discernible residual disease is found and markers are normal. Fibrosis/necrosis, cancer and/or teratoma may be found during this surgical procedure. Unresected teratoma may transform into malignancy and needs to be removed. If no teratoma was present initially, the residual mass was small, or there was a large decrease in size, residual cancer or teratoma is less likely to be found.

18. What acute and long-term toxicities are associated with chemotherapy for testicular cancer?

Acute toxicities: gastrointestinal effects (nausea and vomiting), renal effects (decreased creatinine clearance and tubular loss of sodium, potassium, and magnesium), and bone marrow depression.

Long-term toxicities include the following:
- Bleomycin pneumonitis
  (rarely fatal if < 400 U are given)
- Peripheral neuropathies
- Cisplatin-induced hearing loss
- Sterility
- Secondary acute myelogenous leukemia
  (related to etoposide; typically shows 11q23
  translocation; incidence < 5% at 5 years).

19. If a patient has persistent disease after therapy with BEP, what are the options for salvage treatment?

Patients who fail primary chemotherapy may be salvaged with vinblastine, cisplatin, and ifosfamide (20–45%). Surgery also may have a role. High-dose chemotherapy with peripheral stem cell transplant using etoposide/carboplatin with or without cyclophosphamide or ifosfamide offers a limited potential for cure.

20. What are the significant nursing implications in caring for patients with testicular cancer?

Because all types of testicular cancer require that patients undergo radical inguinal orchiectomy for diagnostic and therapeutic purposes and possibly RPLND for nonseminoma, nurses need to address concerns about body image and fear of sexual dysfunction. Patients are scared of the surgical consequences and toxicities of radiation or chemotherapy. They require careful exploration of fears, explanation, and correction of unfounded concerns and reassurance about positive outcomes. Patients may be so afraid of sexual dysfunction that they refuse potentially curative therapies. Patients need to be prepared about the effect of the orchiectomy on genital appearance and about the possibility of retrograde ejaculation after RPLND. Inform patients about testicular prostheses and, if indicated, make appropriate referrals. (See chapter 48 for information about sexual counseling, retrograde ejaculation, and sperm banking.)

The views contained in this manuscript are solely those of the author and do not reflect the views or policies of Tripler Army Medical Command, the Department of Defense, or the U.S. Government.

REFERENCES

1. Bajorin DF, Bosl GJ: The use of serum tumor markers in the prognosis and treatment of germ cell tumors. Cancer: Principles and Practice of Oncology Updates 6:1–11, 1992.
2. Bokemeyer C, Schmoll H: Treatment of testicular cancer and the development of secondary malignancies. J Clin Oncol 13:283–292, 1995.
3. Brock D, Fox S, Gosling G, et al: Testicular cancer. Semin Oncol Nurs 9:224–236, 1993.

4. Droz JP, Kramer A, Rey A: Prognostic factors in metastatic disease. Semin Oncol 19:181, 1992.
5. Fleming I,Cooper JS, Henson DE, et al (eds): AJCC Cancer Staging Handbook. Philadelphia, Lippincott-Raven. 1998
6. Greenlee R, Hill-Harmon MB, Murray T, Thun M: Cancer statistics, 2001: CA Cancer J Clin 51:15–36, 2001.
7. Fox EP, Weathers TD, Williams SD, et al: Outcome analysis for patients with persistent nonteratomatous germ cell tumor in postchemotherapy retroperitoneal lymph node dissections. J Clin Oncol 11:1294–1299, 1993.
8. Hawkins C, Miaskowski C: Testicular cancer: A review. Oncol Nurs Forum 23:1203–1213, 1996.
9. International Germ Cell Cancer Collaboratiave Group: International Germ Cell Consensus Classification: A prognostic factor-based staging system for metastatic germ cell cancers. J Clin Oncol 15:594–603, 1997.
10. Loerher PJ, Einhorn LH, Elson P, et al: Phase II study of cisplatin plus etoposide with either bleomycin or ifosfamide in advanced stage germ cell tumors: An intergroup trial. Proc Am Soc Clin Oncol 12:262, 1993.
11. Munshi NC, Loehrer PJ, Roth BJ, et al: Vinblastine, ifosfamide and cisplatin (VeIP) as second line chemotherapy in metastatic germ cell tumors (GCT). Proc Am Soc Clin Oncol 9:A520, 134, 1990.
12. Sesterhenn IA, Weiss RB, Mostofi FK, et al: Prognosis and other clinical correlates of pathologic review in stage I and II testicular carcinoma: A report from the Testicular Cancer Intergroup Study. J Clin Oncol 10:69–78, 1992.
13. Stephenson WT, Poirier SM, Rubin L, et al: Evaluation of reproductive capacity in germ cell tumor patients following treatment with cisplatin, etoposide, and bleomycin. J Clin Oncol 13:2278–2280, 1995.
14. Steyerberg EW, Donohue JP, Gerl A, et al: Residual masses after chemotherapy for metastatic testicular cancer: The clinical implications of the association between retroperitoneal and pulmonary histology. J Urol 158: 474–478, 1997.
15. Unger PS: Testicular cancer. In Wood ME (ed): Hematology/Oncology Secrets, 2nd ed. Philadelphia, Hanley & Belfus, 1999, pp 305–311.
16. Williams SD, Birch R, Einhorn LH, et al: Treatment of disseminated germ-cell tumors with cisplatin, bleomycin, and either vinblastine or etoposide. N Engl J Med 316:1435–1440, 1987.

36. CANCER OF UNKNOWN PRIMARY SITES

Jamie S. Myers, RN, MN, AOCN, and Kelly Pendergrass, MD

1. What are cancers of unknown primary sites, and how often do they occur?

Cancers of unknown primary sites (CUPs) are malignancies that present as a metastatic lesion for which the primary malignancy cannot be identified. Estimates of the incidence of CUPs vary from 3–10% of cancer diagnoses. For certain categories of CUPs it is estimated that the primary site becomes obvious during the patient's lifetime in 15–20% of cases. Even at autopsy, the primary site cannot be identified in 20–30% of patients with CUP. CUPs may occur in metastatic sites not expected for the site of origin.

2. How are CUPs categorized?

There are four major categories of CUPs. They are: (1) poorly differentiated neoplasm, (2) well-differentiated and moderately well-differentiated adenocarcinoma, (3) squamous cell carcinoma, and (4) poorly differentiated carcinoma (with or without features of adenocarcinoma). These categories are important to the clinical evaluation and management of the disease, and may be predictive of the response to treatment.

3. How do the clinical evaluations differ for the various categories of CUPs?

Poorly differentiated neoplasm: About 5% of oncology patients will present with an initial diagnosis of poorly differentiated neoplasm by initial light microscopy. Most patients' diagnoses can be further defined into a general histologic category of neoplasm (e.g., carcinoma, lymphoma, melanoma, and sarcoma) by conducting further specialized pathologic studies such as immunoperoxidase staining, electron microscopy, and/or genetic analysis. Until a general category of neoplasm can be determined, it is very difficult to make treatment decisions. Correct histology allows for a more rational and potentially effective treatment plan.

Well-differentiated and moderately well-differentiated adenocarcinoma (also referred to as ACUP): This is the most common category of CUP and represents about 60% of the cases. The most common types of cancer in this category are lung and pancreas (40%). Gastrointestinal cancers (stomach, colon, liver) also occur relatively frequently. Cancers of the breast, prostate, and ovary are more rare. Patients tend to be elderly with metastatic tumors at multiple sites (e.g. lymph nodes, liver, lung, and bone). These patients typically have a poor prognosis with a median survival of 3–4 months. Clinical evaluation should include a thorough history and physical (H&P) to include patterns of tobacco use, complete blood count (CBC), liver function tests, serum creatinine, prostatic acid phosphatase, prostate-specific antigen (PSA), urinalysis, chest radiograph, mammogram, and computed tomography (CT) of the abdomen and pelvis. Women with axillary node presentation may have a primary breast cancer. Lymph node biopsy, Her-2-neu, and estrogen/progesterone receptor (ER/PR) status should be performed even when mammography is negative. Elevated PSA levels, and/or osteoblastic bone metastases, may indicate a primary prostate cancer in men (about 3% of cases), in spite of an unusual metastatic pattern. Radiolabeled imaging such as the Prostascint scan (Indium-111 Labeled Capromab Pendetide) targets specific proteins on the surface of prostate cancer cells and may be a valuable tool for recognizing primary prostate cancers. Breast, prostate, and ovarian cancers may respond to hormonal therapy and be more amenable to treatment than tumors of gastrointestinal origin.

Squamous cell carcinoma: This category represents about 5% of cases of CUP.

Cervical lymph nodes are the most common metastatic site for middle-aged or older patients. Most patients have a history of alcohol and/or tobacco use. Upper or middle cervical nodes may indicate a head and neck primary.

Evaluation should include panendoscopy with biopsies of any suspicious lesions. Positron emission tomography (PET) scanning has been shown to be a valuable tool for the identification of primary tumors, as well as occult metastatic disease.

Lung cancer should be suspected when lower or supraclavicular nodes are involved. Evaluation should include chest CT and examination of the head and neck. If these are negative, fiberoptic bronchoscopy is indicated.

Inguinal lymph nodes may indicate a genital or anorectal primary. Evaluation should include digital rectal exam and anoscopy.

Poorly differentiated carcinoma: About 30% of CUP cases fall into this category. Approximately ⅓ of these cases have some features of adenocarcinoma. The patients are typically younger than those in the other categories and demonstrate a rapid progression of symptoms and tumor growth. Predominant sites of involvement are the lymph nodes, particularly in the retroperitoneum and mediastinum. Clinical evaluation should include H&P, CBC, liver function tests, serum creatinine, human chorionic gonadotropin (HCG) and alpha-fetoprotein (AFP), and CT of chest and abdomen. Elevations of HCG and AFP with a mediastinal or retroperitoneal presentation are suggestive of a germ cell tumor. It is hypothesized that some highly responsive tumors are marker negative germ cell tumors not identifiable by present pathologic methods. There is some indication that genetic analysis of the i(12p) marker chromosome may be a useful diagnostic method for patients suspected to have midline germ cell tumors. These are neuroendocrine tumors that may respond favorably to treatment with chemotherapy. NeoTect (Technetium-99m depreotide) scanning may be used to identify small-cell and non–small-cell lung primaries that overexpress somatostatin.

Clinical Evaluation for Carcinoma of Unknown Primary Site

CUP CATEGORY	RADIOGRAPHIC TESTS/ EXAMS	LAB TESTS	PATHOLOGIC STUDIES
Adenocarcinoma			
Well/moderately differentiated	CT abdomen	AFP CEA CA 19-9	Mucin stain
	Women: Mammography	Serum CA 15-3 Serum CA 125 CA 27-29	ER/PR receptors HER-2-neu expression
	Men: Prostascint scan	Serum PSA	PSA stain
Squamous carcinoma			
Cervical nodes	Panendoscopy PET scan		Genetic analysis Keratin
Supraclavicular nodes Inguinal nodes	Bronchoscopy Pelvic/rectal exam Anoscopy		
Poorly differentiated carcinoma			
With or without adenocarcinoma	CT of chest/abdomen NeoTect scan	Serum HCG Serum AFP	Immunoperoxidase stains Electron microscopy Genetic analysis

4. How are treatment decisions made for CUPs?

Treatment decisions are based on the most likely primary site for the CUP as indicated by the cell type (e.g. adenocarcinoma versus squamous cell carcinoma), geography of presentation (e.g. axilla versus cervical lymph nodes), risk factors (such as use of alcohol or tobacco), and tumor markers (i.e., elevated PSA, CA 15-3, or HCG/AFP). The patient's performance status and any comorbidities are taken into consideration before considering aggressive treatment versus supportive care.

5. Are some subsets of CUPs more responsive to treatment than others?

Yes. There are subgroups within the categories that have a greater chance of treatment response. About 10% of patients in the well-differentiated or moderately well-differentiated adenocarcinomas category may respond. For example, presentation of a woman with peritoneal carcinomatosis may suggest an ovarian or endometrial cancer. These women may benefit from platinum/taxane-based chemotherapy after aggressive surgical cytoreduction. Axillary lymph node presentation in women who are ER/PR positive and have no other sites of metastases may behave like a stage II breast cancer. These women may be successfully treated with loco-regional radiation therapy. It is also advantageous for women with positive axillary lymph nodes to receive systemic treatment with chemotherapy and/or hormonal manipulation. PSA elevations and/or osteoblastic bone metastases in men may indicate prostate cancer that will respond to an empiric trial of hormonal therapy.

The most responsive subgroups to treatment, however, occur in the poorly differentiated carcinoma category. Within this category, patients with elevated HCG or AFP and a mediastinal or retroperitoneal mass typically present as having a germ cell tumor and can be successfully treated, and even cured, with a chemotherapy regimen of paclitaxel, carboplatin, and etoposide. Favorable prognostic factors include tumor location, limitation to one or two sites of metastases, younger age, and negative smoking history. Electron microscopy will detect neurosecretory granules in 10% of patients. These patients can be treated for neuroendocrine carcinoma of unknown primary site. The response rate to a platinum agent and etoposide ranges as high as 77%. Thymomas (primary tumors of the thymus gland) may also be the primary site in this category. These too respond to platinum-based therapy. Many clinicians believe that all patients with poorly differentiated carcinomas should be considered for treatment with platinum-based chemotherapy.

6. What treatment is recommended for patients who do not fall into the favorable subsets?

For 90% of patients in the well-differentiated and moderately well-differentiated adenocarcinoma category, chemotherapy has not yielded much success. A variety of single agents have been tried (5FU, cisplatin, methotrexate, doxorubicin, mitomycin C, vincristine, semustine). Combination regimens have included 5FU, doxorubicin, mitomycin-C (FAM), 5FU and leucovorin, as well as platinum-based regimens. Paclitaxel may be a useful drug because it has activity in many solid tumors (lung, head and neck, breast, ovary, esophageal, and urothelial neoplasms). Other potentially active agents include docetaxel, irinotecan, and gemcitabine.

Patients with squamous cell carcinoma and a head and neck presentation may be treated with radiation therapy and/or combination chemotherapy. Although radical neck dissection occasionally yields the primary tumor in 20–40% of patients, it is avoided when possible due to the devastating cosmetic and functional effects on patients' quality of life. Patients with suspected lung cancer primaries may be candidates for chemotherapy.

7. How do I discuss this diagnosis with my patients and their families?

Discussing a cancer diagnosis can be difficult enough without having to deal with the fact that you are not sure where the cancer started. Educating patients and families that the treatment recommendation is being made based on the most likely primary site requires patience and the development of trust. Ideally the topic of CUP is brought up during the clinical evaluation as the work-up proceeds without a definitive primary being identified. Once all the test results are in, an important function of the oncology nursing role is to participate in the physician/patient/family conference as the diagnosis and treatment options are discussed. This enables the nurse to hear exactly what treatment options are presented and observe the patient/family reaction to the diagnosis of CUP. It will then be a little easier to answer questions and provide emotional support and education about the treatments, expected side effects, and possible toxicities.

8. What educational resources can be recommended to patients and families with CUP?

Patients who have access to the internet may be interested in the OncoLink website (http://oncolink.upenn.edu). This site is sponsored by the University of Pennsylvania Cancer

Center and provides links to multiple websites with cancer-based information. As patients browse this site they can select from disease-oriented menus that include a section for "Adult Cancers." This is further subdivided into "Miscellaneous" and "Other Diseases," which include information about CUPs. Patients can then select from the following options:

- A search engine for protocols
- Frequently Asked Questions section about the miscellaneous and other disease entities
- Subscription to *Rare Cancer*, a newsletter
- Subscription to ACUP, a support group for CUPs of adenocarcinoma cell types
- The National Cancer Institute's Physicians Data Query (PDQ) in either physician or patient format.

Patients and families with CUPs may also benefit from a variety of the NCI sponsored educational materials related to cancer in general and various treatment options such as:

- *Taking Time*
- *Eating Hints*
- *Chemotherapy and You*
- *Radiation Therapy and You*
- *What Are Clinical Trials All About?*

REFERENCES

1. Abdel-Rahman H, Shi R, Mansour R, et al: Metastatic cancer of unknown primary site: Identification of favorable clinical subsets [abstract 2279B], ASCO, 2000. http://www.asco.org/prof/me/html00abstracts/misc/m_2279 B.htm
2. Briasoulis E, Kalofonos H, Bafaloukos D, et al.: Carboplatin plus paclitaxel in unknown primary carcinoma: Phase II Hellenic cooperative oncology group study, J Clin Oncol 18:3101–3107, 2000.
3. Greco FA, Erland JB, Patton JF: Carcinoma of unknown primary site (CUPS): Long term follow-up after taxane-based chemotherapy [abstract 2279A], ASCO, 2000. http://www.asco.org/prof/me/html00abstracts/misc/m_2279A.htm
4. Greco FA, Hainsworth JD: Cancer of unknown primary site. In DeVita VT, Hellman S, Rosenberg SA (eds): Cancer: Principles & Practice of Oncology, 5th ed. Philadelphia, Lippincott-Raven, 1997, pp 2423–2443.
5. Greenlee RT, Hill-Harmon MB, Murray T, Thun M: Cancer statistics, 2001. CA Cancer J Clin 51:15–36, 2001.
6. Jungehulsing M, Scheidhauer K, Damm M, et al: 2(F)-fluoro-2-deoxy-D-glucose positron emission tomography is a sensitive tool for the detection of occult primary cancer (carcinoma of unknown primary syndrome) with head and neck lymph nodes manifestation. Otolaryngol Head Neck Surg 123:294–301, 2000.
7. NCI/PDQ Physician Statement: Carcinoma of unknown primary—updated 06/2000. http://oncolink.upenn.edu/pdq_html/1/enl/103331-1.html.
8. Sumi H, Ito K, Minami H, et al: Treatable subsets in cancer of unknown primary origin [abstract 2279D], ASCO, 2000. http://www.asco.org/prof/me/html00abstracts/misc/m_2279D.htm.

V. Symptom Management

37. CONSTIPATION

Leslie Tuchmann, RN, MS, HNC

1. Define constipation. How common is it in patients with cancer?

Constipation is defined as a decrease in frequency of defecation accompanied by difficulty and discomfort. Some define constipation as the passage of fewer than three stools per week. As a subjective symptom, assessment must take into account the patient's previous elimination pattern. In comparison, obstipation is a more severe or intractable constipation characterized by no bowel movement and large volumes of stool throughout the bowel. Constipation occurs in approximately one-half of patients with cancer and in over three-fourths of terminally ill patients. It is more common in women and elderly patients.

2. How are the causes of constipation classified?

Primary: related to extrinsic factors, such as lifestyle factors. Examples: age, inadequate privacy or time to defecate, low-fiber diet, depression, dehydration, decreased activity and exercise, weakness and poor muscle tone, lack of energy to defecate.

Secondary: related to another primary problem or disease process, such as cancer. Examples: tumors that compress spinal nerve roots innervating the bowel; spinal cord compression at T8–L3; cauda equina compression from epidural metastases; metabolic effects (hypercalcemia, hypokalemia, uremia, hypothyroidism); and diseases other than cancer (e.g., diabetes).

Iatrogenic: resulting from the use of pharmacologic agents or medical interventions (probably the most common type in patients with cancer). Examples: opioids, radiation therapy complications, surgical anastomosis (which may lead to narrowing of the colon lumen from scarring), and barium enemas.

3. What are the major consequences of constipation?
- Abdominal discomfort/pain
- Anorexia, nausea and/or vomiting
- Rectal fissures and tears
- Inflammation of hemorrhoids
- Rupture of the bowel
- Obstruction
- Reluctance or refusal to take opioids because of constipating effects, which results in poor pain control and decreased quality of life

4. What factors should be included in assessing the potential for and evaluating the severity of constipation?
- Comprehensive history and physical examination, including extent of the patient's cancer and understanding of past and current therapy
- Number of impactions since diagnosis
- Previous pattern of bowel elimination (particularly in past 2 weeks): frequency, amount, timing
- Last bowel movement: when, amount, consistency, color, presence of blood
- Abdominal discomfort: pain, distention, bloating, cramping, nausea, vomiting, excessive gas, rectal fullness

- Type of diet, appetite
- Amount of fluids and what type (normal fluid intake is 2 quarts/day)
- Previous regular laxative or enema use and its effect
- Present medications: dosages and frequency
- Whether symptom is a recent change
- Patient's understanding and compliance with fluid, fruit, and fiber intake (recommend 30–40 gm of fiber /day)
- Exercise, functional status, and level of mobility

5. List the basic elements in the evaluation of constipated patients.

1. Assessment of abdomen for bowel sounds, tenderness, masses, or palpable stool-filled colon
2. Evaluation of perineal region (rectal or stoma exam is indicated to rule out hemorrhoids, fecal impaction, or rectal malignancy)
3. Hemoccult test (positive result may be an early warning of an intraluminal lesion)
4. Laboratory tests (electrolytes, complete blood count, renal and liver tests, levels of thyroid-stimulating hormone) to assist in metabolic evaluation
5. Radiographs in both supine and upright positions (to differentiate between mechanical obstruction and decreased motility due to an ileus)
6. Ultrasound and/or computed tomography scan of abdomen and pelvis (if an extraluminal site is suspected)
7. Barium enema and endoscopy (if intraluminal site is suspected)

6. How is constipation best managed?

Prevention is the key to effective management of constipation. It is important to identify the cause and its relationship to cancer and to reverse the cause if possible. Treatment may involve nonpharmacologic and pharmacologic interventions.

7. What nonpharmacologic interventions help to prevent constipation?

Teaching patients and families the following interventions can be helpful; most people are unaware of how these factors relate to constipation.

1. **Increase fiber in the diet.** Warn patients that they may experience abdominal discomfort, flatulence, or erratic bowel habits in the first few weeks. Tolerance develops, and such effects can be minimized by slowly titrating fiber upward, starting with the addition of 3–4 gm of fiber/day and increasing to 6–10 gm/day.

2. **Increase fluid intake.** Increasing fluids may be difficult for patients experiencing nausea, vomiting, anorexia, and/or fatigue. However, an increase of approximately 6–8 glasses of water/day (1–2 L) helps to keep stool soft. Suggest carrying a water bottle at all times to sip fluids (especially between meals). Coffee, tea, and grapefruit juice usually are discouraged because they act as diuretics. However, some form of warm liquid before an attempt at defecation may be helpful. Patients have reported that drinking 2–4 ounces of prune juice before meals may be helpful.

3. **Establish a routine.** Regular toilet activities after breakfast are most productive because propulsive contractions in the intestine are strongest. The use of raised toilet seats, footstools, and bedside commodes may be helpful. Ensure privacy.

4. **Increase exercise.** Gastrointestinal motility is diminished by immobility and stimulated by regular exercise (e.g., 30-minute walk/day). Teach patients simple diaphragmatic breathing and abdominal muscle exercises to strengthen and increase muscle tone, which is necessary for defecation.

8. Describe a regimen for fiber titration in constipated patients.

- Take one tablespoon of psyllium in 8 ounces of fluid; follow with 8 more ounces of fluid daily.

- Increase daily amount of psyllium and fluid as needed, using increments of 1 tablespoon; maintain that amount for 3 days before adding more.
- Once the patient reaches the point of maintaining soft, formed stools, continue the fiber dose that the patient is taking at that time.

Caution: This approach may be contraindicated in patients whose constipation results from structural blockage of the bowel because increasing bulky intraluminal contents may increase the obstruction.

From Bisanz A: Managing bowel elimination problems in patients with cancer. Oncol Nurs Forum 24:684, 1997, with permission.

9. **Which home remedies are useful for treating constipation?**
   Anticonstipation fruit paste no. 1:
   Ingredients: 3 cups prune juice
               3 cups applesauce
               ½ cup bran
   1. Mix ingredients together.
   2. Keep in refrigerator.
   3. Take 30–60 ml/day.
   Anticonstipation fruit paste no. 2:
   Ingredients: 1 lb prunes
               1 lb raisins-pitted
               1 lb figs
               4 oz senna tea
               1 cup brown sugar
               1 cup lemon juice
   1. Prepare tea by adding about 2½ cups boiled water; steep for 5 minutes.
   2. Strain tea to remove tea leaves.
   3. Add only 1 pint tea to a large pot; then add fruit.
   4. Boil fruit and tea for 5 minutes.
   5. Remove from heat, and add sugar and lemon juice. Allow to cool.
   6. Use hand mixer or food processor to turn fruit mixture into smooth paste.
   7. Store in glass jars or plasticware, and place in freezer. (Paste will not freeze but will keep indefinitely in freezer.)
   8. Take 1–2 tablespoons/day.

10. **Are prunes or prune juice the best choices for increasing dietary fiber and aiding in constipation?**
    A common misconception in treating constipation is the belief that patients should consume prunes or prune juice as the primary source of increased dietary fiber. In fact, prunes contain only 2 gm of fiber, and prune juice contains very little. Prunes also contain phenolphthalein and may cause cathartic colon (narrowing of the ileum and proximal colon in addition to loss of colonic muscle tone) with prolonged use. Better high-fiber recommendations include wheat bran (in breads and cereals), beans, broccoli, sweet potatoes, carrots, and dried apricots.

Food	Dietary fiber
Wheat bran (3 tbsp)	10 gm
Bran flakes (100 gm)	2.7–6.5 gm
Whole wheat bread (1 slice)	1–2 gm

11. **List the common laxatives and cathartics along with their mechanisms of action, contraindications, adverse effects, and drug interactions.**
    See table on pages 302–305. **Caution:** Because oral laxatives can increase peristalsis, they are contraindicated in patients with possible bowel or actual intestinal obstruction because of the risk of bowel perforation.

12. List helpful hints to optimize the administration of commonly prescribed constipation medicines.

Psyllium, methylcellulose, and polycarbophil. Give with adequate fluids (8 oz) to minimize risk of intestinal or esophageal obstruction. Allow at least 3 hours before and after administration of other drugs to minimize potential interactions. Citrucel is the least gritty of these agents; it is also sodium-free and should be used for patients on a sodium-restricted diet.

Diphenylmethanes. Phenolphthalein is more potent than bisacodyl. Because bisacodyl is packaged as enteric-coated tablets, it should not be given within 1 hour of ingesting milk or antacids; it should be swallowed whole and not chewed. Bisacodyl also has a strong stimulatory effect, which may be helpful for refractory opioid-induced constipation.

Anthraquinones. One Senokot tablet reverses the constipating effect of 120 mg of codeine. Warn patients of urine discoloration (yellowish brown or reddish, depending on urinary pH). Cascara sagrada fluid extract is 5 times more potent than cascara sagrada aromatic fluid extract. Cascara is the mildest form of anthraquinone and rarely causes colic.

Lactulose, sorbitol, and polyethylene glycol electrolyte solutions. Lactulose's sweet taste may be more palatable mixed with fruit juice, water, or milk; it also may be given as an enema. If lactulose is administered through gastric or feeding tubes, it should be diluted in 60–120 ml of water. Chronulac is the preferred form for chronic constipation. Sorbitol is equally effective but less expensive and may be less nauseating than lactulose. GoLytely (8–16 oz/day) is reserved for resistant chronic constipation; it should be used within 48 hours of preparation. Chill before use.

Glycerin. Glycerin suppositories are usually given high in the rectum and held for 15 minutes.

Mineral oil. Mineral oil should be taken on an empty stomach.

Docusate. Surfak (docusate calcium) is preferred over Colace (docusate sodium) for patients with salt and fluid retention. It should be taken with a full glass of water, and total daily fluid intake should be increased.

Magnesium salts. Magnesium salts should be chilled and the taste disguised in fruit juice or a citrus-flavored carbonated beverage. Magnesium citrate is best taken on an empty stomach (e.g., on rising in the morning, 30 minutes before meals, or at bedtime for overnight action.)

13. Which constipation medications should be avoided for daily use in patients with cancer?

Mineral oil, castor oil, and phenophthalein.

14. How do you know which laxative to start with?

A stepwise approach to using laxatives for constipation begins with bulk-forming agents (not recommended in counteracting bowel effects of opioids); then add or change to docusate. Although some providers believe doses of docusate > 200 mg may yield little benefit, the palliative care literature notes use of up to 300 mg 3 times/day with positive effect. If docusate produces no result, add senna or cascara (docusate and senna are frequently used in combination for opioid-induced constipation). If these combinations are ineffective, switch to lactulose or sorbitol. The last step is use of magnesium citrate or GoLytely; however, referral to a gastroenterologist may be indicated before using either agent. Drug and dosage selection should be based on patient condition, drug response, and tolerance of side effects. Once medications have been used at maximal doses with little effect, switch to medications in the next step of the ladder rather than adding several medications from different steps. It is usually best to allow 2 days for the intervention to work. Titrate the regimen to produce a bowel movement every 1–2 days. For patients who have not had a bowel movement in 3 days, a rectal exam is indicated. Digital disimpaction, followed by suppositories or enemas, may be necessary. After success with this type of treatment, the maintenance regimen can be escalated. (See figure on page 304.)

Constipation Medications: Laxatives and Catharctics

	DRUG	MECHANISM OF ACTION
Bulk Formers	Psyllium (Metamucil) Methylcellulose (Cologel, Citrucel) Polycarbophil Onset of effect: 12 hr–3 days	Nondigested plant cell walls absorb water in feces; softens, increases stool size, thus increasing peristalsis; acts in small and large intestines.

Bowel Stimulants	**Diphenylmethanes**
	  Phenolphthalein (in Ex-lax, Feen-a-mint, Correctol, Doxidan)
	  Bisacodyl (Dulcolax): 5 mg enteric-coated tablet orally 1–3 times/day; 10-mg suppository (single dose as needed)
	Onset of effect: 6–10 hr; Rectally: 15–60 min
	
	Anthraquinones
	  Senna (Senokot, X-Prep): 187 mg tablet; daily maximum of 8 tablets or 4 tsp granules (326 mg)/day
	  Cascara Sagrada (aromatic): 5 ml or 1 tablet (325 mg) at bedtime as needed
	  Casanthranol (cascara derivative): 30 mg, usually in combination with docusate
	Onset of effect: 6–12 hours
		Directly stimulates nerve plexus of colon
		Irritates smooth muscle of intestine, stimulating peristalsis
		Phenolphthalein and bisacodyl first metabolized in liver, then colon; effect may be prolonged
		
		Exact mechanism unknown; may stimulate colon and myenteric plexus
		Senna stimulates submucosal nerve plexus and peristalsis in transverse and descending colon, decreases sodium and water absorption; produces semiliquid or formed stool
		Cascara directly irritates intestinal mucosa, results in motility and changes in fluid and electrolyte secretion

Oxidative Laxatives	Lactulose
	  Cephulac: 30–45 ml 3 or 4 times/day or hourly to induce rapid effect in initial phase
	  Chronulac: 15–30 ml/day; may increase to 60 ml/day
	  Sorbitol: 3–150 ml/day (70% solution)
	
	Polyethylene glycol electrolyte solution (Colyte, GoLytely): 8 oz orally every 15 min as tolerated over 3–4 hr until 1 L taken or diarrhea results
	Onset of effect:
	  Lactulose: 24–48 hr
	  Polyethylene glycol: first bowel movement within 1 hr
	Glycerin: rectal suppositories, 1–2/days as needed, or 5–15 ml as enema
	Onset of effect: within 30 min of use
		Lactulose/sorbitol: nonabsorbable sugars; exert osmotic effect mostly in large bowel
		Lactulose also used in hepatic encephalopathy to lower serum ammonia
		
		Polyethylene glycol: catharsis by strong electrolyte and osmotic effects
		
		Lubricates and softens
		Stimulates defecation osmotically; sodium stearate in suppository may irritate rectal membranes

Lubricants	Mineral oil: 15–40 ml/day orally (once or in divided doses); as retention enema: 60–150 ml/day as single dose Onset of effect: within 8 hr	Lubricates intestinal mucosa and feces; softens stool by preventing loss of water from feces

Columns continued on following page

Constipation Medications: Laxatives and Cathartics (Columns Continued)

CONTRAINDICATIONS	ADVERSE EFFECTS	DRUG INTERACTIONS
Intestinal strictures, partial or total bowel obstruction or fecal impaction, phenylketonuria Advanced cancer with early satiety, nausea, anorexia Caution in diabetics due to sugar content	Flatulence, erratic habits, abdominal discomfort or irritation	May decrease effects of tetracycline, anticoagulants, digitalis glycosides or salicylates, nitrofurantoin
Bowel obstruction Phenolphthalein less suitable in cancer patient because major GI peristalsis effect difficult to predict and control Bisacodyl: abdominal pain	Phenolphthalein: diarrhea, cramps, skin reactions, photosensitivity, hypersensitivity-type encephalitis Bisacodyl: cramps, urgency, incontinence	Bisacodyl decreases effect of warfarin
Bowel obstruction	Cathartic colon, may result in intestinal atony Fluid and electrolyte disturbances	Cascara decreases effect of oral anticoagulants
Lactulose/sorbitol: avoid with fecal impaction or intestinal obstruction Caution with severe cardiopulmonary and renal impairment (contraindicated in anuria) May cause elevations in blood glucose levels in diabetics	Lactulose: cramps, flatulence, nausea, vomiting; excessive use may cause electrolyte losses, diarrhea Chronulac: gas from bacterial degradation Sorbitol: edema, nausea, vomiting, diarrhea, abdominal discomfort, potential fluid and electrolyte loss	Decreased effects of neomycin, other anti-infectives, and antacids
GoLytely: do not give with bowel obstruction (high risk for perforation), toxic colitis, megacolon, gastric retention, bowel perforation	Polyethylene glycol: nausea, abdominal fullness, bloating, cramps	Do not give oral medications within 1 hr of GoLytely
Abdominal pain, nausea, vomiting	May cause rectal irritation if used too frequently; headache	
Known reflux, dysphagia (risk of lipid pneumonia or aspiration pneumonitis, especially in elderly)	Excessive use may lead to anal leakage and irritation Chronic use reduces absorption of fat-soluble vitamins Lipid pneumonitis with aspiration	Docusate sodium increases absorption and risk of lipid granuloma of gut wall Alters absorption of antibiotics, anticoagulants, oral contraceptives, digitalis glycosides

Table continued on following page

Constipation Medications: Laxatives and Catharctics (Continued)

DRUG	MECHANISM OF ACTION
Detergent Laxatives Docusate: 50–500 mg/day in 1 to 4 doses Docusate sodium (Colace) Docusate calcium (Surfak) Onset of effect: 24–72 hr	Decreases surface tension and allows water and fat penetration of hard stool Mucosal contact effect decreases electrolyte and water reabsorption in small and large intestines

Saline Laxatives
Magnesium (Mg) salts
  Mg citrate: 1/2–1 full bottle (120–300 ml) orally as needed
  Mg hydroxide (e.g., Milk of Magnesia Regular Strenth): 30–60 ml/day orally or in divided doses
Sodium (Na) salts
  Sodium phosphate
    Fleet Phospho-soda: 20–30 ml as single dose
    Fleet enema: 4.5 oz enema; may repeat
Onset of effect:
  Mg citrate: 30 min–6 hr, depending on dose
  Mg hydroxide: 4–8 hr
  Sodium phosphate: Oral: 3–6 hr
              Rectal: 2–5 min
	Mg increases gastric, pancreatic, small intestine secretion and motor activity of small and large intestines
	Mg and Na salts are poorly absorbed and draw water into lumen, thus increasing stool water content and frequency

Columns continued on following page

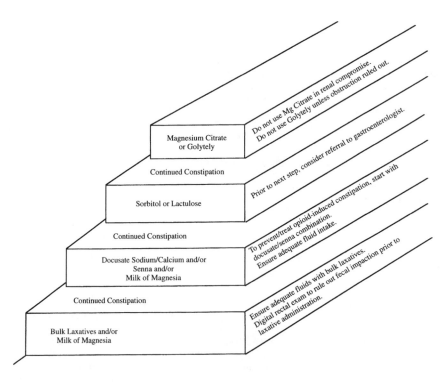

Ladder indicating appropriate steps in the use of constipation medications. Advance to next step after exceeding the upper-limit dose. Allow two days for intervention to work. (Chart created by Thomas Loughney, MD, and Leslie Tuchman, RN.)

Constipation Medications: Laxatives and Catharctics (Columns Continued)

CONTRAINDICATIONS	ADVERSE EFFECTS	DRUG INTERACTIONS
Intestinal obstruction, acute abdominal pain, nausea, or vomiting	Diarrhea, abdominal cramps Prolonged use may lead to dependence or electrolyte imbalance	Increases mineral oil absorption Decreases effect of Coumadin and aspirin
Fecal impaction, intestinal obstruction, nausea, vomiting, abdominal pain Avoid Mg salts in renal failure, myocardial damage, heart block, hepatitis, ileostomy, colostomy	Mg salts: excessive use may cause electrolyte losses, hypermagnesemia, diarrhea, cramps, pain	Effects of Mg counteracted by aluminum salt in many antacids Milk of Magnesia decreases absorption of tetracyclines, digoxin, indomethacin, or iron salts
Avoid Na salts in cardiac or renal disease, hyperphosphatemia, hypernatremia, hypocalcemia; use with caution if diet is sodium-restricted	Na salts: nausea, vomiting, diarrhea, edema, hypoten- sion; excessive use may cause dependence	Na phosphate: do not give with Mg or aluminum-containing antacids or sucralfate; they may bind with phosphate

15. How do opioids affect the bowel?

Opioids are a major cause of cancer-related constipation. Opioid-induced constipation is thought to be dose-related, but variability among patients is considerable. Opioids affect the bowel by activation of specific opioid receptors in both the GI tract and central nervous system. Activation of these receptors results in increased tone and nonpropulsive motility in the ileum and colon, re- sulting in increased transit time and water absorption. Difficult passage of hard dry stool is the end result. Morphine-induced insensitivity to rectal distention further contributes to slowed defecation.

16. How is opioid-induced constipation managed?

The key point is prevention. To prevent opioid-induced constipation, many protocols or algo- rithms use Senokot-S in dose ranges of 1–4 tablets orally at bedtime or twice daily, with individual titration. Oral naloxone continues to be studied as a means to reverse opioid-induced constipation; however, patients need to be monitored for signs of opioid withdrawal and increased pain.

17. Do patients develop a tolerance to the constipating effects of opioids?

Tolerance to this side effect of opioids develops extremely slowly, if at all. It is not uncom- mon for patients to require laxative therapy for as long as they are taking opioids.

18. Why are combination laxatives, such as Senokot-S or Peri-Colace, better than Colace alone for opioid-induced constipation?

Colace softens the stool but usually does not provide the peristaltic stimulation needed to counteract opioid-induced constipation. By combining the softening action of docusate with the peristaltic stimulant effect of the anthraquinone derivatives (e.g., senna concentrate, casanthra- nol), success in managing opioid-induced constipation may be achieved. Patients need to be in- structed to consume adequate amounts of fluids while using these medications. Examples of combination medications include the following:

Senokot-S = senna concentrate and docusate sodium

Peri-Colace = casanthranol and docusate sodium

The following formula is useful for the prevention of opioid-induced constipation:

1 Senokot tablet + 100-mg tablet of Colace per 30-mg tablet of MS Contin

Titrate to effect.

19. Other than opioids, what medications cause constipation?

Numerous medications contribute to constipation. Unfortunately, patients frequently take more than one at a time, further compounding the problem:

- Chemotherapy (vinca alkaloids, cisplatin, etoposide)
- Antiemetics (serotonin antagonists, phenothiazines)
- Anticonvulsants
- Anticholinergics
- Tricyclic antidepressants
- Diuretics
- Calcium channel blockers
- Antiparkinsonian agents
- Iron supplements

20. How do the vinca alkaloids cause constipation?

Vincristine may damage the myenteric plexus of the colon. Severe constipation may occur in up to 35% of patients. It is more common in elderly patients and may lead to bowel obstruction. Constipation has been reported in 20% of patients receiving vinblastine, especially in high doses or with prolonged treatment. Both vincristine and vinblastine may cause neurotoxicity of smooth muscles of the gastrointestinal tract, which may lead to decreased peristalsis or paralytic ileus. The bowel effects of vinca alkaloids may be unaccompanied by peripheral nerve dysfunction. Vinorelbine causes mild-to-moderate constipation with an overall incidence of 34%. Combinations of a laxative and stool softener may be used prophylactically with the vinca alkaloids to avoid constipation.

21. How should constipation be managed in neutropenic or thrombocytopenic patients?

Constipation in neutropenic or thrombocytopenic patients requires an increase in fluids and fiber and management with oral medications. Avoid manipulation (rectal exams, suppositories, enemas) of the anus or stoma in neutropenic patients, because it may lead to anal fissures or abscesses, which serve as a portal of entry for infection. Manipulation also may put the thrombocytopenic patient at risk for bleeding. If the anal area must be manipulated, it should be done gently, using a generous amount of lubricant. The use of suppositories or enemas is contraindicated.

22. What is the origin of laxative misuse?

The belief that one needs to have a "normal" number of bowel movements per day, as well as the myth that laxatives "cleanse the blood" or eliminate "corrupt humors" from absorbed colonic contents, has led to the steady sales of laxative agents. However, as long as the liver is functioning properly, intoxication does not result from intestinal contents. The use of bulk substances as a supplement to low-residue diets is not a problem. However, chronic use of irritant purgatives or cathartics may be dangerous because of potentially serious electrolyte imbalances (e.g., hypokalemia resulting in cardiac arrhythmias).

23. Discuss the physiologic and psychological bases of laxative dependence.

The natural defecation reflex, which empties the large bowel from the descending colon downward, is triggered when the sigmoid colon and rectum are full. The reflex is not triggered again until the colon segments are refilled. Unlike the natural reflex, large-bowel irritant purgatives (anthraquinone derivatives such as senna and diphenylmethane derivatives such as bisacodyl and phenolphthalein) clear the entire colon. As a result, the interval to refill the sigmoid colon and rectum lengthens; in this interval, patients become concerned that they are constipated and believe they need the assistance of a laxative to move their bowels. Thus, they use the laxative repeatedly; repeated use continues to empty the entire colon; and a vicious cycle begins. It is important to instruct patients to expect a "compensatory pause" after discontinuing laxative therapy. In addition, an actual physiologic bowel inertia may result from laxative-induced hypokalemia, leading the person to mistake decreased peristalsis for constipation and to reinitiate laxative therapy.

24. What factors place a patient at risk for high impaction?

Patients with a poor appetite who do not consume adequate food and fluids are at risk for high impaction of the transverse colon.

25. How does the assessment of high impaction differ from that of low impaction?

A thorough history of the patient's current elimination pattern is the most critical indicator of any bowel problem. A digital exam is helpful to detect stool for a low impaction; however, abdominal palpation is better for revealing stool in the upper parts of the colon. (Radiographs can be ordered to differentiate mechanical obstruction from high impaction). A high impaction is likely if the patient reports little fluid intake, anorexia, and no bowel movement for 5–10 days.

26. Describe the treatment for low impaction.

To promote comfort prior to treatment, the patient should be instructed to lie down and to avoid drinking hot fluids or eating which could stimulate peristalsis. To relieve a low impaction, administer an oil retention enema and follow with a manual disimpaction. If a large amount of stool is present, administer a saline-type cathartic (e.g. lactulose) orally along with a low-volume (300 ml) milk and molasses enema every 6 hours until no more stool is obtained.

27. How can high impactions be cleared?

High impactions need to be cleared with oral laxatives (e.g. lactulose) followed by enemas (e.g., low-volume milk and molasses). In administering the enema, it is important to gently introduce the enema tube approximately 12 inches into the colon to reach the stool. **Caution:** Do *not* advance tube beyond resistance. Start administration of enema and release the enema after withdrawing the enema tube ¼ inch from the point of resistance. The lactulose and enema can be repeated every 4–6 hours in the hospital (every 6 hours in the home setting) until the large bowel is completely cleared. **Note:** Patients are predisposed to developing another impaction if enemas are stopped too soon and a lot of stool is left in the colon. Magnesium citrate also can be used to treat a high impaction if the patient is able to tolerate a large volume of fluid and does not have cancer in the trunk of the body.

28. What is the safest way to treat impaction?

The first step in treatment for impaction is softening the stool so that it can be gently removed or passed. Enemas (e.g., oil retention or tap water) or glycerin suppositories assist in lubrication of bowel and softening of stool. Laxatives that stimulate the bowel or cause cramping should be avoided to prevent further damage to the bowel wall. Digital disimpaction, if needed, is best done after lubrication with an enema or glycerin suppository. Because of the discomfort associated with disimpaction, some form of analgesia is recommended before the procedure; a light sedative may be indicated as well.

29. What types of enemas can be used safely in patients with cancer?

Enemas tend to be used for the management of acute constipation or fecal impaction. Use caution in administering enemas because they may place the patient at risk for bowel perforation due to previous bowel wall irritation from impaction and electrolyte imbalance, particularly in the setting of renal failure. Commonly recommended enemas include the following:

1. Tap water or saline enemas
2. Water-soluble lubricant enema. Fill a 60-ml syringe with water-soluble lubricant (Surgilube), replace plunger, and attach rectal tube to syringe. Lubricate tip of tube and place tip inside rectum. Slowly inject, as for retention enema. Retain for one-half hour.
3. Milk and molasses enema
   - To 1 liter of warm water, add 1 cup of powdered milk and 1 cup of molasses or corn syrup.
   or
   - Put 8 oz of warm water and 3 oz of powdered milk into a plastic jar. Close the jar and shake until the water and milk appear to be fully mixed.
   - Add 4.5 oz of molasses, and shake the jar again until the mixture appears to have an even color throughout.

• Pour the mixture into enema bag. Administer the enema high by gently introducing the tube about 12 inches into the rectum. Do not push beyond resistance. Repeat every 6 hours until good results are achieved.

From Bisanz A: Managing bowel elimination problems in patients with cancer. Oncol Nurs Forum 24:683, 1997, with permission.

30. What types of enemas should be avoided?

Fleet enemas are reported to cause tissue necrosis and are not safe in patients with renal or cardiac disease.

Soap suds enemas are no longer used because of the risk of acute colitis (usually self-limiting). More serious potential complications include anaphylaxis, hemorrhage, and rectal gangrene.

31. When is bowel training of use in patients with cancer?

The goal of bowel training is to empty the contents of the large bowel at predictable times every day. This strategy can be effective for cancer patients who are undergoing a rehabilitation program and able to consume adequate food and fluids (i.e., three good-sized meals per day, 30–40 grams of fiber, and 2 quarts of fluids).

32. Describe an appropriate bowel training regimen.

The following regimen requires clearance of the gastrointestinal tract of all stool 3 days before beginning the program. Training to control diarrhea requires that stool be firm. Before initiating the program, it is important to teach sphincter-strengthening exercises to patients with anal sphincter control problems. If dietary intake decreases to one-third of the usual amount, a bowel movement can occur every 3 days without problems. If the diet decreases by one-half of the normal amount, a bowel movement can be expected every other day. If there is no bowel movement in 3 days, intervene to induce defecation.

Generic Bowel Training Program
• Drink 2–4 ounces of prune juice before the meal of choice.
• Eat a big meal (including fruits, vegetables, proteins, fat).
• Drink a hot liquid.
• Insert a bisacodyl suppository. After 2 weeks, substitute a glycerin suppository because the body may not need the stimulative laxative and will respond to the stimulus of the prune juice, big meal, and hot liquid. If the patient does not have a bowel movement with the glycerin suppository, return to the use of a bisacodyl suppository for 1 more week. Then try the glycerin suppository again.

Modifications

If constipation continues, alter the above program to meet individual needs. Make *one* change at a time and continue it for 3 days to determine response:
• Add stool softeners (titrate up to 8 per day).
• Eat 5 prunes at bedtime.
• Increase the fluid intake (titrate slowly upward to need).
• Gradually increase the fiber content of the diet over a period of time (titrate upward to need). If fiber is increased too quickly, cramping and diarrhea can occur.
• Increase physical activity if patient is not active.

For diarrhea or extra stools:
• Decrease the amount of prune juice.
• Cut the bisacodyl suppository in half, and insert only one half of the suppository.

For anal sphincter problems:
• For a tight sphincter, teach the patient to put on a rubber glove and massage around the anal opening to relax the sphincter muscle for easy passage of stool.
• For a weak sphincter, exercises can be prescribed and taught by the nurse:
  1. Tighten the buttock muscles (as if to hold back a bowel movement), hold 5–10 seconds, and release (count one-one thousand, two-one thousand, etc., up to 10-one thousand).
  2. Note the difference between tension and relaxation.
  3. Do 10 repetitions 4 times/day.

If the patient has a problem having stools after every meal and not just the meal chosen for bowel training:

- Start the patient on psyllium, administering 1 teaspoon twice daily, and titrate upward to the amount needed based on individual outcomes.
- Gradually increase the dose by 1 teaspoon every third to fifth day. Rapid increases of fiber can cause cramping and bloating.
- When taking psyllium for diarrhea, do not take fluid as prescribed for constipation.

From Bisanz A: Managing bowel elimination problems in patients with cancer. Oncol Nurs Forum 24:685, 1997, with permission.

REFERENCES

1. Bisanz A: Managing bowel elimination problems in patients with cancer. Oncol Nurs Forum 24:679–688, 1997.
2. Curtiss CP: Constipation. In Groenwald SL, Frogge MH, Goodman M, Yarbro CH (eds): Cancer Symptom Control. Boston, Jones & Bartlett, 1996, pp 484–497.
3. Lacy C, Armstrong LL, Ingrim N, Lance LL: Drug Information Handbook, 3rd ed. Hudson, OH, Lexi-Comp Inc., 1995.
4. Levy M: Constipation and diarrhea in cancer patients. Cancer Bull 43:412–422, 1991.
5. Lin EM: Constipation. In Yasko JM (ed): Nursing Management of Symptoms Associated with Chemotherapy, 4th ed. Philadelphia, Meniscus Health Care Communications, Division of Meniscus Limited, 1998, pp 89–93.
6. Lullman H, Mohr K, Ziegler A, Bieger D: Pocket Atlas of Pharmacology. New York, Thieme, 1993.
7. Portenoy R: Constipation in the cancer patient: Causes and management. Med Clin North Am 71:303–311, 1987.
8. Robinson CB, et al: Development of a protocol to prevent opioid-induced constipation in patients with cancer: a research utilization project. Clin J Oncol Nurs 4:79–84, 2000.
9. Storey P: Primer of Palliative Care. Gainesville, FL, Academy of Hospice Physicians, 1994.
10. Yakabowich M: Prescribe with care: The role of laxatives in the treatment of constipation. J Gerontol Nurs 6(7):4–11, 1990.

38. CANCER-RELATED DIARRHEA

Leslie Tuchmann, RN, MS, HNC, and Constance Engelking, RN, MS, OCN

1. How prevalent is diarrhea in patients with cancer?

Diarrhea related to cancer and/or its treatment occurs in 6% of hospitalized patients with cancer. Cancer-related diarrhea occurs in up to 10% of patients with advanced cancer, 20–49% of patients undergoing abdominopelvic irradiation, 50–87% of patients receiving fluoropyrimidines (e.g., 5-fluorouracil [5FU]) and topoisomerase inhibitors (e.g., irinotecan), 43% of patients undergoing bone marrow transplant, and 80% of patients with carcinoid tumors. Diarrhea is also problematic for a significant number of patients receiving nasogastric feedings, high-osmolar compounds, and antibiotic therapy. As newer antineoplastic agents and higher dosages of drugs and radiation therapy are introduced into treatment regimens, it is anticipated that the number of patients experiencing diarrhea will increase.

2. Describe the impact of diarrhea on patients with cancer.

Diarrhea results in increased morbidity and can be life-threatening as a result of secondary dehydration, metabolic disturbances, infection, and malnutrition. Diarrhea can exert a negative effect on treatment outcomes by necessitating dose reductions and treatment delays, thus limiting the total therapy that patients are able to receive. In one study of 100 patients with colorectal cancer, 56% required modification of the therapeutic regimen and 37% required additional health care resources, including emergency room care (14%), hospitalization (23%), and intravenous fluids (21%). Unfortunately, underreporting by many patients who are worried that the diarrhea will cause their oncologist to stop "life-saving" treatment often leads to more severe diarrhea because of undertreatment. Conversely, when diarrhea has a significant negative effect on quality of life, some patients or their physicians choose to abort anticancer therapy all together. Quality-of-life consequences of diarrhea include irregular sleep patterns, fatigue and discomfort, reduction in performance, disturbance in interpersonal relationships and socialization, altered self-image, travel restrictions, absenteeism from work, hospitalization, and increased family/caregiver burden.

3. How is diarrhea defined and recognized?

Diarrhea is an increase in the liquidity (> 300 ml of stool/day) and frequency (passage of > 3 stools/day). Especially high volumes of stool output, up to 8–10 L/day, may occur in bone marrow transplant patients with graft-vs.-host disease (GVHD). Diarrhea can be acute, with sudden onset and duration of 7–14 days, or chronic, persisting beyond 2 weeks despite treatment. Taking patient variation into consideration, it has been suggested that the definition of diarrhea should indicate that increases in stool loss must be of a sufficient magnitude to constitute a change in the patient's established bowel pattern. Unless the patient is hospitalized, clinicians identify diarrhea by patient self-report. Patients often do not report or underreport diarrhea, because they do not recognize it as a significant symptom, they are worried that treatment will be discontinued, or they plan to self-manage with over-the-counter medications and home remedies. Uncontrolled diarrhea can result in signs of volume depletion (e.g., orthostatic hypotension, decreased skin turgor, dry mouth), significant losses of potassium and bicarbonate, and perianal irritation. Early identification of diarrhea is facilitated when clinicians are aware of patients' risk for the development of diarrhea and ask direct, detailed questions about bowel function during assessment.

4. What pathophysiologic mechanisms produce diarrhea?

The pathophysiology of diarrhea is related to fluid movement, decreased absorption, and/or increased secretion. Balanced transport of intestinal fluid and electrolytes in the bowel is the result of two principal mechanisms: (1) secretion, which is believed to take place in the crypt cells, and (2) absorption, which occurs in the enterocytes lining the wall of the GI villi. Diarrhea occurs when an irregularity in one or both mechanisms disrupts the balance between intestinal secretion and absorption to the extent that the total secretion of fluid and electrolytes overwhelms the absorptive capacity of the bowel. These processes are influenced by a number of mechanical and biochemical factors. Increased secretion may occur in response to the release of endogenous secretagogues (inflammatory mediators, neurotransmitters) and bacterial endotoxins, which overstimulate ion transport processes. Decreased absorption results from defects in villus absorptive processes (e.g., reduced numbers of villi secondary to bowel surgery), osmotically active agents are in the lumen of the bowel (e.g., blood from intestinal hemorrhage, enteral feeding solutions), or intestinal motility is increased. (See table for types of diarrhea and specific causes.)

Pathophysiologic Mechanisms, Causes, and Clinical Manifestations of Cancer-related Diarrhea

TYPE	PATHOPHYSIOLOGIC MECHANISMS	CAUSES	CLINCAL MANIFESTATIONS
Osmotic	Mechanical disturbance. Characterized by large-volume influx of fluid and electrolytes into intestinal lumen that overwhelms absorptive capacity of bowel. Osmotic forces responsible for drawing substrates across the intestinal epithelium are interrupted by direct contact with hyperosmolar stimuli.	Ingestion of hyperosmolar preparations and substances • Nonabsorbable solutes (e.g., sorbitol, magnesium-based antacids) • Enteral feeding solutions Intestinal hemorrhage • Intraluminal blood acts as osmotic substance	Large-volume, watery stools that resolve with withdrawal of causative agent
Malabsorptive	Combined disturbance of mechanical and biochemical mechanisms responsible for maintaining absorptive processes. Secondary to factors that alter luminal and mucosal integrity and nature. Reduction in available mucosa or membrane permeability disrupts enterohepatic circulation of bile salts; unabsorbed osmotically active substances then can enter colon, exerting direct bowel stimulatory effects.	Enzyme deficiencies that prevent complete digestion of fats • Lactose intolerance • Pancreatic insufficiency due to obstruction by cancer or pancreatectomy Morphologic/structural changes resulting in decreased absorptive capacity • Surgical resection of intestine Mucosal changes that alter membrane permeability	Large-volume, foul-smelling steatorrhea-type stools
Exudative	Characterized by discharge of mucus, serum protein, blood into bowel. Results from inflammation, ulceration of bowel mucosa.	Radiation to bowel mucosa: incidence and severity are dose-dependent. Acute effects are caused by depletion of crypt stem cells. Late or chronic radiation enteritis secondary to mucosal atrophy and fibrosis	Variable volume (< 1000 ml/day) but high frequency stools (> 6 stools/day); associated with hypoalbuminemia, anemia from cumulative protein, blood loss
Secretory	Primarily biomechanical disturbance with mechanical responses Characterized by intestinal hypersecretion stimulated by an array of endogenous mediators that exert primary effect on intestinal transport of water and electrolytes, resulting in accumulation of intestinal fluids.	Endocrine tumors can produce excessive quantities of peptide secretagogues • VIPoma, carcinoid, gastrinoma, insulinoma, glucagonoma Enterotoxin-producing pathogens irritate bowel wall, stimulating intestinal secretion. Associated with antibiotic-induced change in microbial flora that permits growth of *C. difficile*.	Large-volume, watery stools (> 1000 ml/day) that persist despite fasting; osmolality equals plasma concentration.

Table continued on following page

Pathophysiologic Mechanisms, Causes, and Clinical Manifestations
of Cancer-related Diarrhea (Continued)

TYPE	PATHOPHYSIOLOGIC MECHANISMS	CAUSES	CLINCAL MANIFESTATIONS
Dysmotility-associated	Mechanical disturbances characterized by deranged intestinal motility resulting in rapid transit of stool through small/large intestine Peristaltic dysfunction (enhancement of suppression) in response to alterations in variety of mechanical stretch or neural stimuli	Clinical problems (e.g., irritable bowel syndrome, narcotic withdrawal syndrome) External factors such as ingestion of peristaltic stimulants (food, fluid, or medication) or psychoneuroimmunologic effects of stress, anxiety, and fear	Frequent small, semi-solid/liquid stools of variable volume and frequency
Chemotherapy-induced	Combined mechanical and biochemical disturbances stimulated by chemotherapeutic effects on bowel mucosa Characterized by cascade of events: mitotic arrest of intestinal epithelial crypt cells followed by superficial necrosis and extensive inflammation of bowel wall; resulting in production of mucosal, submucosal factors (luekotrienes, cytokines, free radicals) that subsequently stimulate oversecretion of intestinal water and electrolytes Destruction of brush border enzymes responsible for carbohydrate and protein digestion further adds to excessive gut-wall secretion.	Chemotherapy-induced gut wall toxicity. Although many agents are associated with diarrhea, most common include • Fluoropyrimidines (e.g., 5-fluorouracil) • Topoisomerase inhibitors (e.g., CPT-11)	Frequent watery to semisolid stools; onset occurs within 24–96 hours after chemotherapy administration

From Rutledge DN, Engelking C: Cancer-related diarrhea: Selected findings of a national survey of oncology nurse experiences. Oncol Nurs Forum 25:862, 1998, with permission.

5. What pharmacologic agents are most often associated with diarrhea in patients with cancer?

The onset, severity, and duration of diarrhea depend on many factors, including the specific agents, whether they are used in combination with other diarrhea-producing drugs or therapies (such as combination chemo- and biotherapy regimens or abdominopelvic radiation therapy), dosage, and schedule of administration.

Chemotherapeutic agents associated with the highest risk for diarrhea are 5FU (especially in high doses or in combination with leucovorin, methotrexate, or interferon), actinomycin D, the topoisomerase inhibitors (irinotecan, topotecan), paclitaxel (Taxol), and high doses of cisplatin or cyclophosphamide. 5FU administered in lower doses as a continuous infusion is associated with a lower incidence of diarrhea than higher doses administered as a weekly bolus. Other agents that cause diarrhea (> 10%) are fludarabine, cytarabine, idarubicin, mithramycin, mitoxantrone, pentostatin, and floxuridine. Diarrhea occurring with administration of 5FU and floxuridine is a sign of toxicity. The standard of care to permit resolution of diarrhea is the temporary discontinuaton of these drugs. With other agents, dose reduction on subsequent cycles or discontinuation may be indicated, depending on the chemotherapy schedule and severity of the patient's diarrhea.

Biotherapy drugs: interleukin-2, interleukin-4, and interferons.

Others: antibiotics, selected cytoprotectants (e.g., mesna), and antiemetics (e.g., metoclopramide). Opiate withdrawal and the overuse of laxatives are also implicated.

6. What is the unique diarrhea-producing mechanism associated with irinotecan? How is it best managed?

Irinotecan produces both an early-onset cholinergic syndrome (during or within 24 hours of drug administration) and late-onset diarrhea (2 –10 days after drug administration). The early-onset cholinergic syndrome is an infrequent response in which diarrhea is generally a sudden occurrence accompanying an array of other symptoms (e.g., abdominal cramping, diaphoresis, flushing, salivation, nasal congestion, rhinorrhea). This effect resolves readily with atropine, 0.25–1.0 mg intravenously or subcutaneously, but requires close patient monitoring.

Late-onset diarrhea occurs most commonly during the second week after treatment with a median duration of 3 days. It may be severe (grades 3 or 4) and last up to 7 days. The more commonly occurring late-onset diarrhea may be related to the accumulation and deconjugation of SN-38 (the active metabolite of irinotecan) in the intestine and its damaging effect on the mucosa. The management of late-onset diarrhea involves recognition of high-risk patients and prophylaxis. Before drug administration patients should be taught to self-administer high-dose loperamide, beginning with a loading dose of 4 mg orally followed by 2 mg at 4-hour intervals.

7. What condition should be ruled out when acute severe diarrhea occurs unexpectedly after administration of the first few doses of 5FU?

Dihydropyrimidine dehydrogenase (DPD) deficiency should be suspected when patients experience sudden onset of diarrhea accompanied by significant mucositis and myelosuppression, This occurs in approximately 3% of adult patients with cancer. DPD is the rate-limiting enzyme that allows clearance of 5FU. Patients who have DPD congenital deficiencies are at risk for severe adverse drug reactions after exposure to 5FU. Recognition of this pharmacogenetic syndrome is essential to prevent the risk of severe and potentially fatal reactions to fluoropyrimidine therapy, such as cerebellar ataxia, encephalopathy, and coma.

8. What specific mechanisms are associated with radiation-induced diarrhea? How does it typically present?

Abdominopelvic, lower thoracic, and lumbar radiation can result in mild-to-severe diarrhea, depending on dose, schedule, and volume of bowel included in the radiation field. Radiation causes inflammation, ulceration, and sloughing of intestinal epithelium, thus shortening the intestinal villi and reducing the functional mucosal surface necessary for the adequate transport of fluids and electrolytes. In addition, lactase, the enzyme necessary for disaccharide digestion, may be decreased or absent, and patients may become lactose-intolerant. Nonabsorbable lactose in the small intestine causes an osmotic fluid shift that results in accelerated movement of contents and cramping abdominal pain. A lactose-free diet may be recommended, but once healing has occurred, the patient may return to a normal diet. Acute enteropathy due to crypt stem cell depletion is an immediate response (within 1–3 weeks) that develops frequently in patients receiving a dose of 45 Gy or greater. In contrast, chronic radiation enteritis, which occurs in 5–15% of patients undergoing abdominopelvic radiation, has an onset of at least 6–12 months or up to years after radiation and results from mucosal atrophy and fibrosis secondary to damaged endothelial cells in the blood vessels and connective tissues. Ischemic enteritis may result from chronic radiotherapy, but this complication is rare with current radiation techniques.

9. What is *Clostridium difficile* diarrhea?

C. difficile diarrhea is an example of infection-induced diarrhea and should be suspected after any antibiotic therapy, particularly ampicillin, cephalosporins, and clindamycin. *C. difficile* makes enterotoxins that produce watery diarrhea associated with pseudomembranous colitis; symptoms range from mild diarrhea to life-threatening illness. *C. difficile* causes > 50% of nosocomial infectious diarrhea. After a patient has tested positive for *C. difficile* and toxin A, precautions should be taken to prevent nosocomial transmission. An important point in treating infectious diarrhea is to avoid anticholinergic agents or opiates because they slow peristalsis and inhibit elimination of toxins from the gastrointestinal system, causing prolonged and severe symptoms. *C. difficile* diarrhea usually is treated with metronidazole or oral vancomycin.

10. What factors in the patient history are important in the assessment of diarrhea?

Usual bowel pattern. Ask patients to describe their normal bowel elimination pattern, including consistency and number of stools per day or week.

Tumor type, location, and extent of disease. Some malignant diseases, such as carcinoid and VIPoma, are specifically associated with diarrhea. Others, such as colorectal and pancreatic cancers, can produce diarrhea as secondary effects.

Coexisting conditions and treatments. Ascertain whether the patient is receiving abdominopelvic radiation therapy or has a history of bowel resection (with or without diversion), irritable or inflammatory bowel syndrome, or other conditions (e.g., neurologic disorder, malnutrition) that may result in or intensify diarrhea.

Medications. Be alert for antibiotics (especially ampicillin, clindamycin, and broad-spectrum antibiotics) that alter normal gastrointestinal flora or inflame the intestinal mucosa, antacids (especially magnesium-containing compounds), antihypertensives, potassium supplements, diuretics, caffeine, theophylline, NSAIDs, antiarrhythmic drugs, and selected chemotherapeutic agents. Other medication-related causes include overuse of laxatives and opioid withdrawal. The temporal relationship of onset and duration of diarrhea to initiation or discontinuation of chemo- and radiotherapy helps to distinguish whether the diarrhea is a response to treatment or due to some other cause.

Dietary pattern. Establish current diet and volume of daily fluid intake. Assess for change in diet habits or pattern, food allergies, or lactose intolerance, and determine consumption of alcohol and sorbitol-based products. Also query the patient about weight trends during the previous few weeks to a month.

Other factors. Determine whether the patient has traveled during the past year, whether family members are experiencing diarrhea, and how diarrhea is typically self-managed at home.

11. What factors in the physical examination are important in the assessment of diarrhea?

Presenting signs and symptoms. Ask patients to describe recent changes and current bowel pattern, including stool character (consistency, color, odor), volume, frequency and associated symptoms (e.g., pain, cramping, flatulence). Visually inspect stool for evidence of blood, pus, or mucous. Patient weight is particularly important when quantification of stool volume is difficult. The presence of fever and bloody diarrhea may point to an infectious cause.

Abdominorectal evaluation. Auscultate for hyperactive or absent bowel sounds, and perform abdominal palpation. A rectal examination also may be indicated to rule out fecal impaction. In patients with stool incontinence or severe diarrhea, inspect anal and peristomal areas for impaired skin integrity.

Hydration status. Assess objective measures of hydration, including thirst level, vein filling and emptying times, skin turgor and resiliency, degree of mucosal moisture (conjunctiva, lips, tongue, oral mucosa), vital signs, intake and output, urine specific gravity and osmolality. Note indicators of dehydration and electrolyte imbalances (e.g. poor skin turgor, dry mucosal surfaces, periorbital edema, highly concentrated urine, changes in mentation, weight loss exceeding 2 lbs/day, tachycardia, and orthostatic blood pressure changes with accompanying vertigo and weakness.

12. What laboratory analyses help in the assessment of diarrhea?

- Serum chemistries help to establish electrolyte abnormalities and the presence of protein/calorie malnutrition (e.g., hypoalbuminemia).
- Complete blood counts provide clues as to whether infection may be responsible.
- To rule out infection, obtain stool cultures for enteric pathogens, including *Shigella, Campylobacter,* and *Salmonella* spp. A stool sample for *C. difficile* is recommended along with samples for ova and parasites. Obtain tests for viral agents (adenoviral, rotaviral coxsackie viruses), particularly in patients with bone marrow transplant.
- Obtain 5-HIAA (serotonin metabolite) when carcinoid is suspected.
- Radiographic evaluation with contrast, endoscopic exploration, and biopsy are reserved for persistent diarrhea that is refractory to intervention or for ruling out conditions requiring tissue diagnosis.

13. What assessment instruments are used most often to evaluate the severity of diarrhea and its impact on quality of life.

Grading the severity of diarrhea and its accompanying symptoms with a standardized format is essential to selecting and modifying the management plan appropriately and to communicating accurate information to other health care providers involved in the care of the patient. Among the number of available assessment tools, the National Cancer Institute (NCI) Common Toxicity Criteria for Grading Severity of Diarrhea is one of the most commonly used tools in the clinical setting. This four-point grading scale measures loose stools per day and accompanying symptoms. Special criteria that consider liquid stools associated with colostomy, GVHD in bone marrow transplant recipients, and pediatric patients are included in the latest revision. The FACT-D (Functional Assesment of Cancer Therapy–Diarrhea)[3] measures quality-of-life dimensions.

14. Summarize the NCI criteria.

National Cancer Institute's Toxicity Criteria for Grading the Severity of Diarrhea

TOXICITY	GRADE 0	GRADE 1	GRADE 2	GRADE 3	GRADE 4
Patients without colostomy	None	Increase of < 4 stools/day over pre-treatment	Increase of 4–6 stools/day or nocturnal stools	Increase of ≥ 7 stools/day or incontinence; or need for parenteral support for dehydration	Physiologic consequences requiring intensive care; or hemodynamic collapse
Patients with colostomy	None	Mild increase in loose, watery colostomy output compared with pretreatment	Moderate increase in loose, watery colostomy output compared with pretreatment, but not interfering with normal activity	Severe increase in loose, watery colostomy output compared with pretreatment, interfering with normal activity	Physiologic consequences requiring intensive care; or hemodynamic collapse
For BMT*	None	> 500 to ≤ 1000 ml of diarrhea/day	> 1000 to ≤ 1500 ml of diarrhea/day	> 1500 ml of diarrhea/day	Severe abdominal pain with or without ileus
For pediatric BMT*		> 5 to ≤ 10 ml/kg of diarrhea/day	> 10 to ≤ 15 ml/kg of diarrhea/day	> 15 ml/kg of diarrhea/day	

BMT = bone marrow transplant.
* Also consider hemorrhage/bleeding with grade 3 or 4 thrombocytopenia, hemorrhage/bleeding without grade 3 or 4 thrombocytopenia, pain, dehydration, hypotension.
Reprinted by permission of Elsevier Science from Kornblau S, Benson AB III, Catalano R, et al: Management of cancer treatment-related diarrhea: Issues and therapeutic strategies. J Pain Symptom Manage 19:118–129, 2000.

15. What are key considerations in constructing the diarrhea management plan?

Critical elements of the diarrhea management plan are identification and elimination of the causative factor. The primary goals in managing diarrhea are to restore and maintain (1) the patient's normal bowel pattern, (2) fluid and electrolyte balance, (3) skin integrity, and (4) comfort and dignity. CID is managed by the selection and combination of pharmacologic and nonpharmacologic interventions that best meet the patient's specific needs and clinical picture.

16. What guidelines are available to manage noninfectious CID?

A clinical treatment algorithm representing "best practice" pharmacologic management of chemotherapy-induced diarrhea was developed by a consortium of physician, nurse, and pharmacy experts (see figure on pages 317 and 318).

17. What drugs are available for management of noninfectious CID?

Although traditional agents may still be used for selected patients, many are being replaced with antidiarrheal drugs that have demonstrated superiority, enhanced tolerability, and lower side effect profiles. For example, the absorbent and adsorbent agents, such as kaolin and pectate, and psyllium derivatives are less commonly used because they are difficult for patients to ingest; create uncomfortable bloating sensations; and have limited efficacy in controlling persistent and moderate-to-severe diarrhea in patients with cancer. Anticholinergics tend to be avoided because of unpleasant drug side effects that may overlap with disease and treatment-induced symptoms, such as drying of mucosal membranes, blurred vision, and urinary retention. Newer agents with broader mechanisms of action are available for diarrhea refractory to conventional approaches or associated with hypersecretory malignancies (i.e., carcinoid or VIPoma).

18. What is the gold standard for managing CID?

The drugs of choice and most commonly used opioid preparations for CID management are diphenoxylate with atropine (Lomotil) and loperamide (Imodium) because they are effective oral preparations with relatively limited side-effect profiles when administered appropriately. Several studies indicate that of the two choices, loperamide is the superior antidiarrheal agent in both efficacy and tolerability for patients with noninfectious diarrhea.

19. What is octreotide?

Octreotide is a synthetic hormone analog that exerts direct action on epithelial cells to suppress gastroenteropancreatic secretion, slow gastric emptying, prolong intestinal transit time, decrease mesenteric blood flow, and stimulate sodium and chloride absorption. Octreotide is available as subcutaneous injection administered 2 or 3 times/day (Sandostatin injection) and as a long-acting depot (Sandostatin LAR Depot) preparation administered as a single monthly intramuscular injection. Octreotide SC dosing begins at 150 μg 3 times/day and can be titrated in increments of 50–100 μg every 8 hours to doses as high as 2500 μg. The effects of octreotide are seen after about 6 hours for the subcutaneous injection and about 11 days for the depot preparation. It may be necessary to hold octreotide if an assessment reveals absence of bowel tones because ileus may occur as a side effect. To avoid constipation and ileus, octreotide should be discontinued as soon as diarrhea resolves.

20. What drugs are currently under investigation for diarrhea management?

Alternative agents under investigation include alpha$_2$-adrenoreceptor agonists (e.g., clonidine), corticosteroids, nonsteroidal anti-inflammatory agents, serotonin antagonists, calcium channel blockers, and leukotriene synthesis inhibitors. Octreotide administration in high dosages (> 500 μg) by continuous intravenous infusion is under study in bone marrow transplant recipients to manage GVHD-induced diarrhea. Octreotide LAR depot preparation is being evaluated as a prophylactic agent in selected subpopulations. Strategies such as pretreatment with sucralfate as a mucosal protectant, cholestyramine to bind bile acids, and glutathione to bind free radicals released as a treatment-induced tissue effect, are under evaluation to prevent and minimize radiation-induced diarrhea.

21. What interventions can help to maintain skin integrity in patients with diarrhea?

Meticulous attention to skin integrity is essential to prevent infection, maintain patient comfort, and preserve dignity. Watery stool contains bile, enzymes, and frequently blood, all of which contribute to skin irritation and breakdown. The following tips should be taught to patients and caregivers to ensure proper care of the skin and mucous membranes:

1. To minimize risk of infection and enhance patient comfort, wash or instruct the patient to wash perineal and rectal areas after each bowel movement with mild soap and water. Rinse well, and pat dry with a soft towel.

2. To minimize risk for skin irritation and breakdown, apply a topical moisture-barrier cream (e.g., A&D ointment, zinc oxide) to promote skin healing. For patients with moderate-to-severe diarrhea, cream should be applied at least $\frac{1}{4}$-inch thick to provide adequate protection against enzymatic activity.

First Report of Diarrhea to Clinician

Evaluate condition of patient

1. Obtain history of onset and duration of diarrhrea.
2. Description of number of stools and composition (e.g., watery, blood in stool).
3. Assess patient for fever, dizziness, abdominal pain, weakness (i.e., rule out risk for sepsis, bowel obstruction, dehydration).
4. Medications profile (to identify diarrheogenic agents).
5. Dietary profile (to identify diarrhera-inducing foods).

Management

1. Stop all lactose-containing products, alcohol, and supplements.
2. Drink combination of 8–10 large glasses of clear liquid per day (water, Gatorade, broth).
3. Eat frequent small meals (bananas, white rice, applesauce, toast, plain pasta).
4. Instruct patient to record the number/volume of stools and report symptoms of life-threatening sequelae.

Treatment

1. Administer standard dose of loperamide: initial dose of 4 mg followed by 2 mg every 4 hours or after every unformed stool.

12–24 hours later

Diarrhea resolved

1. Continue instructions for dietary modifications.
2. Gradually add solid foods to diet.
3. Discontinue loperamide after 12-hour diarrhea-free interval.

Diarrhea unresolved
(see following page)

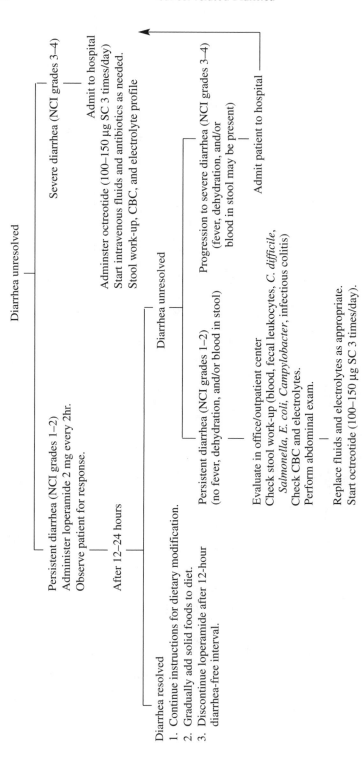

Proposed treatment guidelines for chemotherapy-induced diarrhea. (Reprinted by permission of Elsevier Science from Kornblau J, Benson AB III, Catalano R, et al: Management of cancer-related diarrhea: Issues and therapeutic strategies. J Pain Symptom Manage 19:118–129, 2000.)

Antidiarrheal Agents

DRUG AND DOSAGE	MECHANISM OF ACTION	CONTRAINDICATIONS
Opioids		
Lomotil (2.5 mg diphenoxylate with 0.025 mg atropine sulfate tablet): May load: 10 mg, then 1–2 tablets 3 or 4 times/day. Maximal dose: 20 mg/day.	*All opioids* act as agonists at opiate receptors in smooth muscle of GI tract, reducing secretion and peristalsis. Also increase ileocecal valve and anal sphincter pressure, improving continence.	*All opioids:* parasitic or bacterial infections accompanied by fever, obstructive jaundice
Loperamide: 2-mg capsules. May load: 4–8 mg orally, then 2 mg after each loose stool. Maximal dose: 16 mg/day	*Atropine* (in Lomotil) blocks muscarinic receptors, inhibiting peristalsis and reducing-gastric secretions. It is added for prevention of abuse more than treatment of diarrhea.	*Diphenoxylate* (in Lomotil): advanced liver disease (e.g., cirrhosis); may precipitate hepatic coma
Codeine: 15–60 mg orally every 4–6 hr as needed		*Lomotil and Imodium:* not recommended in children younger than 2 yr
Opium tincture (10% opium liquid: 10 mg morphine/ml with 19% alcohol): 0.3–1 ml every 2–6 hr until controlled. Maximal dose: 6 ml/24 hr		*Paregoric:* convulsive states
Paregoric (0.4 mg morphine/ml with 45% alcohol): 5–10 ml orally 1–4 times/day or 4 ml every 4 hr		
Adsorbents		
Bismuth subsalicylate (Pepto-Bismol): chewable tablets: 262 mg, and suspensions: 262 mg/15 ml or 524 mg/ 15 ml (maximal strength). Usual dose: 524 mg every 30 min up to 5 gm/day	Adsorbs (binds) toxins produced by bacteria and other GI irritants, allowing them to be inactivated or eliminated; direct antimicrobial effect on *E. coli*	Aspirin sensitivity
Kaopectate (5.85 gm kaolin and 130 mg pectin per 30 ml suspension). Usual dose: 2–6 gm every 6 hr as needed	Pectin produces a viscous colloidal solution with both adsorbent and absorbent properties	Obstructive bowel lesions Children younger than 3 yr
Cholestyramine (Questran)	Nonabsorbable resin: adsorbs bile salts/acids, which cause diarrhea by effect on large intestine; adsorbs *C. difficile* toxin.	
Anticholinergics		
Atropine *Dicyclomine* (Bentyl) *Pro-Banthine* (15 mg orally 3 or 4 times/day)	Muscarinic agonists: inhibit GI secretions and peristalsis; decrease spasm of small intestine lining	Closed angle glaucoma Prostate hypertrophy Heart disease Obstructive bowel disease
Somostatin analog		
Octreotide acetate (Sandostatin) 50–200 μg 2 or 3 times/day subcutaneously	Inhibits GI hormone secretion, thus prolonging intestinal transit time and increasing net sodium and water absorption.	

Antidiarrheal Agents (Columns continued)

ADVERSE EFFECTS	DRUG INTERACTIONS	ADMINISTRATION TIPS
Atropine (in Lomotil): limited use due to dry mouth, urinary retention, blurred vision *Imodium:* uncommon effects include cramping, gastric upset, dry mouth, skin rash, dizziness, drowsiness *All opioids:* potential constipation, abdominal and bowel distention, nausea	*Diphenoxylate* (in Lomotil), *codeine, paregoric:* potentiate CNS depressants *Diphenoxylate* (in Lomotil): increases risk of hypertension with monoamine oxidase inhibitors; increases risk of paralytic ileus with antimuscarinics	*Lomotil* favored in partial bowel obstruction due to shorter action *Atropine* useful in diarrhea associated with painful cramping *Imodium* is drug of choice for nonspecific antidiarrheal therapy; unlike codeine and diphenoxylate, it has no central opioid effect at therapeutic doses. Titrated to effect; treat overdose with naloxone. *Opium tincture* for severe diarrhea; prolonged use may result in dependence. Measured by drops; must be diluted in juice or water *Oral equianalgesic doses:* Imodium: 4 mg/day Lomotil: 10 mg/day Codeine: 200 mg/day
Impaction	Potentiates oral anticoagulants and hypoglycemics Reduces uricosuric effects of probenecid and sulfinpyrazone Decreases absorption and bioavailability of tetracyclines Can interfere with radiologic exams because it is radiopaque	Prophylaxis for traveler's diarrhea, but large doses limit utility Useful in secretory diarrhea for enterotoxic bacteria, radiotherapy, prostaglandin-secreting tumors (acts as mucosal antiprostaglandin) Indicated for mild diarrhea
May increase K^+ loss or interfere with absorption of nutrients and drugs	Decreases absorption of many drugs	Indicated for mild diarrhea
Constipation	Binds with and decreases absorption of many drugs (e.g., warfarin sodium, aspirin, thyroxin, digoxin, phenobarbital)	Helpful in radiation-induced diarrhea and ileal surgery Give with meals; use limited by taste; onset of action: 12–24 hr
Decreased memory and concentration. Drowsiness, dry mouth, urinary retention, tachycardia	Antacids interfere with absorption of these drugs	Useful in diarrhea due to peptic ulcer disease or irritable bowel syndrome and refractory diarrhea
Nausea, abdominal cramps, flatulence, steatorrhea. Biliary sludge and gallstones after 6 months. Transient deterioration in glucose tolerance at start		Useful in secretory diarrhea associated with endocrine tumors, AIDS, graft vs. host disease, GI resection, diabetes

3. To relieve pain related to inflammation, use a corticosteroid spray or cream. Suggest frequent sitz baths or bathing in a tub of warm water. A mixture of 1000 ml physiologic bicarbonate, 100 ml of diphenhydramine HCL elixir, and 1 bottle of viscous lidocaine HCL may be used in the sitz bath to relieve pain and itching every 4 hours as needed.

4. To promote healing and treat desquamation, add aluminum acetate solution (Domeboro), 1 package to 1 quart of water, to sitz bath.

5. To prevent further skin irritation, instruct patient to wear loose-fitting cotton clothing and expose affected areas to air as often as possible.

22. What dietary modifications should be recommended to patients with diarrhea?

Dietary modifications are directed at stopping or reducing the severity of diarrhea. The literature is replete with dietary recommendations, although few are evidence-based. Among the most sound recommendations are the following:

1. Change diet to low residue by avoiding foods that stimulate or irritate the GI tract:
   • Whole grain products, dried legumes, nuts, seeds, popcorn
   • Alcohol, caffeine-containing products, and tobacco
   • High-fat spreads or dressings, rich pastries, candied fruits or coconut, chocolate
   • Greasy, spicy (curry, chili powder, garlic), and fried foods
   • Raw vegetables, pickles, relishes, and other high fiber foods
2. Add foods that build stool consistency:
   • Pectin-based foods (bananas, unspiced applesauce, or peeled apples)
   • White rice, plain pasta, baked potato without the skin
3. Increase fluid intake to 3 L/day (i.e., water, weak decaffeinated tea, broths).
4. Eat food at room temperature.
5. Maintain a lactose-free diet or use lactobacillus preparations to aid digestion in lactose-intolerant patients. Patients taking oral nutritional supplements to maintain calorie and protein levels also may benefit from lactose-free preparations (e.g., Vivonex T.E.N., Osmolite). Use lactose-free isotonic (300 mOsm/kg water) enteral feeding formula with dilution to at least 75 mOsm and administer at room temperature.

Note: Patients experiencing nausea and vomiting or significant or refractory diarrhea may require parenteral replacement. Often bowel rest also is recommended to allow the GI tract to heal. Patients are then started on a liquid diet, with a gradual increase in low-residue foods as tolerated (usually proteins first, then fats).

23. Why should water or carbonated drinks not be the primary fluid replacement for patients with diarrhea? What are the better choices?

Water lacks the necessary electrolytes (e.g., potassium) and vitamins. Carbonated caffeine drinks have low electrolyte content and extremely high osmolality, which in fact may worsen acute diarrhea. Better choices for fluid and electrolyte replacement include bouillon, fruitades, cranberry juice, grape juice, Gatorade or other sport drinks, weak tepid tea, and gelatin. Fluids with glucose are useful because glucose absorption drives sodium and water back into the body, supporting oral rehydration therapy. The high osmolality of oral rehydration solutions, such as Pedialyte or Gatorade, may intensify diarrhea by initiating mechanisms responsible for stimulating osmotic diarrhea. Patients should be instructed to vary the type of fluids that they ingest to avoid water toxicity and to discontinue rehydration fluids if diarrhea increases.

24. What "red flags" alert patients with diarrhea and family members to the need for immediate medical assistance?

   • Fever and/or shaking chills (be sure someone at home knows how to take a temperature and read a thermometer)
   • Excessive thirst, rapid pulse
   • Dizziness with or without palpitations
   • Severe abdominal cramping and/or rectal spasm

• Watery and/or bloody stool
• Diarrhea that continues for more than 12 hours despite antidiarrheal treatment

REFERENCES

1. Arbuckle RB, Huber SL, Zacker C: The consequences of diarrhea occurring during chemotherapy for colorectal cancer: A retrospective study. Oncologist 5:250–259, 2000.
2. Berg D: Irinotecan hydrochloride: Drug profile and nursing implications of a topoisomerase I inhibitor in patients with advanced colorectal cancer. Oncol Nurs Forum 25(3):535–543, 1998.
3. Cella DF, Tulsky DS, Gray G, et al: The Functional Assessment of Cancer Therapy scale: Development and validation of the general measure. J Clin Oncol 11:570–579, 1993.
4. Engelking C: Cancer treatment-related diarrhea: Challenges and barriers to clinical practice. In Hubbard S, Goodman M, Knopf MT: Oncology Nursing Updates: Patient Treatment and Support 5(2):1–16, 1998.
5. Engelking C: Cancer-related diarrhea: A neglected cause of cancer-related symptom distress. Oncol Nurs Forum 25:859–860, 1998.
6. Engelking C, Sauerland C: Maintenance of normal elimination. In Bruner DW, Moore G, Haas M (eds): Multidisciplinary Management of Patient Outcomes in Radiation Therapy. Boston, Jones & Bartlett, 2000, pp 530–562.
7. Hassey-Dow K, Bucholtz JD, Iwamoto R, et al (eds): Nursing Care in Radiation Oncology, 2nd ed. Philadelphia, W.B. Saunders, 1997.
8. Ippoliti C, Champlin R, Bugazia N, et al: Use of octreotide in the symptomatic management of diarrhea induced by graft-versus-host disease. J Clin Oncol 15:3350–3354, 1997.
9. Kornblau S, Benson AB III, Catalano R, et al: Management of cancer treatment-related diarrhea: Issues and therapeutic strategies. J Pain Symptom Manage 19:118–129, 2000.
10. Kochman ML, Traber PG: Bowel dysfunction in the cancer patient. In MacDonald JS, Haller DG, Mayer RJ (eds): Manual of Oncologic Therapeutics, 3rd ed. Philadelphia, J.B. Lippincott, 1995, pp 444–449.
11. Levy M: Constipation and diarrhea in cancer patients. Cancer Bull 43:412–422, 1991.
12. Lin EM: Diarrhea. In Yasko JM (ed): Nursing Management of Symptoms Associated with Chemotherapy, 4th ed. Philadelphia, Meniscus Health Care Communications, Division of Meniscus Limited, 1998, pp 95–101.
13. Mercadante S: Diarrhea in terminally ill patients: Pathophysiology and treatment. J Pain Symptom Manage 10:298–309, 1995.
14. Morrison GB, Bastian A, Rosa TD, et al: Dihydropyrimidine dehydrogenase deficiency: A pharmacogenetic defect causing severe adverse reactions to 5-fluorouracil-based chemotherapy. Oncol Nurs Forum 24:83–88, 1997.
15. Rutledge DN, Engelking C: Cancer-related diarrhea: Selected findings of a national survey of oncology nurse experiences. Oncol Nurs Forum 25:861–872, 1998.
16. Skeel RT, Tipton J: Symptom management. In Brain MC, Carbone PP (eds): Current Therapy in Hematology-Oncology, 5th ed. St. Louis, Mosby, 1995, pp 582–584.
17. U.S. Department of Health and Human Services, National Institutes of Health, National Cancer Institute Investigator's Handbook: A Manual for Participants in Clinical Trials of Investigational Agents Sponsored by DCTD, NCI. Bethesda, MD, National Cancer Institute, 1998.
18. Wadler S: Secretory Diarrhea: Induction by Chemotherapy. East Hanover, NJ, Sandoz, 1994.
19. Wright PS, Thomas SL: Constipation and diarrhea: The neglected symptoms. Semin Oncol Nurs 11(4):289–297, 1995.

39. DEPRESSION AND ANXIETY

Barbara I. Damron, RN, PhD

1. What is the prevalence of psychological distress among cancer patients?

In the general United States population, depression and anxiety are the two most common psychiatric problems. The 6-month prevalence of major depression is 3%; of dysthymia (chronic, mild depression), 3%; and of anxiety disorders, 10%. Reported rates of depression or anxiety in patients with cancer vary widely (1–60%). One study reported that 47% of patients with cancer had a diagnosable psychiatric disorder. Adjustment disorders with depressed or anxious mood accounted for 68% of the disorders (13% of patients had major depression and 8% had organic mental disorders).[5]

2. What are the common causes of psychological distress in cancer patients and their families?

- Learning of the diagnosis of cancer
- Painful medical procedures
- Fear of dying from the illness
- Beginning new treatment (surgery, radiation, chemotherapy)
- Arduousness of the treatment
- Threats of disfigurement
- Learning that treatment efforts have failed or of disease recurrence
- Loss of energy
- Managing pain or other symptoms
- New demands on time
- Additional financial expenses
- Social isolation

3. Describe a normal response to the stressors related to the diagnosis and treatment of cancer.

The normal response to the diagnosis and treatment of cancer can include brief periods of denial or despair, followed by distress and a mixture of symptoms, such as depressed mood, anxiety, insomnia, anorexia, and irritability. Patients may have difficulty in performing activities of daily living and may experience recurring thoughts about an uncertain future. These symptoms can last for days to several weeks, after which usual patterns of adaptation and coping return.

Distress is recurrent during frequent crisis points experienced by patients along the cancer trajectory. Normal responses are highly individualized and are affected by many factors, including extent of the disease, presence of side effects, prognosis, past experiences, coping skills, support systems, culture, and religious/spiritual beliefs.

Coping is evidenced as an active, conscious response to stress, with or without unconscious behaviors. Coping efforts are aimed not only at reducing or eliminating stressful conditions but also at minimizing the inherent emotional distress.

About 25% of cancer patients continue to have high levels of anxiety and depression that persist for weeks to months. These disorders are called adjustment disorders with depressed, anxious, or mixed moods, depending on the major symptoms.

4. What are the medical causes of depression that patients with cancer may experience?

- Certain surgeries (e.g., mastectomy, head and neck surgery)
- Radiation therapy and its side effects
- Chemotherapy and its side effects

- Uncontrolled pain
- Hormonal abnormalities (e.g., hyper- or hypothyroidism, adrenal insufficiency)
- Metabolic abnormalities (e.g., anemia, vitamin B12 or folate deficiency, hypercalcemia, sodium or potassium imbalances)
- Medications (e.g., some antibiotics, barbiturates, interferon, interleukin-2, methyldopa, propranolol, reserpine, steroids)

5. Define major depression.

Major depression is a clinical syndrome lasting at least 2 weeks with at least five of the following symptoms:[15]

- Depressed mood most of the day, almost every day
- Markedly decreased interest or pleasure in most activities most of the day
- Significant weight loss/gain or appetite disorder
- Insomnia or too much sleeping
- Psychomotor agitation or retardation
- Inappropriate guilt
- Indecisiveness or difficulty in concentrating
- Recurring thoughts of death, including suicidal ideation

6. Describe how symptoms of depression differ in cancer patients.

The biologic correlates or neurovegetative symptoms, typically used for diagnosing depression in physically healthy adults, are frequently unreliable in patients with cancer. These symptoms (e.g., decreased appetite, insomnia, fatigue, loss of energy, loss of libido, psychomotor slowing) are similar to symptoms caused by many cancer treatments or cancer itself. Patients with cancer frequently have no appetite because of chemotherapy or radiotherapy, sleep poorly because of pain or hospitalization, and are fatigued by cancer or its treatments.

Better indicators of major depression in patients with cancer include a depressed mood that is persistent or worsens, hopelessness, helplessness, worthlessness, despondency, guilt feelings, and suicidal ideation. Depression is treatable and should not be considered normal in most patients with cancer.

7. How is depression diagnosed in patients with cancer?

Depression is best diagnosed with a thorough interview and by asking patients whether they are depressed. In terminally ill patients, it is often difficult to differentiate depression from sadness or the normal grieving that is part of the dying process. Some patients can tell you that they are depressed, whereas others may not be aware of their own depression. The nurse needs to assess constantly the patient's psychological status (mood, severity of depression, and suicide risk), paying attention to cues such as an unexpected decision to discontinue treatment. The patient also should be asked about a personal or family history of depression, bipolar disorders, or substance abuse.

It is particularly important to evaluate carefully whether certain symptoms (e.g., fatigue, insomnia, confusion, decreased libido) are caused by depression, cancer, treatment, drugs, or other medical conditions. For example, mental disorders mimicking depression may be due to metastatic disease or a paraneoplastic syndrome.

8. What is a major risk factor for depression among patients with cancer?

Uncontrolled pain is a major risk factor for depression and suicide among cancer patients. The presence of clinically significant pain nearly doubles the likelihood of a major psychiatric complication of cancer, particularly depressive disorders and confusional states. Any patient experiencing overwhelming physical symptoms and functional limitations should be considered at risk for developing psychologic distress.

9. When should a patient be referred to a psychologist or a psychiatrist?

Whenever the nurse or physician is uncomfortable addressing the patient's psychological needs, a consultation is warranted. Early consultations can be extremely helpful in facilitating the establishment of a supportive relationship for the patient. The following signs are indications for a psychological or psychiatric consultation:

- The patient requests the consultation.
- The patient is suicidal or requests suicide or euthanasia.
- The patient and/or family is experiencing multiple stressors; the family is dysfunctional.
- The patient exhibits signs and symptoms of a depressive disorder, extreme anxiety, or psychosis.
- The patient is not responding to current treatment for depression or anxiety.
- The patient's psychological symptoms interfere with medical treatment.
- The patient is in need of specific psychological therapy, such as biofeedback, hypnosis, or relaxation.

10. How is depression managed in patients with cancer?

Depression in patients with cancer is optimally managed within the context of an interdisciplinary team by a combination of supportive psychotherapy (individual or group), cognitive-behavioral techniques (CBT), and antidepressant medications. Treatment is directed toward helping patients adapt to stresses and strengthening coping abilities.

11. How do cognitive behavioral techniques help patients with cancer?

Nurses trained in CBT can provide useful therapy to patients with depression. Cognitive-behavioral interventions, the most widely adopted and evaluated nonpharmacologic treatment for depression, focus on inaccurate perceptions and assessments that lead to anxious and depressed feelings. These techniques can help patients develop an adaptive perspective and have been shown to decrease depressive symptoms in patients with mild-to-moderate levels of depression. By using CBT, nurses can help patients reframe their situation, using realistically positive perspectives, and therefore alter negative perceptions that impair quality of life.

12. When should antidepressants be considered in patients with cancer?

The use of psychotropic medication should be determined by the patient's level of distress, inability to carry out daily activities, and response to psychotherapeutic interventions. A patient does not have to have a psychiatric diagnosis to receive treatment for psychological distress. According to the American College of Physicians–American Society of Internal Medicine (ACP-ASIM) End-of Life Care Consensus Panel, clinicians should have a low threshold for prescribing antidepressants. Effective psychotherapeutic and pharmacologic therapy can reduce distress, improve quality of life, and even increase survival.[1] When both depression and debilitation are observed in patients with advanced cancer, it may be difficult to determine which condition is primary; thus, a trial of antidepressants is warranted.

13. Which antidepressants are most useful for patients with cancer?

Psychopharmacologic interventions are the mainstay of treating depression in patients with cancer. Clinicians have a wide array of antidepressants from which to choose, including first- and second-generation tricyclic antidepressants (TCAs), heterocyclics, and monoamine oxidase inhibitors (MAOs) as well as newer classes of drugs. The newer classes of antidepressants include selective serotonin reuptake inhibitors (SSRIs), serotonin and noradrenaline reuptake inhibitors, and dopamine antagonists. In addition, drugs such as alprazolam (Xanax), a benzodiazepine, can be used for antidepressant effects in patients with anxiety. Lithium carbonate, an antipsychotic drug, is useful to treat depression in bipolar illness; however it must be used cautiously in patients receiving cisplatin because of the potential for nephrotoxicity.

14. How is the appropriate antidepressant chosen for individual patients?

Antidepressants should be selected according to their mechanism of action, side-effect profile, existing medical problems, nature of the depressive symptoms, and past response to specific antidepressants.

MEDICATION	DAILY ORAL DOSE (MG)	PRIMARY SIDE EFFECTS	COMMENTS
First-generation tricyclics (TCAs)			Onset of action: 2–4 weeks. Administer at bedtime.
Amitriptyline (Elavil)	25–125	Sedation, anticholinergic effects (dry mouth, delirium, constipation), orthostasis	All first-generation TCAs: start at low doses (10–25 mg) at bedtime; slowly increase by 10–24 mg every 1–2 days until effective. Useful for neuropathic pain and as adjunct to opioids. Alternate routes: parenteral or rectal. Not tolerated well in terminally ill patients because of anticholinergic effects. Monitor plasma levels to establish therapeutic dosage.
Doxepin (Sinequan)	25–125	Highly sedating; orthostatic hypotension, intermediate anticholinergic effects; potent antihistamine	
Imipramine (Tofranil)	25–125	Intermediate sedation; anticholinergic; orthostasis	
Desipramine (Norpramin)	25–125	Little sedation or orthostasis; moderate anticholinergic	
Nortriptyline (Pamelor)	25–125	Little anticholinergic or orthostatic effect; intermediate sedation; therapeutic window	
Second-generation TCAs			Generally less cardiotoxic than first-generation TCAs
Bupropion (Wellbutrin)	200–450	May cause seizures in those with low seizure threshold/brain tumors; initially activating. Fewer sexual side effects	Limited role in oncology. Energizing effects may have role for psychomotor retardation in depressed, terminally ill patients. Useful for smoking cessation.
Trazodone (Desyrel)	150–300	Sedating; not anticholinergic; risk of priapism	Highly serotonergic; adjuvant analgesic effect
Monoamine oxidase inhibitors (MAOIs)			
Isocarboxazid (Marplan)	20–40		Use with caution. Avoid tyramine-containing foods.
Phenelzine (Nardil)	30–60		
Tranylcypromine (Parnate)	20–40	Myoclonus and delirium have been reported.	Use of meperidine while taking MAOIs absolutely contraindicated because of potential for hyperpyrexia and cardiovascular collapse.
Serotonin-specific reuptake inhibitors (SSRIs)		SSRIs have few anticholinergic or cardiovascular side effects.	Onset of action: 2–4 weeks. Useful in medically ill patients because of favorable side-effect profile. Beware of possible drug interactions due to inhibition of cytochrome P4502D6. Because SSRIs are strongly protein-bound, consider possiblity of increased levels of other drugs (e.g., warfarin, digoxin, cisplatin, some anticonvulsants).

Table continued on following page

MEDICATION	DAILY ORAL DOSE (MG)	PRIMARY SIDE EFFECTS	COMMENTS
Fluoxetine (Prozac)	20–40	Sexual dysfunction, including anorgasmia; headache, nausea, anxiety, insomnia.	Very long half-life
Sertraline (Zoloft)	50–200	Nausea, insomnia	Useful in medically ill: shorter half-life than fluoxetine and more rapid hepatic and renal clearance.
Paroxetine (Paxil)	10–50	Nausea, somnolence, asthenia	No active metabolites; excreted relatively quickly on discontinuation
Citalopram (Celexa)	20–40	Reportedly fewer GI and sexual side effects; fewer problematic interactions with other drugs	
Heterocyclic antidepressants			
Maprotiline (Ludiomil)	50–75	Side-effect profile similar to TCAs; also increase in seizure incidence	
Amoxapine (Asendin)	100–150	Side-effect profile similar to TCAs; also mild dopamine-blocking activity	Patients taking dopamine blockers (e.g., antiemetics) have increased risk of developing extrapyramidal symptoms and dyskinesias.
Others			
Venlafaxine (Effexor)	225–375	May increase blood pressure. Fewer sexual side effects. Achieves steady state in 3 days.	Inhibits reuptake of both serotonin and norepinephrine. Useful in treatment of hot flashes related to chemotherapy and hormonal therapy (25–37.5 mg/day)
Nefazodone (Serzone)	200–500	Sedating; decreased cardiotoxicity; less reported sexual dysfunction than SSRIs	Affects serotonin, $5HT_3$, and norepinephrine
Mirtazapine (Remeron)	15–45	Sedating at lower doses. Fewer reported GI problems; may cause weight gain. Fewer sexual side effects.	Useful for agitated depression and insomnia

15. How do antidepressants work?

Most antidepressants work by restoring balance between receptors that control neurotransmitter release. For example, amitriptyline inhibits the membrane pump mechanism responsible for uptake of norepinephrine and serotonin in adrenergic and serotonergic neurons, thereby potentiating serotonin and norepinephrine activity. SSRIs selectively inhibit the reuptake of serotonin ($5HT_3$) at the presynaptic neuronal membrane.

16. Are the newer antidepressants more effective than the older TCAs?

Clinicians often believe that the newer antidepressants are more effective with fewer side effects. However, evidenced-based guidelines commissioned by the Agency for Healthcare

Research and Quality recommend that clinicians should consider either TCAs or newer antidepressants (e.g., SSRIs) as equally effective in the treatment of primary care patients with acute major depression or dysthymia.[15] The side-effect profiles of both old and new antidepressants should be reviewed jointly by clinician and patient to accommodate the patient's clinical needs.

17. Do patients with cancer require lower doses of TCAs?

Although the reason is not clear, depressed patients with cancer often have a therapeutic response at much lower doses (10–125 mg orally at bedtime) than other populations (150–300 mg/day). Plasma levels should be monitored to ensure adequate dosing because medically ill patients and those with advanced cancer often have therapeutic plasma levels at modest dosages.

18. Can antidepressants be administered by alternate routes?

Most antidepressants are prescribed orally. For patients who cannot take medications orally, most TCAs are available as rectal suppositories. However, absorption by this route has not been studied in patients with cancer. Some antidepressants are also available in an elixir (amitriptyline, nortriptyline, doxepin, fluoxetine, or paroxetine). Certain tricyclics can be given intravenously. Parenteral administration of TCAs should be considered for patients who are unable to tolerate oral administration because of absence of the swallowing reflex, presence of gastric or jejunal drainage tubes, or intestinal obstruction. Amitriptyline, imipramine, and doxepin can be given intramuscularly (IM). The IM route may cause excessive bleeding in patients with low platelet levels as well as discomfort due to the volume of the diluent. The maximal dose that can be delivered by IM injection is usually 50 mg.

19. How effective are psychostimulants in treating depression in patients with cancer?

The psychostimulants (e.g., dextroamphetamine, methylphenidate, and pemoline) offer an alternative and effective pharmacologic approach to the treatment of depression in patients with cancer. They have a more rapid onset of action than TCAs, and relatively low doses are useful for patients with depressed mood, apathy, decreased energy, poor concentration, weakness, psychomotor slowing, and mild cognitive impairment. These agents stimulate appetite, promote a sense of well-being, improve attention and concentration, and improve feelings of weakness and fatigue in patients with cancer. Psychostimulants are also helpful in countering the sedating effects of morphine.

20. Describe the dosing of psychostimulants in patients with cancer.

Treatment with dextroamphetamine or methylphenidate typically begins with a dose of 2.5 mg at 8:00 AM and at noon. The dosage is slowly increased over several days until a desired effect is achieved or until side effects intervene. Usually a dose > 30 mg/day is not necessary, although occasionally a patient may require up to 60 mg/day. Patients usually are maintained on methylphenidate for 1–2 months; in approximately two-thirds, methylphenidate can be withdrawn without recurrence of depressive symptoms. Patients with recurring symptoms can be maintained on a psychostimulant for up to 1 year without significant abuse problems. Pemoline has the advantage of less abuse potential, mild sympathomimetic effects, and lack of federal regulation through special triplicate prescriptions.

MEDICATION	DAILY ORAL DOSE (MG)	PRIMARY SIDE EFFECTS	COMMENTS
All psychostimulants		May cause nightmares	Onset of action: < 24 hours Administer in morning and at noon. Advantages in patients with cancer: rapid onset, analgesic adjuvant, counter sedation of opiates
Dextroamphetamine (Dexedrine)	2.5–30	Insomnia, anxiety, agitation, restlessness	Energizing, appetite stimulant, promotes sense of well-being, improves feelings of weakness and fatigue.

Table continued on following page

MEDICATION	DAILY ORAL DOSE (MG)	PRIMARY SIDE EFFECTS	COMMENTS
Methylphenidate (Ritalin)	2.5–30	Mild increase in blood pressure and pulse. Confusion in elderly. Possible cardiac complications in elderly or those with heart disease. Rare: dyskinesias or motor tics, mood lability, paranoid psychosis.	Particularly useful in patients with advanced cancer, psychomotor slowing, and mild cognitive impairment.
Pemoline (Cylert)	37.5–150	Liver injury (monitor liver function tests). Use with caution in renal failure.	Onset of action: 1–2 days. Unrelated to amphetamine. Advantges for patients with cancer: mild sympathomimetic effects, lack of abuse potential, available as chewable tablet.

21. How frequently does anxiety occur in patients with cancer?

A number of different types of anxiety syndromes are common in patients with cancer. They appear with and without pain and include reactive anxiety, organic anxiety disorder, phobias, panic, and chronic anxiety disorders. More than two-thirds of patients with cancer who have a psychiatric disorder also have reactive depression or anxiety, which is an adjustment disorder with depressed or anxious mood. About 4–5% of patients with cancer have preexisting anxiety disorders.

22. List the different types of anxiety.

- Reactive anxiety
- Organic anxiety disorders
- Phobias, panic, chronic anxiety disorders

23. What causes reactive anxiety?

Reactive anxiety usually is related to the stresses of cancer and its treatment. It is an exaggerated form of the normal anxious response and is the most common type of anxiety in patients with cancer. Many, if not all, patients experience some anxiety at critical moments during evaluation, diagnosis, and treatment (e.g., various tests, surgery, chemotherapy, awaiting test results). Reactive anxiety is distinguished from typical fears of cancer by the duration and intensity of symptoms and the degree of functional impairment (specifically, interference with treatment compliance). Such anxiety may disrupt the ability to function normally, interfere with interpersonal relationships, and even affect the ability to understand and comply with cancer treatments.

24. What are organic anxiety disorders?

They are anxiety disorders of medical origin. Patients with pain are exposed to multiple potential organic causes of anxiety: medications that produce withdrawal states, uncontrolled pain, infection, some hormone-producing tumors, and abnormal metabolic states. Patients in acute pain and those with acute or chronic respiratory distress often appear anxious.

25. Describe the relationship between cancer and chronic anxiety disorders.

Phobias, panic, and chronic anxiety disorders may predate the cancer diagnosis but can be exacerbated during illness. Occasionally, patients have their first episode of panic or phobia in the cancer setting. A number of variants of anxiety disorders (e.g., panic attack, needle phobia, claustrophobia) can prevent cancer diagnostic work-ups and complicate or halt treatment.

26. What are the common symptoms of anxiety?

Nervousness, fidgeting, palpitations, tremulousness, diaphoresis, shortness of breath, diarrhea, intestinal cramping, numbness and tingling of extremities, feelings of imminent death, derealization or depersonalization, phobias, and fearfulness.

27. What types of psychological treatments are used for anxiety in patients with cancer?

Several psychological approaches—cognitive-behavioral therapy, brief supportive therapy, crisis intervention, insight-oriented psychotherapy, and behavioral interventions—can be used alone or in combination to treat anxiety in patients with cancer. Biofeedback, guided imagery, meditation, progressive relaxation, and hypnosis are behavioral approaches that can be used to treat anxiety symptoms associated with adverse side effects to cancer and its treatment, pain syndromes, awaiting test results, and anticipatory fears.

28. What pharmacologic agents are useful in treating anxiety?

Usually an anxiolytic medication is combined with a psychologic approach. Pharmacotherapy for anxiety in patients with cancer involves the judicious use of the following classes of drugs: benzodiazepines, neuroleptics, antihistamines, antidepressants, and opioid analgesics.

29. List the commonly used benzodiazepine anxiolytics along with dosage, duration of action, half-life, and route of administration.

MEDICATION	DOSAGE RANGE (MG)	DURATION OF ACTION	HALF-LIFE (HR)	ROUTE	COMMENTS
Midazolam (Versed)	10–60/day	Very short-acting	2–7	IV, SC	Used to decrease anxiety in patients undergoing procedures
Alprazolam (Xanax)	0.25–2.0 tid–qid	Short-acting	10–15	PO, SL	Metabolized through oxidative pathways in liver, making it more vulnerable to interference with hepatic damage. Can be absorbed SL in patients with dysphagia.
Oxazepam (Serax)	10–15 tid–qid	Short-acting	5–15	PO	Metabolized by liver and excreted by kidney; safest in patients with hepatic disease.
Lorazepam (Ativan)	0.5–2.0 tid–qid	Short-acting	10–20	PO, SL, IV, IM	Metabolized by liver and excreted by kidney; safest in patients with hepatic disease, lacks active metabolites
Chlordiazepoxide (Librium)	10–50 tid–qid	Intermediate-acting	5–30	PO, IM	
Diazepam (Valium)	5–10 bid–qid	Long-acting	20–70	PO, IM, IV, PR	Can be administered rectally and parenterally to dying patients
Clorazepate (Tranxene)	7.5–15 bid–qid	Long-acting	30–200	PO	
Clonazepam (Klonopin)	0.5–2 bid–qid	Long-acting	30–40	PO	Useful for panic symptoms, insomnia, neuropathic pain, depersonalization in patients with seizure disorders, brain tumors, and mild organic mental disorders.

tid = 3 times/day, qid = 4 times/day, bid = 2 times/day, IV = intravenously, SC = subcutaneously, PO = orally, SL = sublingually, IM = intramuscularly, PR = rectally.

30. How are the benzodiazepines used in the oncology setting?

Benzodiazepines are the most commonly used pharmacologic treatment of anxiety in patients with cancer. They not only decrease daytime anxiety but also reduce insomnia. The dosing schedule depends on tolerance and requires individual titration. The most common side effects are dose-dependent and controlled by titration: drowsiness, confusion, lack of motor coordination, and sedation. All benzodiazepines can cause respiratory depression and must be used cautiously, if at all, in patients with respiratory impairment. The depressant effects are additive or even synergistic in the presence of other drugs, such as antidepressants, antiemetics, and opioids.

The shorter-acting benzodiazepines (lorazepam, alprazolam, and oxazepam) are safest in patients with cancer. However, their disadvantage is that patients often experience breakthrough anxiety or end-of-dose failure. If either occurs, patients should be switched to longer-acting benzodiazepines, such as diazepam or clonazepam. Diazepam can be administered rectally or parenterally to dying patients with dosages equivalent to oral regimens. Rectal diazepam has been used widely in palliative care to control anxiety, restlessness, and agitation associated with the final days of life. Drugs with rapid onset of effect (e.g., lorazepam, diazepam) are most effective for high levels of distress.

31. Besides the benzodiazepines, what other agents can be used to treat anxiety?

1. **Neuroleptics**, such as thioridazine and haloperidol, are useful in the treatment of anxiety when benzodiazepines are not sufficient and when anxiety is accompanied by psychotic symptoms (e.g., delusions, hallucinations).

2. **Hydroxyzine**, an antihistamine, can be quite useful in treating anxious, terminally ill patients with pain because it potentiates the analgesic effects of opioids (100 mg of hydroxyzine given parenterally has analgesic potency equivalent to 8 mg of morphine).

3. **Buspirone** is a useful adjunct to psychotherapy in patients with chronic anxiety or anxiety related to adjustment disorders. The onset of anxiolytic action is delayed compared with the benzodiazepines (5–10 days). Because buspirone is not a benzodiazepine, it does not block benzodiazepine withdrawal; thus, the clinician must be cautious when switching from a benzodiazepine to buspirone. It is best used for elderly patients, patients who have not previously been treated with a benzodiazepine, and patients at risk of habituation with benzodiazepines.

4. **Tricyclic and heterocyclic antidepressants** are the most effective treatment for anxiety accompanying depression and are helpful in treating panic disorder. In dying patients, however, their usefulness is often limited by anticholinergic and sedative side effects and slower onset of action (5–10 days).

32. List the dosage range and route of administration for nonbenzodiazepine anxiolytics.

MEDICATION	DOSAGE RANGE (MG)	ROUTE	COMMENTS
Buspirone (BuSpar)	5–20 tid	PO	Useful adjunct to psychotherapy in patients with chronic anxiety or anxiety related to adjustment disorders. Onset of anxiolytic action is delayed.
Neuroleptics			
Haloperidol (Haldol)	0.5–5 q 2–12 hr	PO, IV, SC, IM	Indicated when an organic cause is suspected or psychotic symptoms such as delusions or hallucinations accompany anxiety.
Thioridazine (Mellaril-S)	10–75 tid–qid	PO	Indicated when an organic cause is suspected or psychotic symptoms such as delusions or hallucinations accompany anxiety.
Trifluoperazine (Stelazine)	1–6	PO, IM	
Chlorpromazine (Thorazine)	12.5–50 q 4–12 hr	PO, IM, IV	Low doses are safe and relatively effective when respiratory distress is a concern.

Table continued on following page

MEDICATION	DOSAGE RANGE (MG)	ROUTE	COMMENTS
Antihistamine			
Hydroxyzine (Atarax, Vistaril)	25–50 q 4–6 hr	PO, IV SC	Mild anxiolytic, mild antiemetic, sedative, and analgesic properties. Low doses are safe and relatively effective when respiratory distress is a concern.
Tricyclic antidepressants			
Imipramine (Tofranil)	12.5–150 hs	PO, IM	Indicated in anxiety accompanying depression, helpful in treating panic disorder; limited use in dying patients because of anticholinergic and sedative side effects.
Clomipramine	10–150 hs	PO	Same as for imipramine

33. Are patients with cancer who take drugs for depression or anxiety at risk for addiction?

Concerns about addiction in patients with no history of drug abuse are exaggerated. Fear of addiction is a factor in the undertreatment of depression, anxiety, and pain. Patients, physicians, and nurses share this fear. Although tolerance and physical dependence commonly occur, addiction (psychologic dependence) is rare in patients with no history of substance abuse.

34. Should cancer patients with a history of substance abuse receive any pharmacologic treatment for depression or anxiety?

Treatment of depression and anxiety should not be neglected in patients with a history of substance abuse. They should be assessed carefully and given the opportunity for treatment with psychological techniques in conjunction with cautious medication use and observation for signs of drug dependence.

35. How common is suicide in patients with cancer?

The literature suggests that suicidal ideation is relatively infrequent in patients with cancer, but they do have a 2.5-10 fold increase in suicide rates compared with the general population. The greatest risk is immediately after diagnosis (within 6 months). Published studies report a 0–17% incidence of suicidal ideation, which is limited to significantly depressed patients. Clinically, however, many health care providers report that thoughts of suicide probably occur quite frequently, particularly in patients with advanced cancer. Suicidal thoughts are often fleeting and may act as an outlet for feelings related to an overwhelming situation. They may be a last attempt at control by the patient who views suicide as a way out. Within the context of a trusting, safe relationship with the nurse, patients may reveal that they have had occasional or even persisting thoughts of suicide as a means of escaping the threat of overwhelming pain or cancer itself.

36. When does suicide most frequently occur in cancer patients?

Patients with advanced illness are at highest risk, perhaps because they have the highest incidence of cancer complications such as pain, depression, and debilitating side effects. Depression is a factor in 50% of all suicides. Patients suffering from depression are at 25 times greater risk of suicide than the general population. The role of depression in cancer-related suicide is equally significant. Many patients with cancer experience hopelessness, which is a key variable that links depression and suicide in the general population.

37. What are the risk factors for suicide in patients with advanced cancer?

- Previous history of suicide attempts
- Family history of suicide
- Preexisting psychopathology

- Few social supports (not married, fewer than 6 friends or relatives, no membership in church or community groups)
- History of substance abuse
- History of recent death of friends or spouse
- Diagnosis of head and neck, pancreatic cancers
- Uncontrolled pain; suffering aspects of cancer
- Advanced illness, poor prognosis
- Depression
- Feelings of hopelessness
- Delirium
- Overwhelming fatigue
- Advanced age

38. How can the nurse assess suicidal risk in patients with cancer?

Nurses must be willing to talk openly about suicide. To do so does *not* mean that the patient is going to commit suicide. No evidence supports the belief that suicidal thoughts are exacerbated by exploration. Warning signs that a patient is considering suicide include actions such as saying goodbye, giving away a treasured object, and wishing to be dead.

The following strategies provide the nurse with a way to initiate a conversation about suicide.[13] Open with a statement: "Most patients with cancer have passing thoughts about suicide, such as 'I might do something if things get bad enough.'"

1. Acknowledge: "Have you ever had thoughts like that? Any thoughts of not wanting to go on or that it would be easier to die?"
2. Plan: "Do you ever think about suicide? Have you ever thought about how you would do it?"
3. Personal history: "Have you ever been depressed or treated for depression?"
4. Substance abuse: "Have you ever had any drug or alcohol problems?"
5. Bereavement: "Have you recently lost someone close to you?"

39. How can the nurse form a supportive relationship with the patient?

Nurses must be aware of their own emotional abilities and limitations to provide the best communication to patients (see Chapter 58). Ways for nurses to form a supportive relationship with the patient include the following:

- Listening
- Projecting an empathetic and welcoming attitude to the patient's concerns
- Reinforcing the patient's strengths
- Facilitating dialogue with family members
- Assuring the patient that what is said in confidence will not be shared unless permission is obtained
- Offering hope that something can be done to make the situation more tolerable

40. Give examples of unsupportive comments to cancer patients.

Usually it is not helpful for the nurse to tell the patient that he or she "knows" what the patient is feeling. Although a sympathetic approach is helpful, for the health professional to assume that he or she can know what the patient is feeling is in fact dismissive of the patient's concerns. Each person's pain, emotional or physical, is unique and highly individualized. It is also not helpful to tell the patient that this is God's will, or to minimize the emotional pain.

REFERENCES

1. Block SD: Assessing and managing depression in the terminally ill patient. Ann Intern Med 132:209–218, 2000.
2. Breitbart W: Psycho-oncology: Depression, anxiety, delirium. Semin Oncol 21:754–769, 1994.
3. Bush N: Coping and adaptation. In Caroll-Johnson R, Gormona L, Bush N: Psychosocial Nursing Care, 35–52, 1998.

 4. Carroll BT, Kathol RG, Noyes R, et al: Screening for depression and anxiety in cancer patients using the hospital Anxiety and Depression Scale. Gen Hosp Psychiatry 15:69–74, 1993.
 5. Derogatis LR, Morrow GR, Fetting J, et al: The prevalence of psychiatric disorders among cancer patients. JAMA 249:751–757, 1983.
 6. Henderson JM, Ord RA: Suicide in head and neck cancer patients. J Oral Maxillofac Surg 55: 1217–1221, 1997.
 7. Katon W, Sullivan MD: Depression and chronic medical illness. J Clin Psychiatry 56(Suppl):3–11, 1990.
 8. Loprinzi CL, Piscansky TM, Fonseca R, et. al: Pilot evaluation of venlafaxine hydrochloride for the therapy of hot flashes in cancer survivors. J Clin Oncol 16:2377–2381, 1998.
 9. Lovejoy N, Tabor D, Deloney P: Cancer-related depression. Part II: Neurological alterations and evolving approaches to psychopharmaclogy. Oncol Nurs Forum 27:795–810, 2000.
10. Lovejoy N, Tabor D, Mattels M, Lillis P: Cancer-related depression. Part I: Neurological alterations and cognitive-behavior therapy. Oncol Nurs Forum 27:667–680, 2000.
11. Myers JK, Weissman MM, Tischler GL, et al: Six-month prevalence of psychiatric disorders in three communities. Arch Gen Psychiatry 41:959–967, 1984.
12. Passik SD, Breitbart WS: Depression in patients with pancreatic carcinoma: Diagnostic and treatment issues. Cancer 78:615–626, 1996.
13. Roth A, Brietbart W: Psychiatric emergencies in terminally ill cancer patients. Hematol Oncol Clin North Am 10:235–259, 1996.
14. Roth A, Massie MJ, Redd WH: Consultation for the cancer patient. In Jacobson JL, Jacobson AJ (eds): Psychiatric Secrets, 2nd ed. Philadelphia, Hanley & Belfus, 2001, pp 412–425.
15. Snow V, Lascher S, Mottur-Pilson D: Clinical guideline. Part 1: Pharmacologic treatment of acute major depression and dysthymia. Ann Intern Med 132:738–742, 2000.
16. Spiegel D: Facilitating emotional coping during treatment. Cancer 66:1422–1427, 1990.
17. Spiegel D: Health caring: Psychosocial support for patients with cancer. Cancer 74:1453–1457, 1994.
18. Spiegel D: Psychosocial aspects of breast cancer treatment. Semin Oncol 24:SI36–SI47, 1997.
19. Trijsburg RW, VanKnippenberg FCE, Rijpma SE: Effects of psychological treatment on cancer patients: A critical review. Psychosom Med 54: 489–517, 1992.
20. Williams JW, Mulrow CD, Chiquette E, et al: Clinical guideline. Part 2: A systematic review of newer pharmacotherapies for depression in adults: Evidence report summary. Ann Intern Med 132:743–756, 2000.

40. FATIGUE

Lillian M. Nail, PhD, RN, FAAN

1. Is fatigue a major problem for patients with cancer?

Cancer treatment-related fatigue (CRF) is the most frequently reported side effect of treatment. All types of treatment produce CRF, and the most severe, dose-limiting form occurs with biologic response modifiers (e.g., interferon, interleukins). The percentage of patients experiencing CRF as a side effect of cancer treatment ranges from < 10% to 100%, depending on the type of treatment, dose of therapy, and method used to measure fatigue. CRF is poorly understood and often ignored in clinical practice. Although many people attribute fatigue to "having cancer," research focuses on fatigue as a treatment side effect, and most studies of fatigue in cancer have been done with patients who have no evidence of disease.

2. Define cancer treatment-related fatigue.

CRF includes sensations of physical tiredness, mental slowness, and lack of emotional resilience. It fluctuates in intensity over the course of the day, often exhibits a pattern that it is tied to administration of treatment, and can be overcome in an emergency. Although patients with CRF may experience muscle weakness, CRF is not synonymous with weakness. In contrast to patients with neurologic problems, patients with CRF may have normal muscle strength and endurance and still experience an overwhelming feeling of tiredness.

3. How is CRF different from the fatigue experienced by healthy people?

In comparison with the fatigue experienced by healthy people, CRF is overwhelming, persistent, and relentless. Fatigue in healthy people is eventually fully relieved by sleep and rest, even if it takes more than one or two nights. In contrast, people with CRF wake up tired no matter how much rest they get. CRF also may cause patients to redefine the level of fatigue that they label as "not tired." Thus, what they formerly viewed as feeling a little tired is now defined as "not tired," and a new sensation of overwhelming fatigue replaces "severe fatigue."

4. What is the impact of CRF?

Patients describe themselves as too tired to do anything, unable to concentrate, frustrated by feeling that they are not themselves, concerned that fatigue means that they are not doing well or that the cancer is progressing, and depressed because of the feeling of tiredness. The limitations imposed by fatigue are dramatic. The person experiencing CRF may not be aware of the magnitude of the negative impact on usual activities until the fatigue resolves.

5. What are the probable causes of CRF?

People with cancer are likely to experience many potential causes of fatigue, such as electrolyte imbalance, poor nutritional status, anemia, hormone shifts, volume depletion, sedation as a side effect of analgesics, hypoxia, and infection. Other contributors include sleep disruption, increased demands for physical activity, emotional strain, interpersonal demands, and increased need for vigilance and concentration. Symptoms, side effects, anxiety, hospital noise, and interpersonal demands at home have the potential to disrupt sleep and rest. Multiple visits to healthcare providers, travel to appointments, physical demands of surgery and other forms of treatment, processing information about treatment options to make an informed decision, establishing relationships with new healthcare providers, explaining the diagnosis and treatment to friends and family members, and monitoring the care provided by others are potential contributors to fatigue that are not fully understood by healthcare providers or friends and family.

6. What physiologic mechanisms are responsible for CRF?

Except for chemotherapy-induced anemia, the physiologic causes of CRF are unknown. Multiple causes are likely, given the variation in the intensity and characteristics of CRF experienced with different types of treatment. Various hypotheses have been proposed, including toxic effects of accumulated products of cell death, neurohormonal changes, depletion of essential neurotransmitters, bone marrow suppression, and accumulation of cytokines. Few of these mechanisms have been studied.

7. How should the nurse assess CRF?

The clinical assessment of fatigue should be modeled on the approach to pain assessment. For example, "On a scale of 0 to 10 where 0 is no fatigue and 10 is the most fatigue possible, how much fatigue have you had today?" Both the time frame (now, today, during the past week, during the past month) and the reference point (highest level of fatigue, lowest level of fatigue, usual level of fatigue) can be altered to accommodate the type of treatment. Patients receiving cyclic chemotherapy often arrive for treatment on a day when they have the lowest level of fatigue during the treatment cycle. Assessment based on the "today" approach does not fully describe their experience after treatment because the peak time of CRF is not captured. Patients assessed on the day of the next treatment should be asked about level of fatigue over the week before the previous treatment as well as "today." The average level of fatigue over each week since the previous treatment also may be assessed to evaluate rate of recovery. Weekly assessment focused on the past week and initiated the second week of treatment is appropriate for most patients receiving radiation therapy.

Potential treatable causes should be evaluated, especially when (1) the pattern of CRF is unusual for the type of treatment delivered, (2) the intensity of fatigue increases suddenly and dramatically, or (3) the impact of fatigue on quality of life is beyond the patient's level of tolerance. In addition to standard laboratory tests and physical examination, daily activity level, sleep patterns, and new demands imposed as a result of cancer should be assessed.

8. What are major barriers to effective management of CRF?

- Assumption by healthcare providers that CRF is the same as the fatigue that all healthy people encounter in day-to-day life
- Lack of knowledge of the underlying mechanisms of CRF
- Erroneous belief that nothing can be done about CRF
- Confusion of CRF with depression
- Failure to appreciate the negative impact of CRF on quality of life

9. What interventions are used to manage CRF?

The approach to managing CRF is multifaceted:
- Assessing level of fatigue
- Delivering preparatory information
- Managing treatable causes
- Controlling symptoms and side effects
- Providing instructions about energy conservation and appropriate exercise
- Promoting sleep and rest
- Evaluating effectiveness of interventions

10. Why should patients get preparatory information?

Preparatory information helps patients (1) to understand that CRF is a side effect of treatment, not an indication that the cancer is progressing; (2) to plan for CRF by using information about onset, pattern, and resolution in planning activities; and (3) to increase confidence in dealing with CRF. Research about informational interventions in patients undergoing stressful medical procedures demonstrates that preparatory information does not cause patients to experience side effects by power of suggestion. Patients who are aware of potential side effects but do not experience them describe themselves as "lucky" and appreciate being prepared.

McHugh, Christman, and Johnson developed specific guidelines for preparatory informational interventions. Their guidelines include objective or factual information about CRF from the patient's perspective rather than value judgments, based on experiences reported by others who have had the same treatment. For example, a message preparing men to receive radiation treatment for prostate cancer included information about the time of day when CRF was likely to occur, the week of treatment when it began, and how long the fatigue persisted after treatment.[20]

11. What are the common treatable causes of fatigue and sleep disruption?

- Pain is an important contributor to fatigue and sleep disruption in patients with cancer. Pain disrupts sleep and rest, increases the energy needed to perform day-to-day activities, restricts mobility, and constitutes an emotional burden. Pain relief should improve fatigue unless the management technique disrupts sleep (e.g., drugs administered every 4 hours around the clock), requires extensive energy investment (e.g., frequent changes of hot or cold packs), or has a sedative effect.
- Symptoms related to tumor involvement (e.g., obstruction, fever, pruritus, coughing, dyspnea)
- Side effects related to therapy (e.g., nausea, vomiting, hot flashes, dry mouth, stomatitis, constipation, diarrhea)
- Urinary frequency, incontinence, retention, spasms, or genitourinary irritation can disrupt sleep as often as every hour.
- Anxiety and depression
- Drugs or other substances that interfere with sleep, such as steroids, sedatives or hypnotics, caffeine or nicotine, and some antidepressants
- Primary sleep disorders (e.g., sleep apnea, narcolepsy, restless legs syndrome)

12. How can patients conserve energy and manage activity?

Although there are no standard guidelines for energy conservation in patients with cancer, they are often advised to conserve energy by decreasing activity. This approach to managing CRF has not been tested, although energy conservation techniques are commonly used by patients with physical illness. The appeal of this approach is derived from patients' perceptions that they have a limited amount of available energy and the assumption that conserving energy allows it to be redirected to other activities.

Current recommendations include assisting patients to prioritize activities by identifying those that are essential and those that are optional. Some essential activities can be delegated to others while the patient maintains involvement in activities that are highly valued. Nonessential activities that are not valued by the patient can be eliminated. Finding different ways to perform activities is also helpful in energy conservation. Simple suggestions, such as sitting in a firm chair with arms to aid getting out of the chair, adding a raised toilet seat in the bathroom, using a wheelchair if walking is difficult, arranging commonly used supplies and equipment within easy reach of a workspace, and sitting rather than standing to perform repetitive tasks, are examples of energy conservation techniques. Physical and/or occupational therapy referrals are important both in evaluating a patient's physical capacity and identifying appropriate energy conservation techniques.

13. How is exercise used in managing CRF?

The conceptual basis for using exercise as a strategy for managing CRF is derived from principles of energetics and muscle physiology. Decreased activity leads to deconditioning, which results in less efficient muscular work. Furthermore, energy use is an important component of energy regulation. No research has explicitly tested the principles behind this concept of the relationship between exercise and CRF. However, research with women receiving adjuvant chemotherapy for breast cancer demonstrates that both supervised and self-administered exercise programs are feasible and safe in this clinical population and suggests that exercise holds promise as a means of preventing or treating CRF.

14. How does sleep disruption contribute to CRF?

In healthy adults, sleep disruption produces varying levels of fatigue, mood disturbance, attention deficit, and daytime performance problems. Inadequate sleep and rest in patients with cancer probably have the same effects. Patients may have difficulty in processing information, adhering to treatment regimens, or implementing self-care instructions. Irritability, depression, and despair are potential consequences of prolonged sleep disruption. Increases in sleep and rest are the most common self-care strategies used by patients with cancer, but they do not fully relieve the symptoms of CRF. The suggestion that sleep and rest may be used to treat CRF is based on a few descriptive studies with cancer patients, findings of the more extensive research on healthy adults, and best clinical judgment.

15. How are sleep disturbances assessed?

• Determine whether the sleep pattern has changed from the patient's precancer pattern.
• Document current sleep patterns by having the patient keep a sleep log to record time to sleep onset, duration of sleep, sleep habits, frequency and reason for awakenings, naps, and use of sleep aids.
• Ask patients about amount and quality of sleep, current medications, and history of sleep disorders.

16. How are sleep disturbances managed?

• Control of pain and other symptoms or side effects of therapy
• Reduction of anxiety (manifested by frightening thoughts, worries, or nightmares) with use of pharmacologic or cognitive/behavioral treatments. Specific cognitive/behavioral treatments, such as biofeedback and relaxation, are established interventions for problems with delayed sleep onset, frequent awakening, and shortened sleep periods.
• Appropriate pharmacologic management (e.g., mild barbiturates, benzodiazepines, antihistamines, chloral hydrate, or antidepressants).
• Appropriate referrals if a primary sleep disorder is suspected.
• Instruction to patients about sleep hygiene.

17. What practical tips may promote sleep hygiene or help patients get a better night's sleep?

• Develop a standard, predictable bedtime ritual.
• Go to bed when drowsy, but do not stay in bed if you are not sleeping.
• Sleep in a dark, well-ventilated, quiet room maintained at a comfortable temperature.
• Avoid stimulants (caffeine, chocolate, nicotine), alcohol, heavy meals, and exercise in the period prior to sleep.
• Avoid disrupting sleep by delegating the care of others to someone else, trying not to ruminate on worries, and turning down telephones.
• Take a warm bath or hot drink before bedtime or get a backrub or massage.
• Ensure comfort by using a mattress and pillow of appropriate firmness and extra pillows for support; by sleeping in comfortable, loose clothing; and by straightening the bed linen.
• Sleep in a familiar environment whenever possible.

18. What drugs interfere with sleep?

Opioids, some hypnotics, and other medications such as hormones, steroids, and nonsteroidal anti-inflammatory drugs may affect the quality of sleep. Any medication that produces respiratory depression may induce the type of breathing problem identified as a cause of chronic insomnia.

19. What medications are commonly used to help sleep?

Expert recommendations for the use of hypnotics include limiting use to relatively brief periods (a few weeks), beginning at a low dose, choosing a drug that does not impair alertness or performance the next day, and considering the duration of action in relation to the specific sleep problem (delayed onset of sleep, frequent awakening, or early wakening). When pain is a problem, adequate analgesia is essential for sleep.

In patients with cancer, adequate symptom management and an environment conducive to sleep form the foundation of sleep promotion. When these interventions do not solve the problem, short-term or intermittent use of pharmacologic agents should be considered. Factors that influence the choice of agent include age of patient, desired duration of effect, nature of the problem, potential side effects, comorbidity, and drug interactions. Benzodiazepines are usually the first class of drugs considered, because they disrupt rapid eye movement sleep less than other hypnotics. Temazepam (15–30 mg for adults; limit dose for elderly patients to 50% adult dose) is the benzodiazepine most often recommended because of its rapid onset, 6–8-hour duration of action, and relatively low incidence of side effects when used in low doses for short periods. Zaleplon (Sonata, 5–20 mg for adults; 5 mg for elderly or debilitated patients), a new nonbenzodiazepine hypnotic from the pyrazolopyrimidine class, has the advantages of a rapid onset of action and a short elimination half-life of approximately 1 hour. Because antihistamines contribute to relief of nausea or itching, diphenhydramine (25 mg) or hydroxyzine (10–100 mg) may be especially useful for some patients.

20. What about depression?

Patients, family members, and care providers often wonder whether CRF is a manifestation of depression. Historically, the diagnosis of depression depends on the presence of vegetative symptoms such as anorexia, sleep disturbance, decreased activity, constipation, and weight loss. All of these symptoms are likely to occur as side effects in patients undergoing treatment for cancer, potentially confounding the diagnosis of depression. Recent revisions to the diagnosis of depression state that symptoms of physical illness and side effects of treatment are not appropriate considerations in making the diagnosis. The incidence of depression in patients with cancer is comparable to that in the general population of the same age when symptom-free measures of depression are used.

In patients with cancer, feelings of sadness and inability to feel pleasure, which are present all or most of the time for several weeks, are the hallmarks of depression. The most important risk factor is a previous episode of depression. Depression in patients with cancer can be treated effectively, but CRF may interfere with attendance at support groups or participation in therapy sessions. However, pharmacologic management is appropriate for many patients if the therapy does not interact with other medications or adversely influence responses to cancer treatment.

21. Do patients with cancer use alternative therapies to treat CRF?

Vitamins, mineral supplements, herbal remedies, and hormones are used by patients with cancer. No published reports confirm the efficacy of any of these agents in preventing or ameliorating CRF. Patients who experience sleep problems may use melatonin as a sleep promoter. Research into the effects of melatonin on sleep and CRF is ongoing, but the results reported at this time are contradictory.

22. What should care providers do about CRF?

- Recognize that fatigue is a side effect of treatment.
- Assess patients for CRF.
- Prepare patients for the experience of CRF.
- Understand that the fatigue experienced by "healthy" people is not the same as CRF.
- Recognize that CRF has a major negative impact on quality of life.
- Pursue treatment to maximize quality of life, including correcting physiologic problems (e.g. chemotherapy-induced anemia, hypothyroidism, infection, dehydration, sleep problems).

REFERENCES

1. Andrykowski MA, Curran SL, Lightner R: Off-treatment fatigue in breast cancer survivors: A controlled comparison. J Behav Med 21:1–18, 1998.
2. Berger A: Patterns of fatigue and activity and rest during adjuvant breast cancer chemotherapy. Oncol Nurs Forum 25:51–62, 1998.
3. Berger AM, Farr L: The influence of daytime inactivity and nighttime restlessness on cancer-related fatigue. Oncol Nurs Forum 26:1663–1671, 1999.
4. Breetvelt IS, Van Dam FS: Underreporting by cancer patients: The case of the response-shift. Soc Sci Med 32:981–987, 1991.

5. Cella D: Factors influencing quality of life in cancer patients: Anemia and fatigue. Semin Oncol 25:43–46, 1998.
6. Cimprich B: Symptom management: Loss of concentration. Semin Oncol Nurs 11:279–288, 1995.
7. Curt GA, Breitbart W, Cella D, et al: Impact of cancer-related fatigue on the lives of patients: New findings from the Fatigue Coalition. Oncologist 5:353–360, 2000.
8. Ferrell BR, Grant M, Dean GE, et al: "Bone tired": The experience of fatigue and its impact on quality of life. Oncol Nurs Forum 23:1539–1547, 1996.
9. Foltz AT, Gaines G, Gullatte M: Recalled side effects and self-care actions of patients receiving inpatient chemotherapy. Oncol Nurs Forum 23:679–683, 1996.
10. Graydon JE, Bublia N, Irvine D, et al: Fatigue-reducing strategies used by patients receiving treatment for cancer. Cancer Nurs 18:23–28, 1995.
11. Hann DM, Garovoy N, Finkelstein B, et al: Fatigue and quality of life in breast cancer patients undergoing autologous stem cell transplantation: A longitudinal comparative study. J Pain Symptom Manage 17:311–319, 1999.
12. Hinds PS, Hockenberry-Eaton M, Gilger E, et al: Comparing patient, parent, and staff descriptions of fatigue in pediatric oncology patients. Oncol Nurs Forum 22:277–289, 1999.
13. Johnson JE: Coping with elective surgery. Annu Rev Nurs Res 2:107–132, 1984.
14. Johnson JE: Coping with radiation therapy: Optimism and the effect of preparatory inventions. Res Nurs Health 19:3–12, 1996.
15. Johnson JE, Nail LM, Lauver D, et al: Reducing the negative impact of radiation therapy on functional status. Cancer 61:46–51, 1988.
16. Kurtz ME, Kurtz JC, Given CW, Given B: Loss of physical functioning among patients with cancer: A longitudinal view. Cancer Pract 1:275–281, 1993.
17. Loge JH, Abrahamsen AF, Ekeberg O, Kaasa S: Hodgkin's disease survivors more fatigued than the general population. J Clin Oncol 17:253–261, 1999.
18. MacVicar MG, Winningham ML, Nickel JL: Effects of aerobic interval training on cancer patients: Functional capacity. Nurs Res 38:348–351, 1989.
19. Massie MJ, Holland JC: Overview of normal reactions and prevalence of psychiatric disorders. In Holland JC, Rowland JH (eds): Handbook of Psychooncology: Psychological Care of the Patient with Cancer. New York, Oxford University Press, 1990, pp 273–383.
20. McHugh NG, Christman NJ, Johnson JE: Preparatory information: What helps and why. Am J Nurs 82:780–782, 1982.
21. Miaskowski C, Lee KA: Pain, fatigue, and sleep disturbances in oncology outpatients. J Pain Symptom Manage 17:320–332, 1999.
22. Mock V, Barton Burke M, Sheehan P, et al: A nursing rehabilitation program for women with breast cancer receiving adjuvant chemotherapy. Oncol Nurs Forum 21:899–907, 1994.
23. Mock V, Piper B, Escalante C, Sabbatini P: National Comprehensive Cancer Network practice guidelines for the management of cancer-related fatigue. Oncology (Huntington) [in press].
24. Nail LM, Jones LS: Fatigue as a side effect of cancer treatment: Impact on quality of life. Qual Life Nurs Chall 4:8–13, 1995.
25. Nail LM, Jones LS, Greene D, et al: Use and perceived efficacy of self-care activities in patients receiving chemotherapy. Oncol Nurs Forum 18:883–887, 1991.
26. Nail LM, Winningham ML: Fatigue and weakness in cancer patients: The symptom experience. Semin Oncol Nurs 11:272–278, 1995.
27. Nicholson AN: Hypnotics: Clinical pharamacology and therapeutics. In Kryger MH, Roth T, Dement WC (eds): Principles and Practices of Sleep Medicine, 2nd ed. Philadelphia, W.B. Saunders, 1994, pp 355–363.
28. NIH Technology Assessment Panel: Integration of behavioral and relaxation approaches to the treatment of chronic pain and insomnia. JAMA 276:313–318, 1996.
29. Pearce S, Richardson A: Fatigue in cancer: A phenomenological perspective. Eur J Cancer Care 5:111–115, 1996.
30. Richardson A: Fatigue in cancer patients: A review of the literature. Eur J Cancer Care 4:20–32, 1995.
31. Richardson A, Ream E, Wilson-Barnett J: Fatigue in patients receiving chemotherapy: Patterns of change. Cancer Nurs 21:17–30, 1998.
32. Schwartz AL: Fatigue mediates the effects of exercise on quality of life. Qual Life Res 8:529–538, 2000.
33. Schwartz AL, Nail LM, Chen S, et al: Fatigue patterns observed in patients receiving chemotherapy and radiotherapy. Cancer Invest 18:11–19, 2000.
34. Vogelzang N, Breitbart W, Cella D, et al: Patient, caregiver, and oncologist perceptions of cancer-related fatigue: Results of a tripart assessment survey. Semin Hematol 34(Suppl 2):4–12, 1997.
35. Winningham M, Nail LM, Burke MB, et al: Fatigue and the cancer experience: The state of the knowledge. Oncol Nurs Forum 21:23–26, 1994.

41. LYMPHEDEMA SECONDARY TO CANCER TREATMENT

Jean K. Smith, RN, MS, OCN

1. Why do we usually think of breast cancer when we hear the word lymphedema?

In the United States, breast cancer and its treatment cause significantly more lymphedema than any other single factor. Increased public interest and media coverage of breast cancer have improved lymphedema awareness and management.

2. What is lymphedema?

Lymphedema is a chronic, abnormal collection of excess proteins, cell debris, fluid, inflammation, and fibrosis in the skin and tissues of a body area. These excesses result from inadequate lymphatic transport capacity. Lymphedema is classified as either **primary** or **secondary**. **Primary lymphedema** is attributed to embryonic developmental abnormalities. **Secondary lymphedema** is acquired through obstruction and/or obliteration of lymphatics. The most frequent cause of secondary lymphedema in developed countries is breast cancer treatment. Filariasis, an infectious disease spread by mosquitoes, causes the vast majority of lymphedema in hot, humid, underdeveloped countries.

3. What causes cancer-related lymphedema?

Cancer surgery, radiation therapy, and cancer metastasis can produce lymphatic injury that progresses to lymphedema. Infection and thrombosis are two common precipitators of lymphedema in cancer patients who have undergone surgery and/or radiation therapy. In addition to breast cancer survivors, lymphedema can occur in patients with prostate, head and neck, pelvic, and skin cancers, and lymphoma, sarcoma, and melanoma.

4. What is the incidence of cancer-related lymphedema?

The literature suggests a 20–30% incidence of lymphedema in breast cancer survivors who have undergone axillary node dissection and/or radiation therapy. The incidence of lymphedema related to other cancers is just beginning to emerge. Lymphedema can develop at any time following cancer diagnosis and treatment and has been reported as late as 30 years after breast cancer surgery. Investigation of the true incidence of lymphedema has not taken place. Such investigation would require lifelong, interval volumetric evaluations of surgical limbs in large samples of patients with each relevant cancer.

5. How is lymphedema diagnosed?

Generally, history and physical assessment are combined with the process of elimination in order to establish a diagnosis of cancer-related lymphedema. The role of imaging for patients with a high risk for or suspected lymphedema is unclear. Imaging has generally been discouraged on the basis that it has little effect on treatment outcomes. There is an increased risk of compromise of lymphatics due to dye-related tissue injury from two common vascular and lymphatic imaging tests: venography and lymphangiography. Thus, when imaging is required, venous ultrasound and/or lymphscintigraphy are generally recommended. Lymphscintigraphy is a nuclear medicine evaluation of lymphatic anatomy and physiology. Currently, use of lymphscintigraphy in lymphedema diagnosis is not widespread because of insufficient research to substantiate a contribution as well as deficiencies in third-party reimbursement and radiologist expertise.

6. How relevant is lymphedema prevention in view of more conservative breast cancer surgeries and sentinel node biopsy?

The trend in the past 20 years has been to forego lymphedema prevention on the basis that conservative breast cancer surgeries have decreased the incidence and severity of lymphedema. A 20% lymphedema incidence for the approximately 180,000 new U.S. breast cancer diagnoses each year represents at least 36,000 lymphedema diagnoses. While this incidence is reduced from the days of the Halsted radical mastectomy, it continues to be substantial. The sentinel node biopsy offers the promise of further reduction in lymphedema incidence but is still controversial in its application as well as its ability to achieve the staging accuracy provided by the standard axillary node dissection. At a minimum, precautions delay the development of lymphatic insufficiency and help reduce the presentation of lymphedema from allergens, infection, and inflammation. Until further research is available, precaution instruction is recommended.

7. What helpful hints can patients be taught to reduce, prevent, or control lymphedema?

Lymphedema is a lifelong risk that is currently manageable but incurable; certain precautions minimize the risk for development and progression.

1. Avoid prolonged limb dependency as much as possible.
2. Clean skin and use oil or skin cream daily.
3. Keep pressure off affected arm or leg. Do not cross affected leg; change position often.
   - Wear loose jewelry, watches, and clothes.
   - Carry bags with unaffected arm.
   - Do not have blood pressure taken on affected arm.
4. Avoid injuries and infection.
   - Use electric razor to shave legs.
   - Wear gloves when gardening and cleaning.
   - Wear thimbles when sewing.
   - Take good care of nails. See a podiatrist for problems. Do not cut cuticles.
   - Use insect repellent and avoid insect bites by wearing protective clothing.
   - Clean any cuts with soap and water followed by antiseptics or antibacterial ointment.
   - Avoid extreme heat or cold on the affected limb.
   - Try to avoid blood draws or intravenous starts on affected arm.
5. Check for changes daily and notify doctor if any of the following symptoms develops:
   - Redness   • Pain
   - Heat   • Swelling
   - Fever
6. Practice drainage promotion exercises (non-rigorous, gentle muscle contractions).

8. How do staff and patients decide when a limb at high risk for lymphedema must be used for intravenous therapy?

Experts recommend affected limbs should not be used for any IV infusions, especially chemotherapy. The reality of patient needs can complicate this recommendation. Development of a set protocol or Lymphedema Prevention Standard of Care is recommended. Suggested criteria include: (1) venipuncture by experienced phlebotomists only; (2) approval process required for use of suggested limb (e.g., by a physician, clinical nurse specialist); (3) central venous catheter considered for any patient requiring more than a few days of IV infusion; (4) established procedure for venipuncture skin preparation and monitoring of infusions when affected limb must be used.

9. Why is infection such a big issue in lymphedema management?

Infection is the most common precipitator of lymphedema in cancer patients and is associated with further compromise of lymphatics. Infections may be acute with dramatic symptoms that require intravenous antibiotic therapy and may progress to life-threatening severity within a few hours. Subclinical infections, which exhibit minimal signs and symptoms, also may be present. Their presence is confirmed when antibiotic therapy results in edema reduction and improved status. Both lymphedema management and control are significantly hindered by the presence of acute and subclinical infections.

10. Is the use of antibiotics for every infection warranted in all patients at high risk for lymphedema?

Antibiotics are recommended prophylactically at the first sign of infection or when a specific injury presents a substantial risk of infection in high-risk patients. Caregivers who have observed the development of severe, life-threatening infection from something as minor as a hangnail recommend antibiotic prevention for everyone because there currently is no way to determine which patients will develop such infections. Patients must be educated about the purpose and possible excesses of prevention as well as the lifelong nature of lymphedema.

11. Is there a relationship between exercise or heavy lifting and lymphedema?

People at high risk for lymphedema have long been encouraged to avoid strenuous, repetitive exercise and heavy lifting with the affected limb. Eighteen recommended steps are available through the National Lymphedema Network (NLN); they are based on case reports and are not likely to be clarified by clinical research. Adherence to activity restrictions must be accompanied by skilled patient monitoring, appropriate staff assistance and support, and consideration of the importance of patient fitness, quality of life, and unique lifestyle situations (i.e., job, home environment).

12. Is lymphedema painful?

Discomfort rather than pain commonly is associated with uncomplicated cancer-related lymphedema. Since cancer metastasis, thrombosis, and infection can cause pain, these conditions always must be ruled out when pain is associated with lymphedema. Surgical complications can result in various pain syndromes such as neuropathies or myofascial restrictions. Ineffective exercising or rehabilitation following cancer surgery and radiation therapy may also be the source of pain. Additionally, pain can be secondary to bursitis, arthritis, tendonitis, fibromyalgia, or other conditions not related to the cancer and its treatment. Pain can usually be managed with nonopioid analgesics; adjuvant drugs such as antidepressants, muscle relaxants, and opioid analgesics; transcutaneous electrical nerve stimulation (TENS); or relaxation techniques.

13. Are there any serious long-term complications for people with lymphedema?

The most common serious complications of lymphedema are cellulitis and loss of limb function. A rare and generally fatal complication associated with long-term lymphedema is lymphangiosarcoma. Less than 1% of patients with lymphedema develop lymphangiosarcoma. The median survival time is 1.3 years. Other serious complications include numerous skin conditions, depression, social isolation, loss of function, loss of employment, disability, and loss of independence.

14. When should a patient be referred for lymphedema treatment?

Whenever patients develop new or increased edema or experience changes in signs and symptoms related to edema, they should be evaluated for infection, thrombosis, and new or metastatic cancer. The presence of these conditions requires appropriate medical attention and resolution followed by appropriate lymphedema management. Since medical management of infection, thrombosis, and cancer can lead to total reduction of the edema, lymphedema management can range from precaution instructions to extensive treatment.

15. How helpful are diuretics in lymphedema management?

Inadequate lymphatic transport capacity is the underlying cause of lymphedema. Diuretics decrease capillary filtration by reducing blood volume rather than improving lymphatic transport. Diuretics can be helpful for minimizing acute symptoms on a short-term basis during acute inflammation, infection, thrombosis, or injury. Long-term use of diuretics is contraindicated because regular reduction of tissue fluid without removal of excess protein, pathogens, and cell debris can result in highly concentrated irritants that cause increased inflammation and stagnation. These conditions are associated with lymphedema progression.

16. How should lymphedema be treated?

Significant treatment diversity and controversy have resulted from the absence of comparative research in lymphedema management. External compression therapy is universally accepted as essential to lymphedema control. For patients with substantial lymphedema, most experts now additionally recommend a combination treatment approach. This multimodality approach, often referred to as "intensive therapy," includes (1) external compression therapy, (2) skin care, (3) exercise, and (4) manual lymphatic therapy. Many titles are used at different treatment centers to describe this European-based approach initially called "combined decongestive therapy" (CDT). Significant volume reductions are common with CDT, but little data exist to quantify long-term results or to compare them with other approaches. Additional research is needed to establish criteria based standards of care. Effective lymphedema treatment additionally requires comprehensive patient support, education, compliance, empowerment in self-care, reimbursement resources, access to crisis intervention, and regular follow-up.

17. What is external compression and how is it provided?

External compression therapy refers to the provision of even pressure to skin surfaces above an area with lymphedema. Several important benefits are provided. Compression support helps restore skin elasticity and prevent additional skin stretching. It also increases the effectiveness of muscle contractions and tissue pressure, both of which stimulate lymphatic circulation. Compression decreases arterial outflow to decrease the fluid load requiring lymphatic transport. External compression also encourages transport of proteins out of tissues and thus decreases tissue fibrosis. Compression products provide protection from abrasions, sunburn, and other such breaches of skin integrity. Several external compression products are available: bandaging (wrapping), garments, custom-made products for various unique lymphedemas, mechanical pumps, and semirigid support products. Nonstretch bandaging must be delineated from Ace-type bandages that provide elastic rather than nonelastic compression. Compression garments are either prefabricated or custom made. Garments include sleeves, gloves, gauntlets, and stockings. Postoperative surgical stockings do not provide sufficient pressure to manage lymphedema. Unique products are now available to assist with head, neck, genital, and trunk edema. Semirigid support products utilize Velcro and foam to provide adjustable, nonelastic support that appears comparable to bandaging but is much easier and more convenient to use.

18. How does exercise help treat lymphedema?

Lymphatic function can be enhanced or hindered by both insufficient and excessive exercise. Muscle contractions stimulate lymphatic contractions resulting in improved lymphatic transport. Deep breathing, which is recommended with exercise, is also useful for improving lymphatic circulation. Rigorous exercise increases arterial inflow, which also increases the lymphatic load. Already compromised, the area with lymphedema is easily overwhelmed by extra fluid, and stagnation increases. Gradual progression of the lymphedema is likely. Use of external compression during exercise often allows greater activity. Signs of excessive exercise include increased edema, tightness, and aching or other discomfort. Since individual patient tolerance for exercise varies immensely, lymphedema patients benefit from cooperating in the development of their individual exercise regimens. They also must monitor for signs of lymphatic overload. Ideally, patients attain the highest possible fitness level without producing lymphatic compromise.

19. Is lymphedema skin care similar to diabetic skin care?

Skin care for both conditions focuses on promoting skin integrity and preventing complications from decreased oxygenation of tissues. Skin care for both conditions is similar: daily cleansing; gentle, thorough drying; lubrication; and monitoring for problems. Bland, nonscented products are recommended. Dermal complications that commonly occur in patients with substantial lymphedema, especially of the lower extremities, include dermatitis, odor, hyperkeratosis, warts, papillomas, lymphorrhea, and infections.

20. What is manual lymph drainage?

Manual lymph drainage (MLD) is a gentle fluid mobilization technique based on principles of lymphatic anatomy and physiology. Excess fluid, proteins, and debris are mobilized out of edematous areas and into areas with healthy lymphatics for return to the blood stream. To obtain maximum benefit, once or twice daily MLD for 4 to 6 weeks along with continual bandaging is recommended (based on the European CDT). Many adaptations of this protocol exist in the U.S. Treatments are time and labor intensive as well as costly. Patients must continue long-term external compression to avoid loss of treatment benefit. Significant edema reduction has been reported in Europe, Australia, and the United States using MLD in combination with the other three modalities of "intensive therapy."

21. What is the role of mechanical pumps in lymphedema treatment?

No research clearly answers this question. Gradient sequential compression pumps became popular in the 1980s. Pumps appear to actually improve venous return rather than lymphatic flow; they do not assist in reduction of tissue fibrosis. Improved venous return reduces the lymphatic load and thus appears useful for patients who have venous congestion associated with lymphedema. Currently, some reputable treatment centers use pumps in conjunction with MLD and external compression. Potential complications include lymphatic injury from excessive pressures (> 40 or 50 mmHg), development of fibrous cuffs at the proximal limb just above the edge of the pump sleeve, genital edema related to use of pumps in the lower extremities, and limb pain. Patients who regularly use pumps must know self-MLD techniques to ensure that fluid leaves the affected limb; self-monitoring skills are also essential.

22. What kind of support is available for people with lymphedema?

The National Lymphedema Network (NLN) has contributed immensely to lymphedema awareness, education, and treatment. This nonprofit organization, located in San Francisco, provides a toll-free hotline, a quarterly newsletter for patients and medical staff, international conferences for patients and caregivers, various low-cost educational materials, and several patient networking programs. Information can be obtained at 1-800-541-3259; website: www.lymphnet.org; or e-mail: nln@lymphnet.org.

REFERENCES

1. Boris M, Weindorf S, Lasinski B, et al: Lymphedema reduction by noninvasive complex lymphedema therapy. Oncology 8:95–106, 1994.
2. Brennan M: The complexity of pain in post breast cancer lymphedema. Natl Lymphedema Net Newslett 11:1–8, 1999.
3. Brennan M, DePompolo R, Garden F: Focused review: Postmastectomy lymphedema. Arch Phys Med Rehabil 77(Suppl 3):95–106, 1996.
4. Brennan M, Weitz J: Lymphedema 30 years after radical mastectomy. Am J Physmed Rehabil 71:12–14, 1997.
5. Foldi E, Foldi M, Clodius L: The lymphedema chaos: A lancet. Ann Plast Surg 22:505–515, 1989.
6. Foldi E: The treatment of lymphedema. Cancer (Suppl)83:2833–2834, 1998.
7. Hull, M.M: Lymphedema in women treated for breast cancer. Semin Oncol Nurs 16:226–237, 2000.
8. Mortimer P, Badger C, Hall J: Lymphedema. In Doyle D, Hank G, McDonald N (eds): Oxford Textbook of Palliative Medicine. Oxford, Oxford University Press, 1998, pp 657–664.
9. Olzewski W: Episodic dermatolymphangioadenitis (DLA) in patients with lymphedema of the lower extremities before and after administration of benzathine penicillin: A preliminary study. Lymphology 29:126–131, 1996.
10. Smith J, Miller L: Management of patients with cancer-related lymphedema. Oncol Nurs Updates 5(3):1–12, 1998.
11. Smith J, Zobec A: Lymphedema. In Ferrell BR, Coyle N (eds): Oxford Textbook of Palliative Nursing. Oxford, Oxford University Press, 2001, pp 192–203.
12. Simon MS, Cody RL: Cellulitis after axillary lymph node dissection for carcinoma of the breast. Am J Med 93:543–548, 1992.
13. Thiadens S: Eighteen Prevention Steps for Lower Extremities. San Francisco, National Lymphedema Network, 1995.

42. MUCOSITIS

Harri Brackett, RN, BSN, OCN

1. Define stomatitis and mucositis.

Stomatitis is an acute inflammation or ulceration involving the oral or oropharyngeal mucosal tissues, whereas **mucositis** is inflammation of any mucosal tissue, including the oral mucosa. Mucositis may progress from dry, red, inflamed, cracked areas to open sores and bleeding ulcers not only in the mouth but also in the esophagus, throughout the gastrointestinal tract, and in mucosal membranes of the vagina and rectum.

2. What causes mucositis in patients with cancer?

Forty percent of patients undergoing cytotoxic chemotherapy experience mucositis. In addition, mucositis is a side effect of head/neck and total body irradiation, surgery of the oral cavity, and some of the biologic response modifiers (Interleukin-2 and lymphokine-activated killer [LAK] cells).

3. Describe the pathogenesis of mucositis.

The mucosal membrane consists of a superficial epthelial layer and its underlying connective tissue. The basal layer of the epithelial lining divides and regenerates every 7–14 days and is susceptible to the systemic effects of chemotherapy and local effects of radiation therapy. Oral complications after cancer therapies result from one of two mechanisms: (1) a direct effect of the drug on the mucous membranes or (2) an indirect result of the drug's myelosuppresive action. Reduced myeloproliferation leads to neutropenia and thrombocytopenia, which in turn lead to opportunistic infection and bleeding of the mucosal area.

4. Which chemotherapeutic agents are associated with mucositis?

Chemotherapeutic agents associated with a high incidence of oral complications are 5-fluorouracil (5-FU) with or without leucovorin, methotrexate, and bleomycin. Other drugs include cytarabine, daunorubicin, docetaxel, doxorubicin, hydroxyurea, mitomycin, mitoxantrone, paclitaxel, vinblastine, vincristine, vinorelbine, and high doses of alkylating agents such as cyclophosphamide.

5. What subgroups of patients are at highest risk for developing oral complications?

Patients exposed to multiple cytotoxic modalities and pharmacologic agents, especially patients undergoing bone marrow transplants and those with hematologic malignancies, have an increased risk of developing stomatitis and mucositis. Forty to 75% of patients receiving 5-FU, particularly those with colorectal cancer, develop stomatitis/mucositis. Other risk factors include age (< 20 years, > 65 years), neutropenia, poor oral hygiene, pretreatment xerostomia, medications (e.g., anticholinergics, phenytoin, steroids), poor nutritional status, and alcohol consumption. Of interest, Dodd et al. reported no significant differences between current smoking status and development of stomatitis. Furthermore, this study also found that stomatitis occurred 7–10 days sooner in patients who had dental care or professional cleaning 2 months prior to chemotherapy.

6. When does mucositis occur?

The effects of chemotherapy on the oral mucosa begin shortly after therapy is started. Because leukocytes and oral mucosal cells have similar rates of renewal, the peak in severity of mucositis usually correlates with that of myelosuppression, and the nadir occurs around day 7–10 of therapy. The condition eventually resolves, usually within 2 weeks. Mucositis associated with radiation therapy begins 1–2 weeks after therapy is started and may persist for many weeks. The intensity and duration of mucositis are influenced by type and dosage of chemotherapy drug or depth of radiation, and number and frequency of radiation treatments.

7. Define xerostomia.

Xerostomia is a Greek term that literally means "dry mouth." Saliva is a natural lubricant that cleans the mouth; assists with chewing, swallowing, and digesting food; acts as a barrier to irritants; protects the teeth; aids taste sensation; and promotes speech. Insufficient or thick saliva predisposes the oral mucosa to bacterial and fungal overgrowth and adversely affects swallowing, eating, talking, taste sensation, and fit of dentures.

8. What causes xerostomia?

Xerostomia typically is associated with an extreme reduction in salivary gland secretion as a result of head/neck irradiation; however, certain chemotherapy drugs, such as doxorubicin, can cause transient mouth dryness. Other drugs that can cause xerostomia include anticholinergics, phenothiazines, tricyclic antidepressants, antihistamines, and antispasmodics. Other medical conditions related to dry mouth include Sjögren's syndrome, oral yeast infections, and gastroesophageal reflux.

9. How is xerostomia treated?

Interventions for xerostomia include use of saliva substitutes; sucking on sugar-free hard candies; frequent sipping, rinsing, and spritzing the mouth with water; and use of a humidifier at night. Some patients have reported that it is helpful to suck on a small pad of butter. Pilocarpine, a cholinergic agonist that is available orally (Salagen), has demonstrated efficacy in relieving symptoms of radiation-induced xerostomia. Amifostine (Ethyol) given as an intravenous infusion before radiation therapy reduces the incidence of acute and late xerostomia.

10. What are the consequences of mucositis?

• Pain	• Ulceration
• Altered nutritonal status	• Xerostomia
• Volume depletion	• Bleeding
• Electrolyte imbalances	• Unpleasant taste (dysgeusia)
• Infection	or absent taste (ageusia)

11. How is mucositis assessed?

The mouth should be assessed daily and after treatment with a tongue blade and light because beginning lesions are difficult to visualize. Carefully inspect all areas of the mouth, including the tongue and beneath the tongue and the sides and roof of the mouth. Look as far back into the throat as possible and in the front and back around the lips. Pay particular attention to the appearance of any lesions and the color of the mucous membranes. Early signs and symptoms of oral mucositis include mild redness and swelling along the gumline and sensations of mild burning and dryness. The presence of redness or white patches indicates a problem. Note the color, amount, and consistency of saliva. Check for swelling, ulcerations, cracks, fissures, and bumps both in the mouth and on the lips. Ask patients if they are having pain, taste changes, swallowing problems, or sore throat.

12. What tools help to assess and document the incidence of mucositis?

In an effort to standardize measurements and descriptions of mucous membrane integrity, several oral assessment tools have been developed to grade the level of mucositis. The University of Nebraska Medical Center's Oral Assessment Guide (OAG) is a commonly used tool with demonstrated validity and reliability. The OAG contains eight categories, each with three levels of descriptive ratings. The eight categories describe quality of the voice, swallow, and saliva, and integrity of the lips, tongue, mucous membranes, gingiva, and teeth. The three descriptive levels rate each category from most normal (1) to most abnormal (3). In addition, the OAG includes a narrative description of each category of assessment. One study of patients who had bone marrow transplants showed that higher OAG scores (increased severity of mucositis) were associated with elevated blood urea nitrogen and creatinine, older age, higher preparative OAG scores, and total body irradiation (TBI).

The U.S. Cancer Cooperative Groups grade stomatitis according to common toxicity criteria (CTC) developed by the National Cancer Institute:

0	None
1	Painless ulcers, erythema, or mild soreness
2	Painful erythema, edema, or ulcers, but patient can eat solids
3	Painful erythema, edema, or ulcers, and patient cannot eat solids
4	Parenteral or enteral support required

13. What do infected lesions look like? How are they treated?

Signs and symptoms of oral infection in immunosuppressed patients may be minimal. Pain and tenderness may be the only symptoms of oral infection. If **odynophagia** (painful swallowing localized to the esophagus) is present, simultaneous involvement of the esophagus must be assumed and systemic therapy is necessary. For example, thrush and odynophagia usually mean candidal esophagitis; oral herpes and odynophagia usually mean herpetic esophagitis. Likewise, bacterial ulcerations and odynophagia, although fortunately rare, may indicate devastating bacterial involvement of the esophagus.

INFECTION	APPEARANCE/SYMPTOMS	TREATMENT
Candida albicans	Cottage cheese-like to pearly white patches may coat tongue, roof, and side of mouth; may be discolored by food or tobacco; scrapes off easily, revealing ulcerated, sometimes bleeding surfaces. Early symptoms: burning sensation or metallic taste	**Topical:** nystatin (Mycostatin) oral suspension, 400,000–600,000 U, swish and swallow 4 times/day; or clotrimazole (Mycelex) troches, 10 mg 5 times/day **Systemic:** ketoconazole (Nizoral), 200 mg/day, or fluconazole (Diflucan), 100 mg/day; amphotericin B may be necessary.
Herpes simplex	Usually appears first on lips as painful, annoying, itchy vesicle. After 6–8 hr, vesicles rupture and become encrusted, painful ulcerations. Lesions may progress to involve other oral mucosa May present as ulcerations only	Acyclovir (Zovirax), 400 mg orally every 8 hr or 5 mg/kg intravenously every 8 hr
Bacterial infection (e.g., *Pseudomonas* and *Klebsiella* spp., *Escherichia coli*	Raised yellow or yellow-white lesions encircled by reddened halo; ulcerated and painful. Fever often present. May present as ulcerations only. Blood cultures may be positive. Tooth pain with manipulation may indicate dental involvement.	Topical or systemic antibiotic therapy based on culture results Empiric therapy should cover *Pseudomonas* spp.

14. How should oral or topical medication be administered?

Fungal infections (50% of oral infections) may be treated with topical agents such as nystatin (Mycostatin) oral suspension or clotrimazole (Mycelex) troches. To facilitate drug contact of topical agents with mucosal surfaces, instruct the patient to do a mouth rinse (normal saline or water) before the medication is given and to avoid eating or drinking for at least 30 minutes after taking the topical agent. The suspension must be swished around the mouth for 5 minutes 4 times/day. It may be spit or swallowed; swallowing is recommended because of coating of the back of the throat, where fungal lesions can hide. Troches need to be sucked and held in the mouth until they dissolve (about 5 minutes). Ketoconazole absorption is greatly enhanced by an acidic gastric fluid and should be taken on an empty stomach. The patient should not be taking antacids, histamine-2 blockers, or proton pump inhibitors (e.g., omeprazole). If hypochlorhydria (inadequate stomach acid) is suspected, absorption can be improved by taking ketoconazole with a cola beverage. Ketoconazole may increase cyclosporine levels. Fluconazole is more expensive, but oral bioavailability is 90% and absorption is not influenced by food or antacid preparations.

For patients with limited oral herpes involvement around the lip area, acyclovir (Zovirax) ointment can be applied topically as needed every 4 hours. Patients should be taught to apply the ointment wearing gloves or using cotton swabs to avoid spread to other areas. Often topical therapy is inadequate and systemic therapy is needed. Acyclovir can be given orally or intravenously.

15. How can oral mucositis be prevented?

There is no standard oral care protocol to prevent mucositis; however, studies show that a protocol emphasizing routine mouth rinsing (regardless of the rinse used), adequate teaching, consistent documentation, and reinforcement of mouth care decreases the incidence of mucositis. Individualized and regular oral care protocols consisting of cleaning, lubricating, and controlling pain are essential. Mouth care should be done hourly to every 4 hours while the patient is awake, depending on the severity of mucositis. Other helpful interventions include:

- Dental evaluation and crucial dental work should be done before chemotherapy is started. Prophylactic cleanings may be helpful, but dental work should be avoided during therapy, unless scheduled when blood counts are normal.
- Dietary intake should emphasize high-protein foods and lots of fluids (> 1500 ml/day) to encourage oral mucous membrane regeneration.
- Oral cyrotherapy (sucking on ice chips) for 5 minutes before and 25 minutes after bolus administration of 5-FU decreases stomatitis.
- Allopurinol mouthwash 4–6 times/day prevents mucositis related to 5-FU.

16. Which is the better rinsing agent—normal saline or sodium bicarbonate?

Frequent oral rinsing of the mouth is encouraged throughout the day, particularly after eating. Because the optimal mouthwash has not been determined, the choice often depends on patient preferences. Commercial mouthwashes should be avoided because their high alcohol content can be irritating and drying to oral mucosa. There is no statistically significant difference in the efficacy of normal saline vs. sodium bicarbonate.

Normal saline controls mechanical plaque. It removes and washes away loose debris while moistening and soothing the oral mucosa. It is generally nonirritating, inexpensive, and readily available. Normal saline is prepared by dissolving 1 tsp of salt in a quart of warm water.

Sodium bicarbonate solution also controls mechanical plaque while neutralizing acidity and decreasing redness. It is prepared by mixing 1 tsp of baking soda in 8 ounces of warm water. Some patients prefer mixing baking soda (1 tsp) and salt (1/2 tsp) together in 1 cup of warm water.

17. Is hydrogen peroxide useful in the treatment of mucositis?

The use of hydrogen peroxide is controversial. Although it loosens debris and mucus and has a good antimicrobial effect, it may cause overgrowth of filiform papillae on the tongue, which enhances growth of candidal organisms. Patients also complain that hydrogen peroxide (1.5% concentration) causes increased thirst, dry mouth, and bad taste. Peroxamint, a mint-flavored solution, may improve the taste.

18. Is chlorhexidine helpful in preventing infection?

Chlorhexidine gluconate, a broad-spectrum antibiotic, binds to glycoproteins coating the oral mucosa and teeth. Chlorhexidine gluconate (0.12%) mouthwash, commercially available as Peridex, has been reported to reduce oral infection in chemotherapy patients with gram-positive (streptococci) or gram-negative organisms, yeast, and fungi. The usual dose is 15 ml, swished 2 or 3 times/day for 30 seconds after brushing teeth. Peridex can be used prophylactically as well as with moderate-to-severe stomatitis. A drawback to chlorhexidine is that it contains 11.6% alcohol glycerin, which leads to drying and burning. Other disadvantages include teeth staining, dysgeusia, need for prescription, and expense.

The use of chlorhexidine mouthwash in the prevention of chemotherapy-induced stomatitis is controversial. One study supported its prophylactic use in decreasing stomatitis in patients undergoing bone marrow transplantation. Another study showed no significant differences in the incidence and severity of mucositis in a large group of patients randomized to the use of mouthwashes containing sterile water or chlorhexidine to prevent chemotherapy-induced oral mucositis. However, all patients in this study were also educated in oral assessment; routine, systematic mouth care; and when to report findings to health care workers. Patients receiving high-dose head and neck irradiation showed little or no reduction in stomatitis because chlorhexidine does not bind directly to epithelial tissues; instead, it binds to negatively charged salivary mucins or glycoproteins, which are decreased by radiation-induced xerostomia.

19. When should a patient use a foam brush?

Toothbrushing with a nonabrasive toothpaste is an effective means of reducing plaque and gingivitis. However, there are times when toothbrushes are not recommended (thrombocytopenia) and not practical because of pain (secondary to ulcerations) or unavailabiltiy of an appropriate (soft-bristled) toothbrush. The use of a foam brush (toothette) soaked in chlorexidine can be as effective in reducing plaque and gingivitis as a soft-bristled toothbrush and even more effective than a foam brush alone.

20. What techniques are recommended for stomatitis prevention and treatment?

- **Alcohol-free chlorhexidine mouthwash.** Though drying and irritating, the purpose of alcohol in mouthwashes is twofold: it serves as a vehicle to dissolve other ingredients and as an antiseptic agent. In a comparison study between commercially available chlorhexidine (Peridex), alcohol-free chlorhexidine, and Listerine mouthwashes, both chlorhexidine solutions were effective in reducing microbial growth, whereas Listerine was less effective.[8]
- **Glutamine** (oral suspension as a swish-and-swallow, 2–4 gm). Glutamine is an amino acid used as a nitrogen and energy source for cells and tissues in the body, especially the intestinal epithelium. In chemotherapy patients, it reduces the severity and duration of mucositis as well as helps to decrease oral pain.[1]
- **Immunomodulatory agents.** Although no benefits were found with granulocyte-macrophage colony-stimulating factor mouthwash, subcutaneous injections of granulocyte-stimulating factor may have promise in the prevention and reduction of the duration of mucositis.
- **Low-intensity laser.** Low-energy laser has been shown to decrease pain and promote proliferation of mucosal cells and wound healing.[17]
- **Sucralfate suspension with cryotherapy**. Sucralfate, a basic albumin salt of sucrose octasulfate, has been approved for the treatment of duodenal ulcers. It adheres to exposed protein in inflamed gastroduodenal mucosa, providing a protective coat against pepsin and a therapeutic benefit locally at the ulcer. In a study by Loprinzi et al., patients received oral cryotherapy for 30 minutes during each dose of 5-FU and then were randomized to receive either a sucralfate suspension or a placebo solution. The study reported no difference in stomatitis severity or duration between the two solutions.
- **Tetrachlorodecaoxide (TCDO) swish-and-swallow mouthwash.** TCDO is a water-soluble, oxygen-containing compound that, in conjunction with hemoproteins, forms a complex in the tissues that activates macrophages and improves oxygenation and granulation. In a recent study, it helped to decrease pain and symptoms of oral mucositis.[16] Further study is needed.
- **Other treatments.** Large, controlled studies are needed to determine the effectiveness of: antibiotics, antifungals, and antivirals; local application of vitamin E; silver nitrate; mucosal barriers such as plastic wrap film; and mouthwashes containing substances such as chamomile, allopurinol, corticosteroids, capsaicin and benzocaine preparations, lidocaine, benzydamine hydrochloride, or Kaopectate.

21. What can be done for vaginal or perianal mucositis?

Patients should be educated to report pain, itching, ulceration, or bleeding and alerted to signs and symptoms of fungal or herpes infections. Management and prevention include frequent and meticulous perianal and vaginal cleansing, especially after voiding. Witch hazel (Tucks) pads may be used for the perianal area if the patient does not have skin breakdowns and can tolerate the potential stinging sensation. Water-soluble lubricants can be applied to prevent dryness and to protect the mucous linings. Sitz baths of warm water may provide comfort to patients without extensive skin breakdown.

22. What helpful hints may be shared with patients?
   1. **Keep mouth moist.**
      - Rinse mouth frequently with water.
      - Use spray bottle and mist often; humidifying the room is also helpful.
      - Use commercially available salivary substitutes or supplements (e.g., Salivart, Oral Balance, Salagen, MoiStir).
      - Apply lip lubricant generously.
   2. **Keep mouth and teeth clean.**
      - Use soft-bristled toothbrushes or sponge-covered oral swabs with nonabrasive fluoride toothpaste to brush teeth 30 minutes after each meal and at bedtime.
      - Follow brushing with routine rinsing. Increase the frequency of rinsing depending on the severity of mucositis (every 2–4 hr as needed is not uncommon).
      - Remove dentures and bridges and clean after meals; do not replace if stomatitis is severe.
      - Avoid alcohol-based mouthwashes and lemon glycerin swabs because of drying and unpleasant taste.
      - Gently floss teeth with unwaxed floss (if platelet count > 20,000).
      - Follow rinsing with the use of a topical anesthetic or topical antifungal as needed (these agents coat better on a clean mouth).
   3. **Maintain integrity of oral mucosa.**
      - Apply liquid from punctured vitamin E capsule to provide natural protective action to mucous membranes and lesions, especially for radiation mucositis.
      - Use sucralfate to help heal and coat oral mucosa (binds to damaged proteins in mucosal surface). Mix 1 tablet in 15 ml water to make a slurry. Swish and spit 3–4 times/day.
      - For mucosal bleeding, apply topical thrombin. Remove dentures or orthodontic retainers. Be aware of secondary infections.
   4. **Follow dietary tips.**
      - Avoid foods that are hot, rough, coarse, highly spiced, or acidic.
      - Avoid temperature extremes of food (hot coffee, ice cream).
      - Avoid citrus juices or foods that irritate the mouth.
   5. **Control pain.**

23. What agents may be used to treat and relieve pain associated with oral mucositis?

Severe pain associated with stomatitis may require systemic opioids such as intravenous morphine, morphine elixir, or nonsteroidal anti-inflammatory drugs (NSAIDs), supplemented with topical anesthetics during more painful times (e.g., during meals or mouth cleansing). Mild oral pain may be controlled effectively with local agents in patients with few ulcerations. Mouth care with oral rinsing should be done first to remove excessive debris. Commonly used topical agents include the following:
   - Xylocaine viscous 2% solution: 5–15 ml; swish and spit every 2–4 hours as needed
   - Diclonine hydrochloride: 5–10 ml; swish and spit every 2–4 hours as needed
   - KBX solution (Kaopectate, Benadryl, xylocaine viscous in equal parts): 5–15 ml; swish for 1 minute, then spit or swallow every 2–4 hours as needed. Xylocaine functions as a topical anesthetic, Benadryl as a short-acting anesthetic. Mylanta may be substituted for Kaopectate.

Each serves as a medium for alkalinizing oral pH, which is usually more acidic in patients with stomatitis.

- Kenalog in Orabase (triamcinolone acetonide): apply paste to mouth or lip sores 2–4 times/day.
- Ulcerease: thick gel that coats, protects, and eases pain.
- Zilactin: topical application to oral and lip lesions (burns on application).
- Oral capsaicin taffy: capsaicin is the active incredient in chili peppers that desensitizes some of the neurons in the pain region. A study by Berger et al. found that patients reported less pain after the initial burning of the candy had faded.

ACKNOWLEDGMENT

The author thanks Janet Kemp, RN, MS, for her contribution to the first edition of this chapter.

REFERENCES

1. Anderson PM, Schroeder G, Skubitz KM: Oral glutamine reduces the duration and severity of stomatitis after cytotoxic cancer chemotherapy. Cancer 83:1433–1439, 1998.
2. Berger A, Eilers J: Factors influencing oral cavity status during high-dose antineoplastic therapy: A secondary analysis. Oncol Nurs Forum 25:1623–1626, 1998.
3. Berger A, Henderson M, Nadoolman W, et al: Oral capsaicin provides temporary relief for oral mucositis pain secondary to chemotherapy/radiation therapy. J Pain Symptom Manage 10:243–248, 1995.
4. Bez C, Federica D, Sardella A, et al: GM-CSF mouthrinses in the treatment of severe oral mucositis. Oral Surg Oral Med Oral Pathol 88:311–315, 1999.
5. Dodd MJ, Larson PJ, Dibble SL, et al: Randomized clinical trial of chlorhexidine versus placebo for prevention of oral mucositis in patients receiving chemotherapy. Oncol Nurs Forum 23:921–927, 1996.
6. Dodd M, Miaskowski C, Shiba G, et al: Risk factors for chemotherapy induced oral mucositis: Dental applications, oral hygiene, previous oral lesions, and histroy of smoking. Cancer Invest 17:278–284, 1999.
7. Eilers J, Berger AM, Peterson MC: Development, testing and application of the oral assessment guide. Oncol Nurs Forum 15:325–330, 1988.
8. Eldridge KR, Finnie SF, Stephens JA, et al: Efficacy of an alcohol-free chlorhexidine mouthrinse as an antimicrobial agent. J Prosth Dent 80:685–690, 1998.
9. Ferretti GA, Raybould T, Brown A, et al: Chlorhexidine prophylaxis for chemotherapy and radiotherapy-induced stomatitis: A randomized double-blind trial. Oral Surg Oral Med Oral Pathol 69:331–338, 1990.
10. Fidler P, Loprinzi CL, O'Fallon JR, et al: Prospective evaluation of a chamomile mouthwash for prevention of 5FU induced oral mucositis. Cancer 77:522–525, 1996.
11. Galbraith LK, Bailey D, Kelly L, et al: Treatment for alteration in oral mucosa related to chemotherapy. Pediatr Nurs 17:233–236, 1991.
12. Johnson JT, Ferretti GA, Nethery WJ, et al: Oral pilocarpine for post-irradiation xerostomia in patients with head and neck cancer. N Engl J Med 329:390–395, 1993.
13. Loprinzi CL, Ghosh C, et al: Phase III controlled evaluation of sucralfate to alleviate stomatitis in patients receiving fluorouracil-based chemotherapy. J Clin Oncol 15:1235–1238, 1997.
14. Madeya ML: Oral complications from cancer therapy. Part I: Pathophysiology and secondary complications. Oncol Nurs Forum 23:801–807, 1996.
15. Madeya ML: Oral complications from cancer therapy. Part II: Nursing implications for assessment and treatment. Oncol Nurs Forum 23:808–819, 1996.
16. Malik IA, Moid I, Haq S, Sabih M: A double blind, placebo controlled, randomized trial to evaluate the role of tetrachlorodecaoxide in the management of chemotherapy induced oral mucositis. J Pain Symptom Manage 14(2):82–87, 1997.
17. Marei MK, Abdel-Meguid SH, et al: Effect of low-energy laser application in the treatment of denture-induced mucosal lesions. J Prosth Dent 3:256–264, 1997.
18. Ransier A, Epstein JB., Lunn R, Spinelli J: A combined analysis of a toothbrush, foam brush, and a chlorhexidine-soaked foam brush in maintaining oral hygiene. Cancer Nurs 18:393–396, 1995.
19. Rutkauskas J, Davis J: Effects of chlorhexidine during immunosuppressive chemotherapy. A preliminary report. Oral Surg Oral Med Oral Pathol 76:441–447, 1993.
20. Skeel RT, Tipton J: Symptom management. In Brain MC, Carbone PP (eds): Current Therapy in Hematology-Oncology. St. Louis, Mosby, 1995, pp 584–586.
21. Skubitz KM, Anderson PM: Oral glutamine to prevent chemotherapy induced stomatitis: A pilot study. J Lab Clin Med 127: 223–228, 1996.
22. Wilkes JD: Prevention and treatment of oral mucositis following cancer chemotherapy. Semin Oncol 25:538–551, 1998.
23. Wojtaszek C: Management of chemotherapy-induced stomatitis. Clin J Oncol Nurs 4:263–270, 2000.

43. NAUSEA AND VOMITING

Rita Wickham, RN, PhD, AOCN

1. How big is the problem of nausea and vomiting (N&V) for patients with cancer?

People with cancer are at risk for N&V from several causes: chemotherapy, radiation therapy, surgery (from anesthesia), and progressive disease. The availability of new antiemetics over the past 10 years has reduced the risk for acute N&V from chemotherapy to approximately 20–40%—even with highly emetogenic chemotherapy. Delayed nausea after chemotherapy may be more frequent. The risk for N&V from radiation therapy ranges from 10–100%, and is related to the site radiated and dose. Postoperative N&V (PONV) can be significant and distressing and is often related to similar patient risk factors such as N&V from other causes. In addition, 50% or more of patients with progressive cancer experience nausea and/or vomiting. The nurse also must consider that other medications or concomitant medical problems may add to N&V in patients with cancer.

2. What are the consequences of poorly managed N&V?

Poorly controlled N&V may lead to negative physiologic and psychosocial effects, thus affecting overall quality of life. For instance, severe vomiting may lead to dehydration and electrolyte imbalance. Rapid weight loss (over one to a few days) signifies water loss. It may be helpful to remember the old saying, "A pint is a pound the world around." That is, the rapid loss of 2 pounds signifies the loss of approximately 1 liter of body water. The nurse should calculate the actual weight loss and the percentage of loss because both reflect fluid volume deficit (FVD). FVD may range from mild (2% weight loss) to severe (8% weight loss). If N&V continue, the patient may not be able to drink liquids. This further exacerbates FVD and may increase the risk for certain chemotherapy toxicities (e.g., renal toxicity from cisplatin, hemorrhagic cystitis from cyclophosphamide).

Sustained nausea also may be associated with anorexia, taste changes, development of food aversions, and weight loss with depletion of body stores of protein and fat (protein-calorie malnutrition). These events further affect quality of life and ultimately may render the person less able to tolerate the rigors of cancer therapy. N&V related to radiation therapy or progressive disease also may interfere with important activities, such as spending time with family and friends, household tasks and outside jobs, leisure activities, and enjoyment of eating and drinking. Patients who have both uncontrolled vomiting and pain typically rate vomiting as the worse symptom.

3.   Are physiology and pathogenesis the same for all instances of N&V?

Despite increasing insight into the physiology of vomiting, all mechanisms of vomiting have not been elucidated, and the understanding of nausea is even less clear. Vomiting occurs when a group of neurons in the brainstem, collectively called the vomiting center (VC), are stimulated. Emetic stimuli do not directly activate the VC; emesis is triggered through one or more incoming pathways (afferents). Afferents implicated in chemotherapy-induced N&V include the vagus nerve and perhaps other abdominal visceral nerves; the chemoreceptor trigger zone (CTZ) in the area postrema; higher brain centers associated with vision, hearing, smell, and memory; and the limbic region, which is associated with emotion. The vestibular apparatus of the middle ear, other neural structures, and visceral organs may play unidentified minor roles.

4. Describe the role of the chemoreceptor trigger zone and higher cortical centers.

The CTZ, which lies close to the VC in the fourth ventricle, is outside the blood-brain barrier and can detect noxious substances in the bloodstream and cerebral spinal fluid. Numerous receptors for neurotransmitters that may play a role in vomiting, including dopamine, serotonin, and histamine, are located in and about the CTZ. Higher cortical centers are important in the development of anticipatory nausea and vomiting, the realization of pain-related N&V, and N&V associated with increased intracranial pressure. The cortex and limbic region are responsible for the emotional responses to N&V, such as anxiety and suffering associated with poorly controlled symptoms.

5. What is the role of the vestibular apparatus (VA)?

The role of the VA is clearly evident to anyone who has experienced motion sickness, Menière's syndrome, or viral infection of the inner ear. Dizziness, nausea, and vomiting follow. The VA may play a minor role in N&V from other causes.

6. Describe the role of serotonin receptors in N&V.

Serotonin receptors, subtype 3 ($5HT_3$), are located along the vagus nerve and play a significant role in helping the body rid itself of substances perceived to be noxious or poisonous, including chemotherapy drugs and products released from damaged cells after abdominal radiation. The vagus lies within the upper gastrointestinal (GI) tract close to enterochromaffin cells, which release serotonin (5HT) in response to toxins in the GI tract or blood stream. When 5HT binds to vagal $5HT_3$ receptors, the message to vomit is transmited to the vomiting center (directly or indirectly through the chemoreceptor trigger zone). $5HT_4$ is a related neuroreceptor that plays a role in gastric stasis and slowed GI transit time and probably has a role in delayed N&V after chemotherapy. In addition, the vagus and/or other visceral nerves also have stretch receptors that respond to compression and stasis, which occur with small bowel obstruction, hepatomegaly, or tumor compression. The neurotransmitters that bind with stretch receptors have not been clearly identified.

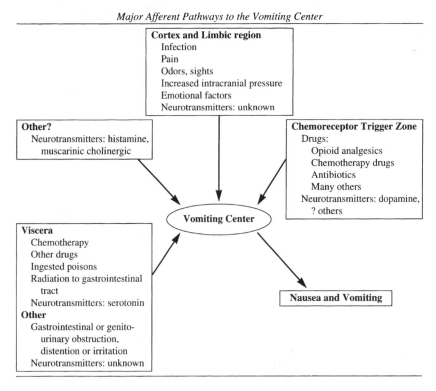

Major Afferent Pathways to the Vomiting Center

Major afferent pathways for nausea and vomiting in patients with cancer include the vagal and visceral nerves, the chemoreceptor zone, and higher brain centers. Neurotransmitters presumed to play the most important role for different pathways are listed, but more than one neurotransmitter may play a role within a given pathway. (From Ettinger DS: Preventing chemotherapy-induced nausea and vomiting: An update and review of emesis. Semin Oncol 22(Suppl 10):9, 1995, with permission.)

7. When are N&V likely to occur after chemotherapy is administered?

Chemotherapy can cause three types of N&V: acute, delayed, and anticipatory. The time frame for acute N&V starts within minutes to hours after chemotherapy administration and resolves within 24 hours. Delayed N&V begins 16–24 hours after chemotherapy and persists for hours to days. Different mechanisms probably are involved in acute and delayed N&V, despite overlap in each phase. For instance, the role of serotonin is most important in acute N&V, wheres other mechanisms probably gain importance in the days after chemotherapy. During delayed N&V, nausea is often worse than vomiting and may have deleterious effects on quality of life. Delayed N&V may persist for one to several days after chemotherapy. In some cases, particularly after cisplatin or cyclophosphamide, delayed nausea and/or vomiting may actually worsen for a day or two before they start to subside.

8. What is anticipatory N&V?

Anticipatory N&V (ANV) result when acute or delayed N&V are not adequately managed. ANV is a classic conditioned response that occurs when patients experience N&V after their first chemotherapy treatment (an unconditioned response). If N&V continue to be poorly controlled, the events surrounding chemotherapy administration (e.g., smells in the clinic, common sights seen at each visit) become stimuli that elicit nausea (a conditioned response). ANV is extremely difficult to manage and may persist for 2–3 years after chemotherapy has been completed. In the past, 25–60% of patients developed ANV within 4 courses of chemotherapy. Now that serotonin antagonist antiemetics are the standard of care for moderately to highly emetogenic chemotherapy, the risk for ANV is lower.

9. Which chemotherapy drugs cause N&V?

Chemotherapy typically has been classified as mildly, moderately, moderately high, and highly emetogenic. Newer and simpler classification schemes are based on a large number of antiemetic studies, including those that examined the efficacy of $5HT_3$ receptor antagonists for chemotherapy. Many studies included large numbers of patients and had sufficient statistical power to provide clinicians with sound evidence to make antiemetic choices for patients receiving chemotherapy. The classification proposed by the American Society of Clinical Oncology (ASCO) is outlined below.

Classification of the Acute Emetogenic Potential of Chemotherapeutic Agents

High risk: > 99%
  Cisplatin

High risk (noncisplatin): 30–90%

Carboplatin	Dacarbazine	Epirubicin	Lomustine
Carmustine	Daunorubicin	Idarubicin	Mechlorethamine
Cytarabine	Doxorubicin	Ifosfamide	Streptozocin
Dactinomycin			

Intermediate risk: 10–30%

Docetaxel	Irinotecan	Paclitaxel	Thiotepa
Etoposide	Mitomycin	Teniposide	Topotecan
Gemcitabine	Mitoxantrone		

Low risk: < 10%

Bleomycin	Fluorouracil	Mercaptopurine	Vincristine
Busulfan	Hydroxyurea	Methotrexate	Vindesine
Chlorambucil	L-Asparaginase	Thioguanine	Vinorelbine
Fludarabine	Melphalan	Vinblastine	

Most data from Gralla RJ, Osoba D, Kris MG, et al: Recommendations for the use of antiemetics: Evidence-based, clinical practice guidelines. J Clin Oncol 17:2871–2994, 1999.

10. What other factors may affect the emetogenic potential of chemotherapeutic drugs?

The ASCO and other guidelines are intended to aid clinicians in making reasonable decisions about antiemetics for chemotherapy but do not supplant clinical judgment, which is critical because of the following factors:

- Inherent differences in particular patients or clinical situations
- Other factors that may alter the risk for N&V (e.g., gender, age, other illnesses, other medications)
- Patient preference (e.g., route of administration)

Other factors not specifically addressed in the guidelines that may be important include chemotherapy dose (i.e., low-dose cytarabine is not highly emetogenic whereas high-dose cytarabine often is) and administration schedule (i.e., a large single dose vs. lower divided doses vs. continuous infusion over several days.) Continuous infusion over several days may cause less vomiting but greater nausea. Virtually all chemotherapy agents that are at least intermediately emetogenic can cause some degree of delayed N&V.

11. Does radiation therapy cause less N&V than chemotherapy?

Radiation therapy is a local treatment, and side effects are related to the irradiated site. Cellular byproducts of radiation therapy may stimulate enterochromaffin cells to release 5HT; thus, patients whose radiation field includes the GI tract are at greatest risk for experiencing N&V. Approximately 60–90% of patients who receive total body irradiation (TBI) in preparation for stem cell transplant or hemibody irradiation to the upper body for pain control or to a large volume of abdominal tissue experience N&V. A smaller number who receive radiation therapy to the chest (~20%) or to the head (~10%) experience N&V. In rare instances, patients who receive radiation to other parts of the body experience N&V. The mechanisms in such cases are unknown but may be related to anxiety and anticipation. Vomiting after radiation occurs within minutes when stem cell transplantation preparatory doses are given and within a few hours after lower doses. N&V may persist for several hours after each treatment. ANV may occur if symptoms are not well controlled. Premedication with a $5HT_3$ antagonist (i.e., ondansetron [Zofran], 8 mg orally or intravenously; granisetron [Kytril], 1 mg orally; or dolasetron [Anzemet], 50–100 mg orally) is indicated for patients who receive radiation therapy to the chest, abdomen, or pelvis because of the high risk for N&V.

12. How common are postoperative N&V?

PONV are not as common as in the past because newer anesthetics are less emetogenic than older ones, but 20-30% of patients still experience significant problems. Women, chidren, and patients with other risk factors (e.g., abdominal surgery, prior surgery with poorly controlled PONV, high anxiety, obesity) may be at increased risk. In addition, opioid analgesics can cause N&V, and delayed return of bowel motility may exacerbate nausea. As a result, postoperative recovery and hospital discharge are delayed. Patients who are at high risk should receive a prophylactic antiemetic before surgery or intraoperatively. First-line antiemetics for PONV are either a $5HT_3$ antagonist (e.g., ondansetron, 4 mg intravenously or 8 mg orally; dolasetron, 12.5 mg intravenously or 100 mg orally) or droperidol, 0.625–1.25 mg intravenously. Alternative antiemetics may include metoclopramide or phenothiazines (e.g., prochlorperazine, chlorpromazine, promethazine). $5HT_3$ antagonists have a more favorable side-effect profile; they are virtually nonsedating.

13. What other causes should the nurse consider when assessing N&V in patients with cancer?

Because N&V may be multifactorial, in-depth nursing assessment is critical. Causes of N&V may include cancer effects on the GI tract (e.g., bowel obstruction, hepatomegaly, stomach cancer, adhesions, ileus, severe constipation) and central nervous system (meningeal or brain metastases that increase intracranial pressure) as well as metabolic abnormalities and paraneoplastic syndromes (e.g., hypercalcemia, hypernatremia, syndrome of inappropriate secretion of antidiuretic hormone [SIADH]). Furthermore, patients may experience nausea secondary to inadequately controlled moderate-to-severe pain, or their nausea may be caused by opioid or other analgesics. Similarly, nausea may be a symptom of infection as well as a side effect of antibiotics or other medications. A single antiemetic, therefore, will not be effective for N&V due to all causes. Antiemetic selection should be based on presumed causes and probable neurotransmitters.

14. In planning interventions for N&V, what patient-related factors should the nurse consider?

The factors that seem to be most predictive of difficult-to-manage N&V from treatment or disease include gender and age. A history of alcohol intake, motion sickness, hyperemesis with pregnancy, and high level of anxiety also may be influencing factors. Patients who experienced inadequate control of N&V with previous chemotherapy may be fearful of and expect N&V with new therapy. Anxiety, past motion sickness, and hyperemesis with pregnancy do not always accurately predict poorer antiemetic control but may be important for certain patients. N&V are often easier to control in patients with a history of regular alcohol use (1–5 alcoholic drinks/day). The nurse must attentively assess and document N&V and patient satisfaction with antiemetic control. Collaboration with the physician to change antiemetics or add other antiemetics for patients whose initial antiemetics are not effective is critical.

15. Explain the effects of gender on chemotherapy-induced N&V.

Even when the best available antiemetic regimens are used, up to 50% of menstruating women have inferior control of chemotherapy-induced N&V compared with men. Increased risk for N&V may be related to female hormones because prepubescent girls and boys have similar rates of N&V and antiemetic control, as do postmenopausal women and older men.

16. How does age affect chemotherapy-induced N&V?

Patients older than 50 years have less N&V than patients younger than 50, and antiemetic control may be superior in older than in younger patients.

17. What questions should the nurse ask when assessing the potential for chemotherapy-related N&V and evaluating the severity of posttreatment N&V?

In addition to considering chemotherapy emetogenicity and inherent patient factors, the nurse also should ask the patient how bothersome N&V were with past chemotherapy and whether they have had N&V secondary to motion sickness or hyperemesis with pregnancy. Such factors may increase the likelihood of chemotherapy-related N&V for some patients. With the first course of a new chemotherapy regimen, the nurse should ask the patient the following questions about 24 hours after chemotherapy:
- Did you vomit/throw up? If so, how many times?
- How much nausea have you have in the past 24 hours? (Use a 0-to-10 or none–mild–moderate–severe scale.)
- How much did nausea and/or vomiting interfere with activities important to you?
- What, if anything, made the nausea and/or vomiting worse?
- Were you able to take your antiemetic(s)? How well do you think it (they) worked?
- Did you have side effects from the antiemetics that were unacceptable to you?
- Did you try anything that made the nausea and/or vomiting better?

18. Are all antiemetics the same? Can they be used interchangeably for cancer and therapy-related N&V?

Antiemetics may be broadly classified as serotonin ($5HT_3$) antagonists, dopamine (D_2) antagonists, and antiemetics with other effects. $5HT_3$ antiemetics are the "cleanest" and have little binding at other receptors. D_2 antagonists often have some binding at other receptors, which may add to therapeutic effect but more often causes side effects. For instance, both chlorpromazine and prochlorperazine are phenothiazines. Chlorpromazine binds similarly to dopamine (D_2), histamine (H_1), and alpha-adrenergic (α_1) receptors. H_1 and α_1 effects include sedation, anticholinergic effects, dizziness, and orthostasis. Prochlorperazine, on the other hand, has a higher affinity for D_2 receptors and a lesser effect at H_1 and α_1 receptors. Chlorpromazine should not be used if sedation is undesirable but may be a reasonable choice for a terminal patient with intractable symptoms in whom sedation would be beneficial. In choosing antiemetics, knowledge of which receptors are the main site of action helps to target management.

Antiemetics by Classification

CATEGORY	EXAMPLES	DOSES	INDICATIONS/COMMENTS
Serotonin antagonists	Ondansetron (Zofran)	Oral: 8–24 mg once or in divided doses IV: 8 mg once	Highly emetogenic chemotherapy: acute and delayed N&V
	Granisetron (Kytril)	Oral: 1–2 mg once IV: 1 mg once	Whole-body radiotherapy, or chest, abdomen, pelvis
	Dolasetron (Anzemet)	Oral: 100 mg once IV: 100 mg once	Prophylaxis for PONV (smaller doses may be effective)
			Do not administer PRN or as continuous infusion
			Not as effective for N&V due to opioids
			If trial of $5HT_3$ antagonist is not effective, switching to second $5HT_3$ antagonist may improve efficacy
Corticosteroids	Dexamethasone (Decadron)	Oral: 4–18 mg (single dose before chemotherapy; divided doses for delayed N&V and terminal disease IV: 10–20 mg before chemotherapy	For immediately emetic chemotherapy and delayed N&V Effective for N&V of unknown causes/related to terminal disease May be effective for PONV
	Methylprednisolone (Solu-Medrol, others)	Oral or IV: 40–140 mg before chemotherapy	
Dopamine antagonists			
Substituted benzamide	Metoclopramide (Reglan)	Oral: 10–20 mg 3–4 times/day Parenteral: 1 mg/hr continuous IV or SC infusion	Delayed N&V N&V related to progressive disease (except from GI obstruction) No indication as first-line antiemetic for chemothearpy
Phenothiazines	Prochlorperazine (Compazine)	Oral: 10 mg every 4–6 hr, 15–30 mg time-released spansules every 8–12 hr Rectal: 25 mg every 12 hr IV: 5–10 mg every 6 hr	Delayed N&V Radiation therapy N&V from progressive disease Do not administer by continuous SC infusion; very irritating
	Thiethylperazine (Torecan)	Oral: 10–25 mg every 4–6 hr Rectal: 50–100 mg every 6–8 hr IM: 12.5–50 mg every 3–4 hr	
	Chlorpromazine (Thorazine)	Oral: 25 mg 3 times/day IM: 25 mg; increase carefully	Chlorpromazine is very sedating; use in terminal disease when sedation is desirable
Butyrophenones	Haloperidol (Haldol)	Oral: 2.5–5 mg every 4 hr Parenteral: 0.5–2 mg IM/IV every 4–8 hr; 0.7–1 mg/hr continuous IV or SC infusion	Delayed N&V PONV N&V of progressive or terminal disease Can be adminstered by continuous SC infusion
	Droperidol (Inapsine)	0.625–1.25 mg IV every 2–4 hr	Droperidol rarely used for delayed N&V due to chemotherapy—highly sedating
Cannabinoid	Dronabinol (Marinol)	Oral: 2.5–5 mg 3 times/day	Chemotherapy: only when other antiemetics not effective N&V from progressive disease May enhance appetite Side effects include sedation and dysphoria; start low and increase slowly

Table continued on following page

Antiemetics by Classification (Continued)

CATEGORY	EXAMPLES	DOSES	INDICATIONS/COMMENTS
Anxiolytic	Lorazepam (Ativan)	Oral: 0.5–1 mg sublingually or swallowed IV: 0.5–1 mg	No effective antiemetic action if used alone Can decrease anxiety and increase personal control May decrease ANV May be useful in terminal disease
Anticholinergic	Scopolamine (Transderm Scop)	Patch every 72 hr 0.6 mg every 6 hr SC, IM, IV	Radiation therapy if other antiemetics are not effective N&V from progressive disease Apply patch to upper chest (not behind ear)
Others	Benzquinamide (Emete-Con) Trimethobenzamide (Tigan)	IM: 50 mg every 4 hr Oral or rectal: 100–200 mg every 4–6 hr	Progressive disease when other antiemetics are not effective Indicated only as last line; poor efficacy

IV = intravenously, N&V = nausea and vomiting, PONV = postoperative nausea and vomiting, PRN = as needed, SC = subcutaneously, IM = intramuscularly, ANV = anticipatory nausea and vomiting.

19. Which antiemetics should be used for chemotherapy-related N&V?

The antiemetics used for acute and delayed/persistent N&V may vary. Current antiemetic recommendations base choices on the most emetogenic agent that the patient receives (see question 7). Patients whose risk is high (30–100%) should receive a 5HT$_3$ antagonist plus a corticosteroid (usually dexamethasone) on the day of chemotherapy. Dexamethasone alone (4–8 mg orally) usually is recommended for moderately emetogenic chemotherapy (10–30% risk), but prochlorperazine (10 mg orally every 4–6 hr) may be an acceptable alternative. When the risk for N&V is < 10%, routine antiemetics are not recommended. Inherent differences (e.g., female gender, young age, previous N&V) may predispose patients to a greater risk for N&V. Such patients should be treated as if they were receiving more emetogenic chemotherapy. In addition, patients who receive emetogenic chemotherapy over several days should receive a 5HT$_3$ antagonist antiemetic plus dexamethasone on each day of chemotherapy. According to current antiemetic recommendations, no patients at risk for N&V should receive antiemetics that are less effective than 5HT$_3$ antagonists (e.g., metoclopramide, D$_2$ antagonists, cannabinoid).

Antiemetics to Prevent Acute Nausea and Vomiting Due to Chemotherapy

EMETOGENIC POTENTIAL	ORAL ANTIEMETICS	IV ANTIEMETICS
High (30–100%)	Ondansetron, 12–24 mg *or* Granisetron, 1–2 mg *or* Dolasetron, 100 mg *plus* Dexamethasone, 10–20 mg or 8 mg × 2 (± lorazepam, 0.5–2 mg; may repeat) (± prochlorperazine, 10 mg every 6 hr)	Ondansetron, 8 mg *or* Granisetron, 1 mg *or* Dolasetron, 100 mg *plus* Dexamethasone, 8–20 mg
Moderate/intermediate (10–30%)	Dexamethasone, 4, 8, or 20 mg ± ondansetron, 16 mg *or* Prochlorperazine, 10 mg every 6 hr	Dexamethasone, 20 mg *or* Prochlorperazine, 10 mg every 4–6 hr
Low (< 10%)	No routine antiemetics *or* Dexamethasone, 20 mg *or* Prochlorperazine, 10 mg every 6 hr	No routine antiemetics *or* Dexamethasone, 20 mg *or* Prochlorperazine, 10 mg every 6 hr

20. Discuss the role of metoclopramide.

Intravenous, high-dose metoclopramide should be reserved for patients who do not have satisfactory control of N&V with at least one of two different $5HT_3$ antiemetics because metoclopramide (and other dopamine antagonists) can cause significant side effects, including sedation and extrapyramidal symptoms (EPS). Metoclopramide usually is combined with other drugs (lorazepam, diphenhydramine, or benztropine) to prevent EPS, but added drugs may cause significant sedation. Most patients abhor feeling "zoned out" or like they "lose days" from their lives. In addition, sedation from metoclopramide plus diphenhydramine may increase elderly patients' risk for falls and requires that someone accompany the patient to the doctor's office or clinic.

21. What is the role of $5HT_3$ antiemetics in delayed N&V?

$5HT_3$ plays less of a role in delayed N&V than in acute N&V, when other mechanisms undoubtedly come into play. Few patients have control of delayed N&V with $5HT_3$ antagonists, and rates of complete control of delayed symptoms are similar with $5HT_3$ antagonists and other antiemetics. Dexamethasone plus oral metoclopramide for 2–4 days or a $5HT_3$ antagonist antiemetic for 2–3 days is recommended for moderately to highly emetogenic chemotherapy predicted to cause delayed N&V. Such chemotherapy agents include cisplatin, cyclophosphamide, dacarbazine, doxorubicin, mechlorethamine, carboplatin, and cytarabine.

22. What factors are important in considering the cost of antiemetics for chemotherapy?

Because similar percentages of patients achieve adequate control of N&V with ondansetron, granisetron, and dolasetron, practice sites usually choose to use one or two based on the cost to the institution, local availability, and ease of use. Availability of $5HT_3$ antagonists may depend on the treatment site—that is, hospital, where costs are bundled, vs. clinic, which can bill for antiemetic treatment. The nurse should assess the patient's response to the antiemetic (control of nausea and vomiting, side effects, and overall satisfaction with antiemetics). In addition, assessment must continue during the period of delayed/persistent N&V to ascertain whether a $5HT_3$ antagonist is most appropriate for a given patient and how many days it should be continued.

Several considerations are important in the overall calculation of antiemetic costs. If less-than-optimal antiemetics are used, the nurse is ethically bound to advocate for the patient, particularly because poorly controlled N&V translate into negative quality of life and increased risk of N&V with further chemotherapy. Less effective regimens, such as metoclopramide plus diphenhydramine, are complex and time-consuming and require several hours of nursing time and use of treatment facilities. If this regimen does not control N&V, the patient may need to return to the clinic or hospital for intravenous fluids and antiemetics.

23. What are the optimal doses of ondansetron, granisetron, and dolasetron? Should intravenous formulations be administered to all patients?

The lowest effective dose of any $5HT_3$ antagonist should be administered as a single dose before chemotherapy (or radiation therapy). Oral $5HT_3$ antagonists are as effective as intravenous formulations because binding of the antiemetic to the 5HT receptor occurs at vagal terminals, which lie in the crypts of the GI mucosa close to the enterochromaffin cells. There is general consensus about antiemetic recommendations for chemotherapy. For typical doses, see the table with question 18.

24. The house staff physician has ordered ondansetron (Zofran), 16 mg in 50 ml normal saline, to be infused over 15–30 minutes every 4 hours for 3 days after cisplatin therapy. What is the problem with this order?

$5HT_3$ antagonists differ from other antiemetics in that their effectiveness depends on initial binding of all 5HT receptors involved with N&V rather than maintenance of drug serum level. Binding affinity is high and persists for approximately 16–24 hours. Therefore, repeated, as-needed, and continuous infusions of $5HT_3$ antagonists are not indicated. Similarly, if the total dose is divided into smaller doses and administered at intervals over several hours (i.e., every 4 or 6 hours), the patient is less likely to achieve complete control of N&V. Tight binding to receptors does not occur with other antiemetics, which must be administered on a regular basis to maintain an adequate serum level of drug.

25. What are the side effects of the $5HT_3$ antagonists?

The most common side effects of ondansetron, granisetron, and dolasetron are mild headache during and after administration and asymptomatic, transient, and clinically inconsequential electrocardiogram changes (e.g., minor prolongation of the ST segment). Headache may be relieved by slowing the rate of intravenous administration or by giving acetaminophen. Few patients feel dizzy or lightheaded, sleepy, or nervous. Constipation is possible, especially if a $5HT_3$ antagonist is given for several doses, as with multiday chemotherapy or radiation therapy. The nurse should assess the patient's usual bowel habits, teach the patient to report subjective awareness of constipation, and initiate a prophylactic bowel program (i.e., stool softener plus laxative) when necessary.

26. Why is dexamethasone recommended as an antiemetic?

Dexamethasone has remarkable efficacy to decrease N&V due to chemotherapy, some instances of disease-related nausea, and PONV. There is less information about methylprednisolone, but it seems to be similarly effective. The mechanism of action is not known, but compelling evidence indicates that dexamethasone is effective to control acute and delayed N&V. The added benefit of dexamethasone over a single antiemetic (including a $5HT_3$ antagonist) is 25–30%. Dexamethasone is almost 50% more effective than placebo and may be superior to $5HT_3$ antagonists for delayed emesis. No evidence suggests that higher doses are more effective than low doses or that intravenous administration is superior to oral doses. A typical dose of dexamethasone is 10–20 mg intravenously or 8 mg orally. Dexamethasone has mild and generally tolerable side effects and is considered safe when used for short periods before and 2–5 days after chemotherapy.

27. What about using other drugs to enhance antiemetic regimens?

Antiemetic regimens combining drugs with different mechanisms of action clearly lead to better control of N&V than single antiemetic agents. However, older regimens also included drugs to counter adverse effects of antiemetics. Therefore, a phenothiazine or lorazepam may add antiemetic benefit, but doses and rationale for use should be considered carefully. For instance, smaller rather than larger doses of a phenothiazine, such as prochlorperazine, should be used to avoid distressing side effects.

Lorazepam has modest antiemetic activity at best but may be useful to decrease anxiety and provide a sense of control to some persons. Lorazepam is sedating, which may or may not be a desirable effect. Sublingual administration bypasses the GI tract and the first-pass effect in the liver, providing rapid transport of drug to the bloodstream. Small doses (e.g., 0.5 mg) may be taken and repeated until the desired effect is reached.

28 What are extrapyramidal symptoms (EPS)?

Dopamine antagonists (metoclopramide, phenothiazines [e.g., prochlorperazine, thiethylperazine, chlorpromazine], and butyrophenones [haloperidol, droperidol]) are associated with EPS, which may occur immediately after administration of large intravenous doses of antiemetic or hours after oral administration. Some patients experience worsening symptoms with repeated administration of oral dopamine antagonists. The concomitant use of more than one drug with dopamine antagonist activity can increase the risk for EPS.

Two types of EPS are akathisia and dystonia. Akathisia, which is sometimes called the "dancing feet syndrome," is the most common and can cause a broad range of uncomfortable, disconcerting symptoms. Mild akathisia causes patients to feel anxious or jittery, moderate akathisia leads to difficulty in sitting still, and patients with severe akathisia cannot sit or lie still at all. Dystonia is less common, involving contraction of muscle groups in the head and neck (torticollis or opisthotonus). Dystonia is frightening because patients may feel they cannot breathe.

29. How are EPS managed?

Akathisia and dystonic reactions can be prevented or treated with lorazepam (Ativan), diphenhydramine (Benadryl), and benztropine (Cogentin). Benztropine, 1 or 2 mg intravenously, rapidly reverses dystonia and may be repeated if dystonia does not resolve with the first dose; it does not cause sedation.

30. What are the benefits of using prochlorperazine (Compazine) sustained-release spansules rather than regular tablets?

Regular antiemetic administration is important for optimal control of N&V in most instances. The duration of action for prochlorperazine tablets is 4–6 hours, whereas sustained-release Compazine spansules are released into the bloodstream over 12 hours. Spansules are easier to administer regularly in adequate doses for many patients. The risk of side effects, such as EPS, may increase with repeated administration.

31. What should be done if the antiemetics fail?

The first step is to make sure that the patient was able to take the prescribed doses. The nurse can do a telephone follow-up the day after treatment and suggest that the patient complete an antiemetic diary. These strategies can lead to timely changes in antiemetic regimens. Antiemetic cost may be an important consideration, particularly for oral $5HT_3$ antagonists, if the patient does not have prescription coverage or if the patient's plan limits $5HT_3$ antagonist use. Medicare now pays for prophylactic intravenous or oral doses for the expected period of acute N&V. In some instances, when a first $5HT_3$ antagonist is not sufficiently effective or causes intolerable side effects, trial of a second $5HT_3$ antagonist may be warranted before switching to another, less effective class of antiemetics.

32. Which antiemetics can be administered by continuous subcutaneous infusion (CSQI)? When should this method be considered?

CSQI of antiemetics is not indicated for N&V due to chemotherapy, and generally is reserved for patients with progressive or terminal cancer. Metoclopramide and haloperidol are especially useful for patients with nausea that precludes oral intake or deteriorating level of consciousness. Neither drug is irritating to subcutaneous tissues, as are other antiemetics. In addition, both metoclopramide and haloperidol are compatible with morphine, which may be important for patients with progressive cancer.

Ambulatory infusion pumps are ideal for CSQI of antiemetics, which are started at a low dose and titrated upward as needed to control vomiting. Metoclopramide is concentrated at 1 mg/ml, and the infusion is begun at 0.4–0.5 ml (0.4–0.5 mg) per hour. Similarly, haloperidol is concentrated at 1 mg/ml, and the infusion is begun at about 0.7 or 0.8 ml/hr. The upper chest and abdomen are appropriate sites for CSQI. After the site is prepared, a 25–27-gauge winged needle or small-gauge intravenous catheter is inserted subcutaneously. The needle is changed every 3–7 days, depending on if the patient is hospitalized or at home. A few patients develop cutaneous erythema and subcutaneous induration at the needle site, which preclude use of CSQI.

33. What other management strategies might be helpful to control N&V from cancer?

Antiemetics should be chosen that target the cause of N&V in each patient. Thus, if a patient is experiencing bowel ostruction, a phenothiazine (e.g, prochlorperazine), a butyrophenone (haloperidol), or dexamethasone may be useful. On the other hand, metoclopramide, which increases GI motility, should not be used for frank obstruction but is useful if N&V are related to GI stasis. Scopolamine patches may be helpful for N&V due to obstruction, opioids, or other causes. Transdermal administration eliminates the need for oral or parenteral administration. Scopolamine patches should be applied to the upper chest (not behind the ear) because of the high blood flow to this area. Antihistamines (promethazine, diphenhydramine) may be helpful for patients with motion-induced increased intracranial pressure, GI obstruction, or GI compression, whereas anxiolytics (e.g., lorazepam) may be helpful for N&V accompanied by agitation or other emotional factors. In all cases, therapeutic effects must be balanced against adverse effects, which may include sedation, anticholinergic effects (e.g., dry mouth), and, on rare occasions, EPS. Benzquinamide (Emete-Con) is a useful second-line antiemetic because it does not have dopamine antagonist activity and can be used when other antiemetics cause side effects or are not effective.

34. Which antiemetics have a limited role for controlling N&V in patients with cancer?

Trimethobenzamide (Tigan) is a benzamide (as is metoclopramide) that is generally considered to be useless. It does not cause EPS, probably because of the small dosage, which is not highly effective. Long-term use may cause EPS and opisthotonus. In general, antihistamines are not first-line antiemetics. For instance, hydroxyzine (Vistaril, Atarax) is not very useful as an antiemetic, and repeated parenteral administration is painful and may cause sedation. Promethazine (Phenergan), like Vistaril, is irritating to tissue and causes dry mouth and other anticholinergic side effects; it is imited to second- or third-line antiemetic use.

35. What about marijuana for N&V?

Initial interest in marijuana as an antiemetic was based on the observation that some patients who smoked marijuana while receiving emetogenic chemotherapy experienced decreased N&V and increased appetite. Tetrahydrocannabinol (THC) was subsequently isolated as the active ingredient and became commercially available as dronabinol (Marinol). Dronabinol acts at cannibinoid receptors (CB1 or CB2) located in the central nervous system (cortex, motor system, limbic system, and hippocampus). Marinol is rarely used as an antiemetic for therapy or palliative care because more potent antiemetics with fewer side effects are available. In addition, it is available only for oral administration (the gel cap can be broken and the liquid inside released into the mouth), is expensive, and may cause the patient to feel dysphoric or confused (especially debilitated and elderly patients). However, dronabinol may be useful for selected patients as a second- or third-line antiemetic or used in addition to other antiemetics.

Some people claim that smoking marijuana is more effective than taking a Marinol tablet. According to current recommendations, short-term use of smoked marijuana (< 6 months) can be tried with medical supervision only for patients with intractable nausea or pain if no other antiemetics have been effective. One concern about this treatment is that smoking marijuana can lead to inhalation of harmful substances.

36. How can a nurse administer needed antiemetics to patients who do not have venous access devices and cannot take oral drugs?

Compounding pharmacists can formulate antiemetics into suppositories. For example, Benadryl (25 mg), Decadron (4 mg), and Reglan (20 mg) (BDR) suppositories (or Benadryl and Reglan only) may be useful in the palliative care setting. If the patient who cannot take oral antiemetics and is cared for at home finds the rectal route of administration acceptable, BDR suppositories (or other medications formulated for rectal administration) may be more convenient and less expensive than parenteral medications. Suppositories usually are administered every 4–6 hours as needed for N&V.

Hospice nurses have found that rectal or vaginal administration of oral tablets is another useful alternative strategy. Rectal absorption is comparable to oral absorption in producing adequate serum levels of antiemetic. If two or more tablets are administered, they can be placed inside a gel capsule. Diarrhea, bleeding, and infection may limit rectal and vaginal administration.

37. What complementary measures are helpful for N&V?

Complementary measures may decrease N&V and enhance personal control but should not be considered alternatives to antiemetics. Nurses often recommend that patients limit food intake on the day of chemotherapy. Modifying dietary intake also may decrease the risk for developing food aversions. In addition, nonpharmacologic measures such as relaxation, imagery, or hypnosis may benefit patients who have developed anticipatory nausea. Nursing research has shown that regular, aerobic exercise may decrease chemotherapy-related nausea. Not all patients are able to exercise regularly, but nurses should offer support and encouragement to those who want to try.

38. What is the role of acupuncture?

Acupuncture can decrease N&V, but few people have access to a trained acupuncturist. An acupressure band may be helpful for patients who have nausea secondary to chemotherapy, PONV, motion sickness, morning sickness from pregnancy, or other causes. Two types of devices are available: an inexpensive band with a small button that is placed snugly over the acupuncture point for N&V and a more expensive electonic device that is battery-powered and stimulates the same point. The point is along the median nerve above the wrist (about 3 fingerbreadths above the lowest wrist crease between the radial and middle tendons of the dominant arm). Of interest, the second device is available in two forms: an expensive prescription device for patients undergoing chemotherapy and a much less expensive over-the-counter device for travelers. Acupressure bands may enhance antiemetic control. Relief occurs within 1 hour of applying the band and may persist as long as it is worn.

39. What herbal preparations may be used to decrease nausea?

Ginger is the best known and is superior to placebo to decrease N&V due to chemotherapy, motion sickness, or morning sickness with pregnancy. Ginger can be consumed as dried or fresh ginger root made into a tea, ginger ale, or ginger tablets. Concern that ginger may interfere with platelet aggregation has been allayed by animal studies, which show that huge amounts must be consumed to induce antiplatelet action. The nurse should remind the patient to inform healthcare providers of all medicine and herbs that they take. Herbal alternatives to ginger include chamomile, marshmallow, peppermint, and slippery elm.

REFERENCES

1. American Society of Health-System Pharmacists Commission of Therapeutics: ASAP therapeutic guidelines on the pharmacologic management of nausea and vomiting in adult and pediatric patients receiving chemotherapy or radiation therapy or undergoing surgery. Am J Health-Syst Pharm 56:729–764, 1999.
2. Ernst E, Pittler MH: Efficacy of ginger for nausea and vomiting: A systemic review of randomized clinical trials. Br J Anaesth 84:367–371, 2000.
3. Gralla RJ, Osoba D, Kris MG, et al: Recommendations for the use of antiemetics: Evidence-based, clinical practice guidelines. J Clin Oncol 17:2871–2994, 1999.
4. Ioannidis JPA, Hesketh PJ, Lau J: Contribution of dexamethasone to control of chemotherapy-induced nausea and vomiting: A meta-analysis of randomized evidence. J Clin Oncol 18:3409–3422, 2000.
5. Morrow GR, Roscoe JA, Hickok JT, et al: Initial control of chemotherapy-induced nausea and vomiting in patient quality of life. Oncology 12:32–37, 1998.
6. Watson SJ, Benson JA, Joy JE: Marijuana and medicine: Assessing the science base: A summary of the 1999 Institue of Medicine Report. Arch Gen Psychiatry 57:547–552, 2000.
7. Wickham R: Nausea and vomiting. In Groenwald S, Frogge MH, Yarbro CH, Goodman M (eds): Cancer Symptom Management, 2nd ed. Boston, Jones & Bartlett, 1999, pp 228–263.

44. NUTRITIONAL SUPPORT

Colleen Gill, MS, RD, Barbara Eldridge, RD, LD,
and Deborah Rust, RN, MSN, CRNP, AOCN

> I wish someone had told the secret to me, that I could do anything I wanted to do.
> *A patient after diagnosis of cancer*

1. Describe the incidence and significance of malnutrition.

From 40–80% of all patients with cancer experience some degree of malnutrition, which is a major cause of morbidity and mortality. Severe protein-calorie malnutrition is the single most common paraneoplastic syndrome resulting from cancer and its treatment. Protein-calorie malnutrition occurs when macronutrient intake cannot meet the body's metabolic needs. Results include progressive weight loss, muscle wasting, skin breakdown, poor wound healing, potential intolerance to therapy, endocrine abnormalities, electrolyte and fluid imbalances, and inadequate immune function.

2. What causes cancer cachexia?

Cancer cachexia is characterized by inadequate nutritional intake to meet physiologic and metabolic needs. Severe progressive, involuntary weight loss; weakness due to loss of muscle mass; anorexia; early satiety; immunosuppression; increased basal metabolic rate; and serum protein depletion can result. The cause of cancer cachexia is not entirely understood, and it can manifest in patients with either metastatic cancer or localized disease. The degree and rate at which cachexia develops are determined by a complex mixture of tumor, host, and treatment variables that are multifactorial and additive in effect:

- Taste changes: cancer may cause elevated thresholds for sweet and lowered thresholds for bitter tastes; treatment may create mouth blindness and alterations in taste.
- Altered hypothalamic control of appetite with brain metastasis or lesions.
- Abnormal neurotransmitter concentrations, changing levels of tryptophan and serotonin, with profound anorexia.
- Psychological and emotional impact of disease, depression, and anxiety.
- Pain from tumor, surgery, mucositis, or esophagitis.
- Local mechanical interference from the tumor or treatment side effects may lead to early satiety, nausea and vomiting, diarrhea, malabsorption, and problems with chewing and swallowing.
- Cachectin, or tumor necrosis factor (TNF), a protein substance or cytokine mediator that creates abnormalities in substrate metabolism and appetite.

3. When should nutritional intervention occur?

Ideally, all patients with cancer should be screened and assessed for nutritional risk at the time of diagnosis and re-evaluated throughout the course of treatment and recovery. Because malnutrition is a common result of cancer and its treatment, "catch-up" or regaining weight is more difficult than maintaining the status quo. Preventive or early intervention must be the primary goal. Whether in the hospital or clinic setting, nurses spend the most time with patients and thus are essential in identification of patients who develop problems with eating. Even if a full nutritional assessment is needed, intervention should not be delayed. Try to provide the patient with the appropriate written materials immediately.

Teaching should focus on what the patient really needs to know; typically patients can remember only 3 or 4 points at a time. Add information in short follow-up sessions, incorporated into routine care, and involving family members whenever possible.

4. How can patients be quickly assessed for nutritional risk?

The Patient Generated–Subjective Global Assessment (PG-SGA), developed by Detsky and adapted by Ottery and colleagues, is inexpensive and easy to use in multiple clinical settings. Patients and/or caregivers fill out sections about weight history, food intake, symptoms, and functioning. A health care team member evaluates weight loss, disease, metabolic stress; performs a nutrition-related physical examination; and generates a score that is used to determine nutrition risk and appropriate intervention.

Scored Patient-Generated Subjective Global Assessment (PG-SGA)

Patient ID Information

History

1. Weight *(See Table 1 Worksheet)*

In summary of my current and recent weight:

I currently weigh about _____ pounds
I am about _____ feet _____ tall

One months ago I weighed about _____ pounds
Six months ago I weighed about _____ pounds

During the past two weeks my weight has:

☐ decreased (1)   ☐ not changed (0)   ☐ increased (0)

2. Food Intake: As compared to my normal, I would rate my food intake during the past month as:
☐ unchanged (0)
☐ more than usual
☐ less than usual (1)
   I am now taking:
     ☐ *normal food* but less than normal (1)
     ☐ little solid food (2)
     ☐ only liquids (3)
     ☐ only nutritonal supplements (3)
     ☐ very little of anything (4)
     ☐ only tube feedings or only nutrition by vein

3. Symptoms: I have had the following problems that have kept me from eating enough during the past two weeks (check all that apply):
☐ no problems eating (0)
☐ no appetite, just did not feel like eating (3)
☐ nausea (1)   ☐ vomiting (3)
☐ constipation (1)   ☐ diarrhea (3)
☐ mouth sores (2)   ☐ dry mouth (1)
☐ things taste funny or have no taste (1) ☐ smells bother me (1)
☐ problems swallowing (2)   ☐ feel full quickly (1)
☐ pain; where? (3)
☐ other** (3)
   ** Examples: depression, money, or dental problems

4. Activities and Function: Over the past month, I would generally rate my activity as:
☐ normal with no limitations (0)
☐ not my normal self, but able to be up and about with fairly normal activities (1)
☐ not feeling up to most things, but in bed less than half the day (2)
☐ able to do little activity and spend most of the day in bed or chair (3)

Additive Score of the Boxes 1-4 ☐ **A**

The remainder of this form will be completed by your doctor, nurse, or therapist. Thank you.

5. Disease and its relation to nutritional requirements *(See Table 2)*

All relevant diagnoses (specify) _____

Primary disease stage (circle if known or appropriate)   I   II   III   IV   Other _____

Age _____

Numerical score from Table 2 ☐ **B**

6. Metabolic Demand *(See Table 3 Worksheet)*
☐ no stress   ☐ low stress   ☐ moderate stress   ☐ high stress

Numerical score from Table 3 ☐ **C**

7. Physical *(See Table 4 Worksheet)*

Numerical score from Table 4 ☐ **D**

Global Assessment *(See Table 5 Worksheet)*
☐ Well-nourished or anabolic (SGA-A)
☐ Moderate or suspected malnutrition (SGA-B)
☐ Severely malnourished (SGA-C)

Total numerical score of boxes A+B+C+D ☐
(See triage recommendations below)

Clinician Signature _____ RD RN PA MD DO Other ___   Date _____

Nutritional Triage Recommendations: Additive score is used to define specific nutritional interventions including patient & family education, symptom management including pharmacologic intervention, and appropriate nutrient intervention (food, nutritional supplements, enteral, or parenteral triage). First line nutrition intervention includes optimal symptom management.
0-1   No intervention required at this time. Re-assessment on routine and regular basis during treatment.
2-3   Patient & family education by dietitian, nurse, or other clinician with pharmacologic intervention as indicated by symptom survey (Box 3) and laboratory values as appropriate.
4-8   Requires intervention by dietitian, in conjunction with nurse or physician, as indicated by symptoms survey (Box 3).
≥ 9   Indicates a critical need for improved symptom management and/or nutrient intervention options.

© FD Ottery, 2000

From Detsky A, McLaughlin J, Baker J, et al: What is subjective global assessment of nutritional status? J Parent Ent Nutr 11:8–13, 1987, with permission.

Tables & Worksheets for PG-SGA Scoring

The PG-SGA numerical score is derived by totaling the scores from boxes A-D of the PG-SGA on the reverse side. Boxes 1-4 are designed to be completed by the patient. The points assigned to items in boxes 1-4 are noted parenthetically after each item. The following worksheets are offered as aids for calcuating scores of sections that are not so marked.

Table 1 - Scoring Weight (wt) Loss

Determined by adding points for subacute and acute wt change. **Subacute:** If information is available about weight loss during past 1 month, add the point score to the points for acute wt change. Only include the wt loss over 6 months if the wt from 1 month is unavailable. **Acute:** refers to wt change during past two weeks. Add 1 point to subacute score if patient lost wt; add no points if patient gained or maintained wt during the past two weeks.

Wt loss in 1 month	Points	Wt loss in 6 months
10% or greater	4	20% or greater
5-9.9%	3	10 -19.9%
3-4.9%	2	6 - 9.9%
2-2.9%	1	2 - 5.9%
0-1.9%	0	0 - 1.9%

Points for Box 1 = Subacute + Acute = [   ] A

Table 2 - Scoring criteria for disease &/or condition

Score is derived by adding 1 point for each of the conditions listed below that pertain to the patient.

Category	Points
Cancer	1
AIDS	1
Pulmonary or cardiac cachexia	1
Presence of decubitus, open wound, or fistula	1
Presence of trauma	1
Age greater than 65 years	1

Points for Box 2 = [   ] B

Table 3 Worksheet. Scoring Metabolic Stress

Score for metabolic stress is determined by a number of variables known to increase protein & caloric needs. The score is additive so that a patient who has a fever of > 102 degrees (3 points) and is on 10 mg of prednisone chronically (2 points) would have an additive score for this section of 5 points.

Stress	none (0)	low (1)	moderate (2)	high (3)
Fever	no fever	>99 and <101	$\geq$101 and <102	$\geq$102
Fever duration	no fever	<72 hrs	72 hrs	> 72 hrs
Steroids	no steroids	low dose (<10mg prednisone equivalents/day)	moderate dose ($\geq$10 and <30mg prednisone equivalents/day)	high dose steroids ($\geq$30mg prednisone equivalents/day)

Points for Table 3 = [   ] C

Table 4 Worksheet - Physical Examination

Physical exam includes a subjective evaluation of 3 aspects of body composition: fat, muscle, & fluid status. Since this is subjective, each aspect of the exam is rated for degree of deficit. Definition of categories: 0 = no deficit, 1+ = mild deficit, 2+ = moderate deficit, 3+ = severe deficit. Degree of muscle deficit takes precedence over fat deficit. Rating of deficit in these categories are *not* additive but a used to clinically assess the degree of deficit (or presence of excess fluid).

Fat Stores:

orbital fat pads	0	1+	2+	3+
triceps skin fold	0	1+	2+	3+
fat overlying lower ribs	0	1+	2+	3+
Global fat deficit rating	**0**	**1+**	**2+**	**3+**

Fluid Status:

ankle edema	0	1+	2+	3+
sacral edema	0	1+	2+	3+
ascites	0	1+	2+	3+
Global fluid status rating	**0**	**1+**	**2+**	**3+**

Muscle Status:

temples (temporalis muscle)	0	1+	2+	3+
clavicles (pectoralis & deltoids)	0	1+	2+	3+
shoulders (deltoids)	0	1+	2+	3+
interosseous muscles	0	1+	2+	3+
scapula (latissimus dorsi, trapezius, deltoids)	0	1+	2+	3+
thigh (quadriceps)	0	1+	2+	3+
calf (gastrocnemius)	0	1+	2+	3+
Global muscle status rating	**0**	**1+**	**2+**	**3+**

Point score for the physical exam is determined by the overall subjective rating of total body deficit; again muscle deficit takes precedence over fat loss or fluid excess.

No deficit	score = 0 points
Mild deficit	score = 1 point
Moderate deficit	score = 2 points
Severe deficit	score = 3 points

Points for Worksheet 4 = [   ] D

Table 5 Worksheet PG-SGA Global Assessment Categories

Category	Stage A Well-nourished	Stage B Moderately malnourished or suspected malnutrition	Stage C Severely malnourished
Weight	No wt loss **or** Recent non-fluid wt gain	~5% wt loss within 1 month (or 10% in 6 months) No wt stabilization or wt gain (i.e., continued wt loss)	a. > 5% loss in 1 month (or >10% loss in 6 months) b. No wt stabilization or wt gain (i.e., continued wt loss)
Nutrient Intake	No deficit **or** Significant recent improvement	Definite decrease in intake	Severe deficit in intake
Nutrition Impact Symptoms	None **or** Significant recent improvement allowing adequate intake	Presence of nutrition impact symptoms (Box 3 of PG-SGA)	Presence of nutrition impact symptoms (Box 3 of PG-SGA)
Functioning	No deficit **or** Significant recent improvement	Moderate functional deficit **or** Recent deterioration	Severe functional deficit **or** recent significant deterioration
Physical Exam	No deficit **or** Chronic deficit but with recent clinical improvement	Evidence of mild to moderate loss of SQ fat &/or muscle mass &/or muscle tone on palpation	Obvious signs of malnutrition (e.g., severe loss of SQ tissues, possible edema)

Global PG-SGA rating (A, B, or C) = [   ]

From Detsky A, McLaughlin J, Baker J, et al: What is subjective global assessment of nutritional status? J Parent Ent Nutr 11:8–13, 1987, with permission.

5. Why is weight loss such a critical marker?

Substantial weight loss and poor nutritional status have been documented in over 50% of cancer patients at the time of diagnosis. The prevalence of weight loss and malnutrition varies greatly across specific cancer types. Any weight loss before or during treatment can adversely affect nutritional reserves. Weight maintenance during cancer treatment, regardless of the extent of overweight, is recommended. Do not rely on weight alone in monitoring patients, because changes in edema or ascites can falsely obscure true weight loss. Unintentional weight loss reflects underlying problems that must be addressed to prevent malnutrition. Use the following formula to calculate percent weight loss.

$$\text{Percent weight loss} = \frac{\text{Usual weight} - \text{current weight}}{\text{Usual weight}}$$

Patients were noted to have statistically increased risk of mortality and morbidity with the following unintentional weight losses:

% Weight Loss From Baseline

TIME COURSE	SIGNIFICANT (%)	SEVERE (%)
1 week	≤ 2.0	> 2.0
1 month	≤ 5.0	> 5.0
3 months	≤ 7.5	> 7.5
6 months	≤ 10.0	> 10.0

6. What laboratory value is used most commonly to measure malnutrition and assess nutritional risk?

Serum proteins are markers of the body's ability to make new proteins. **Albumin** is the most commonly checked; the test is relatively inexpensive if added to a panel of laboratory values. With a half-life of 20 days, the serum albumin level reflects the availability of protein within the past month. Albumin is measured as gm/dl; thus, fluid status must be taken into account during interpretation. The value is falsely low in patients who retain fluids and falsely elevated in volume-depleted patients. Albumin, like all serum proteins, is manufactured in the liver; any liver dysfunction depresses its level. Values are laboratory-specific; check the normal range at your institution.

Normal	> 3.4
Mild depletion	2.8-3.4
Moderate depletion	2.2-2.7
Severe depletion	< 2.1

7. What other laboratory values are helpful?

Other serum proteins, such as **prealbumin** (which has a half-life of 3–5 days) and **transferrin**, can provide more recent snapshots of protein status; however, they may be less readily available as part of laboratory panels. Fluid status and liver function abnormalities also must be taken into account in interpreting levels of these proteins. In addition, transferrin is inversely related to iron reserves and status and thus may be falsely elevated in anemic patients.

Cholesterol levels drop when caloric intake decreases. A low cholesterol value can substantiate suspicions of eating problems and inadequate intake.

Urinary urea nitrogen (UUN) is assessed from a 24-hour collection of urine in which the grams of nitrogen excreted from protein are measured, added to normal losses, and subtracted from nitrogen intake. Increasing negative values reflect the breakdown of lean body mass (LBM); in other words, muscle tissue is being used for calorie and protein needs.

Hematocrit and **total lymphocytic count** (TLC) are frequently invalid because of the effects of cancer and its treatment. However, recent retrospective studies indicate that patients with anemia and decreased hematocrit levels may have statistically worse local-regional control and survival after treatment.

Absolute neutrophil count (ANC) is an indication of immune function. Patients receiving high-dose chemotherapy and/or total-body irradiation may experience immunosuppression (ANC < 500) and are at significant risk for infection. Patients should be advised to consume a diet that minimizes pathogenic organisms and should be instructed in food safety to ensure proper food consumption, preparation, handling, and storage.

8. How can surgery exacerbate nutritional status?

Surgery requires the intake of adequate calories and protein for wound healing and recovery. Most side effects are temporary and resolve within a few days after the surgical procedure, but in some instances surgical interventions have long-lasting nutritional implications. The most commonly experienced side effects include loss of appetite, fatigue, and pain. Surgeries involving the alimentary tract have specific nutritional sequelae, depending on the area of surgical intervention. Potential problems include chewing or swallowing difficulties, aspiration, dumping syndrome, and malabsorption.

9. How can chemotherapy affect nutritional status?

Chemotherapy side effects can result in nausea and vomiting, taste changes, and anorexia. Some regimens have the additional effect of creating severe mucositis, further compromising the ability to eat.

10. Discuss the potential effects of radiation therapy on nutritional status.

The effects of radiation therapy are specific to the region that is irradiated. In addition, chemotherapy agents may be given in combination with radiation therapy because of their radiation-enhancing effects. Patients receiving multimodality therapy may experience side effects sooner and with greater toxicity. Nutritional concern increases when the gastrointestinal tract is included in the irradiation field. Nausea and vomiting, mucositis, taste changes, swallowing, dry mouth, diarrhea and malabsorption, gastritis, and radiation enteritis are possible side effects. Early enteral nutritional support by means of percutaneous endoscopic gastrostomy (PEG) should be considered whenever extended mucositis, dysphagia, or odynophagia is anticipated. The PEG tube may be more acceptable to patients because it can be concealed, whereas a nasogastric tube cannot.

11. How long do the nutritional effects of various cancer therapies last?

Although most side effects of surgery, chemotherapy, and radiation therapy resolve soon after treatment is completed, some patients may not develop certain side effects until several weeks, months, or even years after the prescribed therapy. Continued assessment and re-evaluation of the most appropriate nutrition intervention and side effect management are essential.

12. What supportive medications affect nutrition in patients with cancer?

- Steroids: sodium retention and hypertension, increased protein and calcium needs, potassium wasting, glucose intolerance; loss of muscle mass.
- Cyclosporine: renal insufficiency, magnesium and potassium wasting, weight gain, increased triglyceride and cholesterol levels. Grapefruit or grapefruit juice may interfere with its metabolism, increasing serum levels of the drug potentially into toxic ranges.
- Thiazide and loop diuretics: loss of electrolytes; potassium replacement needed.
- Bactrim: increased folate needs; deficiency affects dividing cell lines such as bone marrow. Supplement with folinic acid if counts drop. Possible decrease in absorption of vitamin K.
- Antibiotics: may increase nausea, creating a baseline "grungy feeling" that is difficult for many patients.
- Linezolid: intake of foods high in tyramine can result in increased blood pressure levels and headache.
- Amphotericin: impairs renal function, creating electrolyte abnormalities, and causes significant nausea, which often reduces oral intake by one-half.
- Opioids: possibly sedating and may interfere with normal meal patterns as well as cause constipation, nausea, and vomiting.

13. What treatment-related medications affect nutrition in patients with cancer?

- Procarbazine: monoamine oxidase inhibitor. Foods high in tyramine should be avoided because they may elicit a hypertensive crisis.

- Vincristine sulfate and vinblastine sulfate: can cause significant constipation.
- Methotrexate: ingestion of foods high in folic acid and folic acid supplementation may reduce its effectiveness; decreases absorption of vitamin B12, fat, D-xylose; change in taste acuity.
- Interferon: increases anorexia, fatigue, and nausea
- Interleukin-2 (IL-2): weight loss or weight gain, hypotension, fatigue, and capillary leak syndrome.
- Cisplatin: may cause decreased serum magnesium, potassium, and zinc; metallic taste.
- 5-Fluorouracil (5FU): may cause taste alterations. Patients should avoid pyridoxine supplements.
- Tamoxifen citrate: may cause edema and fluid retention.

14. What are the most important goals in nutritional management of patients with cancer?
1. To prevent or reverse nutrient deficiencies
2. To preserve lean body mass
3. To minimize nutrition-related side effects
4. To maximize quality of life

15. What three guiding principles have been identified for nutritional management?
1. **Calories.** The first and foremost requirement of the body is adequate calorie intake. The body has an obligatory requirement for energy and will go to any lengths to meet that need, including autocannibalism (breaking down its own tissue).
2. **Protein.** After adequate calories, the body must have enough protein for regeneration and synthesis to limit breakdown of muscle mass. Until adequate calories are obtained, however, protein will be burned as calories to meet the body's basal metabolic needs. Excessive protein is not beneficial and may stress the renal and hepatic systems.
3. **Medications.** The patient needs adequate medications to support nutritional goals (e.g., antiemetics, antidiarrheals, supplements of pancreatic enzymes, medications for pain control).

16. How common is anorexia?
The simple loss of hunger or appetite takes away the primary incentive that most of us have to eat at regular intervals. Although seemingly more benign than overt nausea and vomiting, anorexia is in fact the most common cause of decreased intake that leads to loss of fat and muscle reserves, resulting in weight loss and wasting. Patients may lack the internal clock (hunger) that reminds them to eat, often exacerbated by negative experiences around eating, fatigue, and depression. Most patients simply eat less often and therefore consume fewer calories.

17. The patient with anorexia often says, "I just don't have an appetite. Nothing sounds good." How can you help?
If the anorexia is of short duration (e.g., only a few days after chemotherapy cycles), patients often can maintain weight and lean body mass with increased intake between cycles. When weight loss begins or persists despite early interventions, the patient should be referred to an oncology dietitian. Provide information about appropriate behavioral changes, ways to maximize nutritional intake, and liquid nutritional supplements.

18. What behavioral changes may help patients with anorexia?
1. Increase frequency of meals and snacks, taking advantage of the patient's best mealtimes (often earlier in the day).
2. Divert attention with social activity or television during mealtimes.
3. Arrange for help with meal preparation as needed.
4. Plan ahead for low-energy days.

19. How can nutritional intake be maximized?
The caloric density of the foods that the patient eats should be increased to provide the most calories in the smallest volume of food. One of the key concepts that must be communicated to the

patient is the idea of adjusting priorities to the current situation. Friends and family may be following a low-fat, high-fiber diet to minimize risk of cancer, but in patients with cancer, weight loss compromises immune function. Fat and sugar may be negatives in the well person, but they are critical components in achieving adequate nutritional support for many patients with cancer. Patients may be taught strategies to add calories to their favorite foods.

Adding Calories to Favorite Foods

When dealing with problems that make eating difficult, it is always a bonus to pack calories into the smallest volume possible. Fat and sugar may not seem "healthy," but it is important to understand their use as part of a transitional period that requires extraordinary measures. *This is hardly a time when you will suddenly learn to like foods that you have never liked.* It is possible, however, to add calories to favorite foods, even if they are traditionally low in calories.

Milk/dairy
- Good alone, but go up one level in fat content (e.g., from skim to 2%)
- Add Carnation Instant Breakfast (CIB)
- Make milk shakes
  1 cup ice cream (high calorie, of course)
  1 package CIB
  4 oz half and half
  Flavoring:
  $\frac{1}{2}$ tsp almond or peppermint extract
  $\frac{1}{2}$ cup fruit

Eggs
- Mix grated cheese or cream cheese into scrambled eggs; it softens texture, too
- Melt cheese on fried eggs
- Eggs Benedict
- Use extra mayonnaise in egg salad, deviled eggs

Breads/cereals
- Add fruit, raisins, or nuts to cereals
- Top with sugar, half and half
- Add CIB to hot cereal, top with syrup
- Eat croissants, pastries
- Top pancakes, French toast, or waffles with syrup or fruit and whipped cream
- Eat fruit and nut breads with cream cheese
- Top crackers with cheese or nut butters

Salads/vegetables
- Regular, not low-fat, salad dressings
- Top with cheese, meat, nuts, avocado, egg
- Dips or peanut butter on raw vegetables
- Add margarine/sauces to cooked vegetables

Meats/main dishes
- Breaded and fried meats vs. baked or broiled
- Add gravies
- Mix nonfat dry milk into hamburger patties, meatloaf, or casseroles
- Add extra cheese to pizza, macaroni and cheese, spaghetti, other casseroles
- Add sour cream
- Add mayonnaise, cheese, avocado, or bacon to sandwiches

Soups and stews
- Make soups with milk instead of water
- Add chopped cooked meats

Fruits/desserts/snacks
- Add sour or whipped cream or coconut to fruit salads
- Snack on dried fruits, add to cereals
- Spread peanut butter on fresh fruit
- Fruit in heavy syrup has twice the calories
- Eat dessert with whipped cream or a la mode
- Eat chips with dip
- Nuts provide great calories, great snacks

Extras that count
- Butter   45 cal/tsp
- Sour cream   70 cal/tbsp
- Whipped cream   60 cal/tbsp
- Cheese   100 cal/oz
- Cream cheese   100 cal/oz
- Mayonnaise   100 cal/tbsp
- CIB   130 cal/package
- Avocado   55 cal, $\frac{1}{6}$ medium
- Nuts   160–190 cal/oz
- Peanut butter   90 cal/tbsp

20. Discuss the role of liquid nutritional supplements.

Start with the higher-calorie versions (355 vs. 250/can), which can be diluted if necessary. Most sales representatives are willing to leave trial packs of supplements that allow patients to try several alternatives and decide which they like (or at least tolerate). Consider chilling supplements to enhance flavor. Be positive about supplements; a single negative comment may eliminate the patient's willingness to try. Questions 39 and 40 review these options.

21. What medications are useful as appetite stimulants?

Anticachectic drugs are used to improve intake or correct metabolic abnormalities that prevent effective utilization of intake. Patients must be counseled that, although the drug may make it easier to increase intake, they must also continue previous efforts.

- Steroids, although initially used to enhance appetite, have not been consistently effective in patients with cancer. Of greater significance, their side effects, which include increased muscle breakdown and fluid retention, are counterproductive in this population.
- Cyproheptadine hydrochloride (Periactin) is an antihistamine that stimulates appetite as a side effect in cancer-free populations (anorectic and elderly patients).
- Dronabinol (Marinol), a synthetic cannabinoid, increases appetite but usually results in little weight change. It may cause dizziness and sedation. Older patients may not appreciate its association with marijuana or the slight mood-alterating side effect. Recommended dose: 2.5 mg twice daily.
- Marijuana helps to control nausea and increase appetite in many patients, but there are significant concerns: (1) it is not legal in many states, and (2) the risk of smoking (anything) may exacerbate the pulmonary toxicity of some chemotherapy regimens.
- Metoclopramide (Reglan), although well-known as an antiemetic, may be useful for patients experiencing early satiety because it increases GI transit time and has been shown to be most useful in patients with GI cancers. It may have a negative effect if it increases losses with diarrhea.
- Pentoxifylline (Trentol) suppresses TNF in patients whose baseline levels are elevated and thus improves weight gain.
- Megestrol acetate (Megace) increases appetite and lean body mass and decreases breakdown of fat reserves. Recommended dose: 800 mg/ml. The oral suspension is easier than taking 20 (40-mg) tablets and has the added benefit of being significantly less expensive. The recommended regimen starts at 800 mg/day for 24 days to establish efficacy. If it has not been effective during this time, therapy can be discontinued. If appetite has increased, the dose may be reduced gradually to a lower level that remains therapeutic. Side effects include mild edema and, rarely, deep vein thrombosis.

22. What medications may be used to enhance lean body mass?

Medications showing promise in controlled clinical trials in patients with cachexia due to cancer or AIDS for maintenance and rejuvenation of lean body mass include the following:

- Oxandrolone (Oxandrin), an oral anabolic agent. Dosage: 2.5 mg tablets, 2–4 times/day; maximal dose = 20 mg total for adults, 0.1 mg/kg total daily dose for children.
- Juven, a nutritional supplement that contains HMB (a metabolite of the amino acid leucine), glutamine, and arginine.

23. How can patients get adequate nutrition when fatigue is the primary barrier?

Encourage patients to save time and energy in preparing meals with the following strategies:

Profound fatigue

1. Adequate uninterrupted rest and sleep should be promoted to improve appetite.
2. Activities should be paced to conserve energy in order to stimulate appetite.
3. Exercise should be encouraged gradually and monitored to stimulate appetite (e.g., walking the dog, going for a short walk).

Moderate fatigue

1. Write out menus and choose foods that can be easily prepared.
2. Build shopping lists from the menu, and avoid multiple trips to the store.
3. Ask friends and family for help. Let them know what you like; you can even offer them the recipe. If you cannot use the food right away, freeze it for another day.
4. Minimize clean-up mess by limiting the number of pans and using disposable dishes.
5. Use convenience foods and take-out restaurants. The less time spent cooking and cleaning up, the more energy can be spent eating!

6. Remind patients to be sure that they are sleeping well and exercising to the best of their ability. Recommend limitation of caffeine at bedtime.

24. The patient with early satiety often says, "I can only eat a little bit." Why?

One of the most commonly reported symptoms is a feeling of early satiety. A family member may notice that meal portions are smaller. Physiologically, atrophic changes have been noted in the gut mucosa of patients with cancer. This atrophy and the metabolic abnormalities that cause wasting of muscle in the gut wall may result in increased transit time and delays in digestion. Other metabolic changes related to TNF may cause continuous stimulation of the satiety center in the brain.

25. How can early satiety be managed?

1. Because patients can tolerate only small volumes of food, getting adequate calories requires taking small volumes more frequently. Patients sometimes understand the concept a little better when it is compared to the "preschooler" schedule for children, who also have small stomachs that need to be filled frequently with mid-morning, mid-afternoon, and bedtime snacks.

2. Carbohydrate-containing beverages are useful as between-meal snacks because they empty out of the stomach quickly. However, beverages should be discouraged before solids at meals because they occupy volume and reduce the amount of food that the patient can eat.

3. Concentrating caloric density is also useful, but the patient needs to monitor whether high-fat foods increase early satiety as a result of slower stomach emptying.

4. Metoclopramide (Reglan) may be helpful in decreasing early satiety when delayed gastric emptying is an issue (and diarrhea is not).

Loss of Appetite and Early Satiety

Plan
- Have small, frequent meals and snacks. Discuss the best times with your family, and agree on a schedule. You can set a timer or alarm clock to remind you to eat if others are not around to remind you.
- Drink liquids between meals to avoid getting filled up at mealtimes. Drinking high-calorie fluids between meals is an easy way to include snacks.
- Keep a list of ideas for snacks and quick meals on your refrigerator for the times when you cannot think of anything.
- Keep snacks easily accessible—on the table next to your bed or chair to lessen the work of eating.
- Take advantage of your "best" mealtimes, usually earlier in the day.
- When looking at various options, keep your expectations reasonable: "What do I think I can tolerate today?" Do not expect foods to have the same attraction that they had before treatment.
- Start out with small portions. They prevent you from being overwhelmed by the task of eating and make you feel successful when you manage to finish.
- Variety is not important on these days. If only one thing appeals to you, it's okay.
- Food restrictions suggested before treatment should not be a priority (e.g., low cholesterol). Eliminate them whenever possible.

Concentrate calories
- Eat foods that are calorie-dense, packing the most calories into a small volume. Limit lower calorie foods and fluids such as water, tea/coffee, or diet drinks.
- If solid foods are not possible, fluids often can make up for the missing calories. Milkshakes, cocoa, floats, chocolate milk, juices, sodas, and soups can make a meal.
- Limit high-fat foods that delay stomach emptying if they cause you to feel full early; however, it will be difficult to increase your caloric intake with a low-fat diet.

Keep food fun
- Maintain the positive aspects of eating: set your table attractively, and avoid eating out of cans and cartons.
- Social diversion helps take your mind off the difficulties of eating. Eat with friends or family. Whenever possible, watch television, listen to the radio, or read a book while you eat. (Children, however, may be overly absorbed with television and videos and forget to eat.)

Table continued on following page

Loss of Appetite and Early Satiety (Continued)

- Regular exercise helps to stimulate your appetite. Marathons are not necessary; just incorporate walking and activity into your day. Exercise also helps to prevent muscle loss.
- Some patients find that a glass of wine 30 minutes before a meal can help, but check with your doctor first.
- Ask your physician about antidepressants if anxiety or depression is a problem.

---

26. Patients experiencing nausea and vomiting often say, "What's the use? It just comes back up." What can you do?

A careful history may elicit specific triggers for the patient's nausea. Identifying the underlying cause of nausea and vomiting helps to determine the appropriate intervention and improves treatment of symptoms.

1. **Dietary strategies** (appropriate food choices decrease the likelihood of emesis):
   - Cold clear liquids are often the first foods tolerated. Begin with popsicles, sherbets, sorbets, frozen ices, Jello, and beverages; establishment of tolerance before advancing increases the patient's willingness to increase intake slowly. Gradual incorporation of soft, smooth foods such as ice cream, milk shakes, puddings, hot cereals, and soups is usually tolerated next, although some patients best tolerate lower-fat options.
   - Dehydration alone can cause increased nausea and vomiting; adequate intake of fluids is important.
   - Vitamin tastes from many supplements may increase nausea, but Scandishakes are usually better tolerated because they can be made with a juice base (the recipe is included in question 39).
   - Small, frequent meals reduce distention and reflux.
   - Cold or room-temperature foods decrease aroma-related nausea. Nurses should remove the lids to hot foods outside the room to decrease odors for patients.
   - Avoid fatty, fried foods that delay stomach emptying if the patient experiences increased nausea and vomiting with such foods.
2. **Behavioral strategies** (simple changes around eating times may decrease nausea):
   - Rest after eating, avoiding excessive movement and exercise.
   - Keep the head elevated to allow gravity to work against reflux. The stomach empties fastest when the patient lies on his/her right side.
   - Avoid gagging activities (mouth care, pills) immediately after eating. Foods with increased texture can stimulate the gag reflex; soft foods and fluids are better tolerated.
   - Relaxation techniques, including guided imagery, may be beneficial.
3. **Supportive drug therapy** that includes the timely and consistent use of antiemetics (e.g., ondansetron hydrochloride, prochlorperazine, dronabinol, scopolamine), prokinetics (metoclopramide), and anxiolytics (lorazepam).
   - An initial continuous dosage plan is best, even after the patient seems to have improved.
   - Doses can be weaned gradually to determine whether the patient is doing well because of the medication or no longer needs it.
   - Prevention is crucial. As-needed dosing of secondary antiemetics or anxiolytics must be explained to patients because they may not be aware of the need to request them.
4. **It is helpful to teach patients that unless they lose their meals immediately after eating, they are deriving some benefit from them.** The stomach empties into the intestinal tract in about 2 hours; thus, even if the food stays down for only 1 hour, approximately one-half of its nutrients are available to the body. When initiation of emesis is not meal-related, we can reasonably recommend that the patient keep trying to eat. Vomiting occurs independently of intake, and some nutrients will be retained.

27. What can you do for patients who refuse to try foods that previously caused vomiting?

One of the unique experiences in cancer care is watching a patient throw up at the sight of foods (or even people) that she or he associates with chemotherapy and vomiting. Recent clinical trials indicate that food aversions may develop as early as within 48 hours of the first treatment. Carried to extremes, this pattern of behavior results in a remarkably short list of options for feeding the patient. The key is rebuilding positive associations: "I was able to eat it, and didn't throw up." Try a three-step process:

1. **Relaxation therapy.** Arrange consultation with a therapist who can teach patients to recognize impending nausea and to calm themselves before vomiting by using relaxation techniques.

2. **Education.** Explain the typical peak nausea times after chemotherapy, and encourage patients to avoid favorite foods during this period in order to limit development of new aversions.

3. **Reintroduction.** Patients should be encouraged to retry foods that previously were associated with nausea and vomiting when the probability of tolerance without nausea is at its highest, thus building positive associations. Often the optimal time is earlier in the day, but most patients can identify "good times" vs. times when they feel more nauseated and need to stay with "safe" foods. Obviously, a key ingredient is adequate antiemetic medication throughout the reintroduction process.

28. Patients often complain, "Nothing tastes good anymore." How does cancer and its treatment affect taste?

Both tumor and treatments commonly cause serious damage to the cells involved in taste and smell. Taste is perceived through the cells of the tongue, buccal cavity, lips, and cheeks. The tongue is most sensitive to salty and sweet tastes; the palate, to sour and bitter tastes. As with most cells of the GI tract, the cells of the taste bud have a high turnover rate, with an average life span of 10 days. Drug therapy, radiation, and chemotherapy have the potential to affect cell turnover rate. The enteral nervous system also is involved in taste sensation; thus, tumors affecting the cranial nerves also affect taste. Certain chemotherapy agents (methotrexate, cisplatin, cyclophosphamide, vinca alkaloids) may cause a metallic taste. The common problems of decreased saliva production and mucositis also affect taste. Patients with cancer often complain that food is absolutely tasteless (ageusia, or mouth blindness) because of widespread damage to tastebuds or that food has an "off" taste (dysgeusia) due to changes in balance among the taste centers.

29. How can you help patients with ageusia or dysgeusia?

The best advice is to encourage foods with enhanced flavors rather than the bland foods usually suggested. The obvious exception is the patient with mucositis, in whom tart and spicy foods irritate the oral mucosa. Patients should also be instructed in oral care and encouraged to rinse and clean their mouths frequently throughout the day. Regular rinsing with saline or baking soda can help to keep the mouth clean, remove oral food residue and thick mucous secretions, and maintain the mouth at a pH less conducive to microbial growth.

Overcoming Taste Problems

Elimination of problematic tastes
- Good mouth care and rinsing the mouth with a solution of salt, baking soda, and warm water before eating help to eliminate bad tastes.
- Drink fluids with meals to rinse away bad tastes. Fruit-flavored drinks such as Hi-C, Koolaid, or Gatorade are well tolerated; coffee and tea frequently are not.
- Use plastic eating utensils and glass or plastic cooking containers if you notice a metallic taste while eating.
- If red meats seem bitter, substitute chicken, dairy, pork, fish, and eggs as protein sources.
- Minimize odors that can affect taste by drinking fluids cold and with a straw and by choosing cold foods such as chesse, milk shakes, cold cuts, tuna and egg salad.
- Hard candies and fresh fruit eliminate bad tastes in the mouth and leave a more pleasant taste.
- Retry foods. What tastes "off" this week may work next work.
- Eat foods cold or at room temperature.

Table continued on following page

Overcoming Taste Problems (Continued)

Enhancement of flavors
- Use more strongly seasoned foods, such as Italian, Mexican, curried, or barbequed foods, unless you have mouth sores. Stronger flavors increase the probability that you will sense the taste.
- Tart foods help to overcome metallic tastes. Use lemon, citrus or cranberry juices, and lemon drops.
- Marinate food in wine, fruit juice, soy or teriyaki sauce, Italian dressing, or barbeque sauce.
- Sauces and gravies help to spread taste through the mouth and add calories too.
- Eat meats with something sweet, such as applesauce, jelly, glazes, or cranberry sauce.
- Salt decreases the excessive sweetness of sugary foods.

Dry mouth
- Choose moist foods, adding sauces, gravies, fat, and other lubricants whenever possible. Dry foods such as bread, crackers, or dry meats are not well tolerated alone.
- Use tart substances such as lemon juice, or suck on hard candies (especially sugarless lemon drops) to stimulate maximal production of saliva.
- Drink lots of fluids (juices, broth soups, and fruit-flavored beverages); switch to liquid diet if necesssary.
- Sucking on ice chips keeps the mouth lubricated.
- Rinse your mouth frequently with a saline solution.
- Artificial saliva may be helpful, but some patients complain that such products are thick and have a sticky consistency.
- Regular mouth care is essential with decreased saliva to prevent cavities, gum disease, or mouth ulceration.

© Colleen Gill MS, RD, University Hospital, Denver, CO. May be reproduced for patient use only.

30. What can you suggest to patients who are sensitive to smells?

Smells alone can be a primary trigger for nausea, preventing the patient from attempting to eat a meal or snack. Simple management of food choices, preparation, and service can minimize this problem:
- Choose cold foods, which lack the volatile compounds that reach the nose.
- Caretakers can reduce smells in meal preparation by using fans, covered pans, microwaves, or outdoor grills.
- Meals from take-out restaurants or friends can reduce the smells of preparation for the patient.
- Dietary staff and nurses serving meals can reduce odors in patients' rooms by uncovering the trays in the hallway before entering.

31. A patient with mouth or throat sores often says, "It hurts to eat." What can you do?

Mouth and Throat Sores

Whether caused by radiation, chemotherapy, oral infections, or graft vs. host disease, pain is often the final straw when added to the traditional problems associated with eating. Avoidance of foods that increase pain helps to prevent a total breakdown in eating.

Helfpul
- When solids are not tolerated, use a liquid diet, including Carnation Instant Breakfast, commercial supplements, pasteurized egg nog, milk shakes, and blenderized foods.
- Cook foods until tender and soft in texture.
- Eat soft foods at room temperature or lukewarm rather than hot (e.g., soups, mashed potatoes, eggs, quiche, cooked cereals).
- Dry foods can be soaked in liquids or covered with gravies or sauces.
- Cold foods are tolerated by many patients (e.g., milk shakes, cottage cheese, yogurt, watermelon, Jello, soft canned fruits, baby food).

Table continued on following page

Mouth and Throat Sores (Continued)

Helfpul *(continued)*
- Try frozen foods, although a few patients cannot tolerate extreme cold temperatures (e.g., popsicles, ice cream, frozen yogurt, slushes/ices).
- Fruit-flavored beverages or nectars are tolerated much better than acidic juices.
- Drink through a straw to bypass mouth sores.
- Tilt your head backward or forward to help with swallowing.
- Small, frequent meals limit the irritation to a sore mouth.
- Maintain good mouth care to prevent infection. Brush and rinse with a salt/baking soda solution several times a day. Avoid commercial mouthwashes that contain alcohol.
- Take pain medications as needed to control pain and make eating possible. Liquid solutions that anesthetize the mouth are helpful to some patients when taken before eating.

Harmful
- Tart or acidic foods such as citrus fruits and juices, tomato, or pickles will burn.
- Salty foods and drinks, including broth, may be irritating.
- Strong flavorings and spices, such as peppers, chili, nutmeg, and cloves, will burn and irritate sensitive tissues. No Italian, Mexican, or other spicy foods. Use seasonings sparingly.
- Rough or coarse foods will scratch (e.g., raw fruits and vegetables, dry breads, cereals, chips).
- Alcohol and tobacco irritate tissues.
- Hot foods or drinks burn already damaged surfaces.

32. A patient with diarrhea often says, "It just goes right through me." What can you recommend to manage diarrhea and identify malabsorption?

Like the tastebuds, the cells of the GI tract turn over rapidly and are more vulnerable to the effects of chemotherapy and radiation. Many health care professionals were trained to "rest the gut" while using oral rehydration solutions (e.g., Pedialyte); recent research, however, has shown that this strategy leads to more weight loss without shortening the duration of diarrhea.

Medications
- Medications that use soluble fiber or clay to absorb water in the stool, such as Kaopectate or Pepto Bismol, may be helpful. Medications that slow motility (Lomotil, tincture of opium, Imodium) should not be used until bacterial overgrowth (e.g., *Clostridium difficile*) and infection have been ruled out.
- If possible, hold medications that can exacerbate or cause diarrhea, including oral magnesium supplementation and metoclopramide (antiemetic).
- Gray or tan, greasy-looking stools that float in the toilet may indicate fat malabsorption. Although not typical in patients with cancer, patients with pancreatic cancer sometimes experience this condition and may benefit from pancreatic enzyme supplementation before meals.

Dietary modifications
- Complex carbohydrates (fruits and starches) are particularly well absorbed and beneficial to gut healing. However, high-fiber sources such as bran, whole grains, raw fruits and vegetables, nuts, dried beans and legumes, should be limited.
- Diarrhea is a marker of GI damage; food safety precautions are recommended to limit introduction of pathogenic organisms.
- Patients should avoid gastric irritants, such as caffeine, pepper, and alcohol. These substances also can be irritating to rectal and anal tissues.
- Damage to the GI tract may severely limit the absorption of lactose. The lactase enzyme is easily lost and leaves the carbohydrate available for breakdown by normal gut flora. Their metabolic byproduct is gas, which creates the bloating and cramping and, ultimately, the diarrhea associated with lactose intolerance. Alternatives to milk products include soy milk, lactose-free supplements, sorbet, and soy based frozen desserts. Lactase tablets (available over the counter) may be used if milk products are highly desired; lactose-free milks are available in the dairy section.

- Fluid replacement is essential because of increased losses in the stool. Patients should drink an additional cup of fluid for every episode of diarrhea. Nonacidic juices and nectars often work well. Fruit-ade drinks, especially those without carbonation (e.g., Hawaiian Fruit Punch), are especially well tolerated. Sport drinks (e.g., Gatorade) can help to replace lost electrolytes. Some patients find that it helps to avoid liquids at meal times, to limit liquids with high sugar content, and to drink fluids at room temperature.
- If a patient experiences stool losses at >1000 ml/day, they should receive zinc supplementation to cover losses in the stool (12–17 mg/1000 ml stool volume).

Total parenteral nutrition (TPN): When diarrhea continues despite diet modifications and appropriate medications, the GI tract may well be sufficiently impaired to meet criteria for the consideration of TPN.

33. How can I help the patient with an overly helpful caregiver?

Family and friends are often heavily invested in helping to ensure adequate nutrition for the patient, perhaps because this is one area in which they feel competent. Unfortunately, when the patient is less than cooperative in complying with their direction and help, some caretakers react by exerting increased pressure and encouragement. This predictably brings patients, at least mentally, back to their childhood when they were forced to eat foods that they did not want. In general, patients eat less when they are pressured. You can help relationships that are heading for control battles with the following strategies:

1. Suggest that the patient and caretakers discuss appropriate meal and snack schedules in advance as well as a list of foods acceptable to the patient. Friends and family can shop for foods, remind the patient at the agreed times, ask the patient what he or she would like to try, and prepare it. The control of what and how much the patient eats must remain with the patient, because the consequences are the patient's alone.

2. Encourage the evaluation of progress over a week's time, not day to day. Remind family that everyone has a variable appetite, but healthy people are not obsessed with the variations. Patients with cancer also have "good" and "bad" days. If the family expects that every day will be better than the day before, the tendency to push food on "bad" days will increase. This pattern, unfortunately, adds to the patient's list of food aversions because forced foods are more likely to be associated with feeling badly.

3. Discuss the reality of "force feeding": it never works. Eating is one area over which the patient exerts total control; others cannot do it in their behalf. In fact, if others attempt to take responsibility for their eating, some patients simply give up the responsibility altogether—a set-up for failure. The patient must be educated about the consequences of weight loss—loss of strength and quality of life—so that they are motivated to eat to their best ability.

34. What other significant psychological issues surround eating?

Weight loss. One of the most frequent comments from patients, especially women in general and men who have had prior weight problems, is that "It doesn't matter. I can afford to lose a few pounds." Although some are open enough to joke about their "cancer diet," others are affected on a more subliminal level. For most of their life they have tried to avoid eating too much or to lose a few pounds. Changing engrained thoughts requires education about changing priorities and the effect of weight loss on strength and muscle mass.

Weight gain. Patients with breast cancer and patients undergoing treatment regimens that include steroids may gain weight during treatment. Patients can become increasingly alarmed and frustrated, especially when friends or family question the gain: " I thought cancer patients lost weight?" Clinicians need to be sensitive to patient concerns as they seek nutritional guidance to control unwanted weight gain.

Expectations from food. Of necessity, food has been part of our life since birth. Simple observation of the various ethnic preferences shows that the foods to which we are exposed determine what we eventually like or dislike, what "sounds good" to us. Globally, eating has always been a self-reinforcing activity: food tastes good, so we want more of it. For patients with cancer, such expectations are no longer fulfilled. It is important to help patients to realize that eating is part of treatment. Rekeying expectations to "What do I think I can tolerate?" may help significantly.

Depression. The depression that frequently accompanies cancer can significantly limit patients' ability to motivate themselves to overcome eating problems. Achieving adequate intake may require antidepressant therapy in some patients.

35. What additional considerations are necessary for pediatric patients?

Although most issues apply equally to adult and pediatric patients, four areas of difference warrant special attention:

1. The child is still growing. Optimal nutrition is even more critical to ensure that body and brain growth and development are not significantly impaired during the treatment process.

2. Getting more calories into children is complicated by their increased propensity for nausea, vomiting, and taste changes because of the youthfulness of sensory receptors.

3. Depending on age and maturity, many children cannot conceive of delayed gratification. This difference is crucial, because we often ask patients with cancer to eat without incentives—and often despite significant disincentives. Working closely with the family to establish a reward system for eating helps to address this issue. In working with adolescents, control issues can be especially important to review with parents and patient.

4. Working with children with cancer can be challenging because of their apprehension about unfamiliar routines and caregivers and their fears of cancer treatment procedures. Parents also can feel overwhelmed by the demands of their child's therapy and side effects that their child may experience.

36. When are commercial supplements helpful?

Many patients with cancer find it easier to drink their calories because fluids do not require the energy of chewing, rarely stimulate the gag reflex, and generally empty out of the stomach more quickly, resulting in fewer complaints of early satiety. Most fluids are relatively low in protein, however, and therefore are not complete nutritional sources. Many complete nutritional products are now on the market, but cost containment generally restricts hospitals to one or two options within a category. Some formulas are meant for oral intake and others solely for tube feeding (unflavored). Specific contents are detailed in information provided by the manufacturer.

37. Why are tube feedings preferred over total parenteral nutrition (TPN)?

Tube feedings have a lower risk of infection, require less medical assistance, create less disruption of normal eating patterns, and are significantly less expensive. The classic phrase, "When the gut works, use it!" is based on these advantages as well as the knowledge that the GI tract nourishes itself from the inside as nutrients travel through it. GI health, therefore, is maintained far better with enteral feedings than with TPN, even when calories are equal. A nighttime tube feeding may improve the patient's quality of life by allowing a more normal lifestyle during the day and by lessening the pressure on the patient to "force feed" the total requirement of calories. Severe mucositis can prevent both oral nutrition and placement of a nasogastric feeding tube, requiring gastrostomy tube placement.

38. Summarize the benefits and risks of lactose-containing supplements.

Benefits include decreased cost, improved taste for many patients more familiar with milk products, and less of a vitamin aftertaste. The major risk is lactose intolerance.

39. What lactose-containing supplements are available?

- Flavored packets of instant breakfast powder, generally found in the cereal aisle, provide 250–280 calories when added to 8 oz milk (2% or whole) as well as 12 gm of protein.
- Scandishake (Scandipharm) initially was used for patients with cystic fibrosis and increased calorie needs. It is now popular among patients with AIDS or cancer and is available in sugar-free and lactose-free formulas as well. Scandishake provides 440 calories and may be added to 8 ounces of milk (total of 600 calories) or 6 ounces of juice and ice (total of 500 calories). The juice version is particularly well tolerated by patients with cancer, because tart

juices counteract the sweet taste that many do not tolerate. Although this product contains a significant amount of calories, it also contains 21 grams of fat and may not be indicated for patients experiencing early satiety. However, much of the fat is medium chain triglycerides, which generally are better absorbed.

40. What types of lactose-free supplements are available?

- Lactose-free supplements containing intact proteins from soy isolates or calcium caseinate provide 9–11 gm of protein and 250 calories per 8 oz. Examples include Ensure, Boost, Osmolite, Resource, and Nutren.
- Higher calorie versions (355 cal or more/8 oz) with increased protein include Ensure Plus, Resource Plus, Boost Plus, Nutren 1.5 or 2.0, Deliver 2.0, and Magnacal. The 2 cal/ml options generally are not as well tolerated. All options require additional fluids to meet hydration needs.
- Higher protein versions with standard 250 calories for patients with increased protein needs include Osmolite HN, Boost High Protein, and Ensure High Protein.
- Fiber-containing versions are often helpful in limiting diarrhea as well as constipation. Examples include Jevity, Ultracal, Nutren with Fiber, and Fibersource. Ensure with Fiber is an oral supplement that may be preferred by patients because it tastes less sweet. These products are also beneficial for patients with poor appetites and oral intake secondary to pain and constipating drugs for pain management.
- Clear-liquid, high-protein beverages such as Enlive or Resource Fruit Beverage are good choices for variety and for patients who find "milk-type" beverages too heavy and/or distasteful. Patients experiencing nausea, diarrhea, or fat intolerance often find these formulas more acceptable. They generally contain 160–180 calories per 8 oz. and 4–8 gm of protein, with no fat.
- Predigested supplements provide a peptide-based diet that can be beneficial for patients with impaired GI function. Examples include Sandosource Peptide, Peptamen, and Peptamen VHP. They contain more fat than the truly elemental formulas, although primarily in the form of medium-chain triglycerides, which are more easily absorbed.
- Elemental supplements provide protein that is hydrolyzed to free amino acid form for absorption with minimal digestion. Fat is provided at very low levels that nonetheless meet the need for essential fatty acids. Vivonex Plus occasionally is associated with increased diarrhea. Current research indicates that peptide-based formulas may be better absorbed than strictly elemental formulations.
- Immune-enhancing supplements are supplemented with large amounts of key nutrients that modulate the inflammatory, metabolic, and immune processes. Recent studies have shown that the malnutrition occurring in 30% of patients undergoing GI surgery results in increased risk of perioperative complications. Impact and ImmunAid have been shown to decrease infectious complications and hospital length of stay.

41. How can nutrition be reinstated after the gut has not been used?

Lack of enteral intake, required to nourish mucosal cells, results in significant mucosal atrophy within days. The villi decrease in height and number, and the rate of mucosal cell turnover also decreases. In this setting, instituting enteral intake too rapidly may result in diarrhea and abdominal cramping. An isotonic, semi-elemental formula may be needed initially, but the problem is best overcome by slowly reinstituting feeding, titrating the rate of feeding upward over several days at a pace determined by the patient's tolerance. The diarrhea and cramps are not dangerous; antidiarrhetics such as Imodium may be tried if the diarrhea is not severe. The problem of mucosal malnutrition and diarrhea should be temporary. Some clinical trials indicate that the use of glutamine supplementation (10 grams 3 times/day) may be beneficial in refeeding of the gut. In addition, delayed emptying of the stomach can be a problem, leading to high residuals and intolerance. Reglan or IV erthromycin may be needed as a prokinetic agent. Erythromycin is especially effective and is indicated over Reglan when loose stools are already present.

42. How are enteral feedings instituted?

If the gut is functional, enteral tube feedings should be used. The nasogastric or nasoduodenal (Dobbhoff) tube is used most often if the tubefeeding is expected to be short term. For long-term feeding, especially in a patient who cannot take food orally for more than 1 month, a tube placed directly into the stomach (via percutaneous endoscopic gastrostomy [PEG]) or small bowel may be used.

43. How do I choose among the various types of enteral solutions?

Several factors should be kept in mind: functional capacity of the gut, tube size, the patient's metabolic status, and cost. The primary food of enterocytes is the amino acid glutamine, which can be added in powdered form to most nutritional supplements. Blenderized formulas have the advantage of lower cost; however, they are mainly suitable only for large-diameter tubes, such as the PEG tube. Commercial milk-based products such as Carnation Instant Breakfast may serve most patients' needs, but if mucosal damage is severe, a lactose-free formula will be better tolerated.

44. When is TPN appropriate?

TPN may be used when the gut is not functional because of cancer or its treatment. Common reasons for implementation include extensive GI surgery, bowel obstruction, or severe malabsorption. Prolonged oral or esophageal mucositis may be an indication for short-term TPN, but if long-term support is needed, physicians should consider placement of a gastrostomy tube.

45. What are the disadvantages of TPN?

TPN involves much higher costs ($300–500/day); without insurance, it is usually not financially feasible at home since TPN for > 3 months may exceed the patient's lifetime insurance benefits. Patients on TPN are also at increased risk of infection unless blood sugar levels are well controlled. One study showed a 5-fold increase in infection if blood sugar levels were above 200. TPN has not been shown to be beneficial for patients with cancer unless they are severely malnourished or the gut is not functional. It should be initiated only when problems prevent adequate oral intake for > 10 days, the patient has a life expectancy of at least 40 days, and central line access can be established.

46. What are appropriate nutritional goals in the outpatient setting?

Prompt nutritional screening and assessment (i.e., PG-SGA) can identify outpatients at nutritional risk. Patients then need to receive appropriate nutritional counseling and management of treatment-related side effects. Patients receiving aggressive cancer therapy also need aggressive nutritional intervention to help them maintain quality of life. Goals include:

- Weight maintenance or maximal weight loss within ½-1 pound/week to minimize loss of lean body mass and to spare dietary protein for needed tissue repairs.
- Adequate hydration: approximately 1 ml/calorie needed = 30 ml/kg adjusted ideal weight.

47. What should I say to patients who ask about using complementary and alternative medicine such as nutrition and vitamins as adjuvant therapy?

After cancer diagnosis, patients often are highly motivated to seek information about diet, vitamin and mineral supplements, and nutritional complementary and alternative medicine (CAM) therapies. Ironically, just when patients have the greatest motivation and most questions, we have the least definitive answers for them. Less than 10% of current research has focused on nutrition and cancer survivors; most research has involved cancer prevention. Patients are offered an overload of information from well-meaning friends and family, gathered from a variety of sources. This deluge can be confusing and at times overwhelming to patients as well as health care professionals. Patients should be encouraged to discuss CAM use and nutritional questions and concerns. Health care professionals should ask all patients about CAM use so that they can guide the patient, emphasizing possible benefit as well as any potential harm. A nonjudgmental approach increases the patient's receptivity to the information provided.

48. Summarize the guidelines for a healthy diet in patients with cancer.

During all phases of cancer treatment and survival, the principles outlined in the American Cancer Society's Guidelines on Diet, Nutrition, and Cancer Prevention serve as the basis for a healthy diet:

1. Choose most of the foods that you eat from plant sources.
   - Eat five or more servings of fruits and vegetables each day.
   - Eat other foods from plant sources, such as breads, cereals, grain products, rice, pasta, or beans, several times a day.
2. Limit intake of high fat foods, particularly from animal sources.
   - Choose foods low in fat.
   - Limit consumption of meats, especially high-fat meats.
3. Be physically active, and achieve a healthy body weight.
   - Be at least moderately active for 30 minutes or more on most days of the week.
   - Stay within your healthy weight range.
4. Limit alcoholic beverages, if you drink at all.

Patients should be encouraged to consume a nutritionally adequate diet that contains recommended amounts of the essential nutrients, including protein, carbohydrate, fat, vitamins and minerals, and water. During times of illness and recovery from cancer treatment, nutritional needs are often increased and patients should be counseled to consume additional nutrient dense foods to ensure adequate nutrition and weight maintenance.

49. Describe the proper use of dietary supplements.

As a rule, vitamin, mineral, and dietary supplements should never replace whole foods. Components of foods often act synergistically in providing their benefits. In focusing on a single ingredient, a patient may be missing others of equal importance. In fact, the use of supplements and single nutrients at doses higher than the recommended daily allowances and the new dietary reference raises safety concerns related to toxicity and the possibility of adverse interactions with prescribed anticancer therapies. A daily multivitamin without iron can help to ensure adequate coverage when intake is limited.

50. What organizations can help professionals find answers to nutritional questions?

- American Institute for Cancer Research
  1759 R. Street NW
  Washington, DC 20069
  Hotline: 800-843-8114 (9 AM-5 PM EST). A registered dietitian is available to answer questions.
  aicrweb@aicr.org
  http://www.aicr.org
  Free materials for the consumer and health care professional offer practical information about cancer prevention, particularly through diet and nutrition.
- American Cancer Society
  2599 Clifton Road, NE
  Atlanta, GA 30329-4251
  1-800-227-2345
  http://www.cancer.org
  Offers a variety of printed materials and educational programs. Summary of current research for diet and cancer survivors is included in, *Nutrition: During and After Cancer Treatment: A Guide for Informed Choices for Cancer Survivors.*
- American Dietetic Association
  216 West Jackson Blvd, Suite 800
  Chicago, IL 60606
  1-800-877-1600
  http://www.eatright.org

Offers information and assistance in nutritional issues for consumers and health care professionals.

- National Cancer Institute
9000 Rockville Pike
Building 31, Room 10A18
Bethesda, MD 20892
Hotline: 800-4-CANCER (422-6237) (9 AM–7 PM EST). Spanish-speaking assistance is available.
http://www.icic-nci.gov/nci-icic-html
Free single copy of *Eating Hints for Cancer Patients: Before, During, and After Treatment.* Additional information is included in booklets about chemotherapy and radiation treatment.

51. What additional sources are available on the Internet?
- American Botanical Council
http://www.herbalgram.org
1-800-373-7105
- Food and Drug Administration
http://www.vm.cfsan.fda.gov
1-800-322-0178
- Herbs Research Foundation
http://www.herbs.org
(303)449-2265
- Home Food Safety
http://www.homefoodsafet.org
- International Bibliographic Information on Dietary Supplements (IBIDS)
http://dietary-supplements.info.nih.gov/databases/ibid.html
1-301-435-2920
ODS@nih.gov
- Office of Complementary and Alternative Medicine (NIH)
http://www.altmed.od.nih.gov
1-800-531-1794
- Oncolink (sponsored by the University of Pennsylvania Cancer Center)
http://www.oncolink.upenn.edu

52. List selected written resources of particular value.
Bloch A (ed): Nutrition Management of the Cancer Patient. Rockville, MD, Aspen Publishers, 1990. Management of nutrition needs of cancer patients across the continuum of care.

Bloch A (ed): Oncology: Diet & Nutrition Patient Education Resource Manual. Gaithersburg, MD, Aspen Publishers, 2000. Ready-to-use materials at two literacy levels, in Spanish and English, for adult and pediatric populations. Includes information about the development of effective nutritional education materials as well as nutritional assessment and education tracking forms.

Cassileth BR: Alternative Medicine Handbook. New York, WW Norton, 1998. A comprehensive guide to alternative medicine for clinicians and consumers.

McCullam P, Polisena C (eds): Clinical Guide to Oncology Nutrition. Chicago, American Dietetic Association, 2000. A comprehensive resource by registered dietitians with expertise in oncology nutrition.

Melina V, Davis B, Harrison V: Becoming Vegetarian: A Complete Guide to Adopting a Healthy Vegetarian Diet. Toronto, Macmillan Canada, 1999. Step-by-step information on how to eat a nutritious, well-balanced vegetarian diet.

Pierce A: American Pharmaceutical Practical Guide to Natural Medicines. New York, Stonesong Press, 1999.

Sarubin A: Health Professional's Guide to Popular Dietary Supplements. Chicago, American Dietetic Association, 2000. A complete resource that provides clinicians with resources on popular supplements, including vitamins, minerals and herbals.

Weihofen D: Cancer Survival Cookbook. Minneapolis, MN, Chronimed Publishing, 1998. Snack and recipe ideas from a registered dietitian working in oncology nutrition.

REFERENCES

1. Allison G, Dixon T, Eldridge B, et al: Nutrition implications of surgical oncology. In McCallum PD, Polisena CG (eds): Clinical Guide to Oncology Nutrition. Chicago, American Dietetic Association, 2000 pp 79–89.
2. American Cancer Society Guidelines Advisory Committee: Guidelines on diet, nutrition, and cancer prevention: Reducing the risk of cancer with healthy food choices and physical activity. CA Cancer J Clin 46:325–341, 1996.
3. Baltzer L, Berkery R: Oncology Pocket Guide to Chermotherapy, Revised Edition. St. Louis, Mosby, 1995.
4. Block AS: Defining and applying supportive nutrition. Nutr Oncol 2:5–6, 1995.
5. Cohen D: Nutrition Support of the Cancer Patient. ON-Line Newletter, Oncology Nutrition Dietetic Practice Group, Spring 2000.
6. Cunningham R: The Anorectic-Cachetic Syndrome in Cancer. Bristol-Myers Squibb Oncology/Immunology Monograph, 1997.
7. Detsky A, McLaughin J, Baker J, et al: What is subjective global assessment of nutritional status? J Parent Ent Nutr 11:8–13, 1987.
8. Eldridge B: Chemotherapy and nutrition implications. In McCallum PD, Polisena CG, eds. Clinical Guide to Oncology Nutrition. Chicago, American Dietetic Association, 2000 pp 61–69.
9. Eldridge B, Rock C, McCallum P: Nutrition and the patient with cancer. In Coulston AM, Rock CL, Monsen ER (eds): Nutrition in the Prevention and the Treatment of Disease. San Diego, Academic Press, 2001, in press.
10. Heys S, Walker L, Smith T, Eremin O: Enteral nutritional supplementation with key nutrients in patients with critical illness and cancer. Ann Surg 229:467–477, 1999.
11. Kennedy LD: Common supportive drug therapies used with oncology patients. In McCallum PD, Polisena CG (eds): Clinical Guide to Oncology Nutrition. Chicago, American Dietetic Association, 2000, pp 168–181.
12. Langstein H, Norton J: Mechanisms of cancer cachexia. Hematol Oncol Clin North Am 5:103–123, 1991.
13. McMahon K, Decker G, Ottery F: Integrating proactive nutritional assessment in clinical practices to prevent complications and cost. Semin Oncol 25:20–27, 1998.
14. McCallum P: Patient generated-subjective global assessment. In McCallum PD, Polisena CG (eds): Clinical Guide to Oncology Nutrition. Chicago, American Dietetic Association, 2000, pp 11–23.
15. Nelson K, Walsh D, Sheehan F: The anorexia-cachexia syndrome. J Clin Oncol 12:213–225, 1994.
16. Polisena C: Nutrition concerns with the radiation therapy patient. In McCallum PD, Polisena CG (eds): Clinical Guide to Oncology Nutrition. Chicago, American Dietetic Association, 2000, pp 70–78.
17. Riddle S: Drug interactions: Examining the impact of botanicals and dietary supplements. Supportline, Publication of Dietitians in Nutrition Support 22(5), October 2000.
18. RTOG 9903: A randomized phase III trial to assess the effect of erythropoietin on local-regional control in anemic patients treated with radiotherapy for carcinoma of the head and neck. Protocol available at www.rtog.org.

45. ORGAN TOXICITIES AND LATE EFFECTS: RISKS OF TREATMENT

Brenda Ronk, RN, MS, OCN

1. Define late effects of therapy.

Late effects are toxicities caused by cancer therapy that appear months to years after treatment. They may be mild, severe, or life-threatening.

2. How do late effects differ from acute toxicities?

Late effects often occur in tissues with slowly proliferating cells, such as the heart. Acute toxicities tend to occur in tissues with rapidly proliferating cells, such as bone marrow and mucous membranes of the gastrointestinal tract. They occur during or shortly after treatment. Some drugs cause specific toxicities only when given in high doses or in combination with other chemotherapy agents or radiation therapy.

Some acute and late toxicities are well-defined and predictable, whereas others are unpredictable and vary with dose, duration of treatment, method of administration, and the status of the patient. (Refer to Chapter 7 for common toxicities of chemotherapy.)

3. What is the most common dose-limiting toxicity of chemotherapy?

Depression of bone marrow stem cells or peripheral blood cell lines is caused to some degree by almost all chemotherapy agents. The acceptable degree of myelosuppression depends on the type of cancer, the duration of myelosuppression, treatment goals, and patient status. Neutropenia occurs before thrombocytopenia and anemia because the half-life of granulocytes is much shorter (6–8 hours) than the half-lives of platelets (5–7 days) and red cells (approximately 120 days). The nadir of myelosuppression for most chemotherapy drugs generally is between 7 and 14 days. The nitrosureas cause a late thrombocytopenia 4 to 6 weeks after administration, and drugs such as ifosfamide and mitoxantrone are relatively platelet sparing. Drugs that usually do not cause bone marrow depression include steroidal hormones, bleomycin, vincristine, and L-asparaginase.

4. What are the most common late effects of cancer treatment on the major organ systems? How are they managed or prevented?

Selected Late Effects of Therapy

ORGAN SYSTEM	LATE EFFECT	CAUSATIVE TREATMENT	MANAGEMENT
Cardiovascular	Cardiomyopathy	Anthracycline chemo-therapy; risk increases with mediastinal irradiation	Prevention by limiting dosage to lifetime maximum Treatment of congestive failure (diuretics, digitalis, diet modification)
	Pericarditis	Mediastinal irradiation	Treat pericardial effusion if necessary
Pulmonary	Pulmonary fibrosis	Lung irradiation Some chemotherapeutic agents, especially in high doses	Avoid other respiratory irritants Corticosteroids may be beneficial For drug-induced toxicity, avoid high concentrations of oxygen

Table continued on next page

Selected Late Effects of Therapy (Continued)

ORGAN SYSTEM	LATE EFFECT	CAUSATIVE TREATMENT	MANAGEMENT
Musculoskeletal	Kyphosis, scoliosis	Radiation therapy in childhood	Orthopedic rehabilitation
	Fibrosis, joint immobility	Radiation therapy for head and neck cancers, sarcoma	Physical therapy
	Shortening of a growing bone	Radiation to long bones in childhood	Counseling about unequal length of limbs
Gastrointestinal	Chronic enteritis	Radiation therapy to pelvis	Symptomatic treatment with antidiarrheals, low residue diet
Neurologic	Peripheral neuropathy	Cisplatin (usually higher doses), vinca alkaloids	Effect may be permanent
	Orthostatic hypotension due to autonomic nervous system defects	Vinca alkaloids	Teach patient to change positions slowly
	Cataracts	Cranial irradiation High-dose corticosteroids	Surgical correction
	Hearing loss (high-frequency range)	Cisplatin	Audiology consultation Fit with hearing aid

5. Which chemotherapeutic agents are cardiotoxic?

Doxorubicin, daunorubicin and, to a lesser degree, idarubicin, epirubicin, and mitoxantrone may cause cardiac damage, commonly manifested as myocardial depression or congestive heart failure (CHF). At a cumulative dose of 450–550 mg/m^2, the incidence of CHF related to doxorubicin is only 0.1 to 0.2%, whereas it increases to 30% for doses above 550 mg/m^2.

5-FU has been implicated as causing myocardial ischemia, particularly when given as a continuous infusion or in combination with cisplatin. Cyclophosphamide normally has no cardiac effects at standard doses but can be cardiotoxic at high doses. Paclitaxel causes asymptomatic bradycardia, and its safety in patients with significant preexisting cardiac problems is still being investigated.

6. How can cardiac toxicity be prevented?

Numerous studies have documented that lifetime doses of anthracyclines (daunorubicin, doxorubicin) above 450–550 mg/m^2 are likely to produce cardiac symptoms. Generally, total lifetime doses of anthracyclines are maintained at these limits. Dosing depends on current cardiac status, age of the patient, and amount of chest irradiation. Often, left ventricular ejection fraction (LVEF), which is the portion of blood in the ventricle that is ejected during systole, is measured in patients before therapy with high doses of anthracyclines. LVEF can be measured by performing a multigated acquisition (MUGA) blood pool scan, a radionuclide imaging study of ventricular function. Normal LVEF is > 50%. Measurement of LVEF before treatment assists in making decisions about chemotherapeutic agent and dosage for persons with impaired cardiac function.

Because of the importance of dose-intensive therapy in prolonging disease-free survival, alternatives and modifications for current therapy have been developed. One such alternative is mitoxantrone, an anthracycline analog that may produce less cardiotoxicity than doxorubicin. Mitoxantrone may be substituted for doxorubicin for patients at risk for cardiac compromise. A second method of reducing cardiac toxicity is use of dexrazoxane, a cardioprotective agent that is given intravenously 30 minutes before administration of an anthracycline. Dexrazoxane (Zinecard) is currently used in patients who have already received some doxorubicin and need to continue therapy. Varied administration schedules of doxorubicin have also been used to prevent cardiac toxicity. Doxorubicin by continuous infusion or on a weekly schedule in lower doses produces less toxicity than the traditional higher dose given every 21 days. Cardiotoxicity can also be reduced by administering doxorubicin over 30 to 45 minutes instead of as a bolus infusion.

7. What is radiation recall?

Radiation recall is severe erythema, pain, blistering, or ulceration in areas previously irradiated. Radiation recall occurs 3 to 7 days most commonly after infusion of dactinomycin, doxorubicin, daunorubicin, or bleomycin. Other agents include mitoxantrone, idarubicin, mitomycin, 5-FU, methotrexate, cyclophosphamide, and paclitaxel. Dry or moist desquamation is another common cutaneous toxicity experienced by patients receiving chemotherapy agents before, concurrently, or after radiation.

8. A 26-year-old woman who has undergone autologous bone marrow transplant for Hodgkin's disease presents with dyspnea and dry cough 4 months after discharge from the transplant unit. Which long-term effect is likely to produce these symptoms?

A frequent effect of high-dose chemotherapy is pulmonary toxicity. In treatment regimens for bone marrow or peripheral stem cell transplant, cyclophosphamide, carmustine (BCNU), and busulfan are commonly responsible. Bleomycin and methotrexate also may produce acute or chronic pulmonary toxicity. Dyspnea that worsens with exercise, dry cough, and decreased diffusion capacity on pulmonary function testing are hallmark signs. Often open lung biopsy is necessary to distinguish pulmonary toxicity from metastatic disease or an infectious process.

9. What is the treatment for pulmonary toxicity?

Corticosteroids may be of some benefit in many cases of pulmonary toxicity. Often after an aggressive course of gradually tapered steroids, pulmonary symptoms resolve. However, severe cases may be disabling or life-threatening.

10. Why are patients with pulmonary toxicity cautioned about using oxygen?

Oxygen must be used judiciously in patients with pulmonary toxicity, especially if the toxicity is produced by bleomycin or BCNU. In such patients, high-concentration oxygen may cause acute respiratory failure that requires mechanical ventilation and exacerbates lung injury. Oxygen may be used during anesthesia as long as the patient receives the least amount needed to produce an oxygen saturation of > 90%. Patients who have received high doses of chemotherapeutic agents or who have experienced pulmonary toxicity should carry identification describing their pulmonary condition and the risk of oxygen administration.

11. In what ways may cancer therapies affect the sexual and reproductive functions of men and women?

Chemotherapy, radiation therapy, and hormonal therapy may have permanent and significant effects on sexual and reproductive functioning, which are summarized in the table.

Changes to Sexual and Reproductive Function after Cancer Treatment

TREATMENT	EFFECT

Chemotherapy
  Busulfan
  Chlorambucil
  Cyclophosphamide
  Nitrogen mustard
  Nitrosureas
  Procarbazine
	Amenorrhea, ovarian failure, decreased or absent production
	  of sperm, decreased libido

Table continued on next page

Changes to Sexual and Reproductive Function after Cancer Treatment (Continued)

TREATMENT	EFFECT
Radiation therapy	
External beam	Ovarian failure, decreased or absent production of sperm, impotence, erectile dysfunction, decreased libido
Brachytherapy	Vaginal stenosis
Hormonal therapy	
Estrogens	Gynecomastia
Androgens	Masculinization (in women)
Antiandrogens	Decreased libido, impotence, erectile dysfunction

12. What are some dermatologic toxicities caused by chemotherapy?

Dermatologic effects include rashes (docetaxel, idarubicin), hyperpigmentation (hydroxyurea, methotrexate), nail thickening or banding, acral erythema, phlebitis, chemical cellulitis, radiation recall and enhancement, photosensitivity, reactivation of UV light-induced erythema (methotrexate), seborrheic inflammation or actinic keratoses (dacarbazine, dactinomycin, doxorubicin, cisplatin, cytarabine), scleroderma-like changes, and vasculitis (cytarabine, hydroxyurea, methotrexate).

13. Do hyperpigmentation and photosensitivity induced by 5-FU, bleomycin, or methotrexate ever resolve?

Hyperpigmentation, photosensitivity, generalized skin darkening, dermatitis, and nail changes are usually of short duration (during the course of treatment) and diminish gradually once therapy has stopped.

14. What is "hand-foot syndrome"?

Palmar–plantar erythrodysesthesia (acral erythema) syndrome, referred to as hand-foot syndrome, is a painful erythema of the palms, fingers, and soles of the feet that may progress to bullae or vesicular formation and desquamation before healing spontaneously within a week. Patients with this condition frequently require opioids for pain relief. The condition may respond to pyridoxine treatment and cooling. Acral erythema is induced by standard and high-dose cytarabine, hydroxyurea, continuous infusion 5-FU, bleomycin, doxorubicin, methotrexate, high-dose etoposide, thiotepa, and docetaxel.

15. What are some hepatotoxic effects of chemotherapy and which drugs usually require dose modification with hepatic dysfunction?

Hepatotoxic effects of chemotherapy agents include hepatocellular injury, necrosis, venoocclusive disease, and reactivation of chronic hepatitis B virus infection. Combination chemotherapy and high-dose regimens used for autologous bone marrow transplantations have enhanced the potential for hepatotoxicity, particularly hepatic venoocclusive disease. At conventional doses, venoocclusive disease has been associated with cytarabine, dacarbazine, 6-mercaptopurine, and 6-thioguanine. If there is evidence of hepatic impairment or abnormal liver function tests (e.g., bilirubin > 1.5 mg/dl), the following agents should be held or reduced: doxorubicin, daunorubicin, vinblastine, vincristine, cyclophosphamide, methotrexate, 5-FU, and paclitaxel.

16. Can chemotherapy affect vision or cause other ocular complications?

Although relatively uncommon, the incidence of ocular complications has increased in accordance with increased patient survival and high-dose chemotherapy regimens. Ophthalmologic side effects include decreased or blurred vision (cisplatin, cyclophosphamide, cytarabine, mitomycin C, methotrexate); eye pain (busulfan, cytarabine, methotrexate); papilledema (cisplatin); altered color vision (cisplatin); conjunctivitis (cytarabine, 5-FU, methotrexate); tear duct stenosis and increased lacrimation (5-FU, doxorubicin, methotrexate); photophobia (cytarabine, methotrexate);

optic neuropathy or blindness (vincristine); photopsia (paclitaxel); and cataracts (busulfan). Conjunctivitis related to high-dose cytarabine may be reduced effectively with prophylactic glucocorticoid eye drops, as well as artificial tears, which probably decrease toxicity by diluting intraocular drug concentrations.

17. How can sexual and reproductive changes be prevented or managed?
In chemotherapy and radiation therapy, older age at time of treatment is more likely to cause permanent infertility. Sperm banking and in vitro fertilization may make conception possible in some patients. In women receiving pelvic irradiation, the ovaries may be surgically moved behind the uterus (oophoropexy) to shield them from the beam. Changes in sexual functioning require open and sensitive discussion of the issue, with exploration of possible solutions or modifications in activity.

18. What is the most frequent long-term effect of radiation therapy to the head and neck?
Xerostomia (dryness of the mouth) is the most frequent chronic effect of radiation to the oral cavity. Radiation, both external beam and implanted, may produce permanent injury to the acinar cells of the salivary glands. The small amount of saliva that is produced is thick and ineffective at performing the normal salivary functions: lubricating the mouth, providing a buffer for acids, and washing food and organisms from the teeth and gums. Chronic xerostomia is a highly distressing condition. Swallowing dry foods and taking pills become difficult, and the patient frequently awakens at night with dry mouth. Artificial saliva products are available. Some patients may find relief with pilocarpine hydrochloride. Many patients find that water, hard candies, or lozenges are equally effective in relieving the sensation of dryness.

19. How is dental caries related to radiation therapy? How can they be prevented?
Inadequate production of saliva increases the risk of dental caries, because there is too little saliva to clear bacteria from the mouth. In addition, patients undergoing radiation therapy may also have poor oral hygiene if they experience mucositis. Despite instructions to perform meticulous mouth care, patients may not be compliant if pain due to mucositis is poorly controlled. These factors contribute to the development of dental caries, which may create a problem for several years. Dental caries is prevented by the following methods:
1. A thorough dental evaluation before the start of therapy, with diseased teeth repaired or extracted
2. Meticulous oral hygiene with frequent saline rinses, gentle toothbrushing, and fluoride application
3. Provision of adequate analgesia for oral care to be performed
4. Prompt treatment of any infection in the oral mucosa
5. Prevention of further irritation to the oral mucosa by avoiding the use of alcohol and tobacco.

20. A 10-year-old girl who underwent total body irradiation during a bone marrow transplant for acute lymphoblastic leukemia developed a cataract 3 years later. How does her cataract compare with a cataract in an elderly person?
Physiologically, the girl's cataract is exactly the same as a non–radiation-related cataract and should be surgically removed in the same manner. The lens of the eye is sensitive to radiation, more so in children than in older persons. Cataracts may result from cranial or ocular radiation therapy, especially at higher doses. They often present several years after treatment.

21. How is the gastrointestinal tract affected by radiation therapy to the pelvis?
Proctitis and enteritis, which may be acute effects of radiation therapy, also may become chronic effects if the mucosa is permanently damaged. Radiation may produce shortening of the intestinal villi and thus prevent adequate absorption. Acutely injured mucosa may become atrophied, thickened, or ulcerated. Proctitis or small bowel enteritis results, causing diarrhea with cramping. This chronic condition is physically and psychologically debilitating. A few individuals also experience fecal incontinence. Nurses may assist patients to cope with this problem by instructing them

about low residue diets and use of antidiarrheals. Steroid enemas are sometimes used. If conservative measures fail, a colostomy may be required.

22. How are the late effects of therapy different in children?

Because children undergo such rapid growth and development, effects on their developing tissues are different from those seen in mature tissues. Children often receive treatment to the central nervous system (total body irradiation, brain irradiation, intrathecal chemotherapy) for leukemia or brain tumors. The most serious long-term effects are seen in children under the age of 3 years, when brain development is rapid. Such patients may later manifest intellectual deficits, as well as attention and memory problems. CNS treatment also may affect endocrine function because of damage to the hypothalamic–pituitary axis. Frequently seen are growth impairment with growth hormone deficiency and delayed or arrested development of secondary sexual characteristics. Children may need exogenous hormones to produce normal growth and maturation.

Common Late Effects of Treatment of Childhood Cancer

Short stature	Dental caries
Intellectual deficits	Cataracts
Delayed sexual development	Kyphoscoliosis
Secondary malignancies	Skeletal growth retardation

23. What are secondary malignancies?

Secondary malignancies are cancers caused by damage to the DNA of normal cells exposed to chemotherapy and radiation therapy. The most common secondary malignancy is acute myeloid leukemia due to therapy with an alkylating agent for Hodgkin's disease, non-Hodgkin's lymphoma, and multiple myeloma. Agents that may cause secondary malignancies include nitrogen mustard, procarbazine, melphalan, cyclophosphamide, busulfan, chlorambucil, and thiotepa. Radiation-induced sarcomas have been known to occur in patients treated for Hodgkin's disease and non-Hodgkin's lymphoma. The period of highest risk for developing secondary leukemia is 2–10 years after treatment. Secondary leukemia is one of the most serious long-term effects of therapy, because it generally has a poor prognosis.

24. What late psychosocial effects may be seen in patients after treatment for cancer?

Numerous psychosocial changes may be experienced by patients who have received cancer treatment. Often they live with the fear of recurrence of cancer and death. Any change in health status may produce worry about cancer recurrence. Changes may occur in relationships with family, friends, coworkers, and sexual partners. Persons who are healthy after recovering from cancer and its treatment may still be perceived as ill or disabled, creating relationship stress and feelings of isolation. Disabilities and physical changes may require adjustment in lifestyle, employment, or family role.

REFERENCES

1. Byrne J: Long-term genetic and reproductive effects of ionizing radiation and chemotherapeutic agents on cancer patients and their offspring. Teratology 59:210–215, 1999.
2. Coia LR, Moylan DJ III: Introduction to Clinical Radiation Oncology. Madison, WI, Medical Physics Publishing, 1991.
3. DeVita VT Jr, Hellman S, Rosenberg SA (eds): Cancer: Principles and Practices of Oncology, 6th ed. Philadelphia, Lippincott Williams & Wilkins, 2001.
4. Green DM: Effects of treatment for childhood cancer on vital organ systems. Cancer 71(Suppl 10):3299–3305, 1993.
5. Lockwood KA, Bell TS, Colegrove RW Jr: Long-term effects of cranial radiation therapy on attention functioning in survivors of childhood leukemia. J Pediatr Psych 24:55–66, 1999.
6. Moore IM, Hobbie W: Late effects of cancer treatment. In Yarbro CH, Frogge MH, Goodman M, Groenwald SL (eds): Cancer Nursing: Principles and Practice, 5th ed. Boston, Jones & Bartlett, 2000, pp 597–615.
7. Perry MC (ed): The Chemotherapy Source Book, 2nd ed. Baltimore, Williams & Wilkins, 1996.
8. Ruccione K, Weinberg K: Late effects in multiple body systems. Semin Oncol Nurs 5:4–13, 1989.

46. PAIN MANAGEMENT

Diana Ruzicka, RN, MSN, CNS, AOCN, Rose A. Gates, RN, MSN, CNS/NP, and Regina M. Fink, RN, PhD, AOCN

1. What is cancer pain?

As defined by McCaffery, "Pain is whatever the experiencing person says it is, existing whenever the experiencing person says it does." It is "an unpleasant sensory and emotional experience associated with actual or potential tissue damage, or described in terms of such damage" (IASP, 1979). Unrelieved pain affects quality of life in all dimensions, including physical, psychological, and spiritual well-being, and social concerns. Cancer patients have multiple sources and sites of pain due to:
- Direct tumor involvement and related pathology (65–80% of patients)
- Anticancer therapy and invasive diagnostic or therapeutic procedures (25% of patients)
- Unrelated to cancer or therapy; prior or concurrent painful conditions (3–10% of patients)

2. Can cancer pain be controlled?

Pain is well controlled by oral analgesics in 90% of patients with cancer. Unfortunately, about 25% of all patients with cancer die with unrelieved pain because of patient, provider, and family misconceptions and fears. Adequate pain control is further complicated by regulatory agencies that scrutinize professional licensure and restrictively regulate controlled substances. To address issues related to the undertreatment of cancer pain, position papers, educational materials, and guidelines have been developed by various organizations (e.g., state cancer pain initiatives, Oncology Nursing Society, American Society of Clinical Oncology, and the American Pain Society). Management of cancer pain requires a multidisciplinary approach. As with other symptoms, the best way to treat pain is to treat the cause. Surgery, radiation, and chemotherapy may be used to control the pain by removing or shrinking the tumor. Drugs (nonopioids and opioids) remain the mainstay of pain treatment.

3. How do the types of pain differ?

Pain is classified as nociceptive (traveling along normal nerve conduction pathways) or neuropathic (caused by damage to the central or peripheral nervous system). Nociceptive pain may be further divided into somatic and visceral.

TYPE OF PAIN	DESCRIPTORS	ETIOLOGY	TREATMENT
Somatic (well localized)	Achy Throbbing Dull	Originates at peripheral nerve endings Bone and spine metastases Cutaneous or deep tissue inflammation or injury	Opioids ± nonsteroidal anti-inflammatory drug Muscle relaxants Pamidronate Strontium 89
Visceral (poorly localized)	Squeezing Pressure Cramping Distention	Originates in deep organ; often referred to dermatomes innervated by same fibers Bowel obstruction, stretching, or infection Blood flow occlusion	Opioids (caution with bowel-obstructed patients)
Neuropathic	Burning, "fire" Shooting Numbness Radiation "Electrical sensation"	Nerve damage by tumor or fibrosis of nerve plexus Postherpetic neuralgia Peripheral neuropathies secondary to tumor, radiation fibrosis, or chemotherapy	Antidepressants Anticonvulsants Benzodiazepines ± opioids

4. How is pain assessed?

Patient assessment needs to be ongoing, individualized, and documented so that everyone involved has an understanding of the problem. Pain should be reassessed during each follow-up visit, by every shift during hospitalization, or after every intervention. Recent studies of health care professionals identified poor pain assessment, lack of knowledge, and insufficient time as the greatest barriers to adequate pain treatment. In 2001, the Joint Commission for the Accreditation of Healthcare Organizations (JCAHO) implemented new standards, making pain the fifth vital sign. (*Note:* Vital signs are neither sensitive nor specific indicators of chronic pain.) In addition to assessment of pain characteristics, psychosocial and thorough physical and neurologic evaluations are necessary, as is a review of other symptoms (e.g., anxiety, nausea, insomnia, constipation, anorexia). Cultural and ethnic backgrounds also may influence pain expression and behavior; however, patients should not be stereotyped. An easy way to assess pain is to incorporate the **WILDA** strategy:

Pain Assessment Guide

Words to describe pain

aching	throbbing	shooting
stabbing	gnawing	sharp
tender	burning	exhausting
tiring	penetrating	nagging
numb	miserable	unbearable
dull	radiating	squeezing
crampy	deep	pressure

Pain in other languages

itami	Japanese
tong	Chinese
dau	Vietnamese
dolor	Spanish
doleur	French
bolno	Russian

Intensity (0–10)

If 0 is no pain and 10 is the worst pain imaginable, what is your pain now? . . . in the past 24 hours?

Location

Where is your pain?

Duration

Is the pain always there? (persistent)
Does the pain come and go? (breakthrough)
Do you have both types of pain?

Aggravating and alleviating factors

What makes the pain better?
What makes the pain worse?

How does pain affect

sleep	energy	relationships
appetite	activity	mood

Are you experiencing any other symptoms?

nausea/vomiting	itching	urinary retention
constipation	sleepiness/confusion	weakness

Things to check

vital signs, past medication history, knowledge of pain, and use of noninvasive techniques

© Regina Fink, University of Colorado Hospital, 1996.

Three commonly used assessment scales are shown below. The Numeric Pain Intensity (0–10) Scale is useful in the clinical setting for patients older than 5 years. Ask the patient, "If 0 is no pain and 10 is the worst pain imaginable, what is your pain right now?" The Faces Pain Rating Scale is appropriate for children older than 3 years and for patients with language barriers. The Verbal Descriptor Scale has six numerically ranked choices of word descriptors, including no, mild, moderate, severe, very severe, worst possible pain. Each adjective is given a number that indicates the patient's pain intensity.

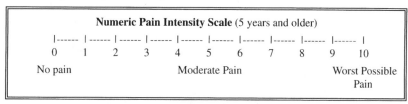

Faces Pain Rating Scale

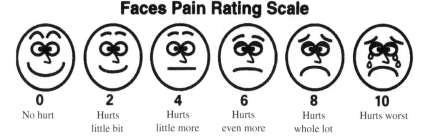

Explain to the child/adult that each face is for a person who feels happy because he has no pain (hurt) or sad because he has some or a lot of pain.

Face 0 is very happy because he doesn't hurt at all.   *Face 6* hurts even more.
Face 2 hurts just a little bit.   *Face 8* hurts a whole lot.
Face 4 hurts a little more.   *Face 10* hurts as much as you can imagine, but you don't have to be crying to feel this bad.

Ask the child/adult to choose the face that best describes how he is feeling. **Recommended for persons aged 3 or older**. (From Wong D, Whaley L: Clinical Handbook of Pediatric Nursing, 2nd ed. St. Louis, Mosby, 1986, p 373, with permission.)

5. How can you assess pain in the cognitively impaired and nonverbal patient?

The patient's self-report is the gold standard even in nonverbal or cognitively impaired patients. However, instruments that rely on verbal self-report may not be appropriate for use in nonverbal, cognitively impaired, delirious, or dying patients. Based on behaviors observed by nurses, an objective nine-item scale for assessing discomfort is used in patients with Alzheimer's disease.[13] Further research is needed to determine the generalizability of this scale and others for use in oncology patients. Key nonverbal indicators include noisy breathing; negative vocalizations (e.g., moaning, groaning); absence of a contented look; looking sad, frightened or tense; facial grimacing; fidgeting or increased restlessness; and absence of relaxed body posture or guarding of a body part.

6. How often should pain be assessed?

The frequency of assessment is determined by the clinical situation. According to the JCAHO, patients have the right to appropriate assessment and management of pain. An initial screening assessment identifies patients in pain. Patients should be assessed at least once a shift (or every 8 hours); if pain has been reported, it should be assessed at least every 4 hours. If a patient has severe pain requiring upward titration of analgesics, pain assessment should be completed frequently (e.g., every 15 minutes). Pain should be assessed approximately 15–30 minutes after administration of a parenteral medication and 60 minutes after oral medication. If pain is well controlled, pain intensity should be assessed routinely along with vital signs. Record the results of pain assessment in a way that facilitates regular reassessment and follow-up.

7. Should placebos be used to assess pain?

No. According to the Oncology Nursing Society's Position Statement on the Use of Placebos, "Placebos should not be used (a) to assess or manage cancer pain, (b) to determine if the pain is 'real,' or (c) to diagnose psychological symptoms, such as anxiety associated with pain. Nurses should not administer placebos in these circumstances even if there is a medical order." Placebos are appropriate in the context of controlled studies when patients have given informed consent. Because placebos involve secrecy, ethical tenets of truth-telling and patient autonomy are violated. Use of placebos can destroy a therapeutic relationship if the patient becomes aware of their use. Placebos may mimic drug effects, make symptoms worse, produce side effects and directly affect body organ functions. Placebos may be highly effective, as demonstrated by studies in patients with postoperative pain. About 30–35% of patients in control groups reported pain relief from placebos. Instead of labeling patients who respond to placebos as "fakers" or "addicted," the mechanism of the placebo response should be examined.

8. How do you deal with physicians, nurses, or patients who are afraid of addiction?

First, describe the difference between physical dependence, tolerance, and addiction (psychological dependence). Then quote studies reporting the low incidence of addiction among patients taking opioids to relieve pain. Emphasize that the incidence of addiction is < 1% in patients without a previous history of addiction. For patients afraid of addiction, ask whether they would take the drug if they were not having pain. If they say "no," then reassure them that they are not going to become addicted if they use pain medications for the right reason.

9. Are patients with cancer addicted when they keep asking for more pain medicine?

No. They are probably exhibiting signs of tolerance, an involuntary response in which the patient requires higher doses of opioids to provide the same analgesic effect. It is important to determine whether disease progression is responsible for an increased opioid requirement. The exact mechanisms for tolerance are still unknown. Because of incomplete cross-tolerance, opioid rotation (switching from one opioid drug to another) is usually recommended to treat tolerance as well as increasing the drug dose or decreasing the interval between doses. An important factor under investigation in the treatment of opioid tolerance is the variation in the affinity of opioids for both opioid receptors (mu, delta, kappa) and nonopioid receptors. For example, opioid rotation from morphine to methadone may be effective because methadone can interact with both opioid and nonopioid receptors.

10. Do signs of withdrawal mean the patient is addicted?

No. The patient is probably showing signs of **physical dependence**, which develops when patients take opioids for an extended period (usually 1 week or more). Like tolerance, physical dependence is a normal body response. If an opioid is abruptly stopped, the patient may experience withdrawal symptoms: nervousness, sweating, anxiety, chills alternating with hot flashes, salivation, lacrimation, rhinorrhea, diaphoresis, piloerection, nausea, vomiting, abdominal cramps, or insomnia. Reassure patients that physical dependence is not unique to opioids. For example, an abstinence syndrome occurs when patients abruptly stop taking long-term steroids. Opioids should be tapered gradually, like steroids. In contrast, **addiction** or **psychological dependence** is an abnormal behavior involving an overwhelming desire to obtain the medication for its psychological effects. Addiction rarely occurs in patients with cancer. Most patients would prefer not to take the medication and not to have the pain.

11. What are some common patient and family concerns about pain medication?

It is important to solicit patients' and families' worries about pain control and medications to legitimize and clarify their concerns. Patients may fail to report pain in the desire to be "good" patients or because of the following common myths about opioids:

• If I take pain medicine (opioids) regularly, I will get hooked or addicted.
• Pain is inevitable. I just need to bear it.

- If the pain is worse, it must mean my cancer is spreading and nothing more can be done.
- I had better wait to take my pain medication until I really need it or else it won't work later.
- My family thinks I am getting too spacey on pain medications. I'd better hold back.
- If it's morphine, I must be getting close to the end.
- If I take my pain medication before I hurt, I will end up taking too much. It's better to hang in there and tough it out.
- I'd rather have a good bowel movement than take pain medication and get constipated.
- I don't want to bother the nurses or physician. They're busy with other patients.
- Good patients avoid talking about pain.

12. How do you know which analgesic to use when a patient is experiencing pain?
The analgesic must be selected according to the type and severity of pain as well as the appropriate route of administration. (*Note:* The intramuscular route is not recommended for management of cancer pain.) Successful relief of cancer pain requires around-the-clock dosing with as-needed doses for breakthrough pain. The choice of drug also should be based on the patient's previous experience with the medication, age, physical condition (e.g., renal and hepatic function), response to the prescribed regimen, provider recommendations, and possible interactions with current therapies.

A step-wise approach, as suggested by The World Health Organization (WHO) analgesic ladder, provides a convenient method for starting analgesics. Each step describes analgesic interventions appropriate to pain intensity. The ladder originally was proposed with three steps, as depicted; however, a two-step approach is currently considered more appropriate for patients with cancer. The first step includes NSAIDs, and the second step combines steps 2 and 3 from the previous ladder with emphasis on use of noncompounded opioids (e.g., analgesics not combined with acetaminophen or aspirin).

The World Health Organization (WHO) analgesic ladder:

Step 1   For mild pain (intensity = 1–3), start with nonopioid drugs such as acetaminophen or NSAIDs (e.g., ibuprofen). Add adjuvant drugs if indicated (e.g., tricyclic antidepressant, anticonvulsant).

Step 2   If pain persists, add an opioid for mild-to-moderate pain (intensity = 4–6), such as hydrocodone or low-dose oxycodone (5 mg) plus aspirin or acetaminophen with or without adjuvant drugs.

Step 3   If pain persists or increases, switch to an opioid for moderate-to-severe pain (intensity = 7–10), such as oxycodone, morphine, hydromorphone, fentanyl (transdermal), levorphanol, or methadone with or without a nonopioid and with or without an adjuvant drug.

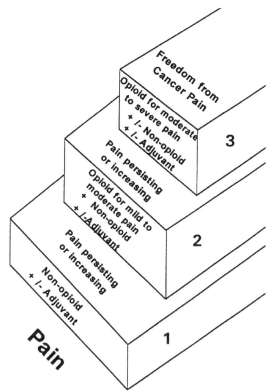

Compounded opioids are limited by the analgesic ceiling effect of acetaminophen (doses > 1000 mg add minimal analgesia) and its ceiling for toxicity (dose should not exceed 4 gm/day because of potential liver necrosis or toxicity). Chronic use of 5–8 gm/day for several weeks or 3–4 gm/day for a year has resulted in liver damage.

13. Explain the use of NSAIDs in controlling pain.

NSAIDs may relieve bone pain or generalized musculoskeletal pain by decreasing subperiosteal swelling around nerve endings and inhibiting prostaglandin synthesis. Although NSAIDs may be given in higher than recommended doses, they have a ceiling effect; that is, increases above a certain dose do not provide additional analgesia.

The selection of NSAIDS is influenced by side-effect profile, patient preference, and cost (over the counter NSAIDs, such as ibuprofen, are most economical). The use of NSAIDs in patients with cancer is limited by concerns about side effects, such as platelet dysfunction, nephritis, fluid retention, and gastrointestinal tract bleeding or ulceration. NSAIDs must be used with extreme caution in patients with thrombocytopenia or poor renal function. Patients should be assessed for potential hypersensitivity reactions; patients with a history of aspirin or NSAID allergy, rhinitis, nasal polyps, or asthma are susceptible to development of severe respiratory reactions. (*Note:* Monitor serum levels of blood urea nitrogen [BUN] and creatinine. Instruct patients not to take on an empty stomach.)

Nonacetylated salicylates are often recommended because they do not affect platelet aggregation profoundly or clinically alter bleeding time; however, their analgesic effect may not be strong enough for patients with more intense pain. NSAIDs such as nabumetone (Relafen) cause less gastric distress. For chronic use of NSAIDs, histamine-2 blockers or prostaglandin analogs may be used to decrease the potential for gastric ulceration.

NONOPIOID ANALGESIC	DOSE
Acetaminophen (Tylenol) or acetylsalicylic acid (aspirin)	325–1000 mg every 4–6 hr (maximal daily dose: 4 gm)
Choline magnesium trisalicylate (Trilisate)	1000–1500 mg 3 times/day (maximal daily dose: 4500 mg)
Salsalate (Disalcid)	1000–1500 mg every 8–12 hr (maximal daily dose: 4000 mg)
Ibuprofen (Motrin)	200–800 mg every 4–6 hr (maximal daily dose: 3200 mg)
Naproxen (Naprosyn)	375–500 mg every 8–12 hr (maximal daily dose: 1500 mg)
Nabumetone (Relafen)	1000 mg in 1 dose or 2 divided doses; may increase up to 2000 mg/day

14. What are COX-2 inhibitors? How do they work?

The COX-2 inhibitors (celecoxib [Celebrex] and rofecoxib [Vioxx]) are NSAIDs that selectively block the cycloxygenase-2 (COX-2) enzyme without blocking COX-1 enzymes, which protect gastric mucosa. The advantage of COX-2 inhibitors over other NSAIDS is reduction of pain and inflammation with decreased potential for gastrointestinal toxicity and platelet inhibition. Genetic differences in patients may influence the COX-2 selectivity of these drugs. Of interest, celecoxib has antiangiogenesis properties and is under study for a role in tumor suppression. These drugs are not risk-free. COX-2 inhibitors can cause edema and have potential drug interactions. They should be used cautiously in patients taking anticoagulants and may compromise renal function in patients with renal insufficiency. As with other NSAIDs, patients need to be monitored for adverse effects and given information about potential drug interactions, toxicities, and precautions.

15. Describe the appropriate dosing of celecoxib and rofecoxib.

Celecoxib is FDA-approved for osteoarthritis (100 mg twice daily or single dose of 200 mg) and rheumatoid arthritis (100–200 mg twice daily). It is contraindicated in patients with sulfonamide allergies. **Rofecoxib** is available in tablets and oral suspension. It is indicated for the treatment of acute pain in adults, osteoarthritis, and primary dysmenorrhea. Because of its interaction with methotrexate, rofecoxib may cause methotrexate toxicity. The dosage for acute pain in adults is 50 mg/day. (To date, the use of rofecoxib has not been studied in acute pain for more than 5 days). The pain-relieving efficacy of a single oral dose of 50 mg is similar to that of three daily doses of 800 mg ibuprofen and may provide more pain relief than the combination of codeine, 60 mg, with acetaminophen, 600 mg.

16. How are tricyclic antidepressants used to control pain?

Tricyclic antidepressants relieve neuropathic pain by blocking the reuptake of the neurotransmitter serotonin, which is released by the pain-modulatory systems that descend from the brainstem to the spinal cord. Accumulation of serotonin and norepinephrine at the synapse inhibits transmission of pain impulses. Amitriptyline also has morphine-sparing effects by increasing the plasma concentration of morphine. Dose-related side effects of the tricyclics include sedation, orthostatic hypotension, and anticholinergic effects, particularly dry mouth. Uncommon, serious side effects include cardiac arrhythmias, obstipation, and urinary retention. Desipramine and nortriptyline are less sedating and may produce insomnia; they can be given during the day. Tricyclic antidepressant dosages to control pain are much lower (e.g., 10–50 mg/day) than those needed to treat depression (e.g., 100–150 mg). Although it takes weeks for a therapeutic antidepressant effect with tricyclics, the onset of analgesia is much sooner (usually 1 week). Pain can be reduced by the next morning after taking 1 dose of amitriptyline. To increase patient compliance and decrease side effects, start with low doses (10 mg in elderly or frail patients) and gradually titrate upward. (*Note:* To prevent confusion in patients, avoid increasing at the same time that opioids are increased.) After symptoms are controlled, titrate dosage downward to the lowest level that maintains pain relief. (Refer to Chapter 39 for more information about antidepressants.)

ANTIDEPRESSANT	DOSE
Amitriptyline (Elavil)	Start 10–25 mg at bedtime; increase gradually to 50–150 mg
Doxepin (Sinequan)	Start 10–25 mg at bedtime; increase gradually to 75–150 mg
Desipramine (Norpramin, Pertrofane)	Start 25 mg; increase by 25–50 mg every 3–4 weeks; maintenance dose: 25–150 mg/day
Nortriptyline (Aventyl, Pamelor)	Start 10–50 mg; increase by 10–25 mg every 3–4 weeks; maintenance dose: 10–150 mg/day
Imipramine (Tofranil)	Start 10–25 mg; maintenance dose: 20–150 mg/day
Trazodone (Desyrel)	Start 50 mg; maintenance dose 50–200 mg/day

17. How are anticonvulsants used to control pain?

Anticonvulsants (e.g., phenytoin, carbamazepine, clonazepam) stabilize the nerve membrane, prevent depolarization. and block transmission of pain impulses. They are indicated for trigeminal and postherpetic neuralgias, lancinating pains (e.g., electrical, shooting), and nerve injury caused by cancer or cancer treatment. (*Note:* Phenytoin and carbamazepine should be initiated at low doses and titrated upward according to patient response and plasma levels. Dosing follows antiseizure guidelines.)

- **Phenytoin and valproic acid** are best for continuous neuropathic pain. Plasma levels of phenytoin should be monitored for therapeutic and toxic concentrations. Side effects include skin rash, ataxia, and liver function abnormalities. (*Note:* Be aware of drug interactions; e.g., phenothiazines and trazodone increase phenytoin levels, whereas phenytoin increases the metabolism of meperidine and methadone).
- **Carbamazepine** is best for lancinating or shooting pain. Because carbamazepine may cause bone marrow depression (e.g., aplastic anemia), continuous hematologic monitoring is necessary (e.g., baseline and follow-up complete blood counts). Plasma drug levels also should be monitored for therapeutic and toxicity concentrations. Other common side ef-

fects include sedation, vertigo, or confusion. (*Note:* Like phenytoin, carbamazepine is metabolized by the liver and associated with multiple drug interactions; e.g., carbamazepine levels are increased with propoxyphene and decreased with doxorubicin and cisplatin).
- **Gabapentin** is an amino acid anticonvulsant that may increase the rate of synthesis and accumulation of gamma-aminobutyric acid (GABA) or its binding to an unknown receptor in brain tissue. GABA is the main inhibitory pathway in the body. The two types of receptors, GABA-A and GABA-B, are equally distributed throughout the central nervous system. Because gabapentin has relatively mild side effects and has been highly effective, it is probably preferred for use in patients with cancer. Dosing should start at 100 mg/day and be titrated upward according to patient tolerance. Common side effects include blurred vision, dizziness, confusion, and mild generalized edema. When discontinuing gabapentin, taper slowly (10% of the daily dose/day over 10 days) because patients may experience side effects such as anxiety, stomach cramps, and sweating.
- **Clonazepam**, which binds to GABA-A, is effective in controlling neuropathic pain. It is also excellent for use in patients with cancer as an antianxiety agent with the added benefit of reducing pain.

ANTICONVULSANT	DOSE
Carbamazepine (Tegretol)	Start with 100 mg/day; increase by 100 mg every 4 days to 500–800 mg/day.
Phenytoin (Dilantin)	Start with 100 mg/day; increase by 25–50 mg every 4 days to 250–300 mg/day.
Clonazepam (Klonopin))	0.5–6 mg/day in 2 or 3 divided doses.
Valproic acid (Depakote)	250–2000 mg/day at bedtime or in 3 divided doses; titrate upward by 5–10 mg/kg; maximal dose: 40 mg/kg day.
Gabapentin (Neurontin)	300–2400 mg/day in divided doses; mean dose: 1000 mg/day

18. When are local anesthetics indicated?

Local anesthetics may produce analgesia by stabilizing the nerve cell membrane and inhibiting depolarization and transmission. They also may inhibit the release of neurotransmitters centrally. They are effective for lancinating neuropathic pain and various neuralgias. Patients may be given an IV trial of lidocaine. If the IV lidocaine is effective, the patient may respond to mexiletine (oral form of lidocaine) or other oral neuropathic agents. During IV administration, the patient should be observed for slurred speech (a sign of toxicity) and the dose adjusted accordingly. Anecdotally, a cream compounded with a mixture of lidocaine 5% and ketamine 10% has been effective in reducing painful peripheral neuropathy.

LOCAL ANESTHETIC	DOSE
Lidocaine	1–5 mg/kg of 0.1% solution by slow IV infusion over 10–60 minutes; total dose of 50–300 mg.
Mexiletine	150–200 mg (2–3 mg/kg) 2 or 3 times/day; increase by 50 mg every 2 weeks as needed. Maintenance dose: 150–400 mg 3 or 4 times/day. Maximal dose: 1200 mg/day.

19. How do corticosteroids decrease pain?

Corticosteroids help to reduce pain due to perineural edema, visceral organ distention, infiltration of soft tissues, and bone pain in advanced disease. They are part of the emergency management of spinal cord compression and increased intracranial pressure.

CORTICOSTEROID	DOSE
Dexamethasone	4 mg orally 3–4 times/day
Prednisone	10 mg orally 3 times/day; maximal dose: 20–80 mg/day

20. How is pain due to muscle spasms treated?

Baclofen, cyclobenzaprine, and methocarbamol are skeletal muscle relaxants. Common side effects are sedation, confusion, or muscle weakness. These drugs are often used in combination with rest or physical therapy. Of these, baclofen is used most often as an adjuvant analgesic for management of cancer pain. Other useful agents include quinine sulfate, dicyclomine, oxybutynin chloride, and diazepam. Calcium supplementation is effective when crampy pain is due to calcium deficiency.

- **Baclofen**, which binds to GABA-B receptors, is indicated primarily for spasticity but is also effective for neuropathic pain, organic headache, trigeminal and postherpetic neuralgias, and fibromyalgias. Baclofen is comparable to diazepam but less sedating.
- **Quinine sulfate** is effective for nocturnal leg cramps. It increases the refractory period of skeletal muscles by direct action on muscle fiber, decreases excitability of the motor endplate, and affects distribution of calcium within the muscle fiber. *Note:* Quinine is associated with thrombocytopenia, neutropenia, and hemolytic uremic syndrome.
- **Dicyclomine** acts on smooth muscles of the gastrointestinal tract. It is effective for abdominal cramps (colorectal cancer) and irritable bowel syndrome.
- **Oxybutynin chloride** has direct effects on the bladder. Belladonna and opium suppositories (B&O Supprettes) are also effective for bladder spasms.
- **Diazepam** is used as an acute antianxiety agent but is also an excellent antispasmodic. Side effects include sedation, decreased muscle tone, and hypotension.

RELAXANT/ANTISPASMODIC	DOSE
Baclofen (Lioresal)	5 mg 2 times/day to 20 mg 3 times/day; increase by 5 mg every 3 days to maximum of 80 mg/day
Cyclobenzaprine (Flexeril)	10 mg 3 times/day; range: 20–40 mg/day in 2–4 divided doses; maximal dose: 60 mg/day
Methocarbamol (Robaxin)	Initially 1500 mg 4 times/day for 2–3 days; maintenance dose: 4–4.5 mg/day in 3–6 divided doses
Quinine sulfate	260–300 mg at bedtime
Dicyclomine (Bentyl)	10–20 mg 3 or 4 times/day to maximum of 40 mg 4 times/day orally or 20 mg every 4–6 hr intramuscularly
Calcium	500 mg/day
Oxybutynin chloride (Ditropan)	5 mg 2 or 3 times/day; maximal dose of 5 mg 4 times/day
Diazepam (Valium)	2–10 mg orally or intravenously 2 or 3 times/day

21. What is capsaicin? How is it used?

Capsaicin (Zostrix), a cream made from cayenne pepper, depletes and prevents reaccumulation of substance P in peripheral sensory neurons. Capsaicin (0.025%) has been reported to be effective in some patients with chemotherapy-induced neuropathies and chronic postherpetic neuralgia, but it should not be applied to open lesions. It has also been of benefit to patients with postmastectomy pain. A thin film is applied to the affected area of intact skin 3–5 times/day. Fewer applications per day may decrease efficacy. Onset of action may take 14–28 days. Treatment should be continued to provide an adequate trial and to achieve optimal clinical response. Patients need to be warned about transient burning that occurs with application but decreases within several days. To ease or prevent the burning sensation, opioids should be administered during this initial period. Investigators at Yale University have made a candy containing cayenne pepper that reduces the pain of oral mucositis in patients undergoing chemotherapy:

Cayenne Candy for Oral Mucositis

1. Place in a heavy pan large enough to allow for foaming:
   2 cups brown sugar   2 tbsp water
   1/4 cup molasses   2 tbsp vinegar
   1/2 cup butter   1/2 tsp cayenne pepper (McCormick brand)
2. Stir mixture, except for pepper, over low heat until sugar is dissolved.

3. Boil gently, stirring frequently until the mixture reaches the hard crack stage (300°F, the temperature at which a spoonful of candy separates into hard and brittle threads when dropped into cold water).

4. Add the cayenne pepper toward the end of the boiling process.

5. Drop candy from a teaspoon onto a buttered slab or foil to form patties. Makes about 1 pound.

For additional recipes, contact Ann Berger, M.D., Supportive Care Services, PO Box 20851, New Haven, CT 06520-8050.

22. What agents are used for metastatic bone pain?

- Radiation therapy is the mainstay for palliation of localized bony metastases. Wide-field and hemibody irradiation has been used for diffuse bony metastasis.
- Strontium 89 (Metastron), a radiopharmaceutical that follows the same biochemical pathways as calcium, has been used for pain due to diffuse bony metastasis from breast or prostate cancer. Patients need to be warned about possibility of flare pain for a few days after administration. Response can take as a long as 2–3 weeks; patients must remain on analgesics during that time.
- Samarium-153 and Rhenium-186 (pending FDA approval) are phosphinate chelates that have demonstrated 65–80% efficacy in international clinical trials for the management of metastatic bone pain.
- Bisphosphonates may be helpful in bone pain associated with hypercalcemia. Pamidronate (Aredia) inhibits accelerated bone resorption. Pamidronate is given as a 90 mg intravenous infusion over 2 hours approximately every 4 weeks.
- Calcitonin inhibits osteoclastic bone resorption by the tumor and also has been reported to be effective for bone pain and phantom limb sensation. It is given in doses of 4 IU/kg every 12 hr. The dose may be increased to 8 IU/kg every 12 hr if no response is seen in 2 days. If this regimen produces no response in 2 days, the dose may be increased to 8 IU/kg every 6 hr.

23. How do you switch from one opioid to another?

An equianalgesic chart is used to help convert medication dosages from one route to another and from one drug to another, with morphine as the prototypical opioid. The equianalgesic doses are approximate doses that provide similar analgesia. Doses should be adjusted to the patient's age, condition, and pain intensity. In patients with hepatic or renal impairment, opioids should be initiated at one-fourth to one-third of the usual dose and slowly titrated upward. There is no ceiling effect for opioids used to treat severe pain. The correct dose is whatever dose it takes to relieve the patient's pain without adverse side effects. For opioid-tolerant patients, the new opioid may need to be decreased by 25–50% of the equianalgesic dose. *Note:* Frequent dose adjustments may be necessary when converting from an opioid with a short elimination half-life to one with a long half-life.

Equianalgesic Reference Guide

OPIOID AGONISTS	PARENTERAL (mg)	ORAL (mg)	COMMENTS
Morphine	10	30	Active glucuronide metabolites that are more potent with longer half-lives than morphine. Injection; immediate-release tablets, 10, 15, 30 mg; and rectal suppositories, 5, 10, 20, 30 mg. Morphine solution contains 10 or 20 mg/5 ml; morphine concentrate contains 20 mg/ml.
Morphine controlled-/ sustained-release tablets	—	30	Do not crush. Give every 8–12 hr, not PRN. MS Contin, 15, 30, 60, 100, and 200 mg, or Oramorph SR, 30, 60, and 100 mg
Morphine sustained-release capsules	—	30	Give once daily (every 24 hr), not PRN. Kadian, 20, 30, 50, 60, and 100 mg. Capsules may be opened and given via G-tube or sprinkled over food.

Table continued on following page

OPIOID AGONISTS	PARENTERAL (mg)	ORAL (mg)	COMMENTS
Hydromorphone (Dilaudid)	1.5	7.5	No clinically active metabolites. Injection; tablets, 2, 4, 8 mg; liquid, 1 mg/ml; rectal suppository, 3 mg; and high-potency injection, 10 mg/ml.
Fentanyl (Sublimaze IV, Actiq OT)	100 μg (0.1 mg)	1000 μg OT	Drug of choice for renal or liver disease. Injection: 50 μg/ml. Actiq, oral transmucosal (OT) fentanyl, approved for breakthrough pain; 200, 400, 600, 800, 1200, and 1600 μg units.
Transdermal fentanyl	—	—	May cause less constipation than oral sustained-release opioids. Transdermal (Duragesic) patches, 25, 50, 75, and 100 μg/hr. Change patch every 48–72 hr. Approximate equianalgesic conversion: divide total 24-hr oral morphine dose (mg) by 2 to get fentanyl dose in μg/hr. Reaches therapeutic serum level 12–16 hr after initial application; lasts about 17 hr after removal.
Levorphanol (Levo-dromoran)	2	4	Half-life = 12–16 hr; accumulates on days 2–3. Consider dose reduction after 12–24 hr. Approximate maintenance dose may be one-twentieth the oral morphine dose. Tablets, 2 mg; injection, 2 mg/ml.
Methadone (Dolophine)	10	20	Half-life = 24–36 hr; accumulates on days 2–5. Consider dose reduction after 12–24 hr. Maintenance dose of oral methadone may be one-tenth the equianalgesic dose of oral morphine. Tablets, 5 or 10 mg; oral solution, 5 or 10 mg/5 ml and 10 mg/ml; and injection, 10 mg/ml.
Meperidine (Demerol)	75	300 NR	Normeperidine (toxic metabolite) accumulates with repetitive doses, causing CNS excitation. Avoid use for chronic pain, longer than 48 hr, and doses > 600 mg/24 hr. Contraindicated in patients with impaired renal function.
Oxycodone (Roxicodone, Percocet, Tylox, Roxicet, Percodan)	—	20	Immediate-release tablets, 5, 15, and 30 mg (Roxicodone); elixir, 5 mg/ml; and concentrate, 20 mg/ml. Oxycodone, 5 mg, with acetaminophen, 500 mg (Roxicet, Tylox), acetaminophen, 325 mg (Percocet), or aspirin, 325 mg (Percodan).
Oxycodone controlled-release tablets	—	20	Do not crush. Give every 12 hr, not PRN. Oxycontin, 10, 20, 40, 80, and 160 mg.
Codeine	130	200 NR	Used for mild to moderate pain. Tablets, 15, 30, 60 mg; Tylenol #3 = codeine, 30 mg, + acetaminophen, 300 mg; Tylenol #4 = codeine, 60 mg, + acetaminophen, 300 mg. Tylenol-codeine elixir contains acetaminophen, 120 mg, + codeine, 12.5/5 ml
Hydrocodone (Vicodin, Lortab)	—	30? NR	Used for mild to moderate pain. Vicodin = hydrocodone, 5 mg + acetaminophen, 500 mg ; Vicodin ES = hydrocodone, 7.5 mg + acetaminophen, 750 mg. Vicoprofen = hydrocodone, 7.5 mg + ibuprofen, 200 mg.
Oxymorphone (Numorphan)	1	—	Rectal suppository, 5 mg = IM morphine, 5 mg.

NR = not recommended at that dose. Equianalgesic doses are estimates. All doses must be titrated to individual response, age, condition, and clinical situation. Rescue dose for breakthrough pain is calculated as 10–20% of 24-hr dose. For a single IV bolus, use ¼ to ½ the intramuscular dose. Unless otherwise stated, half-lives of opioids range from 2–3 hr.

Adapted from Gates RA, Fink RM, Slover R: Analgesic Reference Guide. University of Colorado Health Sciences Center, 1998.[18,20]

24. Give an example of switching from one opioid to another, using an equianalgesic chart.

To convert 6 mg of oral hydromorphone every 3 hr to oral, continuous-release morphine:

1. Calculate the 24-hr dose of medication that the patient currently receives:

    6 mg × 8 (every 3 hr) = 48 mg hydromorphone/24 hr

2. Review the equianalgesic chart for equivalence guidelines:

    7.5 mg oral hydromorphone is equivalent to 30 mg oral morphine.

3. Equation: $$\frac{30 \text{ mg oral morphine}}{7.5 \text{ mg hydromorphone}} = \frac{X \text{ morphine}}{48 \text{ mg hydromorphone}}$$

4. Cross-multiply to solve for X:

    48 mg hydromorphone × 30 mg morphine = 7.5 mg hydromorphone × X mg morphine
    1440 mg = 7.5X   1440/7.5 = X   X = 192 mg oral morphine

5. Divide the dose by the number of administration times per day to obtain the interval dose. Continuous-release morphine is dosed every 12 hr.

    192 mg/2 = 96 mg orally 2 times/day (100-mg tablet or three 30-mg tablets)

6. In addition to the scheduled dose, order as-needed doses for breakthrough pain; for example, morphine elixir (20 mg/ml), 20–40 mg orally every 2–4 hr as needed.

25. How do you calculate the dose of medication for breakthrough pain?

Breakthrough pain refers to an exacerbation or transitory flare of pain, which occurs in about 65% of patients who take regularly scheduled analgesics for stable or baseline pain. The recommended breakthrough dose should be 10–20% of the 24-hr dose administered every 2–4 hours or more frequently, as needed.

26. What is the relevance of plasma half-lives and steady states in opioid dosing?

The half-life is the time taken for a drug to reach half of its plasma concentration. For all drugs and routes of administration, usually 4–5 half-lives are necessary to reach steady state; therefore, dose changes should not be made until steady state is achieved. This approach is often not possible in patients with increasing levels of pain. In such patients, it is more advantageous to use opioids with short half-lives for breakthrough pain. Drugs with long half-lives may result in delayed or prolonged side effects, particularly in elderly patients or patients with liver or renal impairment. Half-lives for commonly used opioids are listed below:

Opioids with short half-life	Opioids with long half-life
Morphine (2–3.5 hr)	Methadone (24–36 hr)
Hydromorphone (2–3 hr)	Levorphanol (12–15 hr)
Oxycodone (2–3 hr)	Propoxyphene (12 hr)

27. What are the possible complications or side effects of opioids used to treat pain?

- Sedation
- Respiratory depression
- Nausea and vomiting
- Constipation
- Ileus
- Pruritus

28. How is sedation managed?

Tolerance to sedation usually develops within 3–5 days with repeated doses of opioids. In addition to caffeine drinks (tea, coffee, coke), antisedatives such as dextroamphetamine and methylphenidate are helpful. Antisedatives should be given in the morning or early afternoon. Dextroamphetamine and caffeine also increase analgesia when combined with other opioid or nonopioid analgesics. Doses of remedies for sedation include the following:

Caffeine	100–200 mg/day (1.0–1.5 mg/kg in children)
Dextroamphetamine (Dexedrine)	2.5–10 mg orally (0.05–0.1 mg/kg in children)
Methylphenidate (Ritalin)	2.5–10 mg orally (0.1–0.2 mg/kg in children)

29. How is respiratory depression managed?

High-dose opioids given to an opioid-naive patient may cause respiratory depression; however, tolerance to respiratory depression develops with repeated doses over several weeks.

Pain acts as an antagonist to respiratory depression. Morphine doses as high as 10,000 mg/day have been reported. The risk of respiratory depression in a patient receiving chronic opioid therapy is < 1%. Oversedation usually can be managed by holding or not giving the opioid dose and stimulating the patient. Naloxone (Narcan), an opioid antagonist, should be administered only to patients with significant respiratory depression or apnea. In the rare instance that naloxone is indicated, the following regimen is appropriate: (1) dilute 1 ampule (0.4 mg/ml) with 9 ml of normal saline, and (2) administer 20 mg (0.02 mg or 0.5 ml) every 3 minutes to desired effects. The goal is to reverse the respiratory depression or sedation without reversing the analgesia.

30. How are nausea and vomiting managed?

Nausea and vomiting due to stimulation of the chemoreceptor trigger zone usually resolve in 48–72 hr. Antiemetics, such as oral Compazine spansules, 15–30 mg every 12 hours for the first 3–5 days, help to prevent nausea and improve patient acceptance.

31. Describe the management of constipation.

Unfortunately, tolerance to constipation does not develop. All patients receiving opioids should be placed on a prophylactic bowel regimen consisting of both stool softener (e.g., docusate sodium, l00–300 mg/day) and laxative (e.g., senna, 2–6 tablets twice daily). (Senokot-S is a combination of senna and docusate sodium.)

32. How is ileus reversed?

Ileus induced by opioids has been reversed with continuous infusion of metoclopramide and oral naltrexone.

33. Describe the management of pruritus.

Pruritus due to IV or oral opioids is associated with histamine release and may be treated with Benadryl. Pruritus from epidural opioids is not due to histamine release but may result from binding of the opioid to the trigeminal nerve as it spreads rostrally (e.g., facial itching); it is also treated in many institutions with Benadryl, 25–50 mg IV. Mild pruritus may be treated with cool compresses or lotion. Narcan and Nubain (mixed agonist/antagonists) have been used to reverse pruritus due to spinal opioids; however, analgesia also may be reversed. Naltrexone (a long-acting formulation of Narcan) has been recommended with epidural morphine to prevent pruritus. Other causes of pruritus (e.g., drug allergy) should be ruled out. Doses for treatment of pruritus are listed below:

Benadryl	12.5–25 mg IV, orally every 6 hr
Narcan	20 μg IV; may repeat to desired effect
Nubain	2.5–5 mg IV every 4–6 hr
Naltrexone	5 mg orally

34. What drug:drug interactions are causes of concern with opioid use?

Because patients with cancer experience multiple symptoms and receive numerous drugs, nurses need to be constantly aware of potential clinical and physical interactions and incompatibilities. Fortunately, opioids such as morphine are physically compatible with many supportive care drugs.

1. **Any medication that causes sedation** must be used cautiously with opioids. The phenothiazine antiemetics (promethazine, droperidol, prochlorperazine), muscle relaxants (baclofen, cyclobenzaprine), benzodiazepines (diazepam, midazolam), alcohol, clonazepam, and phenytoin also cause sedation. When such drugs are given with opioids the patient should be monitored closely and the opioid dose may need to be decreased to prevent oversedation and respiratory depression. *Note:* It is safe for patients in pain to take an opioid dose along with a regularly scheduled sleeping pill.

2. **Monoamine oxidase (MAO) inhibitors** (e.g., phenelzine [Nardil], tranylcypromine [Parnate]) may produce severe, fatal reactions when given in combination with opioids. In addition, concomitant use of MAO inhibitors and tricyclic antidepressants may result in death.

3. **Phenytoin sodium** is physically incompatible with the following opioids: fentanyl citrate, hydromorphone hydrochloride, methadone hydrochloride, and morphine sulfate.

35. How should opioids be tapered to prevent an abstinence or withdrawal syndrome when they are no longer needed?

The rate of tapering may vary with individual patients; however, the following approach is often used:

- Decrease the 24-hr total dose by 50%, and administer as divided doses on schedule for 2 days.
- Decrease the dose by 25% every 2 days thereafter until the total daily dose is equivalent to 30 mg of oral morphine/day or 0.6 mg/kg/day in a child.
- After 2 days on this final dose, stop the medication. If the patient is anxious or nervous, a clonidine patch (changed every 7 days), 0.1–0.2 mg/day, may be used to lessen or prevent anxiety, tachycardia, sweating, and other autonomic symptoms.

36. How do you switch to a fentanyl patch?

A fentanyl patch is a transdermal system that delivers fentanyl over 72 hours. Patches deliver 25, 50, 75, and 100 μg/hr. It takes 48 hours to achieve a steady-state blood concentration after the patch is placed. Equianalgesic charts are available with ranges of oral morphine equivalent to fentanyl patches of various strengths; however, the following formula is a simple method of calculating approximately equivalent doses:

1. Convert the 24-hour dose of current opioid to the equianalgesic dose of oral morphine, using an equianalgesic chart.

2. Divide the result by 2 to equal the dose of fentanyl in μg/hr. For example, an opioid converted to 180 mg of oral morphine/24 hr is divided by 2 to equal 90 μg or a 100-μg patch.

3. Because the patch takes approximately 9–16 hours to provide analgesia, an additional analgesic is needed. If the patient is converted from continuous-release morphine, the last 12-hr dose may be administered at the same time as the patch is applied because it may take longer than 17 hours for the patch to be out of the patient's system. If the patient was receiving a short-acting analgesic, continue this medication for the next 12 hours.

4. Calculate an appropriate dose of oral medication for breakthrough pain. This dose may be 10–20% of the 24-hr equivalent of continuous-release oral morphine. For example, the breakthrough dose for a 50-μg fentanyl patch should be 10–20 mg of immediate-release morphine (50 μg = 90–100 mg of oral morphine/24 hr).

37. What are special considerations for using fentanyl patches?

- Patients must have adequate fat stores to absorb and retain the medication to enable the patch to last 72 hr. In emaciated patients, the patch may need to be changed more frequently because of more rapid absorption.
- Increased absorption in febrile patients may result in oversedation.
- To secure the patch in place for diaphoretic patients, apply a transparent dressing over the patch.
- For itching at the site of application, a steroid inhaler can be sprayed over the site with complete drying prior to placing the patch. (Creams should not be used on sites of application because they can affect drug absorption).

38. What is the fastest acting oral opioid?

Oral transmucosal fentanyl citrate (OTFC; Actiq) is a solid formulation of fentanyl citrate that is indicated only for breakthrough pain in patients with cancer who are tolerant to opioid therapy for underlying continuous pain. OTFC is available as a raspberry-flavored lozenge on a stick in dosages of 200, 400, 600, 800, 1200, and 1600 µg. Treatment usually is begun with the 200 µg dose and then titrated to effect.

The oral mucosa is highly vascularized and permeable to the analgesic effects of fat-soluble fentanyl, allowing rapid absorption and analgesia (within 5 minutes). Patients should not bite or chew the lozenge; Actiq should be placed in the mouth between the cheeks and gum and moved around the buccal mucosa for 15 minutes until done. Upon consumption, 25% of the unit is absorbed buccally. The remaining 75% is swallowed and absorbed gastrointestinally, and one-third of this amount becomes systemically available, bypassing hepatic metabolism. Thus, patients get immediate relief yet may not have full analgesia for up to 45–60 minutes later.

39. What safety and disposal tips must be discussed with patients who use Actiq?

1. Keep Actiq in a locked cabinet.

2. If any medicine remains on the handle, use hot water to melt it; alternatively, put any unused Actiq into a storage bottle out of children's reach.

3. Do not flush the unused Actiq in its entirety (using wire-cutting pliers, the medicine end may be removed and flushed).

40. How do you start a patient-controlled analgesia pump?

An intravenous patient-controlled analgesia (PCA) pump allows the patient to self-administer a predetermined dose of analgesic at a specified interval. In addition, a basal infusion can be programmed into most pumps.

1. Calculate the equianalgesic IV dose of agent that the patient currently receives.

2. Divide the 24-hr dose by 24 to obtain the hourly or basal dose.

3. Set the hourly rate (mg/hr), PCA or bolus dose, and interval.

4. If the patient has uncontrolled or increased pain, administer a loading dose to control the pain before starting the PCA. Loading doses should be individualized. A good starting loading dose is equal to one-third, one-half, or one full hour total of the patient's normal maintenance (hourly plus PCA or as-needed doses).

In contrast to patients with acute postoperative pain, patients with chronic cancer pain require that most of the analgesic dose be programmed into the hourly PCA infusion so that pain is prevented (similar to around-the-clock oral dosing). The PCA (breakthrough) dose is usually one-half of the hourly infusion rate set at every 6–15 minutes. Thus, if the equianalgesic dose of IV morphine was 6 mg/hr, the pump may be set at the following values: continuous infusion, 3–6 mg/hr, and PCA dose, 1–3 mg, with a 15-minute lockout. However, if the patient's pain is not well controlled by the oral dose, the hourly and PCA dose may be set higher. The patient should be reassessed frequently, and the continuous rate should be increased based on the patient's response. The table below lists starting dosages for commonly used PCA opioids; after the initial setting, however, the dose should be titrated to effect.

DRUG	CONCENTRATION	PCA DOSE	CONTINUOUS INFUSION	ONSET (MIN)	PEAK (MIN)
Hydromorphone (Dilaudid) (adults)	0.2 mg/ml	0.2 mg	0.2–0.4 mg/hr	5	10–20
Hydromorphone (Dilaudid) (children)	0.2 mg/ml	0.003–0.0045 mg/kg	0.0015–0.003 mg/kg/hr	5	10–20
Morphine (adults)	1 mg/ml	1 mg	1–2 mg/hr	10–20	15–30
Morphine (children)	1 mg/ml	0.02–0.03 mg/kg	0.01–0.02 mg/kg/hr	10–20	15–30
Fentanyl	10 µg/ml	10–25 µg	10–25 µg/hr	1	1–5

41. Can a PCA pump be used in patients without venous access?

A PCA pump also can be used to deliver analgesics subcutaneously. Although morphine and fentanyl can be used, hydromorphone (Dilaudid) is ideal for this purpose because it provides a high concentration of medication (high-potency preparation, 10 mg/ml) in a low volume. Butterfly (25–27 gauge) or special needles for subcutaneous administration may be used (e.g., a 27-gauge, ¼-inch needle with extension tubing). The site is covered with a transparent dressing, and the needle needs to be changed every 3–7 days with routine inspection of the site for erythema, swelling, or tenderness.

42. How effective is sublingual morphine?

For patients who cannot swallow, morphine concentrate (20 mg/ml) is ideal for sublingual administration. Drug bioavailability is estimated at 20–30%. Problems with sublingual morphine include sour taste, dry mouth, and bitter taste. Also available are 30-mg soluble sublingual morphine crystals. Sublingual morphine is an excellent medication in patients who are at the end of life to alleviate symptoms of dyspnea or air hunger. Titration is key.

43. Is morphine still the gold standard for cancer pain?

Morphine is still the standard of comparison for opioids used to treat severe pain. However, as knowledge about pain physiology and pharmacology translates into better analgesics or new formulations of opioids with fewer side effects, morphine may not continue to be the drug of choice. Morphine has several active metabolites, including morphine-3-glucuronide (M3G) and morphine-6-glucuronide (M6G). M3G has no analgesic activity, antagonizes morphine's analgesic effect, may induce allodynia and hyperalgesia, and causes CNS excitation. M6G has greater affinity for mu receptors than morphine and is responsible for respiratory depression and gastrointestinal toxicities (e.g., nausea). Morphine can be eliminated in patients with renal disease, but its metabolite M6G can accumulate because of decreased clearance and prolonged elimination half-life. Because of problems related to morphine's active metabolites, the trend may be to use semisynthetic opioids, such as fentanyl, hydromorphone, and oxycodone. For example, oxycodone has gained popularity since its availability as a continuous-release tablet (Oxycontin) that can be given twice daily (every 12 hours). A continuous-release, once-daily formulation of hydromorphone may soon be available.

44. What opioids are available in rectal suppositories?

Morphine (5, 10, 20, 30 mg), hydromorphone (3 mg), and oxymorphone (5 mg) are available in rectal preparations. Several of the immediate-release oral preparations can be crushed and diluted or crushed and placed in a gel suppository shell and administered rectally. Although sustained-release compounds are not to be crushed, rectal administration in whole form has been reported with good results.

45. What are the uses for nebulized morphine?

Inhaled or nebulized morphine has been used as a treatment for terminal patients with pulmonary metastases to decrease air hunger and to treat dyspnea related to end-stage cancer, chronic obstructive pulmonary disease, and congestive heart failure. Approximately one-third or less of nebulized morphine is bioavailable. Although there are no controlled studies, other opioids, such as fentanyl and hydromorphone, have been nebulized.

To administer nebulized morphine, dilute 2–5 ml of preservative-free parenteral morphine with sterile water or normal saline, and nebulize via face mask for 15 minutes every 4 hours. Nebulized doses of morphine range from 5 to 25 mg and are not adequate for analgesia.[21]

46. Can any long-acting opioids be used in a gastrostomy or nasogastric tube?

A once-daily, sustained-release oral morphine (Kadian) is available in capsule form. Kadian's efficacy is not destroyed by breaking the capsule and sprinkling it over food (e.g., applesauce) or administering it via an enteral feeding tube (e.g., gastrostomy, nasogastric tube).

47. Does methadone or levorphanol have a place in the management of cancer pain?

Yes. In the hands of experienced clinicians, methadone (Dolophin) and levorphanol (Levodromeran) are highly effective synthetic opioids for relieving moderate-to-severe cancer pain. However, their use has decreased with the availability of continuous-release opioids. Both have prolonged half-lives and can be complicated to titrate. Caution is necessary in elderly patients and patients with major hepatic or renal failure or dementia. They are good alternatives if the patient is allergic to morphine.

48. What are the advantages of methadone compared with morphine?

- Higher oral bioavailability
- Incomplete cross-tolerance with other opioids
- No active metabolites
- Lower cost

Methadone may have other clinical advantages because it also blocks the NMDA (n-methyl-D-aspartate) receptor involved in pain processing. Compared with other opioids, methadone demonstrates better control of pain with a neuropathic component, perhaps because of its affinity for opioid and nonopioid receptors.

49. What are the disadvantages of methadone?

The major disadvantages of methadone are the risks of drug accumulation related to an unpredictable and long half-life and possible complications related to the clinician's inexperience with the drug. In switching from another opioid to methadone, it is also complicated to determine accurate doses according to equianalgesic guides based on single-dose studies. Effective doses of methadone vary from 3% to 68% of the calculated equianalgesic dose. Typically, the ratio of morphine to methadone is 1:1 for parenteral dosing and 3:1 or 3:2 for oral dosing. However, one study[24] reported that the oral methadone-to-morphine ratio may be more like 1:5. Other studies suggest that the maintenance doses of oral methadone may be one-tenth the equianalgesic dose of oral morphine.[20] Thus, it is extremely important that methadone doses be carefully individualized according to patient response.

50. Why is meperidine not recommended for use in patients with cancer?

Meperidine (Demerol) is not indicated for treatment of cancer pain or chronic pain because of its toxic metabolite, normeperidine, which has a 15-hour half-life. Normeperidine accumulation causes CNS excitability and seizures; patients with compromised renal function are definitely at risk. As recommended by the American Pain Society, meperidine doses should not exceed 600 mg/24 hours and should not be used longer than 48 hours for acute pain in patients without renal or CNS disease.

51. When is tramadol used for cancer pain?

Tramadol (Ultram) is an opioid for mild-to-moderate pain; its additional analgesic effect is related to its inhibition of serotonin and noradrenaline reuptake. Tramadol is not chemically related to morphine but is thought to bind weakly to mu opiate receptors. It is not currently scheduled by the Drug Enforcement Administration. Tramadol, 50 mg, is equianalgesic to codeine, 30 mg, plus acetaminophen, 300 mg; 100 mg is comparable to aspirin, 600 mg, plus codeine, 60 mg. Normal doses are 25–100 mg, administered orally every 4–6 hours, not to exceed 400 mg/24 hours. Patients older than 75 years should not exceed a total daily dose of 300 mg. Tramadol is effective for patients with early bone or neuropathic pain and has been used primarily to treat chronic pain.

Tramadol (50–100 mg) can be used in patients with cancer when nonopioids alone are not effective and as an early opioid substitute for analgesics such as Tylenol #3 (acetaminophen and codeine). Higher doses of tramadol (300–600 mg/day) also have been reported to be safe and effective for relief of cancer pain. It is not a good choice for breakthrough pain in patients receiving opioids because it may compete for the same binding site and act as a significantly weaker mu agonist. Common side effects include dizziness, nausea, constipation, and somnolence. *Note:* Usually acetaminophen, 650 mg, is given with each dose of tramadol (a combined formulation may soon be available).

52. Can opioids be used topically?

Contrary to previous belief that opioids act only on the central nervous system, opioid receptors have been identified in peripheral tissues such as immune cells, nerves, lungs, and cardiac muscle. This discovery has implications for various applications of opioids, including topical administration or injections into peripheral tissues. Application of morphine in topical gels over painful pressure sore ulcers and injections of morphine into knee joints have been proved to produce analgesia. Topical or peripheral use of opioids has the advantage of few or no systemic effects. Further research is needed to explore this area before topical opioids are commercially available.

53. What is Brompton's cocktail?

Brompton's cocktail, devised at Brompton's Hospital, was used in early hospices in England for cancer pain. The cocktail consists of the following: morphine hydrochloride, 15 mg; cocaine, 10 mg; alcohol 90%, 2 ml; chloroform water, 15 ml; and syrup, 4 ml. Before World War II, the alcohol and syrup were replaced by gin and honey. A solution allows easier titration of the analgesic; however, if side effects develop or increase, it is difficult to determine which component is responsible. Brompton's cocktail has been replaced with other liquid preparations (morphine sulfate elixir).

54. What is the difference between intrathecal and epidural administration?

Intrathecal administration. The subarachnoid fluid is bounded by the dural ligament (ligamentum flavum). Intrathecal or subarachnoid catheters are placed into the subarachnoid space, and medications are delivered directly into the spinal fluid. Because medication delivered intrathecally does not have to diffuse across the dural ligament, smaller doses are required.

Epidural administration. Epidural catheters are placed just outside the dural ligament. Medication is delivered into the epidural space, which is a potential space located below the ligamentum flavum and above the dura mater. The medication diffuses across the dura mater and arachnoid mater into the cerebrospinal fluid, where it binds with opiate receptors to block pain transmission. Epidural catheters are at greater risk than intrathecal catheters for compression of flow due to tumor growth.

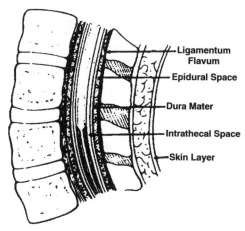

Lateral section of the spine. (From St .Marie B: Management of Cancer Pain with Epidural Morphine. St. Paul, MN, Pharmacia Deltec, 1994, with permission.

55. When should epidurals be considered for cancer pain?

The epidural route can be used to administer opioids alone, local anesthetics alone, or an opioid/local anesthetic combination. Epidurals should be considered to provide analgesia in the following settings:

1. Whenever pain is not adequately controlled by other routes.
2. When the dose of oral or intravenous opioids reaches a point at which side effects become a significant issue. Epidural analgesics are associated with fewer side effects (e.g., sedation) be-

cause the IV dose of morphine may be reduced by $\frac{1}{10}$ and the oral dose by $\frac{1}{30}$. When the intrathecal route is used, the amount of morphine is even less: the IV dose is reduced by $\frac{1}{100}$ and oral dose by $\frac{1}{300}$.

3. For neuropathic pain, such as tumor invasion of a nerve plexus or nerve root and scarring from radiation therapy. Neuropathic pain is effectively treated with epidural or intrathecal placement of local anesthetics and clonidine, an alpha$_2$ agonist, approved by the FDA for epidural administration. When used with opioids, clonidine helps to decrease neuropathic pain.

56. What effect do catheter placement and opioid choice have on epidural pain relief?

The lipid solubility of opioids is one of the major properties that influence receptor binding, systemic uptake, and rostral spread. Increased lipid solubility shortens the time needed for drug transfer through lipid barriers of blood vessels and cell membranes, resulting in a more rapid onset and shorter duration of action. The most lipophilic (lipid-soluble) opioids are sufentanil and fentanyl. Morphine is the most hydrophilic opioid. Other opioids, such as hydromorphine, have intermediate lipid solubility. Because of its high lipid solubility, analgesia related to fentanyl is more segmental in nature; thus, it is more important for the epidural catheter to be placed close to the site or dermatomal area of pain.

57. What are the advantages and disadvantages of the spinal delivery of pain medications?
Advantages
- Direct delivery to involved receptors (allows use of less medication and effective control of intractable pain)
- Less sedation
- Ability to use a combination of agents with minimal side effects
- Effective control of neuropathic pain (e.g., intrathecal methylprednisolone for intractable postherpetic neuralgia)

Disadvantages
- Initial high cost if a completely implantable system is used
- Risk of infection leading to epidural abscess with risk of nerve damage and paraplegia
- Risk of meningitis with intrathecal catheters
- Greater incidence of pruritus

58. What nondrug modalities are used to control pain?

Nondrug modalities include physical and psychosocial interventions, which should be introduced early to augment, not replace, pharmacologic therapy for pain management. The success of several of these modalities requires an understanding of the mind/body connection and depends on a therapeutic relationship between the nurse or health care provider and patient. Physical modalities used to reduce pain in patients with cancer include cutaneous stimulation (heat, cold, massage, vibration), exercise, immobilization, transcutaneous nerve stimulation (TENS), reflexology, therapeutic touch, and acupressure or acupuncture. Psychosocial interventions help patients to gain a sense of control by using cognitive techniques that affect how pain is interpreted and behavioral techniques that provide the patient with skills to cope with and modify responses to pain. Examples of psychosocial interventions include relaxation and imagery, meditation and deep breathing, distraction and reframing (replacing negative thoughts with more positive ones), music therapy, humor therapy, psychotherapy, biofeedback, peer support groups, hypnosis, and pastoral counseling.

59. Is heat or cold better in relieving pain?

The use of heat or cold is an individual preference. Use what is most effective for the patient, unless it is contraindicated. Cold may relieve more pain than heat for some conditions, such as painful muscles, because it works faster and the relief lasts longer after the cold is removed. Either heat or cold may be used for aching muscles or spasms, joint stiffness, and back pain. Heat is particularly useful for abdominal cramps, and cold may be more effective for pruritus, muscle spasms, and acute, but not severe, injuries (e.g., minor sports injuries or sprains). Severe pain is best treated by intermittent heat applications or by alternating applications of heat and cold. Cold or heat packs should be sealed, flexible to conform to body contours, and wrapped with a dry or moist cloth. Moist cloths should be used with caution because water permits faster cooling or greater heat intensity. Commercially available (dual controlled heat/cold) or homemade packs (e.g., 1-lb bag of frozen green peas or corn kernels) can be used. (*Note:* Heat should not be used over skin exposed to radiation therapy, and ice should not be used over skin that has been damaged by radiation therapy.)

60. What can be done if a patient feels that the painful site is too tender to tolerate heat or cold application?

By an unknown mechanism, the benefits of heat and cold are not limited to the direct sites of application and may have distant effects. Thus, cold or heat applications can be effective over an opposite site, or the patient can experiment using the cold or heat at various sites distant from the painful area (e.g., between the painful site and brain, acupuncture or trigger points). For example, ice over the unaffected side may reduce pain during a bone marrow biopsy.

61. What is important to know about controlling pain in elderly patients?

In addition to other pain relief barriers, elderly patients fail to report pain because they believe pain is expected with aging. Furthermore, health professionals may believe that elderly patients experience a lower pain level or that they are unable to tolerate high doses of opioids. Assessment is further complicated by sensory or cognitive impairments. The patient should be assessed frequently, and the dosage should be adjusted based on the patient's response. A thorough medication history is essential. Tips for administering or selecting analgesics include:

1. Avoid opioids with long half-lives, such as methadone, propoxyphene (Darvon), or levorphanol. Drugs may have longer half-lives in elderly patients because of decreased renal clearance, decreased hepatic function, and decrease in the ratio of lean body mass to fat.

2. Avoid meperidine because accumulation of its metabolite, normeperidine, is associated with confusion and seizures.

3. Morphine also has active metabolites (morphine 6-glucuronide) that may accumulate, resulting in nausea, confusion, and sedation.

4. Avoid long-term use of NSAIDs.

5. Use steroids cautiously because they aggravate osteoporosis.

6. For a tricyclic antidepressant, consider nortriptyline over amitriptyline because of its lower anticholinergic effects.

7. With both opioids and adjuvant medications, the recommendation is to "start low and go slow." When the equianalgesic chart is used to convert from one agent to another, the dose of the new analgesic should be decreased by 25–50%.

8. Start one medication at a time, and give it a thorough trial before changing or adding a new medication.

9. Keep it simple. Avoid high-technology pumps, especially if the patient lives alone.

10. Provide medication instructions to the patient and a responsible family member verbally and in writing (large print).

11. Assess and treat constipation vigilantly because of elderly patients' decreased mobility, decreased fluid intake, and concomitant use of other medications.

62. How is pain treated in a patient with cancer and a history of substance abuse?

In patients with cancer and a history of substance abuse, pain still should be treated with opioids as indicated. If patients are actively abusing opioid drugs or on a methadone maintenance program, they may require substantially higher starting doses to provide adequate analgesia because of drug tolerance. The dosing interval also may need to be shortened. Morphine, which has a usual duration of action of 3–4 hr, may need to be dosed every 1–2 hr in persons with opioid addiction and a large degree of pharmacologic tolerance.

The use of opioids should be openly discussed with the patient. Patients may fear repeat addiction and should be encouraged to express their concerns. Patients and health care providers should contact the recovery program for advice and collaboration. A patient's wish to decline opioids should be honored. Explicit rules or a contract should be established to guide behavior:

1. Supervision of prescription renewals
2. Procedure to be followed with lost or stolen prescriptions or medications
3. Procedure to ensure that only one clinician is prescribing analgesic medication.

Consequences of failure to conform with rules should be delineated:

1. If drugs are "lost," the patient may be readmitted to the hospital for pain control.
2. The patient may be required to come to the treatment facility to obtain daily doses.
3. If the source of pain is gone, opioids may no longer be prescribed and the patient is referred to a drug treatment program.

Patients should be assessed frequently and prescribed a set amount of opioids. Nonopioid or adjuvant drugs may be helpful in decreasing opioid requirements.

63. Is pain treated in comatose or verbally unresponsive patients?

Yes. Comatose or verbally unresponsive patients should be placed minimally on their baseline level of analgesia, and analgesics should be administered before any painful procedure. Some patients in whom opioids were stopped during a comatose period have reported severe pain after recovering from the coma. Some patients also may experience withdrawal without the ability to express it. Health care providers should pay attention to nonverbal cues (e.g., grimacing, sighs or gasps, frowns). Significant others may be queried about their assessment of the patient's level of pain. Although they are the least sensitive, physiologic measures (elevations in pulse, blood pressure, respiratory rate) may indicate pain.

64. What organizations are available to assist with pain management?

- American Alliance of Cancer Pain Initiatives
  1300 University Ave., Room 4720
  Madison, WI 53706
  608-265-4013; Fax 608-265-4014
  www.aacpi.org
  E-mail: aacpi@aacpi.org
- American Pain Society (APS)
  4700 W. Lake Avenue
  Glenview, IL 60025-1485
  847-375-4715
  www.ampainsoc.org
  Email: info@ampain.soc.org
- American Society of Pain Management Nurses (ASPMN)
  7794 Grow Drive
  Pensacola, FL 32514
  Tel: (888) 34-ASPMN; Fax: (850) 484-8762
  www.aspmn.org
  E-mail: aspmn@puetzamc.com
- City of Hope MAYDAY Pain Resource Center
  City of Hope Medical Center
  1500 E. Duarte Road
  Duarte, CA 91010
  626-359-8111 ext. 3829
  www.cityofhope.org/mayday/default.htm
  E-mail: mayday-pain@smtplink.coh.org
- Pain Management Special Interest Group
  Oncology Nursing Society
  501 Holiday Drive
  Pittsburgh, PA 15220-2749

412-921-7373
www.ons.org
Email: customer.service@ons.org
• International Association for the Study of Pain
IASP Secretariat
909 NE 43rd St., Suite 306
Seattle, WA 98105-6020 USA
Tel: 206-547-6409; Fax: 206-547-1703
www.halcyon.com/iasp
E-mail: IASP@locke.hs.washington.edu

65. What publications are available to assist with pain management?

• Acute Pain Management
Agency for Health Care Research and Quality (AHCRQ)
Management of Cancer Pain
www.ahrq.gov/clinic/cpgonline.htm
• Quality Improvement Guidelines for the Treatment of Acute Pain and Cancer Pain
American Pain Society
www.ampainsoc.org/pub/qi.htm
• Clinical Journal of Pain (Official Journal of the American Academy of Pain Medicine)
• Topics in Pain Management
Lippincott Williams & Wilkins
530 Walnut Street
Philadelphia, PA 19106-3621
Phone: 215-521-8300; Fax: 215-521-8902
E-mail: customerservice@lww.com
www.lww.com/store/
• Journal of Pain and Symptom Management
Includes supportive and palliative care and provides results of important new research
about pain and its clinical management; published since 1988.
www.elsevier.nl/inca/publications/store/5/0/5/7/7/5/index.htt
Elsevier Science
Regional Sales Offic
Customer Support Department
P.O. Box 945
New York, NY 10159-0945
Tel: (+1) 212-633-3730
Toll Free number for North American customers
1-888-4ES-INFO (437-4636); Fax: (+1) 212-633-3680
E-mail: usinfo-f@elsevier.com
• Pain
Official journal of the International Association for the Study of Pain; published since
1975. It publishes original research on the nature, mechanisms, and treatment of pain.
www.elsevier.nl/inca/publications/store/5/0/6/0/8/3/index.htt
• Pain Digest
Springer-Verlag New York Inc.
Journal Fulfillment Services Dept
P.O. Box 2485
Secaucus, NY 07096
Phone 800-SPRINGER; FAX: (1) 201-348-4505
E-mail: orders@springer-ny.com
• Pain Management Nursing
Official journal of the American Society of Pain Management Nurses

W.B. Saunders Company
Periodicals Dept.
P.O. Box 628239
Orlando, FL 32887-4800
1-800-654-2452
www.harcourthealth.com
• Pain Management, 5th ed. ($5.00)
Wisconsin Cancer Pain Initiative
1300 University Avenue
Medical Sciences Center, Rm 3675
University of Wisconsin
Madison, WI 53706
Phone: (608) 262-0978; Fax: (608) 265-4014
• Principles of Analgesic Use in the Treatment of Acute Pain and Cancer Pain, 4th ed.
American Pain Society (address above)
• National Comprehensive Cancer Network (NCCN) Practice Guidelines for Cancer Pain
www.cancernetwork.com
• Journal of Pain
Official journal of the American Pain Society
Department of Pharmacology
University of Iowa
Bowen Science Building
51 Newton Road
Iowa City, IA 52242
319-335-7941; Fax 319-335-7942
E-mail j-pain@uiowa.edu
www.jpain.org.

66. What video resources are available to assist with pain management?
• Physiology and Pharmacologic Management of Pain
Two videos with resource manual (ISBN: 0-683-17357-X)
Judith Paice, RN, PhD
Date: January 1994; price: $325
Lippincott Williams & Wilkins
530 Walnut Street
Philadelphia, PA 19106-3621
Phone: 215-521-8300; Fax: 215-521-8902
E-mail: customerservice@lww.com
www.lww.com/productdetailresults/1,2265,786118732,00.html
• McCaffery Pain Library
Set of eight videos with resource manual (ISBN: 0-683-17164-X)
Date: January 1994, Price $995.00, Lippincott Williams & Wilkins
www.lww.com/productdetailresults/1,2265,780654664,00.html

67. What CD-ROMs are available to assist with pain management and education?
• Pain Management
CD ROM or Online Course (7 CEU)
Author: Susan Pendergrass, MSN, MEd, RNCS, FNP
Date: 1999; price, $89 single learner; organization rates available.
http//www.graphiced.com
Graphic Education, 903 Old Highway 63N, Columbia, MO 65201
Phone: 888-354-6600, 573-449-1200; Fax: 573-449-3344
• Pain Management: Assessment and Overview of Analgesics
CD-ROM for Windows (ISBN: 0-7817-2041-9)

Authors: Margo McCaffery, RN, MS, FAAN, and Chris Pasero, RN, BSN
Date: September 2000; price: $495, Lippincott Williams & Wilkins
First of two programs designed to teach effective management of patient pain in the hospital setting
www.lww.com/productdetailresults/1,2265,546184903,00.html
• Pain Management: The Nurse's Active Role in Opioid Administration
CD-ROM for Windows (ISBN: 0-7817-2042-7)
Authors: Margo McCaffery, RN, MS, FAAN, and Chris Pasero, RN, BSN
Date: October 2000; price: $495
Second of two programs, this CD-ROM is designed to teach effective management of patient pain in the hospital setting
www.lww.com/productdetailresults/1,2265,533405384,00.html

68. What audio tapes/audio CDs are available to assist with pain management education?
• Pain Assessment and Management
Author: Maureen A. Carling, RN
Price list available by E-mail: CarlingMA@earthlink.net
Excellent presentation about pain assessment and treatment based on the description of the pain. Algorithms for pain treatment also available. The author is a freelance pain consultant. 757-220-6640.

The views expressed in this manuscript are those of the author and do not reflect the official policy or position of the Department of the Army, Department of Defense, or the U.S. Government.

REFERENCES

1. Bruera E, Brenneis C, MacDonald RN: Continuous SC infusion of narcotics for the treatment of cancer pain: An update. Cancer Treat Rep 71:953–958, 1987.
2. Chandler SW, Trissel LA, Weinstein SM: Combined administration of opioids with selected drugs to manage pain and other cancer symptoms: Initial safety screening for compatibility. J Pain Sympt Manage 12(3):168–171, 1996.
3. Cherny NI: The use of sedation in the management of refractory pain. Principles and Practice of Supportive Oncology Updates 3(4):1–11, 2000.
4. Coluzzi PH: Effective strategies for managing cancer pain with opioid pharmacotherapy. In Miaskowski C (ed): Helping Patients Manage Cancer Pain: Challenges and Opportunities. Deerfield, IL, Discovery International, 1997.
5. Coyle N, Cherny N, Portenoy RK: Pharmacologic management of cancer pain. In McGuire DB, Yarbro CH, Ferrell BR (eds): Cancer Pain Management, 2nd ed. Boston, Jones & Bartlett, 1995, pp 89–130.
6. Eisenberg E, Berkey CS, Carr DB, et al: Efficacy and safety of nonsteroidal anti-inflammatory drugs for cancer pain: A meta analysis. J Clin Oncol 12:2756–2765, 1994.
7. Ferrell BR, Dean GE, Grant M, Coluzzi T: An institutional commitment to pain management. J Clin Oncol 13:2158–2165, 1995.
8. Ferrell BR, Rhiner M, Cohen MZ, Grant M: Pain as a metaphor for illness. Part I: Impact of cancer pain on family caregivers. Oncol Nurs Forum 18:1303–1309, 1991.
9. Gagnon B, Bruera E: Differences in the ratios of morphine to methadone in patients with neuropathic pain versus non-neuropathic pain. J Pain Sympt Manage 18 (2):120–125, 1999.
10. Gouldlin WM, Kennedy DT, Small RE: Methadone: History and recommendations for use in analgesia. APS Bull 10(5):8–9, 2000.
11. Grond S, Radbruch L, Meuser T, et al: High-dose tramadol in comparison to low-dose morphine for cancer pain relief. J Pain Sympt Control 18 (3):174–179, 1999.
12. Hodgson BB, Kizior RJ, Kingdon RT: Nurse's Drug Handbook 1996. Philadelphia, W.B. Saunders, 1996.
13. Hurley AC, Volicer BJ, Hanrahan PA, et al: Assessment of discomfort in advanced Alzheimer patients. Res Nurs Health 15:369–377, 1992.
14. International Association for the Study of Pain. Pain terms: A list with definitions and notes on usage. Pain 6:249, 1979.
15. Jacox A, Carr DB, Payne R, et al: Management of Cancer Pain. Clinical Practice Guideline No. 9. AHCPR Publication No.94-0592. Rockville, MD, Agency for Health Care Policy and Research, U.S. Department of Health and Human Service, Public Health Service, 1994.

16. Kotani N, Kushikata T, Hashimoto H, et al: Intrathecal methylprednisolone for intractable postherpectic neuralgia. N Engl J Med 343:1514–1565, 2000.
17. Krajnik M, Zylicz Z, Finlay I, et al: Potential uses of topical opioids in palliative care: Report of 6 cases. Pain 80:121–125, 1999.
18. Lichtor JL, Sevaring FB, Joshi GP, et al: The relative potency of oral transmucosal fentanyl citrate compared with intravenous morphine in the treatment of moderate to severe postoperative pain. Anesth Analg 89:732–738, 1999.
19. Masfetter JL, Leahy KM, Koki AT, et al: Antiangiogenic and antitumor activities of cyclooxygenase-2 inhibitors. Cancer Res 60:1306–1311, 2000.
20. Max M, Payne R: Principles of Analgesic Use in the Treatment of Acute Pain and Cancer Pain, 4th ed. Glenview, IL, American Pain Society, 1999.
21. McCaffery M, Ferrell BR, Turner M: Ethical issues in the use of placebos in cancer pain management. Oncol Nurs Forum 23:1587–1593, 1996.
22. McCaffery M, Pasero C: Pain: Clinical Manual. St. Louis, Mosby, 1999.
23. Medical Letter: Drugs for pain 42(issue 1085):73–78, 2000.
24. Mercadante S, Casuccio A, Calderone L: Rapid switching from morphine to methadone in cancer patients with poor response to morphine. J Clin Oncol 17:3307–3312, 1999.
25. Morley JS, Makin MK: The use of methadone in cancer pain poorly responsive to other opioids. Pain Rev 5:51–58, 1998.
26. Omoigui S: The Pain Drugs Handbook. St. Louis, Mosby, 1995.
27. Portenoy RK: Management of cancer pain: Opioid and adjuvant pharmacotherapy. In Portenoy RK (ed): Real Patients, Real Problems: Optimal Assessment and Management of Cancer Pain. Glenview, IL, American Pain Society, pp 5–13, 1997.
28. Portenoy RK, Hagen NA: Breakthrough pain: Definition, prevalence and characteristics. Pain 41:273–281, 1990.
29. Portenoy RK, Payne R, Coluzzi P, et al: Oral transmucosal fentanyl (OTFC) for the treatment of breakthrough pain in cancer patients: A controlled dose titration study. Pain 79:303–312, 1999.
30. Porter J, Jick H: Addiction rare in patients treated with narcotics. N Engl J Med 302:123, 1980.
31. Skobel SW: Epidural narcotic administration: What nurses should know. Oncol Nurs Forum 23:1555–1562, 1996.
32. Spross JA, Curtiss CP, Coyne P, et al: Oncology Nursing Society Position on Cancer Pain Management. Oncol Nurs Forum 25:817–818, 1998.
33. Stein WM: Cancer pain in the elderly. In Ferrell BR, Ferrel BA (eds): Pain in the Elderly. Seattle, IASP Press, 1996.
34. Twillman RK, Long TD, Cathers TA, Mueller DW: Treatment of painful skin ulcers with topical opioids. J Pain Sympt Manage17(4):288–295, 1999.
35. Twycross RG: Strong narcotic analgesics. In Twycross RG (ed): Pain Relief in Cancer. Philadelphia, W.B. Saunders, 1984, pp 109–133.
36. Waldman SD, Leak DW, Kennedy LD, Patt RB: Intraspinal opioid therapy. In Patt RB: Cancer Pain. Philadelphia, J.B. Lippincott, 1993, pp 285–328.
37. Watson CPN, Evan RJ, Watt VR: Postherpetic neuralgia and topical capsaicin. Pain 38:177–186, 1989.
38. Weissman DE, Dahl JL, Dinndorf PA: Handbook of Cancer Pain Management, 5th ed. Madison, WI, Wisconsin Cancer Pain Initiative, 1996.
39. Wolfe MM, Lichtenstein DR, Gurkirpal S: Gastrointestinal toxicity of nonsteroidal antiinflammatory drugs. N Engl J Med 340:1888–1899, 1999.
40. Wong D, Whaley L: Clinical Handbook of Pediatric Nursing, 2nd ed. St. Louis, Mosby, 1986, p 373.
41. World Health Organization: Cancer pain relief and palliative care. Report of a WHO Expert Committee. WHO Technical Report Series 804. Geneva, Switzerland, World Health Organization, 1990, pp 1–75.

47. PALLIATIVE CARE

Sandra Muchka, RN, MS, CS, CHPN, and Julie Griffie, RN, MSN, CS, AOCN, CHPN

1. Define palliative care.

Palliative care is a broad concept, defined by the World Health Organization (WHO) as "the active total care of patients whose disease is not responsive to curative treatment. Control of pain, of other symptoms, and of psychological, social, and spiritual problems is paramount." The goal of palliative care is to promote quality of life and comfort. Death is not hastened, nor is the intent to prolong life.

2. What is the difference between palliative care and hospice care?

The philosophy of hospice care and palliative care is identical, but there are major differences involving reimbursement, eligibility for services, and care settings. In the United States, funding for hospice care is available via the Medicare Hospice Benefit or through private health insurance to patients who have a physician-certified prognosis of < 6 months to live and who are willing to forego life-sustaining treatments. Care is provided by Medicare-certified home hospice agencies with the goal of supporting patients and families at home. Unfortunately, limitations on reimbursement and requirements to forego certain types of therapy restrict the availability of hospice care; approximately 20% of dying patients actually enter a hospice program. Palliative care was developed to "fill in the gaps," to meet the needs of dying patients and families who do not qualify for hospice care and to extend the hospice philosophy into the hospital setting or to a much wider population of patients and care settings than hospice care can provide. Palliative care services are not limited by prognosis, types of treatments offered, or need for a hospice insurance benefit.

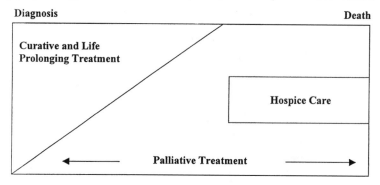

Integrated model of curative and palliative care in patients with chronic illness.

3. Who provides palliative care?

A multidisciplinary team provides palliative care. The team includes a physician, nurse, social worker, chaplain, dietitian, volunteers, and other disciplines as appropriate to meet the needs of the patient and family members. The patient and family are the unit of care. Because the nurse is the provider of direct patient care and the person most frequently in contact with the patient, the role of the nurse is critical.

4. List the elements of a palliative care assessment.

The palliative care assessment begins with a general physical assessment, followed by examination of the following:

1. Distress from physical symptoms. Ask patients:
   - What is their understanding of the cause of the symptom?
   - What is their goal for relief?
   - What are current side effects?
2. Patient goals. Consider:
   - What is important to the patient?
   - How can we help the patient 'live well' in the days ahead?
   - What personal goals does the patient have that healthcare team members should take into consideration?
3. Psychological and spiritual assessment
   - Elicit information about how the patient has coped with stressful situations in the past.
   - Who does the patient turn to for support?
4. Discussion of prognosis. Consider:
   - What is the patient's functional status?
   - Is there major organ failure?
   - Are multiple symptoms present?
5. Support systems and wishes for end-of-life care. Consider:
   - Where does the patient want to be at the time of death?
   - Who is available to assist?
   - What are the capabilities of the caregiver in relationship to the complexity of symptom management needs?

5. Why is information about prognosis important?

Patients and families need prognostic information to plan for the time ahead. The concept of time (months vs. weeks vs. days) should be communicated to the patient if the information is requested. Simply asking, "Do you need to know about time?" can begin the conversation. Prognostic information should be based on functional status, nutritional status, major organ involvement, and number of symptoms.

6. Why is palliative care frequently introduced too late (i.e., in the last days of life)?

Death is a natural part of the life cycle. Contemporary society, including the healthcare system, at times simply refuses to recognize this reality. Health professionals are educated via a curative model of care. Although an abundance of technology has been developed that can do wonderful things, it can also prevent a peaceful death. Death equates with failure for many healthcare providers. Recognizing approaching death is often clouded by discomfort in talking about it.

7. How can we open the conversation about the end of life?

Opening the conversation about dying requires maximizing personal sensitivity and communication skills. Choose a quiet time when the patient is comfortable. Sit down, when culturally appropriate, and make eye contact. Acknowledging that the situation is not going well may open the conversation. Simple statements, such as "Things don't seem to be going as well as we would like," or the question, "How do you think things are going for you?," may open a flood of emotions and concerns. Most oncology patients recognize when they are not getting better and welcome the opportunity to talk about it.

8. Should nurses talk to patients about prognosis?

Recognition of a downhill course may first be apparent to the nurses who see patients on a regular basis. When a patient arrives in a wheelchair after months of being ambulatory, functional status and other prognostic factors should be reviewed. Nurses must be proactive in recognizing functional decline and communicating patients' goals to team members. Patients and nurses can and should discuss disease progression. Many patients have a clear idea of the time frame that is left and need our assistance to ensure that goals are met and family issues are resolved.

9. Why is goal setting important at the end of life?

Goal setting defines the plan of care. For example, if a patient with advanced disease wants only measures that will add to comfort and dignity, cardiac resuscitation does not fall into the plan of care. If identified goals include reconciliation with a family member, escalating analgesic doses that cause sedation may not meet the patient's goals. On the other hand, if all end-of-life goals have been met and the goal is comfort above all, the side effect of sedation may be welcomed.

Patient goals should be considered when the decision is being made to treat or not to treat hypercalcemia. If the cancer is no longer being actively treated, reversal of the hypercalcemic state prolongs the life of the patient, on average, by about 8 weeks. If end-of-life work remains to be done, treatment is appropriate. If end-of-life work and goals have been met, hypercalcemia may be viewed as a part of the dying process and left untreated.

10. When is a family conference appropriate?

A family conference may be convened for the following reasons:
- To review the patient's medical condition and to establish treatment goals
- To clarify care goals
- To make decisions for nondecisional patients
- To resolve patient, family, and/or staff disagreements or conflicts

Guidelines for Conducting a Successful Family Ethics Conference

I. **Why:** clarify goals in your own mind.

II. **Where:** comfort, privacy, circular seating

III. **Who:** legal decision-maker/healthcare power of attorney; family members; social support; key healthcare professionals

IV. **How**
  1. *Introduction*
    - Introduce self and others.
    - Review meeting goals: state meeting goals and specific decisions.
    - Establish ground rules: each person will have a chance to ask questions and express views; no interruptions; identify legal decision-maker, and describe importance of supportive decision-making.
  2. *Review of medical status*
    - Review current status, plan, and prognosis.
    - Ask each family member in turn if he or she has any questions about current status, plan, or prognosis.
    - Defer discussion of decision until the next step.
  3. *Family discussion with decisional patient*
    - Ask patient what decision(s) he or she is considering.
    - Ask each family member the following questions: Do you have questions or concerns about the treatment plan? How can you support the patient?
  4. *Family discussion with nondecisional patient*
    - Ask each family member in turn: What do you believe the patient would choose if he (she) could speak for himself (herself)?
    - Ask each family member: What do you think should be done?
    - Leave room to let family discuss the issues alone.
    - If there is consensus, go to step 6; if no consensus, go to step 5.
  5. *When there is no consensus*
    - Restate goal: What would the patient say if he (she) could speak?
    - Use time as an ally: schedule a follow-up conference the next day.
    - Try further discussion: What values is your decision based on? How will the decision affect you and other family members?
    - Identify legal decision-maker.
    - Identify resources: minister/priest; other physicians; ethics committee.

Table continued on following page

Guidelines for Conducting a Successful Family Ethics Conference (Continued)

6. *Wrap-up*
   • Summarize consensus, decisions, and plan.
   • Caution against unexpected outcomes.
   • Identify family spokesperson for ongoing communication.
   • Document in the chart who was present, what decisions were made, and follow-up plan.
   • Do *not* leave discontinuation of treatment to nursing staff.
   • Continuity: maintain contact with family and medical team; schedule follow-up meetings as needed.
7. *Family dynamics and decisions*
   • Family structure: respect the family hierarchy whenever possible.
   • Established patterns of family interaction will continue.
     Unresolved conflicts between family members may be evident.
     Past problems with authority figures, doctors, or hospitals affect the process.
   • Family grieving and decision-making
     Denial: false hopes
     Guilt: fear of letting go
     Depression: passivity and inability to decide or anger and irritability.

Reprinted with permission of Ambuel B, Ferstenfeld JE. Adapted from Fisher R, Ury W: Getting to Yes. Boston, Houghton Mifflin, 1981; Walker MU: Keeping moral space open: New images of ethics consulting. Hastings Center Report 23(2):33–40, 1993; Bloom M: Family ethics conference. Presented at the 13th Forum for Behavioral Science Education in Family Medicine, Chicago, Illinois, September, 1993.

11. The foundation of excellent palliative care is management of what symptom?

The answer, of course, is pain. Patients consider freedom from pain to be the most important factor at the end of life. Pain is multidimensional and includes physical, psychological, psychosocial, and spiritual dimensions. Many patients have told us over the years that physical pain is often feared more than death itself. Oncology nurses must have well-developed skills in pain assessment, pharmacology, and communication. It is not enough to assess pain; we must know the patient's goals and be able to formulate an analgesic plan based on the WHO Step-Ladder. Analgesic standards are available from the Agency for Health Care Policy and Research, the American Pain Society, and the Joint Commission on Accreditation of Healthcare Organizations (JCAHO).

12. How common is dyspnea in patients with advanced cancer?

Dyspnea is one of the most prevalent symptoms among patients with advanced cancer. It is a subjective sensation defined as the perception of difficulty in breathing or as an uncomfortable awareness of breathing. Some degree of dyspnea occurs in over 70% of dying patients. In patients with advanced, incurable cancer, the sensation of dyspnea ranges from mild breathlessness to a sense of impending death from suffocation. Dyspnea can severely limit function and increase anxiety.

13. What should be included in the assessment of a patient with terminal dyspnea?

Assessment of terminal dyspnea begins with identifying the symptom. Elements of the assessment should include:
• Severity
• Onset
• Factors that exacerbate or relieve dyspnea
• Impact on daily living and quality of life
• Review of oxygen delivery system (Is the oxygen on? Is the tubing kinked?)
• Acute anxiety episode?
• Severe pain?
• Constipation?
• Urinary retention?

Understanding the goals of care is essential to guide the extent of the work-up. For example, if the patient is clearly dying and the goal of care is comfort, pulse oximetry, blood gas, and chest radiographs are not indicated.

14. How is terminal dyspnea treated?
Treatment of dyspnea in a dying patient depends on the goals of care and underlying cause. Dying patients who have severe dyspnea often need aggressive pharmacologic management. Drugs may be sedating, and often a balance needs to be found between symptom management and level of somnolence. The drugs used to treat dyspnea are directed at relieving the sensation of not being able to breathe. The major classes are opioids and anxiolytics. Adjuvant drugs include steroids, sedatives, and/or cough suppressants. It is important to include nonpharmacologic interventions in the treatment plan for terminal dyspnea. Oxygen administration, body positioning, room fans that produce tactile airflow to the patient's face, and relaxation/distraction techniques have been shown to be helpful in conjunction with pharmacologic interventions.

15. Which opioid is most commonly used to control dyspnea? How does it work?
The most commonly used opioid is morphine, which can be administered orally, intravenously (IV), subcutaneously (SC), or via nebulized aerosol. The starting dose of morphine depends on the patient's current and/or prior use. For opioid-naive patients with severe dyspnea, the recommended starting dose is 2–5 mg IV or SC every 5 minutes until symptoms improve.

Morphine affects dyspnea in a number of ways. First, it reduces patients' fears and anxiety. Reduction of anxiety, muscle tension, and restlessness decreases oxygen consumption, which in turn improves oxygenation and increases respiratory comfort. Morphine also improves oxygenation by reducing pulmonary edema through pulmonary vasodilation.

16. Does morphine hasten the patient's death?
A major barrier to providing adequate relief of terminal dyspnea is the fear of using opioids because of the potential for respiratory depression. Ethically, their use is appropriate as long as the intent is to relieve distress rather than shorten life. There is no ethical or professional justification for withholding symptomatic treatment to a dying patient because of fear of potential respiratory depression. It is important to understand the patient's wishes for end-of-life symptom control. Good communication with family and other caregivers about how and why drugs are administered is essential.

17. What are the treatment options for intractable nausea and/or vomiting?
Nausea may represent different sensations to different people. A thorough assessment is necessary to understand what the person is experiencing. Nausea may imply esophageal reflux, inner ear dysfunction, regurgitation, bowel obstruction, or anxiety. As with other symptoms, basic guidelines should be followed in treating nausea and vomiting with medication. If the nausea is continuous, the antiemetic should be scheduled around the clock or administered as a continuous infusion (e.g., chlorpromazine hydrochloride [Thorazine] or metoclopramide [Reglan]). If the nausea is intermittent, the antiemetic can be ordered on an as-needed basis. There is a wide variety of medications for the management of nausea and vomiting. Many times they are used in a trial-and-error fashion.

Medical Management of Nausea and Vomiting

CAUSE	INDICATED DRUG CLASS
Movement-related nausea	Antihistamine
Anxiety	Benzodiazepine
Tumor-related elevated intracranial pressure	Glucocorticoid
Gastric stasis	Metoclopramide
Stimulation of chemoreceptor trigger zone	Dopamine antagonist, serotonin antagonist
Constipation	Laxative

Adapted from Weissman DE, Ambuel B: Improving End-of-Life Care: A Resource Guide for Physician Education, 3rd ed. Milwaukee, Medical College of Wisconsin, 1999.

Nondrug therapies include behavioral treatments such as relaxation, guided imagery, distraction, and music therapy. Nasogastric or percutaneous drainage may be indicated for gastric stasis or obstruction refractory to conservative management.

18. Mr. J. is a 70-year-old man with end-stage lung cancer. The night before discharge home to hospice care the nurse phones the doctor to report that Mr. J. is "confused." What does this report mean?

It is important to understand what "confusion" really means. Mr. J. may be experiencing terminal delirium. Delirium occurs to some degree in virtually all patients before death. The cause is often multifactorial; an exact cause is not established in 40% or more of patients. Possible causes in patients with advanced cancer include drug toxicity, metabolic changes, central nervous system pathology, drug withdrawal, infections, fevers, urinary retention, and/or imminent death.

Potential Causes for Terminal Delirium and Agitation

Metabolic disturbances	Drug withdrawal	Other causes
Hypoxia	Alcohol	Systemic infections
Hypercalcemia	Benzodiazepines	Fever
Hyponatremia	Barbiturates	Heart failure
Hypoglycemia	Steroids	Imminent death
Liver failure	Nicotine	Urinary retention
Renal failure		Constipation
Dehydration		Sleep deprivation
Central nervous system pathology	**Drug toxicity**	Pain
Cerebral metastases	Benzodiazepines	
Infarction	Anticholinergics	
Bleeding	Opioids	
Infection	Steroids	
Seizures	Illicit drugs	
Increased intracranial pressure	Alcohol	

19. What nursing assessment is required in suspected delirium?

1. Complete a history and physical examination, including a Mini-Mental Status Examination (MMSE; see question 20).

2. Distinguish between delirium and dementia. Delirium refers to an altered level of consciousness with reduced attention and memory. Other characteristics of delirium include perceptual disturbances, hallucination, incoherent speech, and altered sleep/wake cycles. Dementia refers to a loss of intellectual function with diminished memory, thinking, and judgment.

3. Assess whether the patient is in danger of harming self or others.

4. Assess whether the cognitive change is distressing to the patient.

5. Review chart and medication record for recent medication changes.

6. Assess for possible physical causes (e.g., fever, urinary retention, impaction).

Depending on the goals of care, further assessment may include a complete evaluation (e.g., brain imaging, spinal tap) to search for the underlying cause.

20. How is the abbreviated MMSE conducted?

Ask the patient the following:

1. Age
2. Birth date
3. Recognition of two persons (e.g., doctor, nurse, family)
4. Hospital or clinic name
5. Address for recall at end of test (e.g., 12 Main Street)
6. Present year
7. Current time (to nearest hour)
8. Name of current president

9. Name of first president or year World War II ended
10. Count backward from 20 to 1
Score: 9–10 = Normal
       8 = Borderline
      < 7 = Cognitive impairment
Adapted from Power D, Kelly S, Gilsenan J, et al: Suitable screening tests for cognitive impairment and depression in the terminally ill: A prospective prevalence study. Palliat Med 7:213–218, 1993.

21. It is determined that Mr. J. is experiencing terminal delirium. What can be done?

Treatment for delirium should encompass a combination of nonpharmacologic and pharmacologic approaches. Nondrug interventions include offering the patient frequent reminders of time and date and providing a quiet, well-lit room. The presence of a family member may help to allay fears and provide patient support. Physical restraints are rarely necessary and should be applied only for a brief time while treatment is initiated.

Drug therapy is indicated for patients with agitated delirium (i.e., those who exhibit restless behaviors such as climbing out of bed or pulling out intravenous lines). The most useful agents include neuroleptics and benzodiazepines. Neuroleptics should be used as first-line agents; haloperidol (Haldol) is one of the most common choices. The recommended starting dose for haloperidol is 1–2 mg orally, subcutaneously, or intravenously every 6 hours; a 1–2-mg dose should be available on an as needed basis. The dose should be titrated to meet the patient's needs.

22. Two months ago Mrs. K., a 54-year-old woman with advanced pancreatic cancer, was told that her survival time was estimated at 3–4 months. She reports a decrease in appetite and weight along with insomnia and increased fatigue. Her family thinks that she is depressed. Do all patients become depressed when they find out that they are dying?

The incidence of depression in patients with cancer ranges from 10–25%. The incidence increases with higher levels of disability, advanced illness, and/or pain. Psychological distress often causes suffering in dying patients. The diagnosis of major depression in a terminally ill patient often relies more on reports of worthlessness, hopelessness, guilt, and suicidal ideation than on the expected changes associated with end of life (e.g., appetite/weight loss, insomnia, fatigue).

Always explore patients' hopes and expectations. Although there may be no hope for a cure, many patients have other hopes, such as avoidance of pain or being at home with their family. Individual and/or group counseling reduces psychological stress and depressive symptoms in patients with cancer. Nonpharmacologic interventions used to treat anxiety and depression include relaxation and distraction techniques. Antidepressants are often the first-line agents for treatment of depression in terminally ill patients. Skillful management of depression relieves suffering and is a core element of the provision of comprehensive end-of-life care.

23. One of the most frequent concerns for patients and families is loss of appetite and/or ability to drink. Does the patient suffer without food or fluids?

Loss of appetite is normal in the days or weeks before death. The loss occurs slowly. Most dying people say that the very thought of eating food is unpleasant. No pain or discomfort is associated with this feeling. After no food intake for 2–3 days, a chemical that suppresses the feeling of hunger accumulates in the blood. The body is shutting down and preparing to die and does not need as much energy from food. Although the feeling of hunger is usually absent in dying patients, the feeling of thirst remains. Thirst may be due to lack of water, or it may be a side effect of drugs used to provide comfort. Sips of water, juice, soda, ice chips, or lemon drops may be used to relieve thirst. A lack of fluids in the final days and weeks of life is not painful.

24. How can you reassure the family if the patient refuses to eat or drink?

It is difficult for family members to watch their loved one appear to "starve to death." Anorexia is troubling because food and drink are culturally considered nurturing and life-sustaining. Starvation in a healthy person is an awful process to watch. The dying person who loses interest in eating is *not* starving; he or she is dying. This difference is important. A disease, such as cancer or Alzheimer's disease, may cause patients to lose their appetite, but it is the disease—not starvation—that leads to death.

25. What are the common causes of pruritus?

Pruritus, which can be among the most irritating symptoms that patients experience, may be caused by many factors. Pharmacologic agents used to treat other symptoms, such as opioids, can cause pruritus. Switching to a different opioid often relieves the discomfort. Other common causes for pruritus include jaundice and uremia.

26. How is pruritus treated?

There is no one outstanding intervention to control itching. For many patients, topical measures such as frequent baths with water at room temperature and a soap substitute or oatmeal powder can be very soothing. Other interventions include drying the skin by patting with a soft towel (no rubbing motion), applying cornstarch lightly to skin folds, and using nonalcoholic lotion after baths. Many medications are also used to control itching. Antihistamines such as diphenhydramine (Benadryl), hydroxyzine (Atarax), and loratidine (Claritin) are commonly prescribed but are frequently ineffective at nonsedating doses. Tricyclic antidepressants are sometimes effective but are frequently too toxic. Naloxone (Narcan), nalbuphine (Nubain), ondansetron hydrochloride (Zofran), and paroxetine hydrochloride (Paxil) also may have some positive effect.

27. Mr. B. is a 60-year-old man with metastatic head and neck cancer. He has a large tumor on his neck that is open, draining, and foul-smelling. He is embarrassed and has asked to have visitors limited because of the odor. What can be done to control the odor?

Odor can be highly distressing for patients and caregivers. Interventions such as frequent dressing changes and Domeboro soaks are effective in decreasing drainage and odor. Another effective treatment is topical 0.75% metronidazole (Flagyl) gel. Other interventions include:

• Cleanse the wound with full-strength chlorhexidene (Hibiclens) for 3 minutes; then rinse.
• Administer an oral antifungal agent.
• Wash the wound with a douche powder (e.g., Massingel, 1 oz in a basin of water).
• Place a dryer fabric-softener sheet over the outside of the dressing.
• Use charcoal-filled dressings.
• Place a pan of charcoal briquettes under the bed.

28. Mrs. K., a 73-year-old woman with metastatic colon cancer, has been on the palliative care unit for 2 weeks. Yesterday she developed hiccups, which have been continuous and distressing. What can be done to relieve her distress?

The incidence of transient or chronic hiccups in terminal disease is unknown. Chronic hiccups are defined as hiccups that last 48 hours or longer or frequently recurring episodes. Complications related to chronic hiccups include fatigue, discomfort, weight loss, sleep deprivation, and depression. Various pharmacologic interventions have been reported; no one medication has been found to be most effective. Case reports support chlorpromazine hydrochloride (Thorazine), baclofen (Lioresal), metoclopramide (Reglan), haloperidol (Haldol), amitriptyline (Elavil), and carbamazepine (Tegretol). The variety of proposed treatments indicates the lack of effectiveness of any one therapy. Nonpharmacologic approaches include interventions that interrupt the vagal and/or phrenic nerve limbs of the reflex arc:

• Gargling
• Sipping ice water
• Swallowing dry bread
• Ingesting a teaspoon of granulated sugar
• Biting on a lemon
• Breath-holding
• Hyperventilation
• Breathing into a paper bag.

29. When pain control results in unacceptable side effects at the end of life, what can be done?

When pain does not respond to traditional approaches, we are challenged clinically, emotionally, and ethically. When interventions no longer provide relief with tolerable side effects or the time frame required for relief is not tolerable, consideration of sedation is appropriate.

Pharmacologic management of sedation at the end of life requires vigilant titration and monitoring. A policy and guidelines for the use of sedation (e.g., benzodiazepines or barbiturates) in this setting can provide support to healthcare providers. Consensus about sedation is essential among healthcare providers, patients, and family members.

30. What have family members suggested that nurses can do to help them when a loved one is dying?

Communication is perhaps the most critical component of palliative care. Family members have made clear that nurses can help them by following three critical guidelines:

1. Facilitate communication between the dying patient and family members.
2. Facilitate communication between the healthcare team and patients and family members.
3. Create an environment conducive to communication.

31. What aspects of the plan of care are important to stop when death is imminent?

When the goal of care is comfort only, all aspects of the patient's care plan should be evaluated to ensure that each aspect adds to the patient's comfort:

• Diagnostic or laboratory tests should be done only if they will provide information that initiates an intervention adding to the patient's comfort. For example, finger sticks to determine blood sugar levels should be stopped when a patient is no longer eating.
• Radiologic tests providing information that will not be used to aid in the patient's comfort should be avoided.
• Implanted defibrillators should be deactivated.
• Routine measurements of vital signs, with the exception of temperature, may be stopped.
• Medications not used for symptom management may be discontinued.

32. Miss V. is dying from metastatic breast cancer to the lung. Her sister comes to the desk crying that Miss V. is struggling to breathe. On entering the room you hear a coarse, rattling sound. Miss V. appears to be struggling but is unresponsive to her surroundings. Should Miss V. be suctioned? What is death rattle?

Death rattle is noisy breathing in terminally ill patients shortly before death as a result of uncleared upper airway or pulmonary secretions. Most likely the patient is unresponsive; family caregivers are usually more distressed than the patient. However, accumulated secretions may lead to dyspnea and restlessness in some patients. Prevention of the death rattle is one argument for not forcing hydration; excessive pulmonary secretions are less likely in dehydrated patients.

Whether to suction the patient is determined by the level of comfort that the family and caregivers perceive in the dying patient. A family member who is distraught that the patient is suffering may be comforted by suctioning. However, suctioning also can cause trauma, bleeding, and shortness of breath. Turning the patient to a lateral position to facilitate drainage of secretions may be helpful. Pulmonary secretions may be minimized by the use of intravenous (IV) atropine. Hyoscine hydrobromide (scopolamine) transdermal patch is also effective to decrease oropharyngeal secretions. One or two patches can be applied every 72 hours. Nursing judgment is critical in determining how the comfort of the patient is affected by proposed interventions. It is important to include family caregivers in the decision.

33. The family tells you that the patient has died. What is expected from the nurse?

Family support is paramount. This moment will be replayed by family members many times over the next few months. Explain what you need to do. Assess the patient to determine if he or she responds to verbal or tactile stimuli. Avoid overtly painful stimuli. Assess heart and lungs for absence of pulse and respiration. Look and listen for spontaneous respiration. Note the time. Advise the physician. Topics of tissue donation, autopsy, and body donation should be reviewed if not previously discussed.

Personal care should be provided for the body. The body should be bathed and dressed. Some family members may wish to assist the nurse. The body should be placed in proper alignment. The temperature in the room may be lowered if it is going to be more than a few hours until the body is removed.

34. Is it important for the nurse to contact family members in the days following the death of the patient?

Family members have many needs after the patient's death. Hearing from the nurse via telephone or written card is helpful and comforting. During contacts with family members, it is appropriate to restate enjoyable memories of the patient, what you found special in the patient, and what you will remember about the family unit. If appropriate, you may want to share information about grief support groups. Referral to a social worker may be appropriate at this time. Family members in hospice programs have the benefit of bereavement follow-up from the hospice agency.

35. How can oncology nurses receive further education about palliative care?

The groups listed below collaborate to help healthcare professionals who want to improve end-of-life care. Many of these organizations also have websites that provide links to affiliated groups and/or educational resources.

American Academy of Hospice and Palliative Medicine: www.aahpm.org

American Alliance of Cancer Pain Initiatives: www.aacpi.org

American Pain Society: www.ampainsoc.org

Center to Advance Palliative Care (CAPC): www.capcmssm.org

Education for Physicians on End-of-Life Care (EPEC): www.epec.net

End-of-Life Physician Education Resource Center (EPERC): www.eperc.mcw.edu/

Growth House: www.growthhouse.org

Hospice and Palliative Nurses Association: www.hpna.org

Innovations in End-of-Life Care: www.edc.org/lastacts/

Last Acts: www.lastacts.org

Medical College of Wisconsin Palliative Medicine Program: www.mcw.edu/pallmed

National Hospice and Palliative Care Organization: www.nhpco.org

Oncology Nursing Society: www.ons.org

REFERENCES

1. American Pain Society: Principles of Analgesic Use in the Treatment of Acute Pain and Cancer Pain, 4th ed. Lakeview, IL, American Pain Society, 1999.
2. Campbell ML: Forgoing life-sustaining therapy: How to care for the patient who is near death. Aliso Viejo, CA, AACN Crit Care, 1998.
3. Cherney N, Portenoy R: Sedation in the management of refractory symptoms: Guidelines for Evaluation and Treatment. J Palliat Care 10(2):31–38, 1994.
4. Griffie J, Muchka S, Nelson-Marten P, O'Mara A: Integrating palliative care into daily practice: A nursing perspective. J Palliat Med 2:65–73, 1998.
5. Jacox A, Carr DB, Payne R, et al: Management of Cancer Pain. Clinical Practice Guideline No. 9. AHCPR Publications No. 94-0592. Rockville, MD, Agency for Health Care Policy and Research, U.S. Department of Health and Human Service, Public Health Service, 1994.
6. Larijani G, Goldgerg M, Rogers H: Treatment of opioid-induced pruritus with ondansetron: Report of four patients. Pharmacotherapy 16:958–960, 1996.
7. Lassauniere J, Vinant P: Prognostic factors, survival, and advanced cancer. J Palliat Care 8:52–54, 1992.
8. Maluso-Bolton T: Terminal agitation. J Hospice Palliat Nurs 2(1):9–20, 2000.
9. Pierce SF, et al: Improving end of life care: Gathering suggestions from family members. Nurs Forum 34(2):5–14, 1999.
10. Power D, Kelly S, Gilsenan J, et al: Suitable screening tests for cognitive impairment and depression in the terminally ill: A prospective prevalence study. Palliat Med 7:213–218, 1993.
11. Shaiova LF: Management of dyspnea in patients with advanced cancer. Principles of Supportive Oncology Updates 2(3), 1999.
12. Steinhauser K, et al: Factors considered important at the end of life by patients, family, physicians, and other care providers. JAMA 284:2476–2482, 2000.
13. Weissman DE: Consultation in palliative medicine. Arch Intern Med 157:733–737, 1997.
14. Weissman DE, Ambuel B: Improving End-of-Life Care: A Resource Guide for Physician Education, 3rd ed. Milwaukee, Medical College of Wisconsin, 1999.
15. World Health Organization: Cancer Pain Relief and Palliative Care. Technical Report Series 804. Geneva, World Health Organization, 1990.
16. Zbigniew Z, Smits C, et al: Paroxetine for pruritus in advanced cancer. J Pain Symptom Manage 16:121-124, 1998.

48. SEXUALITY

Patricia W. Nishimoto, RN, MPH, DNS, COL, AN, USAR

1. Why do nurses need to discuss sexuality with patients?

A diagnosis of cancer and the subsequent treatment have a significant impact on sexuality. To ignore that impact is just as detrimental as ignoring any other side effect, such as stomatitis or diarrhea. The Oncology Nursing Society's standard on sexuality reinforces that sexuality is an integral part of well-being throughout the life span and that nurses need to identify alterations caused by malignancy or treatments to help patients maintain sexual identity. The oncology nurse must recognize that a patient's sexual health is influenced by sexual function before diagnosis, past sexual experiences, other illnesses, medications, stage of disease, religious and cultural background, emotional and psychological status, and relationships with other people.

Too often nurses and other health care professionals ignore the topic of sexual health because they worry that it will embarrass the patient or that it is not clinically pertinent. To speak openly and honestly with patients allows them the ability to make informed decisions about regaining control over their sexual identity.

Sexuality is much more than intercourse; it also encompasses feelings, insights, motivations, thoughts, or behaviors. To define sexuality as coitus ignores the broad spectrum of late night talks, cuddling, how one dresses or sits, self-pleasuring, and the hundreds of ways of expressing intimacy.

2. What should nurses know before discussing sexuality?

It can feel overwhelming even to think of including sexual counseling in clinical practice, but take a deep breath and remember when you began to include other new aspects of care, such as education about chemotherapy. You believed that patients needed to know how the treatment worked and its possible side effects. You should be able to talk with patients about sexually related side effects of chemotherapy, such as decreased vaginal lubrication and the need for additional lubrication to prevent vaginal tears and reduce the risk of infection.

Before beginning a discussion about sexuality, nurses need the recognition that sexuality is a part of nursing care; the desire to provide holistic care; a basic knowledge of sexuality; and knowledge (or access to a resource) of how cancer or treatment can affect sexual functioning. Nurses may gain greater confidence and comfort by attending conferences, reading, role playing, or mentoring with an expert.

When counseling patients about sexuality, nurses should have an open, accepting attitude; ensure time for patients to ask questions and voice concerns; respect the patient's beliefs and practices; avoid making assumptions; and keep in mind that sexuality is highly personal and defined by each individual. Nurses should be careful not to impose their own biases and should be aware of myths; they do not have to be experts in sexual therapy. Many sexual problems require sensitive listening, explanations, and reassurance—the same skills that nurses use daily in clinical practice. Nurses who are uncomfortable about discussing sexual issues can make appropriate referrals or provide written information about available resources. Knowing what, when, and how to inquire about patients' sexual concerns requires awareness, knowledge, skills, and practice.

3. Why do some nurses hesitate to include sexuality counseling as part of holistic care?

Although it is the responsibility of all members of the health care team to address sexuality in their teaching and counseling, the nurse is often the first member of the team to become aware of sexual concerns. Why nurses hesitate is unclear and complex; it may be a refection of their upbringing or cultural background. Many may feel "too busy" or unqualified or believe that it is someone else's responsibility. Others may feel uncomfortable discussing sexuality, believe that it is too private a topic to discuss with patients, or fear that their intervention may be considered sexual harassment.

When nurses are silent about sexuality, patients are given the message that sexuality is not appropriate. Waiting until the patient asks is not realistic. Multiple studies have found that patients are hesitant to ask health care providers about sexuality. Beliefs such as "they are too old, too ugly, or too fat," "cancer ends sexuality," or "focus needs to be on life-or-death issues" can stop the nurse from initiating discussion. Compounding this hesitation may be the lack of support from supervisors or the low priority of sexual concerns in the current atmosphere of health care reform when it is not identified in the critical pathway or is not reimbursable.

4. How can I provide sexual counseling?

Nurses can intervene at the level at which they feel competent. Robinson and Annon developed the **PLISSIT** model to identify four levels of intervention: **p**ermission, **l**imited **i**nformation, **s**pecific **s**uggestions, and **i**ntensive **t**herapy.

5. Explain the importance of permission.

Permission to express sexual concerns or questions legitimizes the topic. A simple way of granting permission is to include sexuality in your teaching handouts about chemotherapy or radiation therapy. Keep brochures or books about sex prominently displayed on your desk or in your bookcase. Seeing such brochures helps to reassure patients that sexuality is a topic of health care concern and that you are open to discussing the issues. Doing so may allow the 16-year-old boy with osteosarcoma to ask if it is "normal" to masturbate or if masturbation caused the cancer. At this level, the nurse needs to know basic physiology, normal cultural beliefs about sexuality, and developmental issues–in other words, information that nurses already have from their scientific background and education. Thus, the nurse can respond by telling the teenager that masturbation *is* normal and that masturbation did *not* cause the cancer.

6. What is meant by limited information?

Limited information is related to the patient's concerns, such as common sexual changes that may occur during or after cancer treatment. When a 36-year-old mother of three children who is receiving chemotherapy after mastectomy comments that she does not "get turned on as often," the nurse needs first to clarify what is meant by "not turned on as often." If it means decreased vaginal lubrication, the nurse gives the patient "limited information" that chemotherapy decreases lubrication and causes fatigue that affects libido. This information may be all that is needed for this patient. Other patients may want to know what to do about the decreased lubrication . The nurse either proceeds to the next level of intervention or refers the patient to someone who can help. At this level, the nurse needs to know how cancer or its treatments can affect sexual functioning.

7. What types of specific suggestions are appropriate?

Specific suggestions help patients to deal with changes in sexuality. For example, the patient may say, "I'm glad to find out that decreased lubrication is normal when you're on chemo. I was worried that maybe it meant I didn't love my husband anymore." If she then asks what to do about the decreased lubrication, the nurse can give a specific suggestion (after assessing the patient's cultural and religious beliefs and current sexual practice), such as using a water-soluble lubricant during intercourse. At this level, the nurse needs a solid knowledge of sexual behaviors and alternatives.

8. Explan intensive therapy.

Intensive therapy usually involves more than four sessions and referral to an advanced practice nurse or other health care provider who specializes in sexual counseling. For example, intensive therapy is needed for the 42-year-old woman diagnosed with cervical cancer who, after repeated gynecologic examinations, begins to relive her rape experiences when she was only 17 years old. At this level, formal advanced practice training and clinical work experience are required.

9. How do I give patients permission to talk about sexual concerns?

The inclusion of open-ended questions or statements about sexuality as part of your routine nursing gives patients permission and opportunity to express concerns. Point out to the patient that you routinely ask questions about sexuality of all your patients to help promote overall health and well-being. Open the door for discussions about sex by prefacing your questions with a comment about sexual concern. It helps to make a statement such as, "Many of our patients who are taking chemotherapy have difficulty having an erection," and then to ask, "Are you experiencing this?" Or simply say, "If you have this happen, our advice is to _____." You may be pleasantly surprised by the response.

The inclusion of sexual information throughout diagnosis, treatment, follow-up, and, when necessary, recurrence and terminal disease reinforces that sexuality is a part of life. In other words, sexuality discussions are not a one-time event but rather a series of conversations that change with situations and conditions. Counseling does not work if you giggle, blush, or run to answer a call light when the patient finally has the courage to ask questions. If you giggle or the patient perceives your comment to be offensive, respond as you usually do when there is a misunderstanding (which happens to all nurses during their career). Express your sincere regret, offer reassurance that no offense was intended, and express hope that the patient understands that your intent is to help. It helps if you have already established a level of rapport, comfort, and trust before openly discussing the emotionally charged topic of sexuality, but sometimes patients are ready to talk before this goal is achieved. By starting with a low-intensity area and then addressing more sensitive areas, you decrease your chance of offending a patient.

10. What are the "three Ls and a P" of sexual counseling?

Language, labeling, listening, and privacy.

11. How is language an important part of sexual counseling?

Some patients may use language that is "raw or earthy," whereas others may use euphemisms or oblique sexual references. If patients use a word that is "dirty," it may be the only term that they know. Do not automatically assume that they are trying to be "gross" or test you. The challenges of language are not one-sided. A nurse who responds to a question of what to do about pain "when we fuck" by giving a long monologue about "strategies to prevent dyspareunia" may get a polite nod followed by the question, "But what do I do so it doesn't hurt?" Nurses need to use appropriate language understood by the patient and not hide behind professional jargon. Thus, it may be better to ask, "What kind of pain do you have when you fuck or have intercourse?" Even if you are uncomfortable using the patient's term, do not embarrass the patient. Repeat the patient's term and then use the term you prefer.

12. Explain labeling and listening.

Labeling can create a sense of hopelessness that sexual functioning will be permanently dysfunctional. Neither nurses nor patients should label behaviors with words such as "impotent" or "weird." Listening is a basic nursing skill, but at first it may be uncomfortable to listen to questions or comments about sex. Nurses must give themselves time to learn.

13. What is the role of privacy?

Privacy includes not asking the patient in front of another health care professional, "Did that lubricant help you and your husband?" Provide a relaxed, private place for discussions. When possible and if desired by the patient, include the significant other in discussions.

14. What questions about sex are most commonly asked by patients with cancer?

Patients may ask questions that to you seem simple and have obvious answers, but they are important and would not be asked if the patient knew the answer. Be careful not to assume that the patient is joking; you may miss an opportunity to intervene. Common questions include the following:

1. Will my partner "catch cancer from me" if we have sex?
2. Will my partner leave me because I have cancer?

3. Will my partner think my [ostomy, mastectomy, surgical scar] is disgusting and be "turned off?"

4. Is _____ normal?

5. Will my partner still love me?

6. Will anyone ever want to date me?

7. Will I still be able to have sex?

15. What should the nurse say if he or she does not know the answer to a specific question?

Nurses need to remember three basic principles: (1) they do not have to know all of the answers; (2) seldom is sexuality an emergency; and (3) it is all right to tell your patient, "That is a good question, and I've never really thought about it. Let me do some reading and talking with our consultant. I can either call you at home or give you the information at your next appointment."

16. How does cancer affect various phases of the sexual response cycle?

1. **Desire**, also called libido, is an interest in sex. Stress alone can decrease androgen, resulting in decreased desire. Preliminary studies indicate that transdermal testosterone patches may benefit women after oophorectomy in many phases of the sexual response cycle (i.e., increased fantasies, increased sexual activity, and higher scores of satisfaction with orgasm).

2. **Excitement**, also called arousal, is influenced by physical state, emotions, body image, anxiety, hormonal functioning, and other physical factors. In patients with cancer, other significant factors include drugs, surgery, and radiation therapy, which may interfere with vasocongestion or muscle tension. Damage to the periprostatic plexus during a radical retropubic prostatectomy may prevent erection. Sometimes even though surgery has occurred, such as a mastectomy, the sensation of nipple erection during the excitement phase may still be present because of phantom sensation.

3. During **plateau**, which is characterized by continued vasocongestion and myotonia, the pulse may increase to 100–175 beats per minute, blood pressure may rise, and the labia may change color. Often people become more attentive or hypervigilant toward their body after a diagnosis of cancer and may misinterpret changes as abnormal (e.g., symptoms of cancer or side effects of treatment). For example, before diagnosis a patient may not have noticed the change in color of the labia, but after diagnosis she pays more attention to her body and misinterprets the color change as something "wrong'" and stops sexual activity.

4. **Orgasm** is associated with a sense of warmth in the pelvis and muscle contractions that last 3–15 seconds. Respirations may increase to 40 breaths per minute, depending on the patient's age. In patients who take tranquilizers as part of treatment, muscle contractions may not be as strong because the drug relaxes pelvic muscles. After a hysterectomy, the loss of uterine contractions may interfere with or prevent orgasm. Orgasm may be affected by an abdominal hysterectomy and damage of the pudendal or pelvic nerve.

5. **Resolution**, also called the refractory period, is the period when respirations, pulse, and blood pressure begin to return to pre-excitement level. After an orchiectomy some men experience scrotal and groin discomfort during resolution.

17. Give specific examples of how symptoms of cancer and its treatment may affect sexuality.

SYMPTOM	EFFECT ON SEXUALITY
Nausea/vomiting	Patients may not want to go out to restaurants or on a date. Use of anti-emetics may decrease sexual desire.
Skin and nail	Body image and self-image may be affected. For example, dry, less pliable skin from radiation treatment may make the patient feel unattractive. If toe sucking is part of usual sexual practice, toenail changes may affect frequency or enjoyment.
Stomatitis	May make kissing painful. If talk is painful, intimate communications with significant other may be difficult. Lesions may occur on vaginal as well as oral mucosa.

Table continued on following page

SYMPTOM	EFFECT ON SEXUALITY
Diarrhea	May affect patient's body and self-image in terms of loss of control. Patients may avoid social situations because of concern about closeness to bathroom. Rectum may become uncomfortable so that anal stimulation is no longer pleasurable.
Neutropenia	Risk of vaginal infections may increase, especially with decreased vaginal lubrication. Anal stimulation may be too risky because of potential for infection. Increased risk of sexually transmitted diseases.
Fatigue	Patients may need to discuss changes in sexual activity or positions during sex to conserve energy or want to change usual times of sexual activity to a time when energy level is highest.
Decreased platelets	Patient may bruise more easily during oral sex or nipple stimulation. Stimulation with nipple or penile rings may damage platelets. If patient engages in bondage and discipline, it may be helpful to change to soft restraints.
Changes in sense of smell	Body smells that used to have aphrodisiac effect may become too strong or unpleasant.
Neuropathy	Loss of sensation may decrease enjoyment of toe and finger sexual play.
Ototoxicity	Hearing the intimate whispers of a significant other may become more difficult and make aural sexual arousal more difficult.
Inability to return to school or work	Loss of mobility and diminished activity may decrease opportunities to meet potential partner and lower self-esteem or cause depression, thus decreasing libido.
Change in weight	Partner may be reminded of life-threatening diagnosis. Examples: discomfort when pelvic bones hit during coitus, clothes that no longer fit.
Decreased hormone levels	Orchiectomy or hormone treatment to decrease testosterone levels for metastatic prostate cancer may affect libido, decrease body hair, or cause testicular/scrotal atrophy. Decreased estrogen in women may decrease vaginal lubrication and cause dyspareunia.
Cardiac/pulmonary toxicity	May affect libido and ability to engage in strenuous sexual activity. Patients may need to change positions or use pillows to conserve energy. Advise patient about what to do if chest pain or shortness of breath occurs.
Alopecia	Single patients may be reluctant to date because of changed body image. Patient's partner may not want sexual contact because alopecia is daily reminder of cancer. Loss of pubic hair may be sexually exciting (increased genital sensation), or it may remind patient or partner of being a child so that sex is avoided because it feels like incest. If eyelashes are lost, patient's constant blinking may "turn off" partner.
Lymphedema	Body image may be affected. Affected limb may become so heavy or so large that it needs to be supported with pillows. Patients may have pain or decreased strength. Joint complications may affect range of motion, which in turn affects position during sexual play. Edema may compress nerves so that tactile sensations and pleasure are decreased. Skin may become fragile.
Pain	In anticipation of pain, a "plan for sex" (e.g., taking a pill 30 minutes before sexual play) may become necessary. Because many people enjoy spontaneous sex, this "plan" may interfere with desire or excitement. Orgasm releases endorphins and may provide pain relief for up to 6 hours.

18. How do changes in fertility affect sexual well-being?

Although reproductive ability is not specifically a sexual function, the meaning of fertility can affect a patient's perception of sexual well-being. Changes in fertility, whether temporary or permanent, may have positive, negative, or no effects on the patient's perception of his or her sexuality. It should not be assumed that infertility will have a negative effect for every patient; the topic needs to be addressed during sexual counseling.

Studies of elderly men after prostate surgery report that fertility is not of importance to men in their 70s or 80s. In the author's study, loss of fertility due to retrograde ejaculation was not a "concern" for many men, but each man commented on it. In fact, 20% of men, whether heterosexual or homosexual, voiced regret about perceived loss of fertility despite no desire to father children. Thus, fertility may be of concern to male patients, no matter what their age or sexual orientation.

19. What factors determine the effect of chemotherapy on fertility?

How chemotherapy affects fertility depends on the age of the patient (50% of women over the age of 35 who receive a single alkylating agent experience permanent infertility), type of chemotherapy agent, total amount of chemotherapy (combination chemotherapy is more likely than single-agent treatment to cause infertility), and whether any other treatment (e.g., radiation therapy, surgery) is given. Of importance is the drug threshold dose. The threshold dose results in permanent sterility regardless of the patient's age.

20. Give examples of chemotherapy drugs that affect fertility.

Drugs that affect both testicular and ovarian function include cyclophosphamide, busulfan, and nitrogen mustard. Chlorambucil, procarbazine, and nitrosoureas affect men, whereas L-phenylalanine affects women. Drugs with probable risk to testicular epithelium but unknown risk to ovaries include doxorubicin, vinblastine, cytosine arabinoside, and cisplatin. Drugs with unlikely risk to fertility for men or women include methotrexate, 5-fluorouracil, and 6-mercaptopurine. Vincristine is unlikely to affect male infertility.

21. How does chemotherapy affect fertility in children?

Although the primary focus of studies on fertility is adults, children also are affected by chemotherapy. For example, chemotherapy seems to have a greater effect on boys when it is given during puberty than when it is given before puberty. Chemotherapy does not seem to affect many prepubertal and pubertal girls because the immature ovary is relatively insensitive to chemotherapy.

22. What issues related to fertility and chemotherapy require further investigation?

How much time it takes for ovarian function to return to normal after chemotherapy and strategies to decrease the risk of infertility. Preliminary studies have looked at the use of oral contraceptives to protect ovarian function, but the results have been conflicting. Women in Australia have the option to freeze ova or embryos before treatment is begun, but ovum banking (cryopreservation) for women is still in the experimental stage in the United States. As a result, fertility issues for women have more to do with prevention by use of drugs less toxic to the gonads or shielding the ovaries during radiation therapy. In some cases the ovaries can be repositioned (oophoropexy) during radiation therapy.

23. How long after therapy completion should a person wait before deciding to have a child?

Although providers agree that pregnancy should be avoided during active treatment, there is no consensus about when it is safe to conceive. In general, most practitioners advise using birth control for a minimum of 6 months after treatment completion. It takes 6 months after treatment completion for men to complete the cycle from stem cell to development of mature sperm. The American College of Gynecologists recommends that most women with carcinomas should wait a minimum of 2 years after treatment completion. It has been reported that babies born within a year after treatment have lower birth weight and may have an increased risk of prematurity. The exception to the two-year waiting recommendation is women with a history of ovarian cancer, who should attempt pregnancy as quickly as possible because of the high recurrence rate.

24. What is sperm banking? What instructions should be provided to patients?

When cancer treatment may affect future fertility, men may choose to bank sperm for later use in artificial insemination or in vitro fertilization. To optimize the success of banking, men need to be able to provide adequate semen for storage. If they have a diagnosis of Hodgkin's disease, non-Hodgkin's lymphoma, or testicular cancer, the sperm count may be too low to bank. It is unclear why these particular diseases seem to cause low counts at diagnosis. Sometimes medications and anesthesia may contribute to the problem. Usually the average ejaculation consists of 2.5–3.5 ml of fluid with 50–80 million motile sperm in each milliliter. Ideally, the greater the number of specimens, the better. It is preferable for specimens to be given every 3 days. Because of the need for immediate treatment, men often have time for only one or two specimens over 2 days.

The following steps usually are taken before sperm banking is done: (1) tests are conducted for sexually transmitted diseases (including HIV and hepatitis); (2) a trial freeze is done on a sperm sample to assess the effects of cryoinjury; (3) an initial sperm analysis is done to determine percent of sperm with normal motility and shape; and (4) informed consent is secured after discussion of possible risks, costs, and benefits. If the patient has a rapidly growing tumor and treatment must be started immediately, sperm banking may be precluded.

25. How successful is sperm banking?

Sperm banking increases a sense of control. In vitro fertilization may be successful with a sperm count of 0.5 million motile sperm per milliliter, but larger numbers of motile sperm increase the success rate. When micromanipulation is used, the probability of pregnancy is 40%. Some men may choose to bank sperm with even lower sperm counts because intracytoplasmic sperm injection uses a single sperm.

26. Does banked sperm increase the risk of congenital deformities?

The risk of congenital abnormalities is reported to be less with thawed sperm than in the general population, even when sperm is stored for 15 years or longer.

27. What other issues are relevant to sperm banking?

Before banking is done, the nurse needs to talk with the patient about religious or cultural beliefs about self-stimulation. If the patient believes that masturbation is "wrong," sperm banking may not be an option. Some banks allow the man to have intercourse with his partner and use sperm collected in a condom, but this technique reduces the amount of sperm collected.

The potential sperm donor should be made aware of the personal financial obligation and legal implications. Sperm banking can be costly, if not covered by insurance. The patient needs to be aware of the costs of the required tests, storage, and artificial insemination. Besides the procedural complications, legal issues have emerged. For example, if the patient dies and the partner uses the sperm for impregnation, questions arise about whether the child is eligible for inheritance, father's military benefits, or other benefits. Some banks have a policy to destroy sperm when the donor dies, but others follow the Uniform Anatomical Gift Act when the donor gives the semen as a gift to his partner. The patient should be informed of all of these implications in order to make an informed decision and may want to consult with a lawyer.

28. What are the most common drugs that cause sexual dysfunction? Describe their effects.

DRUG	EFFECT ON SEXUALITY
Antihypertensive medications	Erection dysfunction, decreased vaginal lubrication. Retarded ejaculation, especially with monoamine oxidase inhibitors.
Antidepressants	May temporarily decrease erections or vaginal lubrication.
Tranquilizers	May decrease anxiety and improve sexual functioning. Retarded ejaculation. Large dose may decrease erection and vaginal lubrication. Relaxation of pelvic muscles may affect orgasm (i.e., loss of muscle tension decreases pleasure of orgasm).

Table continued on following page

DRUG	EFFECT ON SEXUALITY
Recreational drugs (e.g., cocaine, marijuana)	May cause euphoria and increase self-confidence. May increase tactile pleasure or may block sexual arousal and pleasure. May cause extended painful erections or painful ejaculations.
Anticholinergics	Affect arousal (decreased erection and vaginal lubrication).
Opioids	Less pain increases enjoyment of sex. Side effect of constipation may interfere with sexual activity. Long-term opioids may retard ejaculation.
Hormones	May decrease serum testosterone, which can affect sexual desire. Secondary sex changes (deepening of voice, increased facial hair) may affect body image.
Alcohol	Decreases libido. Decreased inhibitions may interfere with use of safer sex and thus increase risk for infection. Decreased vaginal lubrication and erection.
Antiadrenergics	Decrease libido, vaginal lubrication, and erection. May cause retrograde ejaculation.
Endocrine drugs	Hot flashes, dyspareunia due to decreased vaginal lubrication, and mood swings.
Chemotherapy	Alopecia, stomatitis, fatigue, anorexia, decreased immunity, nausea.

29. What factors determine the effect of radiation therapy on sexuality?

Radiation therapy affects patients in different ways, depending on the site of the radiation field, amount of rads delivered, previous level of health, and beliefs about radiation. Patients may have many misperceptions that need to be addressed. A patient may believe that radiation therapy is a "last-ditch effort" and therefore avoid sexual activity because of the belief that "terminally ill people shouldn't do that." Patients may have a total misunderstanding of how radiation works; they may worry that they are "radioactive" and so avoid contact of any kind. Other patients may understand how radiation therapy works, but their partner, who did not come to the clinic appointment, may worry that his "penis will glow in the dark" if they have sex.

30. What sexual side effects of radiaton therapy should the nurse be able to discuss?

- Decreased blood flow to genitals from vascular scarring (erection dysfunction, decreased vaginal lubrication)
- Skin changes (skin becomes too tender for partner to touch; skin texture or color changes)
- Fatigue (possible loss of libido)
- Shortening of vaginal vault
- Vaginal stenosis (causing pain with intercourse)
- Decreased vaginal sensation
- Alteration in sexual patterns
- Concern about bleeding
- Concern about possible recurrence
- Decreased skin sensitivity due to nerve damage
- Pelvic radiation may cause urethral irritation (women may experience pain with penetration or men with ejaculation)
- Infertility (testicular irradiation ≥ 10 Gy may result in irreversible azoospermia)
- Total body irradiation may delay puberty in boys. Young girls may not develop secondary sex characteristics.
- Alopecia in the irradiated field
- Delayed complications (e.g., fistula, rectal or ureteral stricture)

31. How does a laryngectomy affect sexuality?

Frequently, nurses forget to address sexuality when the site of the cancer or treatment does not directly affect a "sexual organ," such as the breast or testicle. Yet sexually neutral sites may have even more effect on sexual functioning. In dealing with the many aspects of treatment for patients with a head or neck tumor that requires laryngectomy, nurses may not be knowledgeable of how sexuality can be affected. The following are a few of the potential effects:

- Patients cannot whisper intimately into partner's ear.
- Partners may find it discomforting to feel the patient's breath on their neck. Wearing a T-shirt or stoma shield may help.
- During oral sex, pubic hairs may get caught in stoma and cause the patient to cough.
- Patient may have increased incidence of halitosis, which may be sexually unattractive.
- Coughing up a "gumba" (increased secretions) can be a turn-off.
- Increased respirations after orgasm may stimulate coughing.
- If patient and partner make love in the shower or hot tub, water may get in stoma.
- Limited neck mobility after radical neck dissection affects positioning during sexual activity.
- Visual appearance may affect ability to attract new partner.
- Body image is radically changed.
- Decreased range of motion of shoulder may affect positions.
- Patients cannot hold their breath at moment of orgasm.
- Patient and partners may be reminded of diagnosis of cancer whenever they see the incision site.

32. What are the special concerns of patients with same-sex partners?

Patients with same-sex partners experience the same physiologic changes from cancer and therapy, but they may be even more hesitant to ask questions. Thus, the challenge to the health care provider is not to learn unique facts about same-sex partners but instead to learn to be open and nonjudgmental so that patients can confide their concerns.

Most books and pamphlets about cancer and sexuality have a heterosexual bias (male and female partners on the covers), and the text refers primarily to "married couples." Opening up is even more difficult when professional or military/legal consequences must be considered. Often we contribute to the bias when we stress the importance of birth control during treatment. This can make the couple feel even more isolated and "invisible" to the provider.

33. How can the nurse combat heterosexual bias?

To combat heterosexual bias, the nurse may ask during the assessment, "Do you have a partner? Is your partner male or female, or do you have both?" Nurses should practice asking such questions until they feel comfortable. Nurses who are comfortable with same-sex issues will be surprised at the information they receive. Visiting policies should be expanded to include non-spouses. Nurses with strong feelings about same-sex partners should use the PLISSIT model (see question 4) and make the appropriate referral.

34. What specific issues may arise with same-sex partners?

As with all patients, cancer and its therapy can suppress bone marrow and compromise the immune system. Thus, nurses must assess specific sexual practices to make suggestions for decreasing the risk of infection or bleeding. If sex toys are used, advise the patient to avoid sharing the toy or to wash the toy carefully with soap and water to decrease the risk of infection. If the patient enjoys anal stimulation (heterosexual as well as homosexual patients may enjoy this because of the multiple nerve endings), caution the patient about how easily rectal tissue can be torn. Tears may result in bleeding and infection (when the patient is myelosuppressed). Although it is best to refrain from anal stimulation during therapy, the patient may choose to continue; in this case, nurses need to help the patient rethink risk-reduction strategies. Examples include liberal use of lubricant and keeping fingernails very short. Nurses who are uncomfortable with this issue should refer the patient.

35. What practical suggestions can nurses make to a patient with a new ostomy before their first postoperative sexual encounter?

- Wear crotchless panties or cummerbund.
- Empty appliance before activity.
- Use picture-frame appliance with tape.
- Cover appliance with a sexy cloth bag.

• Use vaginal lubricant.
• Tight seal decreases risk of odor.
• Towel or lining under the sheet may increase security.
• Use aftershave/cologne to increase confidence.
• Avoid "gassy" food (e.g., onions).
• Avoid "smelly" food (e.g., asparagus).
• Role play what to do if the appliance "slips."

36. What other sexuality-related issues may arise in patients with ostomy surgery?

Ostomy surgery affects body image. The degree of impact depends on the patient's developmental stage, how the partner reacts, and how the patient and partner usually cope with change or crisis. Help patients to communicate their concerns to their partner, or refer them for couple counseling if they so desire.

37. What physiologic changes are associated with ostomy surgery?

Decreased blood flow may affect vaginal lubrication or penile erection. After bladder surgery, it is not uncommon for the vagina to become shorter or narrower, which affects the comfort of normally used positions. Appliance deodorants are available to decrease the smell.

38. What is the value of ostomy support groups?

Tell patients about helpful strategies and encourage them to attend ostomy support groups so that they can discuss their concerns with others. Belonging to a support group provides the opportunity to hear guest speakers discuss sexual issues and to receive ostomy literature with information about sexuality.

39. How should I counsel patients who want to resume sexual activity?

Many nurses avoid this question, because they are concerned that answering it may require a lengthy session. If a patient asks the questions, the nurse's job is already half done, because the nurse has earned the patient's trust. If time is a factor, the nurse should find out what specific concerns the patient has and address those issues. The PLISSIT model (see question 4) is a sound guide. Patients may need only permission to have sexual contact or limited information or specific suggestions about what positions they can use. Most patients do not need intensive therapy, but they may appreciate being told how to obtain a pamphlet or book about sexuality after a diagnosis of cancer.

40. Provide a checklist of possible factors that nurses may want to consider.

• Body image, past sexual history, living arrangements
• Partner's reactions
• Fear of abandonment
• Performance anxiety ("spectator droop" may occur if patients concentrate only on physiologic response)
• Worry about pain. Patients should stop if they have pain. If they do so, their partners will then trust them and not refrain from touching them for fear of causing pain.
• Worry that sexual activity may cause recurrence.
• Nurses and patients alike should expect the unexpected.
• "Use it or lose it." If patients are older, the longer they do not engage in sexual activities, the more difficult (but not impossible) it may be to restart sexual play.
• Let patients role play communication skills.
• Patients should set aside plenty of time to explore; they should not rush. It may be wise to make a date for sex.
• Appropriate timing of activity (after nap, after pain medication, after bath) may increase enjoyment of sex.
• Patients should learn to rest during sexual activity. Sex does not have to be a "marathon" or a "race."

- Inform patients about available resources, including counseling services, books, pamphlets, and support groups.
- Patience (taking one day at a time) and a sense of humor help patients in their exploration of new sexual expressions.
- Skin is the largest sex organ, and the brain is the most important sex organ. Possibilities are limitless.
- Neither the diagnosis of cancer nor treatment side effects dictate what patients can or cannot do. They should use creativity and a sense of play.

41. How can sexuality be approached in patients who have had a mastectomy?

Discharge instructions should include information about the effect of surgery on everyday activities, such as how to wear a seat belt if the belt touches the surgical site. Incorporation into discharge teaching makes sexuality a part of the patient's life without isolating it as a taboo subject. Patients may be asked if they have thought about how they are going to sleep with their partner when they get home. Nurses may find it helpful to share their own experiences in order to promote the patient's comfort. This does not mean that you tell the patient about your entire sex life, but you may try to put her at ease without embarrassment. You are asking intimate questions that they may not have discussed with anyone in the past. Humor can backfire in discussing such a private topic but, depending on the interaction with the patient, may help to defuse the tension surrounding the topic of sex. For example, I ask if the mastectomy affected the partner's favorite breast. I comment that my husband and I sleep spoon fashion and that he tends to sleep holding my right breast. I joke that if my right breast were removed, I would think about putting Velcro on my chest so that he would not fall out of bed.

42. What practical suggestions can be made after mastectomy?

I offer to share the many practical suggestions gleaned over the years from my patients so that the woman can choose the ones that she wants to use. If she is going home with a drain in place, I remark that many women do not choose to have intercourse but do want to be held. Whether or not she chooses to have intercourse, she or her partner may worry about bumping or pulling the drain. Application of extra tape ensures that it is not pulled by mistake. If the woman does not want her husband to look "at such a horrible scar," I discuss body image and mention research with women who had mastectomies. Nurses found that if the woman hides in the bathroom or closet to dress and undress, it may take months or years before she feels comfortable enough to let her partner see the scar. I comment on the wasted anxiety and energy and suggest that it may be better to use the energy to heal themselves and fight the cancer.

43. How may breast cancer therapy affect menstruation?

Chemotherapy and hormone therapy may cause premature menopause. Menopausal symptoms may have a negative impact on sexual well-being, resulting in decreased vaginal lubrication, vaginal atrophy, or decreased androgen (which may decrease libido). In Europe, estrogen is prescribed for many women with breast cancer and menopausal symptoms. In the United States, concern that estrogen may trigger tumor growth, especially if the tumor is hormone-dependent, has discouraged this strategy. Clinical trials are under way to investigate this controversial issue.

44. What other issues may cause concern after mastectomy?

Regardless of gender, age, or cultural background, body image can be a major concern. Loss of a breast can affect posture and result in back pain or clothes that do not fit "right." Weight gain, which is common after a diagnosis of breast cancer, further affects body image and emotional well-being.

Patients who are single and without a steady partner may have many questions about if and when to tell a new partner. Encouraging patients to attend a support group or talk with a "Reach for Recovery" volunteer may help them to decide how to answer such questions. Whether single or in a relationship, patients often have concerns about abandonment. Investigators have found that divorce or separation rates are not higher after a diagnosis of breast cancer.

45. How should the nurse counsel a patient concerned about erectile dysfunction?

The first step is to ask exactly what concerns the patient. Do not automatically assume that you know what the "problem" is but allow the patient to tell you what he perceives. Often patients have tried strategies for erectile dysfunction. Thus, it is important to learn what they have tried and assess its safety. Unsafe techniques include using a vacuum cleaner to "suck" blood into the penis, using a rubber band at the base of the penis to hold blood in place, taping tongue blades to the penis to make it erect, or using "magic" potions that may interact with other medications.

Let him know that it is not uncommon after prostate surgery to have difficulty with erections. Limited information includes that touching will continue to bring pleasure and that an erection or intercourse is not necessary to maintain intimacy. Some men are so focused on the penis and whether it goes up or stays down that they forget about the other 90% of sexuality. This is not to belittle the concern but to remind patients that erection does not equal intimacy.

46. What is the nurse's role if the patient wants to pursue work-up and treatment options?

The nurse should provide anticipatory guidance about what to expect. The work-up includes laboratory tests, a thorough physical examination (including neurologic, peripheral vascular, and pelvic examination), evaluation of erectile function to assess firmness achieved at night, and psychological examination that includes a history of sexual practices. The patient's use of alcohol or tobacco also should be assessed because these products constrict the vascular system.

47. What treatment options are available for erectile dysfunction?

Treatment options are varied and depend on patient's desires and physical condition. Examples include external vacuum constriction devices (which draw blood into the penis to make it erect and have a success rate of approximately 90%), intracavernous injections (vasoactive drugs such as papaverine, prostaglandin E, and phentolamine), counseling, penile arterial reconstruction, and penile prosthesis (malleable rods, hinged prostheses, inflatable prostheses; one-piece, two-piece, and three-piece prostheses). Penile implants are especially helpful for men with venous leak who find the external vacuum unhelpful or unacceptable. When partners are counseled about implants, satisfaction is as high as 80%. The most recent treatment option is sildenafil citrate (Viagra), which is effective in over 50% of all men, no matter what the cause of erectile dysfunction. Because of possible contraindications and/or drug interactions, the nurse should be concerned about the possibility that patients can acquire sildenafil citrate through the internet without appropriate medical supervision.

48. What should a nurse know about sildenafil citrate?

Because the use of sildenifal citrate can be a complex issue, the nurse should be knowledgeable about how it works, contraindications, side effects, and what to teach the patient before suggesting its use. Sildenafil citrate works after a person becomes sexually excited; its does *not* cause engorgement if the person is not sexually excited.

49. What are the contraindications to use of sildenafil citrate?

Sildenafil citrate should not be used by patients taking nitrates or patients allergic to the drug. Because it can interact with other medications, other drug or herbal use should be assessed. Occasionally the dose must be adjusted if the patient is taking certain medications (e.g., protease inhibitors). Sildenafil citrate should be avoided or used with caution in patients with a history of cardiac problems, stroke, hypo- or hypertension, retinitis pigmentosa, kidney disease, liver disease, predisposition to priapism (e.g., sickle cell anemia, multiple myeloma, leukemia), Peyronie's disease, active peptic ulcers, or bleeding disorders. It should not be used if the patient is using any other method to obtain an erection. Patients need to be cautioned not to increase the dose without first talking to a nurse practitioner or physician. They should not lend it to friends or take it more than once daily.

50. Discuss the side effects of sildenafil citrate.

Side effects may include headache, facial flusing, upset stomach, stuffy nose, diarrhea, temporary changes in color vision, light sensitivity, or blurred vision. With proper screening, rarely do users experience heart attack, stroke, irregular heart beats, or death. Because permanent damage can occur, an erection lasting more than 4 hours needs to be reported immediately.

51. Does sildenafil citrate have role in the treatment of women?

Several studies have been conducted with mixed results. At present sildenafil citrate is not recommended for women.

52. What is retrograde ejaculation?

Ejaculate discharges into the bladder instead of the penis. Retrograde ejaculation can result from external radiation therapy as well as retroperitoneal or pelvic surgery that affects the bladder neck. It can affect sexual satisfaction of both partners. Men who are visually oriented may not enjoy it as much when they cannot observe the ejaculation. Their partner may miss the sensation of ejaculate during orgasm.

53. How is retrograde ejaculation treated?

Patient and partner can discuss with the nurse practitioner or physician the use of sympathomimetic drugs, such as ephedrine, that close the bladder neck and allow the ejaculate to go out the penis. These drugs also may be used by the man who desires to regain fertility. If the drug is not effective and retrograde ejaculation continues, sperm sometimes can be retrieved from the bladder. When fertility is an objective, the man may be asked to void immediately after ejaculation, or a catheter may be used to obtain fluid from the bladder. The specimen is then spun down to extract the sperm. Be sure to discuss whether religious or cultural beliefs prevent use of this strategy.

54. How can the nurse deal with religious or cultural taboos about discussing sexuality?

No nurse can learn every religious or cultural taboo, although it is helpful to learn about taboos in certain groups. For example, during the nursing assessment the patient may say that he is Buddhist but grew up in the Catholic religion; thus, his personal beliefs may be a mixture of both. Or the patient may be an Irish-American living in a rural environment, but if his wife is Japanese-American and he grew up in a Polish-American neighborhood, he may have his own unique mixture of beliefs.

Let patients know that sexuality is unique for each person. Acknowledge that you may say something that is either embarrassing or against their beliefs. Remind patient that your comments are not intended to offend, and ask them to let you know if you say or do anything that is offensive. Make it clear that as a nurse you are not embarrassed to ask patients if they have had a bowel movement or what size it was because that is part of nursing care. Therefore, you feel just as comfortable talking about a penis or a clitoris. Probably neither bowel movements nor sexual organs are topics of discussion at church or with friends, but they need to be discussed to give good nursing care.

55. How do you counsel a male patient who experiences painful intercourse?

If a man complains of pain during intercourse, it may be due to skin tears on the penile shaft. Tears may result from steroid use, which increases skin fragility, or the partner's decreased lubrication. Lubricated condoms may be a good strategy because they protect the skin, act as a barrier to decrease possible infection, provide lubrication, and protect the partner from excreted chemotherapy in body fluids the first several days after treatment. Postorchiectomy pain is more likely to occur after ejaculation. Lying in warm bath water can be beneficial. With time (a period of months), most men no longer have pain after ejaculation.

56. How do you counsel a female patient who experiences painful intercourse?

In general, more women than men experience pain with intercourse. Determine when the patient began to have dyspareunia and the cause. If she had a vaginal hysterectomy, she may have increased sensitivity to vaginal barrel distention, especially if she had a postoperative infection. Conversely, the patient may have a loss of vaginal sensation for several months. If she had an abdominal hysterectomy, the small nerves may have been severed, resulting in numbness in the mons for up to 12 months. If the pain is due to a shortened vagina or stenosis from either bladder surgery or radiation, the patient may need to stretch the vagina with dilators.

If the pain is due to decreased vaginal lubrication from treatments, suggest the use of lubricants. Many nurses and physicians offer a sterile lubricant because it is available in the hospital or clinic. I often tease the staff and remind them that the penis is certainly not sterilized before intercourse. Why, then, is sterilized lubrication needed? After several strokes, the jelly "balls" up, just as it would on a T-shirt. Thus, the woman has not only a dry vagina but also little "balls" rolling up and down in her vagina.

57. What types of lubricants may be recommended?

When discussing possible lubricants, keep safety in mind, but remember that the lubricant does not need to be equivalent to a hospital sterile field. Saliva and whipped cream are fine, but they dry quickly and are not really effective.

If the couple uses condoms for birth control, suggest water-soluble lubricants. Many lubricants can be bought in a drug store; patients do not need to go to a "sex shop" unless the experience would be fun for them. It may be embarrassing for patients to buy such products in the drugstore, especially if they know the clerk. Appropriate lubricants include Astroglide (BioFilm, Vista, CA) and Aqualube (Mayer Laboratories, Oakland, CA). Lubricants that help to replenish vaginal moisture but are not intended for use during coitus include Replens (Warner Wellcome, Morris Plains, NJ), Gyne-Moistren (Health Care Products, Memphis, TN), or Lubrin (Kenwood Laboratories, Fairfield, NJ). Nurses may want to keep samples in the clinic so that patient can take them home and try them.

Not all lubricants are comfortable to use. Caution women about lubricants that have perfume or dye, which may be irritating. For example, one type of body lotion feels warm when light air touches it. This sensation may be exciting and pleasurable on external skin but not on mucosa.

If patients are not using condoms or diaphragms, they can use a light vegetable oil for lubrication. It is inexpensive, easily obtained at any grocery store, not embarrassing to buy, edible, and light enough that, even with decreased vaginal lubrication, it flushes out and does not cause infection. Many women taking antiestrogen hormones find this option helpful.

58. Which positions are most comfortable or best to conserve energy?

If a limb was amputated because of cancer, discuss different positions that the patient may use. If patients used to feel muscle tension in the amputated limb during orgasm, they may still have phantom sensation. Multiple books are available with pictures demonstrating the use of pillows and different positions. Visit the library and bookstore so that you can make good recommendations. If the woman had an abdominoperineal resection, talk with her about positions in which her partner's penis does not hit the posterior vaginal wall. Sitting or lying on top may let her feel even more control and pleasure.

59. What other techniques help to conserve energy or enhance comfort during sex?

Patients may want to consider sexual activity in the morning when they are the least tired. (This is a problem if the couple has children who need help in getting up for school or breakfast). To enhance comfort during sex, the patient may want to consider taking a pain medication 30 minutes before having sex, taking a warm bath to loosen tight muscles, using pillows for support, or trying new sexual activities that are less tiring. If a hot tub is available, the water is a good place for sexual play and supports the patient while trying different positions for comfort. There are alternative forms of sexual stimulation, but before extolling the joys of toe sucking, make sure that the patient is interested in discussing options.

When making suggestions, think of how each activity that you suggest can be made safe for patients with specific conditions, such as neutropenia or thrombocytopenia. For example, if a neutropenic patient wishes to suck a partner's toe, you may want to remind the couple to trim the toenail so that it does not accidentally tear oral mucosa and put the patient at risk of infection.

Patients may fatigue easily but miss sexual play and want to explore new options. If their partner is male, the patient can use pillows to get comfortable, rest their head on the partner's belly and chew or mouth gently the partner's penis while listening to music or watching television. If the patient is male and his partner wants to chew on his penis, remind the partner not to do so if the platelet counts are low.

Often we forget to talk about the use of fantasy. Remind patients of the times when they were separated because of work or school and only talked on the telephone. Phone sex is not only fun but expends little energy. It is a great option for the patient who is in reverse isolation for neutropenic fever.

60. What resources are available for learning more about sexuality?

- American Association of Sex Educators, Counselors, and Therapists (AASECT)
  11 Dupont Circle, N.W., Suite 220
  Washington, DC 20036

- Mary-Helen Mautner Project
  For Lesbians with Cancer
  1701 L Street, NW, Suite 1060
  Washington, DC 20036
  (202) 332-5536

- Sex Information Education Council
  of the U.S. (SIECUS)
  130 West 42nd St., Suite 350
  New York, NY 10036-7802
  (212) 819-9770
  http://www.siecus

- United Ostomy Association, Inc.
  19772 MacArthur Blvd, Suite 200
  Irvine, CA 92714
  (800)- 826-0826

- American Cancer Society
  (800)-ACS-2345 or contact your
  local chapter
  http://www.cancer.org

- Planned Parenthood Organization
  810 7th Avenue
  New York, NY 10019
  (212) 541-7800
  http://www.plannedparenthood.org/

- Society for Scientific Study of
  Sexuality
  P.O. Box 29795
  Philadelphia, PA 19117
  http://www.ssc.wisc.edu/ssss/

The views expressed in this chapter are those of the author and do not reflect the official policy or position of the Department of the Army, Department of Defense, or the United States Government.

REFERENCES

1. Adams J, DeJesus Y, Cole F: Assessing sexual dimensions in Hispanic women: Development of an instrument. Cancer Nurs 20:251–259, 1997.
2. Annon JS: Behavioral Treatment of Sexual Problems: Brief Therapy. Hagerstown, MD, Harper & Row, 1976.
3. Blackwell DA, Elam S, Blackwell JT: Cancer and pregnancy: A health care dilemma. J Obstet Gynecol Neonatal Nurs 29:405–421, 2000.
4. Bruner DW, Boyd CP: Assessing women's sexuality after cancer therapy: Checking assumptions with the focus group technique. Cancer Nurs 21:438–447, 1998.
5. Chorost MI, Weber TK, Lee J, et al: Sexual dysfunction, informed consent, and multimodality therapy for rectal cancer. Am J Surg 179:271–274, 2000.
6. Gallo-Silver L: The sexual rehabilitation of persons with cancer. Cancer Pract 8:10–15, 2000.
7. Hordern A: Intimacy and sexuality for the woman with breast cancer. Cancer Nurs 23:230–236, 2000.
8. Miaskowki C, Buchsel P: Oncology Nursing: Assessment and Clinical Care. St. Louis, Mosby, 1999.
9. Padma-Nathan H: The pharmacologic management of erectile dysfunction: Sildenafil citrate (Viagra). J Sex Educ Ther 23:209–218, 2000.
10. Shifren JL, Braunstein GD, Simon JA, et al: Transdermal testosterone treatment in women with impaired sexual function after oophorectomy. N Engl J Med 343:682–688, 2000.
11. Springhouse Physician's Drug Handbook, 8th ed. Springhouse, PA, Springhouse Corporation, 1999, pp 971–972.
12. Sweet V, Servy EJ, Karow AM: Reproductive issues for men with cancer: Technology and nursing management. Oncol Nurs Forum 23:51–58, 1996.
13. Wilmoth MC, Spinelli A: Sexual implications of gynecologic cancer treatment. J Obstet Gynceol Neonatal Nurs 29:413–421, 2000.

49. SKIN BREAKDOWN

Marion Tolch, RN, BSN, CWOCN

1. Why are patients with cancer more at risk for skin breakdown?

Any patient who, because of pain or extensive disease, becomes increasingly chair- or bed-bound is at risk for skin breakdown due to pressure. Additional risk factors include malnutrition and moisture due to incontinence or wound drainage. Because pressure is not the only cause for skin breakdown, it is important not to label all skin breakdown as "pressure ulcers" or "bedsores."

2. What is the best way to identify patients who are at risk for skin breakdown?

Rather than waste preventive resources by assuming that all patients are at risk or relying solely on institutional and clinical judgment, a more consistent, reliable method is to use a tested risk assessment tool. One of the more frequently used instruments, the Braden Scale, has been tested in various settings, uses six subscales (sensory perception, moisture, activity, mobility, nutrition, friction and shear) to assess risk for skin breakdown, and is supported by the U.S. Agency for Health Care Policy and Research (AHCPR). Reliable skin assessment tools help nurses to detect patients at risk for skin breakdown. Initiation of appropriate treatment can decrease hospitalization costs through preventative nursing actions.

3. What standardized protocol is used to prevent skin breakdown?

In 1992, the U.S. Agency for Health Care Policy and Research (AHCPR) published clinical guidelines for prevention and treatment of skin breakdown (pressure ulcers). The prevention guidelines focus on four goals: (1) identifying at-risk patients who need prevention and their specific risk factors; (2) maintaining and improving tissue tolerance to pressure to prevent injury; (3) protecting against the adverse effects of pressure, friction, and shear; and (4) reducing the incidence of pressure ulcers through educational programs. These guidelines are available through the AHCPR Publications Clearinghouse at 800-358-9295.

4. What specific interventions help to maintain and improve tissue tolerance to pressure?

Caregivers should include the following as part of daily care:

1. Inspect skin thoroughly, with particular attention to bony prominences and creases prone to moisture.

2. Clean skin at the time of soiling and at appropriate intervals based on patient's needs.

3. Minimize environmental factors leading to dry skin; use moisturizers if necessary.

4. Minimize skin exposure to moisture, using topical moisture skin barriers and absorbent moisture pads.

5. Use proper positioning, transfer, and turning techniques to prevent friction and shearing damage. Examples include maintaining the head of the bed at the lowest degree possible, based on patient needs, and using devices such as trapezes, transfer boards, and turn/lift sheets to avoid dragging patients over bed or chair surfaces.

6. Identify factors influencing nutritional intake, and offer support and supplements as needed.

5. What interventions help to prevent damage due to pressure?

Pillows should be used generously to keep bony prominences (e.g., ankles, knees) from direct contact with one another. Avoid positioning the patient directly on the trochanter; even the smallest degree of turning may reduce surface pressure. Although heels usually sustain higher surface pressures than other bony prominences, heel pressures can be easily reduced by use of pillows or several thicknesses of flannel blankets under the calves. Uninterrupted periods of sitting should be avoided. When possible, patients should be taught to shift their weight frequently when sitting for extended periods.

6. Can "donuts" be used to prevent pressure ulcers?

Ring cushion donuts are not recommended because they increase venous congestion to the area and are more likely to cause than to prevent breakdown. Soft pillows, foam, or gel pads may be used to reduce pressure for chair-bound patients.

7. Discuss options for reducing surface pressures.

Options range from gel, air, or water mattress replacements or surface overlays to electric air flotation or air-fluidized beds. To date, research has not demonstrated that one approach is statistically more effective than another. Product selection, therefore, should be based on patient needs. For example, because pressure reduction for patients with cancer is frequently a long-term need, it may be more cost-effective to consider purchasing a 5-inch foam mattress replacement than renting an air mattress for months at a time. The Health Care Financing Administration (HCFA), which administers Medicare, has developed coverage criteria for reimbursement of support surfaces. Many health maintenance organizations (HMOs) and insurance carriers also require prior authorization for reimbursement of pressure-reducing surfaces. The nurse should be aware that pressure-reducing surface overlays still require frequent turning or repositioning of the patient to continue to reduce pressure over bony prominences.

8. How can family caregivers help to prevent skin breakdown?

For continuity of care, home caregivers should understand the causes of skin breakdown and the importance of their role in prevention. They should be taught the potential causes of skin breakdown; how to do a thorough skin assessment; proper positioning to decrease risk of pressure breakdown; and the importance of good hygiene in maintaining skin integrity.

As part of the skin assessment, caregivers may be taught how to evaluate an area of reddened skin for blanching. Blanching redness describes an area that becomes white when compressed by a fingertip. Nonblanching redness remains red after finger compression and is usually indicative of impaired circulation or already existing tissue damage.

9. How do I determine the most appropriate treatment for skin breakdown?

Treatment should be based on cause, size, condition, and location of breakdown. For example, treatment of breakdown due to moisture should focus on elimination or reduction of moisture, use of moisture barrier products, and absorbent linen or pads. Treatment of redness due to friction may include use of a protective dressing, such as a transparent dressing or a protective wafer barrier. Friction damage to heels can be alleviated with use of socks. Treatment of larger wounds that involve necrotic tissue (due to pressure) should include elimination of causative factors; debridement of necrotic tissue, if appropriate; cost-effective management of drainage; and protection of the wound base. Many of the occlusive dressings or hydrophilic wound products may not be absorbent enough to be cost-effective for larger wounds.

10. How can I be sure that all caregivers understand the rationale for specific interventions or treatment plans?

In addition to providing appropriate inservices and educational programs about skin assessment and care, it is helpful to provide care options in the form of flow sheets or algorithms that are user-friendly and readily accessible to all caregivers at the bedside. Once the condition of the wound has been confirmed, such algorithms can help the caregiver to identify facility protocols, appropriate care options, and available products for care. Below is an example of an algorithm developed for the assessment and management of moisture and incontinence.

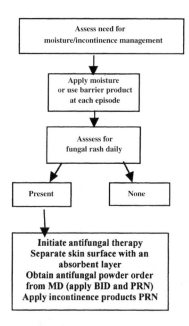

Adapted from Algorithm for skin care, University of Colorado Hospital, 2000.

11. Despite vigilant care, a bedbound patient may still develop a pressure ulcer over the coccyx. What is the appropriate treatment?

The AHCPR guidelines recommend three components for an effective pressure ulcer treatment plan, which should be addressed simultaneously:

1. **Nutritional assessment and support**
   - Low serum albumin (< 3.5) and less than ideal body weight in patients with cancer frequently contribute to skin breakdown.
   - If compatible with patient wishes and overall goal of care, adequate intake and supplements should be encouraged to maintain a positive nitrogen balance (approximately 30–35 calories/kg/day and 1.25–1.50 gm of protein/kg/day).

2. **Management of tissue loads**
   - Use positioning techniques, and avoid pressure to existing ulcer areas and other high-risk bony prominences.
   - Provide pressure-reducing support surfaces (e.g., mattress replacement or chair cushion), taking into consideration ease of use, maintenance requirements, and costs and reimbursement.

3. **Ulcer care**
   - Debride necrotic tissue as necessary, selecting the method most appropriate to the patient's condition and goals. Methods include sharp (scalpel), mechanical (wet-to-dry dressings), enzymatic (ointments), and autolytic (body's own immune system) debridement.
   - For wound cleansing in areas where healthy tissue is present, avoid use of cytotoxic agents such as hydrogen peroxide, Betadine, or Dakin's solution. Normal saline adequately cleans most wounds.
   - Use cost-effective dressings that protect, provide a moist environment, manage exudate, and maintain integrity of surrounding skin.

12. Are any dressings better than others?

Because no one product is appropriate for all wounds, selection should be based on size, condition, amount and type of drainage, and wound location. For example, a transparent dressing or hydrocolloid wafer (e.g., Stomahesive) may be inappropriate for a heavily exudating wound near the rectum but highly appropriate for small superficial breakdown on the outlying buttocks. Dressings that initially seem to be expensive in fact may be cost-effective because they decrease frequency of dressing changes.

13. How are pressure ulcers staged?

Staging of pressure ulcers is based on the degree of tissue damage observed. Wounds with necrotic surface cannot be staged until the necrotic tissue is debrided and the wound base is visible.

Stage I   Nonblanchable erythema of intact skin.

Stage II Partial-thickness skin loss involving epidermis and/or dermis. The ulcer is superficial and presents clinically as an abrasion, blister, or shallow crater.

Stage III Full-thickness skin loss involving damage or necrosis of subcutaneous tissue that may extend down to, but not through, underlying fascia. The ulcer presents clinically as a deep crater with or without undermining adjacent tissue.

Stage IV Full-thickness skin loss with extensive destruction, tissue necrosis, or damage to muscle, bone, or support structures.

14. List important wound care principles and treatment goals.

1. If a blister is intact and noninfected, avoid breaking it and keep it protected.

2. Rule of thumb for cleansing nonnecrotic wounds: if you would not put it in your eye, do not put it in a wound!

3. Use normal saline to cleanse clean, nonnecrotic wounds. Many other products may be appropriate for cleaning necrotic wounds but are cytotoxic for nonnecrotic wounds and may slow healing.

4. Granulation tissue is the "beefy red" tissue seen in partial-thickness wounds and is a sign of tissue regeneration.

5. If a wound is dry, apply a dressing or product to add moisture.

6. If a wound is wet, apply a dressing to decrease moisture but not dry it out.

7. Evaluate the patient for the cause of a rash; open wounds do not have a rash, but the surrounding skin may.

8. Necrotic tissue must be removed before the wound bed can be assessed or healing can occur.

9. As you debride a wound, the wound usually increases in size and moisture; you must adjust your treatment accordingly.

15. Does massage have a role in preventing skin breakdown?

AHCPR guidelines recommend that massage be avoided over bony prominences because of preliminary evidence that it may lead to deep tissue trauma. There is inadequate scientific evidence to support the theory that massage stimulates circulation.

16. Are Maalox and heat lamps still used?

The old Maalox-and-heat lamp recipe for treatment of open wounds is not appropriate. Clinical research has confirmed that the rate of healing is better in a moist environment. Conversely, healing is delayed when the wound bed is allowed to dry. Multiple wound care products that provide a moist environment for wound healing have replaced Maalox and heat lamps.

17. What can be done to secure dressings for patients with tape allergies?

1. Many of the newer tape products are hypoallergenic and less likely to cause skin problems.

2. A liquid sealant on the skin to be taped serves as a barrier to prevent allergies.

3. Pieces of ostomy barrier wafer may be applied to surrounding skin; then tape is applied to the wafer pieces instead of the skin.

4. Tubular stretch net dressing, which comes in many sizes, holds dressings in place and alleviates the need for tape.

18 Are any over-the-counter ointments or creams better than others?

Many good ointments and creams are on the market. The first step in choosing an appropriate product is to determine whether you need a moisture barrier or a moisturizer to maintain skin integrity and reduce friction damage. Label information usually identifies whether a product is a barrier, moisturizer, or both.

19. What are helpful hints for dealing with skin irritation around an ostomy?

The first step is to determine the cause of the irritation; the second step is to deal with the cause. Current ostomy products rarely cause skin allergies; however, an area of irritation that conforms to the outline of the wafer or tape may indicate an allergy. Irritation of the immediate peristomal area may be caused by infrequent pouch changes or too large of a stoma opening in the wafer barrier. In the immunosuppressed patient, a red rash with satellite lesions is suspicious of candidiasis, which is best treated with an antifungal powder (oil-based antifungals interfere with adherence of the pouch to the skin).

20. How is odor managed for a patient with a fungating wound due to necrotic tumor?

Odors from wounds can cause discomfort for both patients and caregivers. Odors result from an overgrowth of bacteria on necrotic and dying tissue. Daily wound cleansing and frequent dressing changes are the best ways to prevent and manage odor and should be emphasized. Many patients avoid this aspect of care because of inadequate pain control or tumor appearance. Cleansing options include a gentle hand-held shower or deodorizing wound cleansers. To keep dressings from sticking to the tumor surface (which causes bleeding and pain on removal), non-adherent dressings or wound gels may be used. In addition, antiseptic and astringent solutions such as Domeboro may lessen odors. Dressings should be adequately secured to keep odorous drainage from seeping through to clothing. When these measures fail, a short course of antibiotics may be used to reduce the anaerobic bacterial burden within the wound. Topical metronidazole also helps to decrease odor and eliminate infection from malodorous cutaneous ulcers.

ACKNOWLEDGMENT

The author thanks Mary Beth Flynn, RN, MS, CCRN, for her thoughtful review of the manuscript.

REFERENCES

1. Baranoski S: Skin tears: The enemy of frail skin. Adv Skin Wound Care 13(3):123–126, 2000.
2. Baranoski S: Wound assessment and dressing selection. Ostomy Wound Manage 41(7A):7S–14S, 1995.
3. Bergstrom N, Braden BJ, Laguzza A, Holman A: The Braden Scale for predicting pressure sore risk. Nurs Res 36:205–210, 1987.
4. Brylinsky CM: Nutrition and wound healing: an overview. Ostomy Wound Manage 41(10):14–24, 1995.
5. Bryant R (ed): Acute and Chronic Wounds: Nursing Management, 2nd ed. St. Louis, Mosby, 1999.
6. Chalk L: Wound prevention and healing: Everyone's problem. Surg Serv Manage 5(11):35–38, 1999.
7. Finley IG, Bowszyc J, Ramlau C, Gwiezdzinski Z: The effect of topical 0.75% metronidazole gel on malodorous cutaneous ulcers. J Pain Symptom Manage 11:158–162, 1996.
8. Hess CT: Fundamental strategies for skin care. Ostomy Wound Manage 43(8):32–41, 1997.
9. Hess CT: Skin care basics. Adv Skin Wound Care 13(3):127–129, 2000.
10. Panel for the Prediction and Prevention of Pressure Ulcers in Adults: Pressure Ulcers in Adults: Prediction and Prevention. Clinical Practice Guideline, Number 3. AHCPR Publication No. 92-0047. Rockville, MD, Agency for Health Care Policy and Research, Public Health Service, U.S. Department of Health and Human Services, 1992.
11. Rijswijk LV: The fundamentals of wound assessment. Ostomy Wound Manage 42(7):40–52, 1996.
12. Treatment of Pressure Ulcers: Clinical Practice Guideline, No. 15. AHCPR Publication No. 95-0652. Rockville, MD, Agency for Health Care Policy and Research, Public Health Service, U.S. Department of Health and Human Services, 1994.

VI. Oncologic Emergencies and Complications

50. CARDIAC TAMPONADE

Dawn Camp-Sorrell, RN, MSN, FNP, AOCN

1. What is cardiac tamponade?

Cardiac tamponade is a life-threatening emergency in which excessive accumulation of fluid or blood between the pericardium and heart prevents an adequate amount of blood from flowing into the heart to fill the ventricles. This excessive volume is usually between 200 and 1,200 ml, with a median volume of 500 ml. The rate of fluid accumulation, as well as the volume, is important in causing tamponade. Cardiac tamponade results from increased intrapericardial pressure, which leads to impaired diastolic filling, and low cardiac output (the amount of blood ejected by the ventricle). As blood is increasingly unable to flow into the heart, the patient exhibits the signs and symptoms of systemic venous congestion. Eventually circulatory collapse occurs.

2. How much fluid does the pericardial sac usually hold?

Under normal conditions the pericardium is a thin, tough, double-layered sac that encloses the heart with two distinct components: (1) visceral pericardium (covers the heart), and (2) parietal pericardium. Approximately 15–20 ml of pericardial fluid is located between the layers to prevent friction between the membranes during contraction and relaxation of the heart.

3. What is pericardial pressure?

Pericardial pressure is a reflection of the ability of the two membranes to adapt to changes in the fluid volume. An increase in the volume within the sac increases pericardial pressure.

4. What are the common signs and symptoms of cardiac tamponade?

Small effusions usually do not cause symptoms. Larger or rapid accumulation of fluid may cause epigastric or retrosternal chest pain that is relieved by sitting up or leaning forward (pain is more severe when the patient is supine); other signs and symptoms include dysphagia, cough, dyspnea, hoarseness, increased jugular vein distention, muffled heart sounds (pericardial effusion), pericardial friction rub (when tumor is present), tachycardia, and pulsus paradoxus.

5. Why do some patients present with symptoms whereas others are asymptomatic?

Symptoms depend on how the condition develops. As small effusions begin, the pericardium stretches gradually to accommodate the fluid pressure within the sac and the patient is asymptomatic. When the effusion progresses, causing an increase in pericardial pressure and a resultant decrease in ventricular expansion and diastolic filling, cardiac output drops, and the patient becomes symptomatic. Rapid fluid accumulation causes a rapid decrease in cardiac output and acute symptoms.

6. List the common causes of cardiac tamponade.

Infection	Heart failure
Primary cancer	Myocardial infarction
Cancer metastasis	Trauma
Central vascular catheter perforation	Drugs (e.g., anthracyclines, anticoagulants,
Autoimmune diseases	hydralazine, procainamide)
Renal failure	Dissecting aortic aneurysm
Chest irradiation	

7. What types of cancer can cause cardiac tamponade?

Autopsies prove that up to 21% of all patients with cancer have metastatic disease to the heart or pericardium. Although all cancer types can affect the heart, specific cancers with higher incidence include lung cancer, breast cancer, leukemia, lymphoma, mesothelioma, sarcoma, and melanoma.

8. Can pleural effusions lead to cardiac tamponade?

Yes. Cardiac tamponade may result from an increase in intrapleural pressure, which may be transmitted to the pericardial space.

9. Can cancer treatments cause cardiac tamponade?

Yes. Radiation affects the fine capillary stroma of the myocardium. Pericardial effusion may occur when up to 45 Gy is administered to the mediastinum. Chemotherapy, especially antitumor antibiotics, may affect the myocardial fibers and thus lead to pericardial effusion.

10. What is pulsus paradoxus?

Pulsus paradoxus results from an increase in intrathoracic pressure and is characterized by an exaggerated inspiratory fall in systolic blood pressure > 10 mmHg or > 10%. Pulsus paradoxus is measured by inflating the blood pressure cuff until no sounds are audible. The patient is asked to breathe in and out normally. During expiration, the cuff is gradually deflated until sounds are audible, at which point the pressure is recorded. The cuff is further deflated until sounds are audible during inspiration, at which point the pressure is again recorded. The difference between the two recorded pressures should be 5–10 mmHg.

11. Can pulsus paradoxus be present in other conditions?

Yes. Pulsus paradoxus may be present in chronic obstructive pulmonary disease, bronchospasm, or marked shifts in intrapleural pressure. Arrhythmias may hamper the measurement.

12. Which tests are used to diagnose a pericardial effusion?

A chest radiograph reveals only an enlarged heart shadow. An echocardiogram, computed tomography (CT), or magnetic resonance imaging (MRI) reveals a large pericardial chest effusion and can be used to estimate the volume of the effusion. The electrocardiogram (EKG) provides limited information, as results can be used to diagnose other cardiac abnormalities. Elevated ST segments, nonspecific T wave changes, decreased QRS voltage, and sinus tachycardia may be seen. A common EKG abnormality is the alternation of amplitude and direction of the P wave and QRS complexes on every other beat (electrical alternans). This abnormal finding is thought to result from variations in the position of the heart at the time of electrical depolarization.

13. Describe the treatment of a pericardial effusion.

The goal of treatment is symptomatic relief. In asymptomatic patients, the treatment may be to observe the patient instead of proceeding with an invasive procedure. In an emergency, cardiac tamponade is usually relieved by pericardiocentesis; a 16–18-gauge needle is placed into the pericardial sac to withdraw fluid. Surgical intervention depends on the cause of tamponade and the patient's overall condition. An indwelling pericardial catheter may be inserted to withdraw fluid or to instill medications. A pericardial window may be made to allow drainage of fluid into the surrounding tissue. A total pericardiectomy may be used if the window is not effective in relieving the tamponade and is indicated if the patient has constriction secondary to radiation therapy.

14. What are the complications of surgical intervention?

Potential complications include puncture of the right atrium, right ventricle, or coronary arteries; infection; dysrhythmia; and pneumothorax. Indwelling catheters may cause infection, catheter blockage, dysrhythmias, and pericarditis.

15. What does sclerosing mean? How is it used to relieve cardiac tamponade?

Sclerosing is a method used to produce an inflammatory response that eventually obliterates the pericardial space. The intent is to prevent reaccumulation of fluid. Several sclerosing agents have been used, including tetracycline, bleomycin, doxycycline, talc, and thiotepa. The patient must be premedicated with analgesics before the procedure, which can be very painful.

16. Is balloon angioplasty also used to treat cardiac tamponade?

Percutaneous balloon pericardiotomy may be used. A balloon is placed across the parietal pericardium. Inflation of the balloon creates an opening into the pericardium that allows internal drainage of the effusion into the pleural space for reabsorption.

17. Should the pericardial fluid be assayed?

To establish the diagnosis of malignancy and to rule out preexisting infection, the fluid should be assayed for lactate dehydrogenase (LDH), protein, specific gravity, glucose, cell count, cytology, and pH; it also should be cultured for bacteria and fungi. Most malignant effusions are serosanguineous or bloody and have malignant cells, alkaline pH, glucose, and increased LDH.

18. What assessment parameters must be included in the care of patients with cardiac effusion?

The assessment should include frequent auscultation of heart sounds and blood pressure; palpation of the apical pulse and peripheral pulses; observation for jugular venous distention; and checking the extremities for cyanosis, coolness, and edema. Up to 12% of patients have reoccurrence of fluid after treatment and therefore should be monitored closely.

19. What is the prognosis for a patient with cardiac tamponade?

Prognosis depends on rapidity of fluid accumulation, stage of disease at time of diagnosis, presence of metastatic disease, performance status of the patient, and effectiveness of treatment. Life expectancy ranges from a few hours to years; the average duration of remission is 4–6 months.

20. Can radiation therapy be used to treat cardiac tamponade?

If cardiac tamponade is of gradual onset and caused by a radiosensitive tumor such as lung or breast cancer or lymphoma, radiation therapy may be the treatment of choice. Usually 200–400 Gy of external radiation is delivered to the heart, pericardial structures, and lower mediastinum. In most patients who have received previous mediastinum radiation (e.g., for Hodgkin's disease), the maximal dose to the pericardial region has already been used.

21. What supportive care strategies can be used?

To ease the patient's suffering, the nurse can provide emotional support, administer oxygen, reposition the patient to enhance circulation, assist with all activities, administer analgesics, encourage relaxation techniques, and administer antianxiety or other medications as prescribed. Infusion of intravenous fluids is initiated to increase systolic pressure, thereby increasing effective ventricular filling pressure. Vasoactive drugs may be ordered to increase heart rate and contractility.

REFERENCES

1. Beauchamp KA: Pericardial tamponade: An oncologic emergency. Clin J Oncol Nurs 2:85–95, 1998.
2. Bishiniotis TS, Antoniadou S, Katseas G, et al: Malignant cardiac tamponade in women with breast cancer treated by pericardiocentesis and intrapericardial administration of triethylenethiophosphoramide (thiotepa). Am J Cardiology 86:362–364, 2000.
3. Keefe DL: Cardiovascular emergencies in the cancer patient. Semin Oncol 27:244–255, 2000.
4. Knoop T, Willenberg K: Cardiac tamponade. Semin Oncol Nurs 15:168–173, 1999.
5. Maher EA, Shepherd FA, Todd TJ: Pericardial sclerosis as the primary management of malignant pericardial effusion and cardiac tamponade. J Thorac Cardiovasc Surg 112:637–643, 1996.

51. DISSEMINATED INTRAVASCULAR COAGULATION

Carol S. Viele, RN, MS

1. What is disseminated intravascular coagulation?

Disseminated intravascular coagulation (DIC) is a process that occurs with generalized activation of the hemostatic system, which results in widespread fibrin formation followed by lysis within the vascular system. DIC may result in consumption of both platelets and clotting factors as well as formation of microthrombi.

2. What causes DIC?

DIC does not occur in isolation; it is always a symptom of underlying disease. Of the many disease processes that can cause DIC, one of the most important is cancer. DIC is the direct response to the presence of specific proteins or procoagulants, which may be secreted by malignant cells. Tissue factor, tumor necrosis factor (TNF), and cell proteases are among the proteins responsible for initiating DIC.

3. What is the mechanism of bleeding in DIC?

Fibrin degradation products and D-dimers are almost always abundant in DIC and frequently clump together. These fragments or clumps, particularly D-dimers, competitively inhibit the formation and action of thrombin by binding to thrombin at its fibrinogen receptor site. These fragment complexes, if soluble, may deposit indiscriminately throughout the vasculature. Others bind abnormally to preexisting, growing microthrombi, weakening clot structure. This is the clotting mechanism of DIC.

The mechanism of bleeding comes from the failure of the clotting cascade, which results in systemic release of fibrinogen, fibrin degradation products, or D-dimers. This release creates a host of circulatory disturbances, including the formation of small fragments that inhibit platelet function, large fragments that induce platelet clumping, and mixtures of soluble fragments that may increase capillary permeability, cause extravascular coagulation, and disturb endothelial activity. The result is significant bleeding throughout the vascular system. Both thrombosis and bleeding occur from many areas at the same time.

4. What types of malignancies are associated with DIC?

Both solid tumors and leukemia have been reported to cause DIC. Patients with mucin-secreting adenocarcinomas, prostate carcinoma, or disseminated carcinomas are at highest risk for developing DIC. In addition, all leukemias, to various extents, may induce DIC. However, promyelocytic leukemia (M3) is almost universally associated with the development of some degree of DIC.

5. What are some other causes of DIC in persons with cancer?

Infection is the most common cause of DIC. Gram-negative organisms triggering sepsis may be the culprit. DIC is also seen in gram-positive bacterial sepsis and viremias, most often involving varicella, hepatitis, and cytomegalovirus (CMV). Patients also may develop DIC from intravascular hemolysis secondary to multiple transfusions of whole blood and transfusion reactions. At times, the administration of chemotherapy may cause destruction of blast cells, releasing substances with procoagulation properties.

6. What is the difference between acute and chronic DIC?

DIC can be divided into acute and chronic forms. Acute DIC develops rapidly over a period of hours. The patient presents with sudden bleeding from multiple sites. It must be treated as a medical emergency. Chronic DIC may be subclinical and develop over a period of months. Eventually, however, it evolves into an acute DIC pattern with hemorrhage or thromboembolic episodes.

7. What are the symptoms of DIC?

The most common sign of DIC is bleeding, usually manifested by ecchymosis, petechiae, and purpura. The patient usually presents with bleeding from multiple sites, including skin, nose, gums, lungs, and central nervous system. This bleeding may range from the continuous oozing of venipuncture sites or wounds to uncontrollable hemorrhage that will lead to shock and death unless intervention is swift and effective. If DIC persists for more than a few hours, hemorrhages may be extensive and involve the pleura and pericardium. When this occurs, patients may complain of dyspnea and chest pain.

8. How is DIC diagnosed?

DIC is diagnosed on the basis of clinical presentation plus laboratory evidence of abnormalities. The activated partial thromboplastin time is a less helpful test for diagnosing DIC except in severe cases because it may be physiologically prolonged in children and masked by elevated factor VIII in adults.

Laboratory Abnormalities Associated with DIC

TEST	ABNORMALITY
Platelet count	Decreased
Fibrin degradation products	Increased
Prothrombin time	Prolonged
Activated partial thromboplastin time	Prolonged
Thrombin time	Prolonged
Fibrinogen	Decreased

9. How is DIC managed?

The overall management of DIC is highly controversial because of the lack of controlled studies. The immediate goal of therapy is to stop the patient from actively bleeding and clotting. However, the most important component in the management of DIC is to treat the underlying disorder. Management of DIC can be divided into two categories: use of blood component therapy and use of medications.

10. Describe the use of blood component therapy.

Platelet concentrates, cryoprecipitate, and fresh frozen plasma are frequently used to attempt to control the bleeding associated with DIC. Patients should not be automatically transfused; transfusion is appropriate only when the diagnosis is well established with documented depletion of factors. The exception, of course, is a life-threatening situation with little time to establish a diagnosis. Replacements for thrombocytopenia include 10 units of random donor platelets or a single unit of donor hemapheresed platelets. Hypofibrinogenemia (e.g., fibrinogen level < 100 mg/dl) may be treated with 8 units of cryoprecipitate. A prolonged prothrombin time due to a factor deficiency may be corrected by administering two units of fresh frozen plasma. Depending on the severity of DIC, replacement therapy may need to be given and repeated every 8 hours, with adjustments for platelet count, prothrombin time, activated partial thromboplastin time, fibrinogen level, and volume status. Replacements are discontinued when levels are normal or near normal.

11. Which medications may be used to treat DIC?

There are a variety of medications that can be used in the management of DIC. The choice of medication depends on the patient's condition.

Disseminated Intravascular Coagulation 451

Heparin. Because the patient with DIC has evidence of clotting in addition to bleeding, heparin is used to prevent further clotting. It is indicated as a treatment for DIC in acute promyelocytic and acute monocytic leukemia during induction therapy. Heparin is also used for DIC-induced thromboembolic complications in large vessels and prior to surgery in patients with metastatic carcinoma. The recommended dose of heparin is 4–5 U/kg/hr by continuous infusion.

Antithrombin III (ATIII). ATIII concentrate has been used as treatment for patients with DIC, either alone or in combination with heparin. To date, no definitive studies have shown a decrease in mortality with use of ATIII.

Fibrinolytic inhibitors. Fibrinolytic inhibitors are used only in the setting of an undeniable threat to hemostasis—that is, bleeding that has not responded to any other measures. The agent most commonly used is epsilon aminocaproic acid (Amicar). Epsilon aminocaproic acid (EACA) is a protease inhibitor that is uniquely reactive with plasminogen activators. It inhibits spontaneous fibrinolytic activity. A standard loading dose of 4–6 gm followed by 6–12 gm/day in divided doses provides sufficient plasma concentration to preserve the fibrin of a hemostatic vascular plug. The adverse effects are gastrointestinal disturbances, muscle necrosis, impotence, and the risk of creating clots in the urinary tract and bladder in patients with renal bleeding and hemorrhagic cystitis.

12. What is the controversy over the use of heparin for DIC?

Heparin may be given to inhibit factors IX and X, enhancing the neutralization of thrombin and halting the clotting cascade. However, hemorrhage is one of the main causes of death in patients with DIC, and heparin may induce bleeding. Heparin therapy is not indicated in patients who bleed in areas that compromise important functions (e.g., intracranial or intraspinal hemorrhage). Heparin therapy should be stopped if the patient has any life-threatening bleeding episode. Sometimes physicians think it is safer to use factor replacement therapy, especially if the underlying cause, such as infection, can be treated successfully.

13. What is the prognosis of patients diagnosed with DIC?

Both DIC and the patient's underlying disorder contribute to the high mortality rate. Mortality is correlated independently with the extent of organ or system involvement. It is also correlated with the degree of hemostatic failure and increasing age of patient at onset. Mortality rates in various studies have been reported to range from 42–86%, whether or not heparin was used to treat DIC.

14. What nursing interventions are important to patients with DIC?

Bleeding is the major symptom associated with DIC. Nurses should assess the patient for any signs or symptoms of bleeding. It is essential that a thorough and organized approach be used when assessing the patient suspected of having DIC with a physical assessment performed at least every 4 hours. Starting with the skin, the nurse should inspect the patient from head to toe, including palms of the hands and soles of the feet, looking for petechiae or bruising. Particular attention should be paid to the sclera and buccal mucosa. The patient should also be asked about vision changes. Blurred, cloudy, or diminished vision may indicate retinal hemorrhage and should be reported to the physician immediately. The nurse also should inspect the oral cavity, evaluating for bleeding, ulcers, or hematomas. A mouth care regimen is imperative for patients with DIC because oral cavity bleeding may be significant. Both nares should be inspected for signs of bleeding; epistaxis may be a significant source of blood loss. The inspection proceeds to the chest, back, abdomen, groin area, and lower extremities. Pressure areas should be inspected closely because they are common sites of petechiae, hematomas, and ecchymoses.

15. What can be done to stop bleeding from a central line site?

Bleeding from a central line site is common until DIC is under control. Many leukemic patients with DIC require central line dressing changes every 2 hours because of bleeding. Pressure should be applied during each dressing change for at least 5–10 minutes to reduce oozing. If pressure is not sufficient, Gelfoam sponges may be used at the exit site to enhance hemostasis.

An alternative method is to apply topical thrombin to the Gelfoam sponges in an effort to control bleeding. Once the bleeding has stopped, do not remove the topical thrombin-soaked sponge until it falls off, or the site may again begin to bleed. The Gelfoam sponge usually falls off when clotting conditions have returned to normal. A patient may lose units of blood from the central line site with close to 100 ml of blood contained within each hematoma.

16. What other critical areas should the nurse assess?

After a thorough inspection of the skin, the nurse should assess the chest cavity, including the heart and lungs, and the abdominal cavity, including the liver, spleen, and bowels. Because patients with DIC may develop diffuse alveolar hemorrhage, listening for rales, rhonchi, or areas of decreased breath sounds is important. Any positive finding, in addition to signs or symptoms of respiratory distress such as dyspnea, shortness of breath, nasal flaring, and increased respiratory rate, should be reported.

17. What other medical emergencies may occur with DIC?

In some patients, cardiac tamponade may result from DIC and thrombocytopenia. This is an obvious medical emergency. Signs of tamponade may be acute in onset and include chest pain and shortness of breath. See chapter 50 for more information on cardiac tamponade. Patients with DIC may have symptoms of abdominal pain due to ischemic bowel. Abdominal examination should include listening for bowel sounds in all four quadrants, noting any areas of decreased or absent bowel sounds. Evaluation also should include palpation and observing for peritoneal signs, indication of rebound tenderness, or a fluid wave due to bleeding in the abdominal cavity. The liver and spleen should be palpated and percussed to determine size and degree of tenderness. Any abnormal findings should be noted and reported to the physician. Urine and stool should be inspected for any sign of blood.

18. How else can the nurse offer support to patients with DIC?

The nurse's role in the care of patients with DIC also includes both patient and family education. Explaining the syndrome, along with the expected treatment, whether it be blood components, heparin, and/or an antifibrinolytic, is important. Patients and families are especially anxious because of the symptoms of DIC. Every effort should be made to explain the cause, treatment, side effects, and goals in the simplest way possible. Explanations should be repeated as often as necessary to reduce anxiety and increase patient understanding. Fear is prevalent because the patient looks quite different from normal, and bleeding is a scary symptom. Many people ask how long the bleeding will last; it is important to be honest and to let them know that bleeding time varies with each individual. The most important nursing intervention is to provide safe care during this stressful time.

REFERENCES

1. Arkel Y: Thrombosis and cancer. Semin Oncol 27:362–374, 2000.
2. Carey M, Rodgers G: Disseminated intravascular coagulation: Clinical and laboratory aspects. Am J Hematol 59:65–73, 1998.
3. Gobel BH: Bleeding disorders. In Groenwald S, Frogge M, Goodman M, Yarbro C (eds): Cancer Nursing: Principles and Practice, 5th ed. Boston, Jones & Bartlett, 2000, pp 869–875.
4. Gobel BH: Disseminated intravascular coagulation. Semin Oncol Nurs 15:174–182, 1999.
5. Hathaway W, Goodnight S: Disorders of Hemostasis and Thrombosis: A Clinical Guide. New York, McGraw-Hill, 1993, pp 219–229.
6. Jandl J: Disseminated intravascular coagulation. In Jandl J (ed): Blood: Textbook of Hematology, 2nd ed. Boston, Little, Brown, 1996, pp 1440–1447.
7. Kurtz A: Disseminated intravascular coagulation with leukemia patients. Canc Nurs 16:456–463, 1993.
8. Linker C: Blood. In Tiennery L Jr, McPhee S, Papadakis M (eds): Current Medical Diagnosis and Treatment. Norwalk, CT, Appleton & Lange, 1994, pp 415–466.
9. Schafer S: Oncologic complications. In Otto S (ed): Oncology Nursing, 2nd ed. St. Louis, Mosby, 1993, pp 376–440.
10. Seligsohn U: Disseminated intravascular coagulation. In Beutler E, Lichtman M, Coller B, Kipps T (eds): Williams' Hematology, 5th ed. New York, McGraw-Hill, 1995, pp 1497–1516.

52. HYPERCALCEMIA OF MALIGNANCY

Gari Jensen, RN, BSN

1. Define hypercalcemia.

Hypercalcemia is a common oncologic emergency in which the serum calcium level is above normal parameters. Although there may be variations among institutions, normal serum calcium is generally considered to be 8.5–11 mg/dl of blood. Hypercalcemia occurs when serum calcium levels exceed 11.0 mg/dl. A serum level of 12–14 mg/dl is considered to be moderate hypercalcemia and may or may not be associated with symptoms. Severe hypercalcemia (> 14 mg/dl) is usually symptomatic. Calcium measurements sometimes are expressed in mmol/L, according to the Système International d'Unités (SIU). The conversion factors are as follows: 1.0 mg/dl = 0.2495 mmol/L or 1.0 mmol/L = 4.008016 mg/dl. Normocalcemia is 2.12–2.74 mmol/L.

2. What causes hypercalcemia?

In the general population, hyperparathyroidism is the most common cause of hypercalcemia. Hypercalcemia caused by cancer is called hypercalcemia of malignancy (HCM) or tumor-induced hypercalcemia (TIH).

3. How common is HCM?

HCM is the most common syndrome associated with cancer and occurs in 10–20% of patients with cancer. The highest incidence is in patients with breast cancer (40–50%) or multiple myeloma (20–50%). HCM also is associated with squamous cell and large cell carcinoma of the lung, squamous cell carcinoma of the head and neck, renal carcinoma, lymphomas, leukemias, and prostate, ovarian, and gastric cancers, but it may be found in any cancer. HCM is usually seen in advanced cancer when tumor burden is heavy.

4. How do patients with HCM usually present?

Because it frequently presents with nonspecific symptoms commonly associated with cancer and its treatment, HCM may be overlooked. The usual clinical picture includes fatigue, lethargy, weakness, nausea and anorexia, constipation, dehydrated appearance, decreased mental functioning, thirst, and polyuria. Patients with mild-to-moderate HCM may be asymptomatic.

5. Why is HCM considered an oncologic emergency?

If HCM goes undiagnosed and untreated, about 50% of cases rapidly progress to renal failure, hypotension, severe dehydration, coma, and death. Patients with chronic HCM are at risk for serious complications from hypercoagulative states and widespread calcifications.

6. How is hypercalcemia diagnosed?

Hypercalcemia can be diagnosed through simple blood tests—either calcium and albumin level or ionized calcium level. Ionized or free calcium is the physiologically active form of calcium circulated in the blood. Of the total serum calcium, only about 50% is ionized; 40% is bound to plasma proteins (primarily albumin); and 10% is bound in complexes with substances such as citrate, phosphate, and sulfate.

7. How is the cause of hypercalcemia diagnosed?

After a state of hypercalcemia is identified, the cause must be determined. In patients with cancer the history is usually sufficient because of the dramatic onset and strong association of HCM with advanced cancer. In hyperparathyroidism the onset is usually gradual and less severe. Assessment of parathyroid hormone level is also useful; the level is elevated in hyperparathyroidism but normal or depressed in HCM.

8. How is ionized calcium calculated?

Ionized calcium can be measured directly, but at many institutions this test is not used because of greater expense, lack of availability, or habit. Traditionally, the serum calcium level is assessed and corrected on the basis of the serum albumin level. The corrected serum calcium is obtained by adjusting the calcium level upward by 0.8 mg for every gram of albumin under 4 gm/dl or downward by 0.8 mg for every gram of albumin over 4 gm/dl:

1. Subtract the albumin level from 4.0.
2. Multiply the difference by 0.8.
3. If the result is a positive number, add it to the serum calcium; if it is a negative number, subtract it.
4. The answer is the corrected calcium.

For example, RG, a 76-year-old African-American man with a history of multiple myeloma, presents with mild confusion and disorientation, lethargy, and decreased appetite. His wife states that his mental status has steadily declined over the past week. Serum calcium level is 11.4 mg/dl, and albumin level is 1.9 gm/dl:

1. $4.0 - 1.9 = 2.1$
2. $2.1 \times 0.8 = 1.7$
3. $11.4 + 1.7 = 13.1$

The corrected calcium level, 13.1 mg/dl, indicates moderate HCM; it is significantly higher than the uncorrected serum calcium level of 11.4 mg/dl.

9. What are the functions of calcium in the body?

Calcium is essential in the formation and maintenance of bones and teeth, contractility of muscle cells, transmission of nerve impulses, and normal clotting mechanisms. It also is involved in cardiac automaticity, many enzyme reactions, white blood cell chemotaxis, and cell-membrane permeability.

10. Describe the effects of excessive calcium.

Excessive calcium depresses neuromuscular function, causes increased contractility and irritability in the heart, interferes with antidiuretic hormone (ADH), promotes blood clotting, and may result in deposition of calcium outside the skeletal system, especially in the kidneys.

11. What are the major mechanisms for regulating calcium?

Calcium is regulated through bone formation and resorption, gastrointestinal (GI) absorption, and urinary excretion. These mechanisms are controlled by three hormones: parathyroid hormone (PTH), vitamin D (cholecalciferol), and calcitonin.

12. Describe the mechanism of bone formation and resorption.

The bones of the skeletal system are the major repository of calcium stores. Depending on need, osteocytes differentiate into osteoblasts or osteoclasts. When serum calcium is elevated, osteoblasts secrete collagen to form a bone matrix in which calcium can be deposited. When serum calcium is low, osteoclasts erode existing bone, resulting in calcium resorption (release) into the serum.

13. How do the GI tract and kidneys regulate calcium?

The GI tract, through the mediation of vitamin D, can increase calcium levels by increasing absorption of calcium ingested through diet. The kidneys are able both to conserve and to eliminate calcium. They also play an indirect role in intestinal absorption by converting vitamin D to its active form.

14. How does PTH control calcium regulation?

PTH has an integral role in calcium regulation through effects on all three of the major mechanisms. Released from the parathyroid gland in response to a drop in serum calcium, it directly acts on bone by stimulating increased osteoclast formation and activity and by inhibiting osteoblasts. PTH also has a direct effect on the kidneys by stimulating increased resorption of calcium and inhibiting resorption of phosphorus. Limiting phosphorus resorption minimizes the formation of hydroxyapatite crystals, the form in which calcium is deposited into bone. PTH indirectly stimulates the GI tract to increase calcium absorption by causing the kidneys to convert vitamin D (cholecalciferol) to its active form, 1,25-dihydroxycholecalciferol.

15. Describe the role of vitamin D in calcium regulation.

Vitamin D has a paradoxical role in calcium regulation. After conversion to its active form, 1,25-dihydroxycholecalciferol, its primary effect is to increase calcium and phosphorus absorption from the intestinal mucosa. It also stimulates resorption of calcium and phosphorus by the kidneys. Bone formation is promoted by the abundance of both calcium and phosphorus. When calcium levels are inadequate, vitamin D stimulates bone resorption and release of calcium into the serum.

16. How does calcitonin affect calcium levels?

Calcitonin is released by the thyroid gland in response to high serum calcium levels. It has an antagonistic relationship with PTH but is of short duration. By inhibiting osteoclast formation and activity, it reduces calcium release into circulation as a result of bone resorption. It also increases osteoblast activity and thereby promotes calcium deposition. In addition to its effect on bone, calcitonin works through the kidneys by inhibiting calcium and phosphorus resorption.

17. What causes HCM?

It was once thought that HCM resulted from release of calcium by bone after its invasion and destruction by cancer cells. A troubling aspect of this theory was that no reliable correlation could be found between amount of bone destruction and level of serum calcium. In fact, hypercalcemia may be present without bone metastases. Understanding is limited, but researchers have identified a number of substances secreted or mediated by cancer cells that cause or have some association with HCM. One of the most significant is parathyroid hormone-related protein (PTH-rP). Others include osteoclast-activating factors (OAFs), transforming growth factors (TGFs), and prostaglandins of the E class (PGEs).

18. Discuss the role of parathyroid hormone-related protein (PTH-rP).

PTH-rP closely resembles PTH. It exerts the same effects on the regulation of calcium but is not regulated by the normal feedback mechanisms that suppress PTH. Whereas in response to hypercalcemia PTH levels decrease, PTH-rP is unaffected and continues to stimulate osteoclast activity and increased calcium resorption by the kidneys. Osteoclast breakdown of bone may enhance the opportunity for cancer cells to attach, invade, and release collagen fragments and degradation products, which may be chemotactic for cancer cells. Spectrum immunoradiologic assays have detected PTH-rP in 80–90% of patients with HCM. It is associated with cancer of the kidney, lung, head and neck, GI tract, and genitourinary system as well as with hematologic cancers.

19. What other factors contribute to the development of HCM?

1. Immobilization results in increased resorption (release) of calcium from bone.
2. Thiazide diuretics decrease renal excretion of calcium.
3. Patients may continue to take calcium supplements and vitamin D without realizing that they are contributing to the development of HCM.
4. Androgens, estrogens, and antiestrogens have precipitated HCM in some cases. The onset is usually dramatic, within the first 2 weeks of therapy.
5. Some breast cancers and lymphomas convert vitamin D to its active state.
6. Granulocyte-macrophage colony-stimulating factor (GM-CSF) may stimulate osteoclast formation after interleukin-1 (IL-1) stimulation.

20. Is dietary restriction of calcium necessary?

Dietary restriction of calcium is usually not necessary because calcium absorption from the GI tract is already decreased by negative feedback mechanisms and frequently by anorexia, nausea, and vomiting.

21. Describe the pathologic process of HCM.

Tumor secretion of PTH-rP and other tumor-derived or tumor-mediated substances causes calcium release from bone secondary to osteoclast activity and increased reabsorption of calcium from the renal tubules. As the calcium load increases, it interferes with the ability of the kidneys to reabsorb sodium, which leads to sodium and water loss through polyuria. Common symptoms of cancer and cancer therapy (nausea, vomiting, and anorexia) contribute to the developing dehydration and are worsened by the effects of rising calcium levels on the GI tract. The dehydrated state becomes self-perpetuating. Immobilization from weakness, fatigue, and bone pain caused by hypercalcemia further increases resorption of bone.

22. What are the signs and symptoms of HCM?

Mental status and vision

Fatigue	Visual disturbances	Lethargy	Somnolence
Weakness	Confusion	Apathy	Stupor
Hyporeflexia	Depression	Restlessness	Coma

Cardiovascular system

Hypertension	Electrocardiographic	Digitalis sensitivity	Heart block
Bradycardia	abnormalities	Hypotension	Cardiac arrest

GI tract

Anorexia	Pain and distention	Adynamic ileus
Nausea and vomiting	Constipation	

Skeletal system

Bone pain	Pathologic fractures

Kidneys

Polyuria/nocturia	Dehydration	Nephrocalcinosis	Renal failure
Polydipsia	Azotemia and proteinuria	Nephrolithiasis	

Systemic symptoms

Ectopic calcification	Metabolic alkalosis	Hypercoagulability	Pruritus

23. What are the three major considerations in planning treatment?

1. **Prognosis.** Controlling the malignancy is the most effective treatment for HCM. When the cancer is treatment-sensitive, aggressive treatment of both cancer and HCM is appropriate. In patients whose disease is refractory to treatment, interventions may be focused on palliation and enhancing quality of life.

2. **Patient's overall condition.** Treatment for cancer and HCM must be modified for patients with underlying medical conditions such as renal and cardiac disease.

3. **Severity of HCM.** The urgency and aggressiveness of treatment should correlate with the severity of HCM and its symptoms to prevent mortality and alleviate suffering. However, in cases of advanced cancer, when end-of-life issues have been thoroughly discussed and defined and treatment of the underlying cancer is no longer pursued, withholding treatment for HCM may be seen as an humane and preferred alternative (because of its rapid progression and decreased state of consciousness) to prolonged suffering and pain.

24. List the four strategies for treatment of HCM.

1. Hydration
2. Elimination of drugs that worsen hypercalcemia
3. Loop diuretics
4. Intravenous bisphosphonate therapy

25. Why is hydration important? How is it achieved?

Hydration is fundamental to treatment, both to correct inherent dehydration and its sequelae and to promote calcium excretion. In mild cases, forced oral fluids (3–4 L/day) may be adequate to lower calcium levels. Interventions for nausea may be required to facilitate this goal. In general, intravenous hydration with normal saline is required. Based on the severity of the hypercalcemia and dehydration as well as the patient's cardiovascular status, 2.5–6 L are given over 24 hours. Because calcium is excreted in parallel with sodium chloride, use of saline promotes calcium excretion in the renal tubules. It is essential to monitor electrolytes carefully, especially magnesium and potassium, because imbalances may lead to cardiac dysrhythmias. A urinary output of 100 ml/hr is desirable after euvolemia has been restored.

26. What drugs worsen hypercalcemia?

Calcium and vitamin D supplements, calcium-based antacids, thiazide diuretics (which decrease renal excretion of calcium), and hormonal therapy.

27. Describe the role of loop diuretics.

Loop diuretics (e.g., furosemide) are initiated after intravascular volume has been restored. They accelerate the elimination of calcium by blocking reabsorption in the loop of Henle and also help to prevent volume overload due to vigorous hydration. Hydration and diuresis eliminate excessive calcium but do not alleviate the cause of the condition—bone reabsorption.

28. Describe the role of intravenous bisphosphonate therapy.

The bisphosphonates have become the standard of treatment for moderate and severe HCM because of their effectiveness and low incidence of side effects. It is thought that they bind to bone matrix, prevent release of calcium, and may exert effects on both osteoblasts and osteoclasts that are beneficial. The bisphosphonates are usually given intravenously because GI side effects prohibit adequate oral dosing.

29. Which bisphosphonates are currently used?

Pamidronate is currently the bisphosphonate of choice. Indications include HCM, osteolytic bone metastasis of breast cancer, and osteolytic lesions of multiple myeloma. Beneficial effects in patients with breast cancer and multiple myeloma include decreased bone pain, improved quality of life, and decreased bone complications. Whether pamidronate can prevent or delay onset of bone metastases is also under study. Pamidronate should be given concurrently with chemotherapy for treatment of multiple myeloma. Further study is needed to evaluate its use in prostate and other cancers that frequently involve bone. Pamidronate is dosed at 60–90 mg intravenously over 2–4 hours every 3–4 weeks. Fatigue, nausea, and transient fever are the most common side effects. Electrolytes should be monitored closely. Pamidronate can cause vein irritation.

Etidronate, dosed at 7.5 mg/kg over 4 hours for 3–7 days, is less effective than pamidronate and no longer widely used. Additional disadvantages are that it must be given with vigorous hydration over multiple days and that it prevents bone mineralization.

Clodronate, commonly used outside the United States, is of intermediate strength between etidronate and pamidronate. Although initially it is given intravenously, oral administration has demonstrated some success for maintenance therapy. New and more potent bisphosphonates, including ibandronate and zoledronate, are under investigation.

30. What other agents are sometimes used as adjuncts?

AGENT	DOSE	ACTION	ADVANTAGES	DISADVANTAGES
Calcitonin	4–8 U/kg every 6–12 hr	Inhibits osteoclasts Increases renal excretion	4–6 hr onset Well-tolerated May decrease pain	1–2 days' duration Relatively weak Rare allergic reactions (1 unit skin test recommended)

Table continued on following page

AGENT	DOSE	ACTION	ADVANTAGES	DISADVANTAGES
Plicamycin (mithramycin)	25 µg/kg	Toxic to osteoclasts	Effective Onset in 1–2 days Up to 2 weeks' duration	Thrombocytopenia Nausea and vomiting Vesicant Renal and hepatic toxicities
Glucocorticoids	Variable	Inhibit reabsorption Increase excretion Decrease GI absorption	Selectively effective	Side effects of steroids
Gallium nitrate	200 mg/m^2 over 24 hr for 5 days	Decreases reabsorption	Effective	5-day dosing Renal toxicity Anemia

31. What specific measures should patients and families be taught ?

1. Report early signs and symptoms, such as decreased or absent appetite, nausea, vomiting, constipation, increased fatigue, weakness, excessive thirst, frequent voiding, dry mouth and skin, and dizziness with position changes.

2. Promote hydration by monitoring intake, encouraging patient to drink 2–3 L (quarts)/day, keeping favorite fluids handy, and reminding the patient to sip. Give antinausea medications as ordered.

3. Help the patient to stay mobile by encouraging standing or walking several times a day or isometric exercises if the patient is unable to bear weight. Support the patient in performing self-care activities as much as possible. Monitor pain medications, and inform the nurse or physician if pain control is not adequate.

4. Promote safety by keeping the environment uncluttered and well-lit and encouraging the patient to use safety aids, such as a walker or cane, to prevent falls. Do not allow the patient to overstress bones, and educate others to be gentle when helping. They should not pull on arms or legs or squeeze ribs. Report bone pain and have it evaluated.

5. Up-to-date internet information can be found on Cancernet, a service of the National Cancer Institute, at http://cancernet.nci.nih.gov or by telephone at 1-800-4-CANCER.

REFERENCES

1. Bilezikian JP: Management of acute hypercalcemia. N Engl J Med 326:1196–1203, 1992.
2. Body JJ, Bartl R, Burckhardt P, et al: Current use of bisphosphonates in oncology. J Clin Oncol 16: 3890–3899, 1998.
3 Body JJ, Coleman RE, Piccart M: Use of bisphosphonates in cancer patients. Cancer Treat Rev 22:265–287, 1996.
4. Kaplan M:Hypercalcemia of malignancy:A review of advances in pathophysiology. Oncol Nurs Forum 21:1039–1056, 1994.
5. Miaskowski C: Oncologic emergencies. In Baird SB, McCorkle R (eds): Cancer Nursing: A Comprehensive Textbook. Philadelphia, W.B. Saunders, 1991, pp 888–889.
6. Theriault RL, Lipton A, Hortobagyi GN, et al, for the Protocol 18 Aredia Breast Cancer Study Group: Pamidronate reduces skeletal morbidity in women with advanced breast cancer and lytic bone lesions: A randomized, placebo-controlled trial. J Clin Oncol 17:846–854, 1999.
7. Wall J, Bundred N, Howell A: Hypercalcemia and bone resorption in malignancy. Clin Orthop Rel Res 312:51–63, 1995.
8. Warrell R: Hypercalcemia. In DeVita V, Hellman S, Rosenberg SA (eds): Cancer: Principles and Practice of Oncology, 6th ed. Philadelphia, Lippincott Williams & Wilkins, 2001, pp 2633–2639.
9. Wickham RS: Hypercalcemia. In Yarbro CH, Frogge MH, Goodman M, Groenwald SL (eds): Cancer Nursing: Princples and Practice, 5th ed. Boston, Jones & Bartlett, 2000, pp 776–791.

53. INFECTIONS IN IMMUNOSUPPRESSED PATIENTS

Robert H. Gates, MD, FACP

1. Are infections an important cause of mortality in patients with cancer?

Yes. Infections are the major cause of mortality in many patients with cancer. Infection has replaced bleeding as the major cause of mortality in leukemia. Data about mortality causes from cancer center statistics vary; however, about 75% of deaths in patients with acute leukemia and 50% of deaths in patients with lymphoma result from infection.

2. What factors place patients with cancer at risk for infection?

Multiple factors place patients with cancer at risk for infection, including factors associated with the cancer itself and factors associated with therapy as well as previous antibiotic therapy.

FACTOR PROMOTING INFECTION	EXAMPLES OF ASSOCIATED ORGANISMS	EXAMPLES OF DISEASE STATES

Diminished antibody response	Encapsulated organisms
	  Pneumococci
	  Hemophilus influenzae
	  Neisseria spp.
	  Staphylococci
	  Streptococci
		Multiple myeloma
		Poor nutrition
		B-cell lymphomas
		Post splenectomy (Hodgkin's disease)
		Myelophthisis

Poor white blood cell function or number	Aerobic gram-positive organisms
	  Staphylococci
	  Enterococci
	Aerobic gram-negative organisms
	  Pseudomonas aeruginosa
	  Enterobacter spp.
	Fungi
	  Candida spp.
	  Aspergillus spp.
	  Fusarium spp.
		Leukemias
		Lymphomas
		Myelophthisis processes
		Chemotherapy
		Radiation therapy

Poor cellular immunity	*Listeria* spp. Herpes group virus *Mycobacterium* spp. Cryptococci *Legionella* spp. *Pneumocystis* spp.	Hodgkin's disease Non-Hodgkin's lymphoma Poor nutrition Chronic leukemias Chemotherapy (especially fludarabine) Steroids
Skin and mucosal defects	Staphylococci *Candida* spp. Herpes group virus Aerobic gram-negative organisms	Chemotherapy Pneumocystis carinii Radiation therapy Vascular access devices

Environmental problems
  Construction
  Poor airflow
  Contaminated water supply
  Raw foods
	Aspergillus spp.
	Mycobacterium tuberculosis
	Legionella spp.
	Aerobic gram-negative organisms
		Organ transplants
		Neutropenia

Table continued on following page

459

FACTOR PROMOTING INFECTION	EXAMPLES OF ASSOCIATED ORGANISMS	EXAMPLES OF DISEASE STATES
Anatomic mechanical problems	Anaerobes Staphylococci Aerobic gram-negative organisms	Lung cancer causing airway blockage Skin or mucosal disruption due to primary or metastatic cancer Bowel obstruction due to primary or metastatic cancer Urinary obstruction due to renal or cervical cancer
Prior infection with organism that has propensity to recur	*Aspergillus* spp. *Candida* spp. Herpes group virus	Not disease-specific

3. What is the most significant predisposing factor to infection in patients with cancer?

Neutropenia. Neutrophils are mature white cells that attack and destroy invading bacteria, viruses, and fungi (particularly *Aspergillus* and *Candida* spp.). The absolute neutrophil count (ANC) is calculated by multiplying the percentage of granulocytes (neutrophils = segments + bands) by the total white blood cell (WBC) count. The risk of infection rises as the WBC count falls, with the greatest risk at neutrophil counts < 500/mm^3. Most serious infections occur with neutrophil counts < 100/mm^3. In addition to presence and degree, duration of the neutropenia is also important. As the duration of neutropenia increases, the risk of infection increases, ultimately reaching 100%. A duration of 3–7 days is much less of a risk than a duration beyond 14 days. Currently, about one-third of neutropenic patients with fever have a microbiologically proven infection (positive cultures), whereas about one-fifth have clinically apparent infection with negative cultures.

4. What are neutropenic precautions?

1. Strict handwashing is the most important precaution.

2. Routine wearing of masks by healthcare providers is not necessary. Providers with a transmissible respiratory disease should not care for the patient. The practice of requiring the patient to wear a mask when leaving the room varies by institution.

3. Ideally, the airflow in the patient's room should be positive compared with the hall. The intent is to avoid exposure to airborne pathogens such as *Aspergillus* spp.

4. The patient's room should not be cleaned in a manner that causes dust to be shed (e.g., from drapes).

5. Sources of gram-negative organisms should be avoided (e.g., live flowers in water, raw food, fresh fruits and vegetables).

5. What else can be done to prevent infections in neutropenic patients?

High-efficiency particulate air (HEPA) filtration is used by many centers for patients who undergo organ transplantation or who are expected to have prolonged neutropenia from therapy. The intent is to remove airborne pathogens such as *Aspergillus* spp.

Immunizations should be up to date, including pneumococcal and *Hemophilus influenzae* vaccines. Special consideration should be given to patients about to undergo elective splenectomy. Such patients should receive the above vaccines as well as meningococcal vaccine.

The use of **prophylactic antibiotics** often depends on institutional practice. Experience with prophylactic agents has been mixed, ranging from spectacular success with acyclovir and ganciclovir in bone marrow transplant recipients to failure with nystatin. Major problems of prophylactic agents are that they promote resistant bacteria and are partially responsible for the emergence of *Staphylococcus epidermidis* and enterococci as significant pathogens in neutropenic patients.

6. Which agents have been used to prevent or delay infection in patients undergoing chemotherapy?

    1. Antibiotics: quinolones, trimethoprim-sulfamethoxazole, oral aminoglycosides, and oral amphotericin B for selective bowel decontamination. The use of trimethoprim-sulfamethoxazole is well established in bone marrow transplant recipients to prevent development of *Pneumocystis carinii* pneumonia.

    2. Antifungal agents: nystatin, clotrimazole, and the imidazoles.

    3. Antiviral agents: acyclovir and ganciclovir.

    4. Isoniazid to prevent reactivation of tuberculosis in patients with a positive tuberculosis skin test, particularly patients with lymphoreticular cancer.

7. What is the source of most bacteria that infect patients with cancer?

    Although some infections are acquired from the environment, about 50% of infections in neutropenic cancer patients result from bacteria that make up the patient's endogenous flora (e.g., *Escherichia coli, Enterobacter* spp., *Klebsiella* spp., other gram-negative bacteria, yeast, anaerobes). A patient's flora may change rapidly on admission to the hospital. In immunosuppressed patients, bacterial flora can change in a matter of hours, quickly resembling the bacteria found in the hospital setting.

8. When is fever in neutropenic patients significant?

    Fever in the presence of neutropenia is always significant and should be treated as a medical emergency. A patient may die within hours if prompt and effective therapy is not begun. In neutropenic patients fever is usually regarded and treated as indicating the presence of bacteria in the blood (bacteremia). Clinical evidence of infection and systemic response are usually equated with sepsis; evidence of organ dysfunction (oliguria, altered mentation) indicates sepsis syndrome. If hypotension is added to the list, the result is severe sepsis. If the hypotension does not respond to fluid resuscitation, septic shock is present. This spectrum of response to infection involves a complex and incompletely understood cascade of events triggered by the presence of bacteria, fungi, or viruses.

    Although there is no universal agreement, most authorities agree that significant fever in the neutropenic patient is a single oral temperature > 38.3° C (101° F) in the absence of a clear cause (e.g., administration of blood products) or the presence of a temperature > 38° C (100.4° F) for 1 hour or more. In certain situations the febrile response may be greatly blunted, absent, or less than expected. Steroid therapy is the most common culprit. Nonsteroidal anti-inflammatory drugs (NSAIDs), old age, renal failure, and overwhelming infection also may blunt the normal fever response. Unfortunately, the absence of fever does not mean that the patient does not have a potentially serious infection.

9. Are all fevers due to infections?

    No. Fevers in patients with cancer are commonly drug-induced or related to the cancer itself (e.g., leukemias, lymphomas, renal cell cancer, liver cancer).

10. What is drug-induced fever?

    Drug-induced fever is caused by the drug itself. Drugs that induce fevers include antibiotics, antifungals (e.g., amphotericin B), allopurinol, biologic response modifiers, and chemotherapy agents (e.g., bleomycin, dactinomycin, gemcitabine). The usual mechanism is production of antibody by the patient's immune system that reacts with the drug to cause fever. The diagnosis of drug-induced fever may be relatively easy or obscure and challenging.

11. What clues point to the presence of drug-induced fever?

    1. Timing of the fever is often a clue. Drug-induced fever may occur with each administration of the drug or after 10–14 days of treatment (a typical time frame for the patient's immune system to develop antibodies to the drug). The time to development of drug fever may be accelerated if the patient has received the drug before and already has developed antibodies.

2. The patient often appears well. The pulse may not be elevated in proportion to the fever. Patients also may appear quite ill, with shaking chills (as in reactions to quinidine).

3. The patient may have a rash (not due to infection) and/or other evidence of drug-induced end-organ dysfunction (e.g., interstitial nephritis or hepatitis).

4. Thorough investigation reveals no other reason for fever.

12. What should be done when the neutropenic patient becomes febrile?

After appropriate cultures are obtained, antibiotic therapy should be promptly ordered and administered, ideally within 1 hour of recognizing the fever. Assessment of vital signs and evaluation of early signs and symptoms of serious infection should proceed without delay. Obtain cultures of blood, urine (even with no signs or symptoms), throat (in presence of abnormal findings), stool (in presence of diarrhea), stool for *Clostridium difficile* toxin assay (with current or recent antibiotics), and cultures of intravenous (IV) line sites with evidence of inflammation. For new skin findings, consider immediate evaluation with biopsy and culture. It is mandatory to obtain a baseline chest radiograph in the presence of signs or symptoms attributable to the lungs. A question of sinus disease should prompt an early CT scan of the sinuses; plain radiographs are often not sensitive enough to pick up early evidence of infection. Brilliant diagnoses usually are made by ordinary people being dull and methodical. Keep in mind that without neutrophils, many of the expected signs and symptoms of inflammation may be minimal or absent.

13. List the early signs and symptoms of serious infection.
- Decrease in mentation
- Decrease in urine output
- Decrease in platelet count
- Decrease or increase in temperature
- Increase in glucose
- Increase in heart rate or respiration

14. What aspects of the physical assessment should receive particular attention?

Skin	Check all current and previous IV sites.
	New rashes: consider drug reaction, blood-borne spread of bacteria or fungi
	Perianal pain or inflammation: consider hemorrhoids, fissure, phlegmon (inflammation of soft tissue due to infection)
Head and neck	Headache, sinus, or jaw pain: consider sinusitis
	Nasal ulcers or mucosal necrosis: consider fungal involvement
	Cotton wool spots in front of retina: consider candidal infection
	Oral mucosal white patches that rub off and bleed: consider candidal infection
	Oral ulcers: consider herpes, gram-negative bacteria, chemotherapy
	Odynophagia (pain when swallowing): with oral ulcers, consider herpes virus; with thrush, consider candidal esophagitis
Lungs	Findings on exam may be minimal; may precede radiographic abnormalities
Abdomen	Rebound tenderness, especially involving the right lower quadrant: consider typhlitis

15. How many blood cultures should be done? How much blood is needed per culture?

Two pairs of aerobic and anaerobic blood cultures are usually enough to obtain a positive result. More than two contributes little to the statistical likelihood of a positive culture but may contribute to anemia. It is important to obtain the amount of blood required by the hospital laboratory. Many culture systems are optimized for a given amount of blood; indeed, the blood itself may help to provide the nutrients that the bacteria need to grow. Too little blood may decrease the yield from the culture.

16. How far apart should blood cultures be done?

The interval between cultures need be only as long as it takes to prepare the second site after the first culture is obtained. Delaying therapy so that a second blood culture can be done in 30 or 60 minutes places the patient at needless risk.

17. Should blood be obtained from venous access devices?

Whether to draw blood through a venous access device (VAD) is controversial but usually done. The advantage is that a positive culture from the VAD may suggest the catheter as the source of infection. The bad news is that it may be a contaminant from the hardware of the VAD. If your institution has the capability, quantification of the number of colony-forming units (CFUs) of bacteria may help to decide whether the positive culture is a contaminant. If both sites yield positive cultures and the central catheter culture has 5 times the number of CFUs as the peripheral catheter, the central catheter is probably the source. If the peripheral catheter culture is negative and the central catheter culture colony count is low (< 100 CFUs/ml of blood), the central culture may represent contamination.

18. What is a Gram stain?

This valuable tool, developed over 100 years ago by Dr. Hans Gram, allows bacteria to be picked out from cellular material and debris under a microscope. It is a basic test that can be done in a few minutes at little cost. The technique consists of several sequential steps with a different staining solution (crystal violet, iodine, acetone-alcohol, or safranin) in each step. It takes advantage of the differences in the way that staining solutions are retained within bacteria. Bacteria that retain the crystal violet-iodine complex appear dark blue or violet. Bacteria that cannot retain this complex are stained by the safranin and appear pink under the microscope. Organisms that retain the stain and appear blue are said to be gram-positive, whereas organisms that do not retain the stain are said to be gram-negative. Examples of gram-positive organisms include staphylococci, streptococci, enterococci, *Listeria* spp., and *Bacillus* spp. Examples of gram-negative organisms include *Escherichia coli, Klebsiella* spp., *Enterobacter* sp., *Pseudomonas aeruginosa*, and *Bacteroides* spp. By making the organism visible, the Gram stain makes it possible to determine the morphology of the bacteria; that is, whether it is a coccus or rodlike.

19. What empirical antibiotics should be prescribed to neutropenic febrile patients?

In the absence of findings that may direct therapy (e.g., pus from a VAD exit site with gram-positive cocci in clusters, which suggest a staphylococcal species), all broad-spectrum regimens (regimens containing antibiotics that are anticipated to be effective against the commonly found gram-negative bacteria) appear to work well. Initial clinical responses vary from 60–80%. This variation is probably due to differences in study design, patient populations in different centers, antibiotic use, and antibiotic susceptibility, according to the institution. Broad-spectrum combination antibiotic regimens may include an extended-spectrum penicillin (e.g., ticarcillin, piperacillin) plus an aminoglycoside (e.g., gentamicin, amikacin) or a third-generation cephalosporin (e.g., ceftazidime).

Most authorities believe that two antibiotics with activity against *Pseudomonas aeruginosa* should be given initially. Clinical trials and experience also support the use of broad-spectrum monotherapy with agents that have antipseudomonal activity (e.g., ceftazidime, imipenem, meropenem). Some physicians prefer two antibiotics when the patient exhibits altered vital signs from infection. The decision usually is determined by the institution's antibiotic susceptibilities. For example, if a patient is on a medical or surgical ward with infection problems from a resistant strain of *Enterobacter* spp., initial therapy should cover the possibility that the patient is infected with this organism. Coverage for staphylococci is not given initially unless there is reason to suspect a source for staphylococci. Other agents may be added as necessary for special circumstances (e.g., to cover anaerobes in the case of suspected typhlitis).

20. What factors should be considered in choosing an antibiotic regimen?

- Patient drug allergies
- Route of administration
- Concomitant drugs
- Suspected organism
- Antibiotic resistance patterns
- Previous antibiotic therapy
- Previous infecting organisms
- Duration of neutropenia
- Patient exposure to pathogens

21. Summarize the most commonly used antibiotics in neutropenic febrile patients.

CLASS	EXAMPLES	SPECTRUM/ACTIVITY	CAUTIONS
Penicillins	Ticarcillin Piperacillin	Streptococci Gram-negative anaerobes	Allergic reactions Potassium loss Rash with allopurinol Drug-induced neutropenia
Cephalosporins	Ceftazidime	Streptococci Gram-negative organisms	Allergic reactions Drug-induced neutropenia

Quinolones	Ciprofloxacin
	Ofloxacin
		Gram-negative organisms
		Legionella spp.
			GI absorption decreased by
			  aluminum, magnesium,
			  iron, zinc, sucralfate
			Red neck, red man syndrome

Aminoglycosides	Gentamicin Tobramycin	Gram-negative organisms	Avoid with cisplatin Avoid with cyclosporine Ototoxicity Nephrotoxicity Avoid with amphotericin B
Sulfonamides	Sulfamethoxazole (with trimethoprim)	Gram-negative organisms *Pneumocystis carinii*	Allergic reactions Marrow suppression
Vancomycin	Vancomycin Teicoplanin	Gram-positive organisms	Red neck, red man syndrome Drug-induced neutropenia
Imidazoles	Ketoconazole	*Candida* spp.	Antacids decrease GI absorption

22. Why is it necessary to review the patient's previous antibiotic regimens?

Prior antibiotics can greatly affect the likely organisms currently infecting a neutropenic patient. If an antibiotic that kills or suppresses one kind of bacteria is given, other bacteria or fungi that are resistant to the agent will try to take over the niche left by the killed bacteria. In treating a patient with a quinolone antibiotic, beware of anaerobic bacteria and yeast. Vancomycin therapy leaves gram-negative organisms without the usual competition from gram-positive organisms. Broad-spectrum antibiotics give a free hand to fungi. Even the imidazole class of antifungal agents (ketoconazole, fluconazole, itraconazole) may allow growth of fungi that are resistant to the imidazoles.

23. How long should antibiotics be continued?

In general antibiotics are continued for the duration of the neutropenia. Guidelines to consider include the following:

No fever and ≥ 500 neutrophils
• No source of infection (stop antibiotics)
• Known source of infection (give course appropriate for source)
No fever and < 500 neutrophils: continue antibiotics for up to 14 days
Fever and ≥ 500 neutrophils: consider changing or stopping therapy after evaluation for:
• Hidden site of infection   • Drug-induced fever
• Abscess or catheter-related infection   • Tumor fever
• Resistant bacteria, fungi, or virus
Fever and < 500 neutrophils: continue antibiotics and consider:
• Fungal superinfection   • Viral infection
• Inadequate antibiotic dosing   • Abscess or catheter-related infection
• Resistant bacteria

24. What is meant by a third- or fourth-generation antibiotic?

The habit of referring to cephalosporins by generation was popularized by pharmaceutical companies and tacitly approved by general use. The habit has evolved into calling an antibiotic with expanded activity the product of a new generation. The generation refers roughly to the order in which the drug was introduced and the range of bacteria against which it is active. The first-generation cephalosporins (e.g., cephalothin, cefazolin) have good activity against *Staphylococcus aureus*. The following generations tend to have less activity against staphylococci. The second- and third-generation cephalosporins (e.g., cefamandole and ceftriaxone, respectively) tend to have increased activity against gram-negative aerobic bacteria. The term fourth-generation is sometimes used to denote the extremely broad-spectrum carbapenem class of beta lactam antibiotics (e.g., meropenem).

25. What is antibiotic lock therapy?

Antibiotic lock therapy is a relatively new approach to the management of an infected catheter line. A small volume of concentrated antibiotic solution is placed in the lumen of the catheter and allowed to remain for hours. The approach is said to work poorly for candidal infections. A variation of this technique uses fibrinolytic therapy locally instilled as an adjunct to antibiotic therapy. The fibrinolytic agent (e.g., concentrated urokinase) is thought to exert its antibacterial effect by dissolving the fibrin layer on the interior of the catheter that promotes adherence of bacteria and development of thrombus. As urokinase is currently unavailable, tissue plasminogen activator (tPA) has been used instead. Initial trials suggest that tPA is at least as effective as urokinase. Caution is indicated in considering this procedure in the presence of an infected thrombus because the potentially large bacterial burden that may be released into the bloodstream may worsen signs and symptoms of systemic infection.

26. Describe the role of colony-stimulating factors.

Granulocyte colony-stimulating factor (G-CSF) and granulocyte-macrophage colony-stimulating factor (GM-CSF) shorten the duration of chemotherapy-induced neutropenia and may enhance the function of neutrophils. Both agents are glycopeptides that stimulate the bone marrow to speed the production and maturation of neutrophils. They are expensive and may cause symptoms such as myalgias. The cost-benefit ratio is best in patients with an expected prolonged duration of neutropenia (> 7–10 days) and high risk of infection with agents such as *Aspergillus* spp. G-CSF is started after chemotherapy and continued until the neutrophil count recovers.

27. Amphotericin B has a bad reputation for side effects and for causing problems with kidney and bone marrow function. Is there any truth to this reputation?

Considerable folklore surrounds the administration of amphotericin B ("ampho-terrible"). Common signs and symptoms include chills and fever, phlebitis, and nausea and vomiting. Renal problems include tubular dysfunction leading to loss of electrolytes (particularly potassium and bicarbonate) and suppression of erythropoietin production by the kidney.

28. Separate fiction from fact in regard to the use of "ampho-terrible."

Fiction: Heparin in the amphotericin B solution decreases the risk of phlebitis.

Fact: Heparin is not proved to prevent phlebitis. It is not needed when amphotericin B is given through a central line. Indeed, even small amounts of heparin may lead to immune-mediated platelet destruction.

Fiction: A test dose of amphotericin B is required to avoid anaphylaxis.

Fact: The "test-dose" practice was adapted as a result of side effects with the administration of early, relatively impure preparations of amphotericin B. In patients who have not received amphotericin B before, the test dose may be safely omitted.

Fiction: Steroids should be added to the amphotericin B infusion to decrease the occurrence of febrile reactions.

Fact: Although steroids are often used, there is little scientific evidence of their efficacy. Some authorities advocate against the routine use of steroids because of the theoretical concern of increasing immunosuppression. If steroids are used, they should be the shortest-lived preparations available (e.g., hydrocortisone succinate). Methylprednisolone should not be used.

Fiction: Amphotericin B is better tolerated if the infusion is given over at least 4–6 hours.

Fact: Although bolus therapy is dangerous, amphotericin B is tolerated by most patients when given over 1–2 hours.

29. What should be done to assist in the administration of amphotericin B?
- Individualize the symptomatic medications to the patient's needs.
- Reassure the patient that administration of the drug usually is better tolerated with time.
- Use meperidine, 25–50 mg intravenously, to terminate chills and fever. Rare intractable chills and fever may be treated with dantrolene.
- To help avoid renal toxicity, maintain adequate volume status. Saline boluses given with the infusions are often used for this purpose.
- Consider using the newer lipid-complexed and liposomal preparations of amphotericin B, which may be better tolerated and have less renal and bone marrow toxicity. Thus larger doses may be given.

30. True or false: A patient who receives vancomycin and experiences flushing, wheezing, and hypotension is most likely allergic to vancomycin.
False. The so-called red neck or red man syndrome (from the flushed appearance of the face, neck, and upper torso) is not, strictly speaking, an allergy. Classic allergic reactions are defined by the presence of an antibody that reacts with the patient's immune system to produce the allergic response. Vancomycin directly causes release of histamine from mast cells; antibodies have no role. The histamine causes the vasodilation, flushing, and wheezing. Because histamine release from mast cells is also important in anaphylactic reactions (IgE-mediated mast-cell degranulation), it is not difficult to understand how the patient's clinical appearance suggests an allergic reaction. The patient is not allergic to vancomycin in this setting. Tolerance to infusions tends to improve with time. Do not infuse vancomycin rapidly unless you have never seen the red neck syndrome and would like to do so. Infusion over 60–90 minutes is recommended.

31. Define typhlitis.
Typhlitis or neutropenic enterocolitis is a necrotizing infection of the bowel secondary to a combination of factors toxic to the intestinal mucosa. The resulting mucosal damage allows bacterial invasion. The infection, usually involving the large bowel (especially the cecum), results in bowel wall edema, thinning, and perforation. The situation is a set up for bacterial translocation in a big way. Typhlitis is particularly common in children. Patients may present with symptoms suggesting appendicitis, such as abdominal pain, nausea and vomiting, and fever.

32. How is typhlitis diagnosed and treated?
Blood cultures may be positive despite administration of effective antibiotic therapy. In the proper clinical setting, the diagnosis may be made by CT scan, which shows a thickened bowel wall. Peritoneal lavage with a positive culture for the same organisms as the blood cultures is confirmatory. Medical therapy includes antibiotics to cover the gram-negative organisms, *Candida* spp., and anaerobic organisms. Laxatives and enemas should be avoided. Surgical intervention may be indicated. Unfortunately, surgery is usually difficult because the patients are critically ill and poor surgical risks.

33. Define ecthyma gangrenosum.
Ecthyma gangrenosum is a skin manifestation of the vascular spread of bacteria, usually gram-negative. *Pseudomonas aeruginosa* is the most commonly involved organism. Other organisms include staphylococci and fungi such as *Aspergillus* and *Alternaria* spp. Blood cultures are often positive for the causative bacteria. Lesions begin as nodular papules that quickly progress to central blebs, then ulcerate with underlying induration and central necrosis. The lesions are usually erythematous, often with a violaceous hue. Not unlike petechiae, they may be somewhat hidden in skin folds, buttocks, and the perineum.

34. What are MRSA and MRSE? Why are they significant?

MRSA is methicillin-resistant *Staphylococcus aureus*. MRSE is methicillin-resistant *Staphylococcus epidermidis*. Penicillins and cephalosporins belong to the beta-lactam class of antibiotics. The beta-lactam antibiotics bind to a receptor in bacteria and interrupt the synthesis of the bacterial cell wall, leading to cell death. Shortly after the introduction of penicillin, many bacteria developed resistance by producing a beta-lactamase enzyme that destroyed a portion of the penicillin molecule (the beta-lactam ring), rendering the antibiotic inactive. Biochemists retaliated by making penicillins that were resistant to the destructive action of this enzyme (e.g., nafcillin, methicillin).

In recent years staphylococci resistant to all antibiotics of the beta lactamase-resistant class have evolved. They have a receptor that is much more difficult for the antibiotics to bind. MRSAs are resistant to all beta-lactam antibiotics (e.g., penicillins, cephalosporins, carbapenems). They are sometimes susceptible to trimethoprim-sulfamethoxazole but usually are treated with vancomycin. Infection with MRSA can be deadly, and the necessity of using more vancomycin has led to increased resistance of other bacteria to vancomycin. A good example of this resistance development is the vancomycin-resistant enterococci, which have become a problem in many medical centers.

35. Define bacterial translocation.

Bacterial translocation is the movement of living bacteria from the gastrointestinal tract to the mesenteric lymph nodes and blood stream and thus to other organs. Every moment of our lives, bowel flora are prevented from translocating or quickly cleared when they try to move across the bowel wall. In the presence of neutropenia and other immunosuppression, life-threatening infections can result from mucosal disruption of the bowel wall caused by chemotherapy, invading organisms, or antibiotic suppression of normal bowel anaerobic bacteria (the predominant normal bowel flora that help to prevent translocation). Gram-negative organisms most likely to translocate include *E. coli, Klebsiella* spp., and *Pseudomonas aeruginosa*. Nutritional counseling may be important. Many authorities believe that fiber ingestion assists in mucosal preservation, thus decreasing the rate at which bacterial translocation occurs.

36. What is low-risk neutropenia?

Low-risk neutropenia is a relative term used to describe neutrophil counts < 500/mm^3 but > 100/mm^3 with an expected duration of < 7–10 days. Such neutropenias are often seen after chemotherapy for solid tumors (as opposed to the neutropenia that follows therapy for leukemias or bone marrow transplant). Patients are considered at low risk because they usually respond well to initial antibiotic therapy. An oral quinolone (e.g., levofloxacin) is often used empirically because of its broad-spectrum gram-negative activity and excellent oral bioavailability.

37. Describe the management of patients with low-risk neutropenia.

Some centers have initiated outpatient therapy for patients with low-risk neutropenia. They are treated entirely as outpatients or have responded well to initial inpatient treatment. Outpatient management should be done only by clinicians experienced in the management of neutropenic fevers. Candidates for outpatient therapy should be symptomatically well without hypotension, have no comorbid conditions (e.g., heart failure, kidney failure, serious chronic obstructive pulmonary disease), a responsive tumor, good outpatient support systems, and easy access for follow-up and readmission.

38. What are the indications to remove an infected VAD?
- Lack of response to appropriate antibiotic therapy after 48–72 hours
- Persistent positive blood cultures
- Deteriorating patient
- Line malfunction
- Infection with organisms poorly responsive to antimicrobial therapy (e.g., *Bacillus* spp., *Corynebacterium* spp., mycobacteria, fungal species)

39. What strategies are used to guide therapy for infected VADs?

Therapeutic strategies are guided by infecting organism and location of infection:

ORGANISM	LOCATION	THERAPY
Staphylococcus epidermidis	Exit site	Medical therapy
	Tunnel	Consider removal
	Port	Remove Huber needle and give antibiotic at peripheral IV site
Staphylococcus aureus	Exit site	Medical therapy
	Line or tunnel	Remove line
	Port	Consider removal
Candida spp.	Exit site	Remove line
	Tunnel	Remove line
	Port	Remove line
Gram-negative organisms	Exit site	Try medical therapy
	Line	Remove line
	Tunnel	50% failure rate with medical therapy

Do *not* lose sight of the patient when applying these or any other guidelines. If the patient is not doing well, even with a site or organism that should respond to medical therapy, remove the VAD. Most febrile neutropenic patients without a VAD infection can be treated successfully without removing the VAD.

40. Allogeneic bone marrow transplants result in severe immunosuppression in recipients. When and what infections are patients prone to develop?

The time of greatest risk for infection in bone marrow recipients can be divided roughly into three phases:

1. The first 30 days after transplant involve the immunosuppressant effects of a pretransplant bone marrow-eradicating regimen of irradiation and chemotherapy. After transplant, immunosuppressive medication (e.g., cyclosporine) is also used. Profound, prolonged neutropenia is present with the possibility of gram-negative and gram-positive infections. Antibiotic treatment promotes candidal infection. A striking concern is the risk for herpes simplex virus in patients who are seropositive before transplant.

2. After the first 30 days, initial engraftment of the transplanted marrow begins. Cytomegalovirus infections replace herpes simplex as the major viral concern, with the potential for severe involvement of multiple organ systems. *Aspergillus* spp. replace *Candida* spp. as the major fungal pathogen.

3. After 90–100 days, bone marrow engraftment is completed. Unfortunately, the immune system does not completely recover for up to 1–2 years. The patient remains at increased risk for infections with organisms that take advantage of poor immunoglobulin function, particularly the pneumococci. Varicella zoster replaces cytomegalovirus as the principal viral pathogen. Another major problem is graft vs. host disease, which can begin during the time of bone marrow engraftment. Graft vs. host disease may require immunosuppressive therapy, which further increases the risk of infection.

41. Why should patients have a dental consultation before they begin chemotherapy?

Before administering myelosuppressive chemotherapy, it is good practice to take care of sites that are actively infected and to consider preventive care for potential sources of infection. A dental site that is a minor problem in normal hosts may become a life-threatening source in neutropenic patients.

42. Does it matter what type of dressing is placed on the exit site of a central VAD?

After reviewing the data from clinical trials, noting the good results from institutions with catheter care teams, and discussing the pros and cons with nurses and physicians, the author recommends meticulous attention to protocol in caring for dressings on the exit site of a central VAD. The kind of dressing is not as important as the attention given by the provider and patient to care of the access line. A reasonable strategy is to use a gauze dressing immediately after line placement and during drainage. After the site is healed or drainage has stopped, a transparent, semipermeable occlusive dressing can be used alone or with gauze. It is also appropriate to use no dressing for tunneled catheters.

43. What is linezolid? How does it work?

Linezolid (Zyvox) is the first commercially available member of a new class of antibiotics, the oxazolidinones. Linezolid acts early to block bacterial protein synthesis by preventing the binding of messenger RNA to the 30s ribosome. This mechanism of action is unique to this class of antibiotics, and cross-resistance to other antibiotics has not been reported. Although linezolid is effective against some anaerobic bacteria, the spectrum of activity is largely against gram-positive organisms, including MRSA and vancomycin-resistant enterococci. Although clinical experience is limited, linezolid appears to be better tolerated and easier to administer than quinupristin/dalfopristin (Synercid), a member of the streptogramin class of antibiotics with similar antibacterial activity. Linezolid is 100% bioavailable, which means it should work well by mouth as well as by intravenous administration. Currently linezolid is marketed for treatment of nosocomial infections due to susceptible organisms.

NOTE

The views and opinions in this chapter are solely the author's and do not reflect the views or the policies of the United States Army, the Department of Defense, or the United States Government.

REFERENCES

1. Brandt B, DePalma J, Irwin M, et al: Comparison of central venous catheter dressings in bone marrow transplant recipients. Oncol Nurs Forum 23:829–836, 1996.
2. Chanock SJ, Pizzo PA: Fever in the neutropenic patient. Infect Dis Clin North Am 10:777–796, 1996.
3. Epstein JB, Chow AW: Oral complications associated with immunosuppression and cancer therapies. Infect Dis Clin North Am 13:901–923, 1999.
4. Greene JR: Catheter-related complications of cancer therapy. Infect Dis Clin North Am 10:255–295, 1996.
5. Hoeprich PD: Clinical use of amphotericin B and derivatives: Lore, mystique, and fact. Clin Infect Dis 14(Suppl 1):S114–S119, 1992.
6. Hughes WT, Armstrong D, Bodey, GP, et al: 1997 Guidelines for the use of antimicrobial agents in neutropenic patients with unexplained fever. Clin Infect Dis 25:551–573, 1997.
7. Jones GR: A practical guide to evaluation and treatment of infections in patients with central venous catheters. J Intraven Nurs 21(5 Suppl):S134–S142, 1998.
8. Karthaus K, Carrarala J, Jurgens H, Ganzser A: New strategies in the treatment of infectious complications in haematology and oncology: is there a role for out-patient antibiotic treatment of febrile neutropenia? Chemotherapy 44:427–435, 1998.
9. Quadri TL, Brown AE: Infectious complications in the critically ill patient with cancer. Semin Oncol 27:335–346, 2000.
10. Wujcik D: Infection control in oncology patients. Nurs Clin North Am 28:639–650, 1993.

54. SPINAL CORD COMPRESSION

Lisa Schulmeister, RN, MN, CS, OCN, and Michael R. Watters, MD, FAAN

1. Why is spinal cord compression an oncologic emergency?

Spinal cord compression is a true neurologic emergency that develops in up to 10% of patients with cancer. Without prompt treatment, the patient may become partially or completely paralyzed. Spinal cord compression is sometimes the first presentation of undiagnosed cancer. The key prognostic factor is the neurologic status of the patient at the time of presentation. Significant neurologic deterioration at diagnosis is associated with a worse prognosis. Therefore, spinal cord compression is an oncologic emergency that requires prompt recognition and emergency treatment to relieve pain and preserve neurologic function.

2. What are the most common cancers associated with spinal cord compression?

Breast cancer is the most common cause of spinal cord compression in women. Other cancers that are commonly associated with spinal cord compression include lung and prostate cancer and multiple myeloma. Less commonly associated cancers include lymphomas, melanomas, renal cell cancers, gastrointestinal adenocarcinomas, and sarcomas. In children, sarcomas, neuroblastomas, and lymphomas have been associated with spinal cord compression.

3. What levels of the spine are most frequently involved?

SPINAL LEVEL	INVOLVEMENT (%)	ASSOCIATED CANCERS
Cervical	10	Lung, breast, kidney, lymphoma, myeloma, melanoma
Thoracic	70	Lung, breast, kidney, lymphoma, myeloma, prostate
Lumbosacral	20	Lung, breast, kidney, lymphoma, myeloma, melanoma, prostate, gastrointestinal

4. How does spinal cord compression occur?

The most common source of spinal cord compression in patients with cancer is metastasis to the epidural space with or without bony involvement. Tumors may also reach the epidural space by direct extension through the intervertebral foramen, particularly lymphomas and nerve sheath tumors. Some primary cancers may occur within the cord itself and may not be associated with pain. Regardless of the route of access, the mass effect of the tumor with associated edema compresses the cord, resulting in ischemia and neural damage. The degree of involvement and speed of compression of the cord explain the wide range of signs and symptoms.

5. What is the first symptom of spinal cord compression?

Because the dura is pain-sensitive, over 95% of patients with spinal cord compression report back pain as the first symptom, preceding other symptoms by weeks to months. The areas most commonly involved are the thoracic, lumbosacral, and cervical spine. However, very early symptoms of spinal cord compression may be nonspecific.

6. How is back pain caused by spinal cord compression characterized?

The pain may be localized or radicular. Local pain usually occurs at the level of the lesion and is said to be dull and constant. The pain is more severe with recumbency and when a patient coughs, bears weight, or uses the Valsalva maneuver. Ideally, the diagnosis will be made while the patient is having only spinal axis pain—before neurologic deficits develop. Among children, the back pain is characterized as severe and persistent and is often accompanied by stiffness of the affected extremities.

7. How does dural pain from tumor compression differ from referred pain of visceral origin or musculoskeletal back pain?

Patients with cancer also may have other sources of back pain. Musculoskeletal pain, by far the more common, is accentuated by movement and improved with rest; it is not associated with imaging changes of spinal metastasis.

Visceral tumor pain may refer to the back, with a constant boring quality that worsens at rest. The pain may have fleeting sharp qualities, cause sleeplessness, and even be improved with activity. This type of pain may be seen in patients with intraabdominal tumors (pancreatic cancer, lymphoma, or sarcoma). Abdominal computed tomography (CT) scan may be diagnostic.

8. What other signs and symptoms are associated with spinal cord compression?

If the epidural lesion is not detected at the painful phase, ischemic and compressive damage to neurons may follow, often initially manifested as weakness (75–85% of cases). Weakness may progress rapidly, adding to the clinical urgency of making a diagnosis. The weakness is typically bilateral and corresponds to the level of spinal cord involvement. Cervical lesions cause quadriparesis, whereas thoracic or lumbosacral lesions cause paraparesis. Other motor signs include spasticity, hyperreflexia, abnormal stretch reflexes, and extensor plantar responses. Sensory loss below the level of cord compression and autonomic dysfunction with impotency and bladder or bowel retention (or incontinence) may result. These deficits may occur in any sequence and progress rapidly.

9. How long is the interval from diagnosis of cancer to presentation with symptoms of spinal cord compression?

The interval from diagnosis to presentation depends on the biologic rate of growth of the cancer and varies from the initial presentation to years later.

10. How is spinal cord compression diagnosed?

1. **Physical examination**. Back pain in any patient with cancer should prompt a rapid evaluation. Palpation with gentle percussion over the vertebral spinous processes often will reveal tenderness at the site of involvement. The neurologic findings follow logically from the extent of compromise of cord function. Weakness, as noted above, is often associated with signs of upper motor neuron involvement (spasticity, hyperreflexia). A change in the patient's sensory exam is usually seen below the level of cord involvement. Decreased rectal tone and a distended bladder signal autonomic dysfunction.

2. **Laboratory results**. In adults, an elevated alkaline phosphatase may suggest bony involvement by the cancer.

3. **Complete spinal images**. *Radiographs* of the spine may reveal erosion of a pedicle, lytic lesions of the vertebral body, or collapse of a vertebral body. Most patients with spinal cord compression eventually have an abnormal radiograph; however, normal spine films do not exclude the possibility of an epidural metastasis, and radiographic changes may not be evident for several months after the presence of a tumor.

Bone scans can be helpful in locating metastasis to the vertebrae but do not differentiate cancer from benign processes such as vertebral collapse or osteoporosis and do not visualize the epidural space or neural elements. Twenty percent of scans reveal lesions missed on plain films.

Myelogram metrizamide CT scans are more sensitive for determining the extent of tumor involvement, particularly in the axial plane. The risks of myelography include neurologic deterioration after lumbar puncture (rare in patients with complete myelographic block) and adverse reactions to contrast agent.

Magnetic resonance imaging (MRI) is currently the imaging modality of choice. Its advantages over myelography include its noninvasive nature and its ability to distinguish prevertebral, vertebral, extradural, intradural, extramedullary, and intramedullary lesions. MRI provides better anatomic visualization with sagittal and axial images of the spinal cord than CT scans. MRI contrast agents are less likely to produce neurologic or systemic adverse reactions and are administered parenterally rather than intrathecally.

4. **Fine-needle aspiration** (FNA) may provide tissue confirmation, especially in patients with metastatic involvement of the dorsal bony elements.

11. How is treatment of spinal cord compression determined?

Once the diagnosis of spinal cord compression is made, the patient is started on cortico-steroids, regardless of further immediate therapy. The type of therapy depends on :
- Primary tumor type and prior treatment
- Level of the myelopathy
- Degree of the spinal block
- Potential for neurologic reversibility

Surgery may be performed for:
- Radiation therapy failure
- Relapse in area of prior radiation therapy (if long survival expected)
- Complete block
- Unstable spine
- Single lesion when complete removal may be possible
- Diagnosis is uncertain
- Mild deficits
- Symptom progression during radiation

Chemotherapy may be given for:
- Cancers that are highly sensitive to chemotherapy or hormones; always given with other modalities

Radiation therapy may be given for:
- Early diagnosis
- Incomplete block
- Severe deficits
- Relapse in area of prior radiation if short survival expected

12. What is the usual first-line treatment for spinal cord compression?

Radiation therapy alone is the usual first-line treatment for ambulatory patients experiencing spinal cord compression, except when there is spinal instability, bony compression, or paraplegia on presentation. In the latter case, surgery is usually performed.

13. How quickly is treatment for spinal cord compression initiated?

Radiation therapy for spinal cord compression is often initiated as an "emergency;" it is not uncommon for radiation therapy to be delivered in the middle of the night or on weekends. Expedient treatment is just as important as timely diagnosis. The mainstay of treatment is radiation therapy with the field extending 1–2 vertebral bodies above and below the compression. The usual dose is 3000–4000 cGy, given in fractionated doses over 2–4 weeks. Patients tolerate the treatment well when pretreated with corticosteroids. Two-thirds of patients remain neurologically stable or improve after radiation therapy treatment, and 67–75% of patients obtain pain relief.

14. Why are corticosteroids given to patients with spinal cord compression?

Corticosteroids are used in conjunction with all of the various treatment options. They are begun as soon as spinal cord compression is suspected to reduce edema and mass effect, which may lessen pain. The appropriate dose recommendations are largely empirical. An intravenous bolus of dexamethasone, 10 mg, is commonly followed by 4–6 mg orally every 6 hours for 2 days; then a slow taper is begun. If a high degree of compression is diagnosed, some providers recommend larger doses with an initial intravenous bolus of 96 mg of dexamethasone, followed by 24 mg orally every 6 hours for 2 days, with a rapid taper. Steroid-related side effects may occur (e.g., hyperglycemia, gastrointestinal bleeding, psychosis) and require specific monitoring.

15. What percentage of patients with spinal cord compression are able to ambulate after pretreatment motor dysfunction?

Pretreatment ambulatory function is the main determinant of posttreatment gait function. About 90% of patients who were ambulatory before treatment remain so; only 10% of patients who were paraplegic before treatment regain the ability to ambulate.

16. What are the options for recurrent disease?

Patients with recurrent disease in an area of prior radiation can be treated surgically if systemic disease is controlled and expected survival is greater than 1 year. Repeat irradiation can be given to patients who are not surgical candidates or whose systemic disease is active or advanced if expected survival is limited. Repeat irradiation may allow preservation of neurologic function. In one series of 54 patients who were ambulatory at the time of repeat irradiation, 75% were still ambulatory on completion of repeat irradiation, and 69% remained ambulatory at last follow-up (median = 4.7 months).

The major risk of repeat irradiation is radiation myelopathy. Despite the high total doses of radiation (median = 5425 cGy), the limited survival (5.1 months) for patients with recurrent disease was too brief for radiation myelopathy to develop, and preservation of ambulation contributed to quality of life. Collateral tissue damage by radiation necrosis in the brain has been limited by the use of stereotactic radiosurgery (x-knife and gamma knife). This technology will be applicable to the spinal cord once stereotactic body frames become available and should reduce the likelihood of radiation myelopathy from initial or repeated spinal radiation.

17. What is the nurse's role in caring for a patient with spinal cord compression?

The major role of the oncology nurse is continual assessment of the patient and prompt notification of changes in pain, sensory, motor, urinary, or bowel function. Because nearly all patients report back pain as their first symptom, pain assessment and treatment are crucial. Methods of pain relief may include nonpharmacologic techniques (e.g., relaxation, massage), nonopioid and opioid analgesics, and adjuvant medications. Analgesics also are sometimes given epidurally. Nearly all patients can achieve pain control with appropriate multidisciplinary pain management.

Another important nursing role is to preserve and maximize the patient's functional status. A bowel and bladder program may be required. It also may be necessary to provide skin care, wound care, and rehabilitation services. The nurse needs to instruct the patient about diagnostic tests, treatment and possible side effects, potential complications, and general safety measures. Emotional support for patient and family is a major focus of care, particularly if spinal cord compression is the presenting sign of a cancer diagnosis. Patients with severe neurologic deficits may require home and hospice care.

ACKNOWLEDGMENT

The authors wish to acknowledge the previous work of Linda Petersen-Rivera, RN, MSN, OCN, for her contribution to the Spinal Cord Compression chapter published in the first edition of *Oncology Nursing Secrets.*

REFERENCES

1. Abrahm JL: Management of pain and spinal cord compression in patients with advanced cancer. ACP-ASIM End-of-Life Care Consensus Panel. American College of Physicians–American Society of Internal Medicine. Ann Intern Med 131:37–46, 1999.
2. Brown PD, Stafford SL, Schild SE, et al: Metastatic spinal cord compression in patients with colorectal cancer. J Neurooncol 44:175–180, 1999.
3. Bucholtz JD: Metastatic epidural spinal cord compression. Semin Oncol Nurs 15:150–159, 1999.
4. Camp-Sorrell D: Spinal cord compression. Clin J Oncol Nurs 2:112–113, 1998.
5. Ciezki JP, Komurcu S, Macklis RM: Palliative radiotherapy. Semin Oncol 27:90–93, 2000.
6. Cowap J, Hardy JR, A'Hern R: Outcome of malignant spinal cord compression at a cancer center: Implications for palliative care services. J Pain Symptom Manage 19:257–264, 2000.
7. Daw HA, Markman M: Epidural spinal cord compression in cancer patients: Diagnosis and management. Cleve Clin J Med 67:497, 501–504, 2000.
8. Garner CM: Cancer-related spinal cord compression. Am J Nurs 99:34–35, 1999.
9. Grattan-Smith PJ, Ryan MM, Procopis PG: Persistent or severe back pain and stiffness are ominous symptoms requiring prompt attention. J Paediatr Child Health 36:208–221, 2000.
10. Helweg-Larsen S, Sorenson PS, Kreiner S: Prognostic factors in metastatic spinal cord compression: A prospective study using multivariate analysis of variables influencing survival and gait function in 153 patients. Int J Radiat Oncol Biol Phys 56:1163–1169, 2000.

11. Karagiri H, Takahashi M, Inagaki J, et al: Clinical results of nonsurgical treatment for spinal metastasis. Int J Radiat Oncol Biol Phys 42:1127–1132, 1998.
12. Khaw FM, Worthy SA, Gibson MJ, Gholkar A: The appearance on MRI of vertebrae in acute compression of the spinal cord due to metastasis. J Bone Joint Surg 81B:830–834, 1999.
13. Kienstra GE, Terwee CB, Dekker FW, et al: Prediction of spinal epidural metastasis. Arch Neurol 57:690–695, 2000.
14. Kovner F, Spigel S, Rider I, et al: Radiation therapy of metastatic spinal cord compression. Multidisciplinary team diagnosis and treatment. J Neurooncol 42:85–92, 1999.
15. Loblaw DA, Laperriere NJ: Emergency treatment of malignant extradural spinal cord compression: An evidence-based guideline. J Clin Oncol 16:1613–1624, 1998.
16. Lu C, Stomper PC, Drislane FW, et al: Suspected spinal cord compression in breast cancer patients: A multidisciplinary risk assessment. Breast Canc Res Treat 51:121–131, 1998.
17. Nygaard IE, Kreder KJ: Spine update: Urologic management in patients with spinal cord injuries. Spine 21:128–132, 1996.
18. Oberndorfer S, Grisold W: The management of malignant spinal cord compression. Spine 25:653–654, 2000.
19. Quinn JA, DeAngelis LM: Neurologic emergencies in the cancer patient. Semin Oncol 27:311–321, 2000.
20. Rathmell JP, Roland T, DuPen SL: Management of pain associated with metastatic epidural spinal cord compression: Use of imaging studies in planning epidural therapy. Reg Anesth Pain Med 25:113–116, 2000.
21. Schiff D, Shaw EG, Cascino TL: Outcome after spinal reirradiation for malignant epidural spinal cord compression. Ann Neurol 37:583–589, 1995.
22. Talcott JA, Stomper PC, Drislane FW, et al: Assessing suspected spinal cord compression: A multidisciplinary outcomes analysis of 342 episodes. Support Care Cancer 7:31–38, 1999.

55. SUPERIOR VENA CAVA SYNDROME

Kelly C. Mack, RN, MSN, AOCN, NP-C, and Carolyn Becker, RN, OCN

1. Define superior vena cava syndrome.

Superior vena cava syndrome (SVCS) is a clinical diagnosis that describes a pattern of physical findings resulting from obstruction of blood flow through the superior vena cava. The resulting engorgement of collateral veins of the thorax, head, and neck produces the classic symptoms.

2. What causes SVCS?

Obstruction of blood flow can be caused by any of the following three factors or a combination thereof:

1. **Compression.** Extrinsic pressure on the blood vessel as a result of tumor or enlarged lymph nodes is the most common mechanism of superior vena cava obstruction.

2. **Thrombosis.** Thrombosis, usually caused by compression by a tumor or central venous catheter or pacemaker wire, is becoming an increasingly common cause of superior vena cava obstruction.

3. **Invasion.** Invasion within the superior vena cava by tumor is an unusual cause.

3. What anatomic mechanism underlies SVCS?

The superior vena cava is the major vessel for drainage of venous blood from the head, neck, upper extremities, and upper thorax. It is located in the right anterior superior mediastinum and is surrounded by rigid structures: sternum, trachea, right bronchus, aorta, pulmonary artery, perihilar and paratracheal lymph nodes, and vertebral bodies. The superior vena cava is a low-pressure, large but thin-walled, easily compressible structure. It is vulnerable to any space-occupying process in its vicinity.

When the superior vena cava is fully or partially obstructed, venous return to the right atrium is diminished, resulting in increased venous pressure behind the obstruction. This increase in venous pressure (venous hypertension) causes venous stasis in the head, arms, and upper chest. Engorgement and dilation of superficial veins result, and extensive venous collateral circulation in the neck and thorax develops in an effort to bypass the obstruction. Other mediastinal structures, such as the bronchi, esophagus, and spinal cord, may be threatened as a result of an enlarging mass within the mediastinum. The symptoms depend on the rate, degree, and location of obstruction; the aggressiveness of the tumor; and the competency of collateral circulation.

4. What are the classic signs and symptoms?

The most common **early** symptoms include dyspnea, orthopnea (ability to breathe easily only in the upright position), and facial edema. A "tight-collar" feeling with fullness in the face and upper extremity swelling is less common. Less frequently, chest pain and dysphagia are experienced. The physical findings are classic and unmistakable. Venous distention of neck, scalp, anterior and posterior chest wall, and shoulders is the hallmark of SVCS. Venous pressures in the upper body and head have been recorded as high as 200–500 cm H_2O. The veins become prominent, dilated, tortuous, and palpable. This sign is more evident when the patient is prone or bending forward. Veins often run a vertical or nearly vertical course. They can be distinguished from the telangiectasias of the elderly in that they are more numerous, widespread, and enlarged. Other features of SVCS include facial and periorbital edema and swelling of the upper extremities, in particular the right arm. Plethora (ruddy, purple-red complexion), cyanosis, and cough are less common but still considered classic features.

Symptoms of **advanced** disease are rare. Examples include hoarseness, stridor, engorged conjunctiva, and symptoms of increased intracranial pressure, such as headache, dizziness, visual changes, changes in mental status, respiratory distress (respiratory rate > 30/min) and seizures.

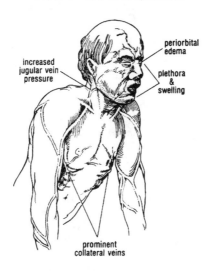

Classic clinical symptoms of SVCS. (From Miller SE: Superior vena cava syndrome. In Polomano RC, Miller SE (eds): Understanding and Managing Oncologic Emergencies. Columbus, OH, Adria Laboratories, 1987, with permission.)

5. What determines the severity of symptoms?

The severity of symptoms is determined by how rapidly the obstruction develops. A slowly developing obstruction allows time for collateral circulation to develop, and the severity of symptoms is lessened. Conversely, rapid onset of symptoms precludes development of collateral circulation and therefore increases circulatory compromise. Regardless of rapidity of onset, all symptoms and physical findings are aggravated by bending forward, stooping, or lying down—anything that increases intrathoracic or intracranial pressure.

6. Who is at risk for developing SVCS?

Up to 97% of all cases of SVCS are caused by cancer. Nonmalignant causes are responsible for only 3–10% of cases. Although these numbers suggest that SVCS is a common disorder, in fact it is relatively uncommon. Only 3–4% of oncologic patients develop SVCS, usually in later stages of disease.

7. What types of malignancies are associated with SVCS?

Lung cancer is responsible for 85% of all cases of SVCS. Small cell carcinoma is the most common histologic type, followed by squamous cell carcinoma of the lung. Cancers arising in the right lung are four times more likely to cause SVCS because the superior vena cava is located in the right lung. Nonetheless, only 6–7% of patients with lung cancer develop SVCS.

Non-Hodgkin's lymphoma is the second most common malignancy to cause SVCS. Between 7–20% of all patients with non-Hodgkin's lymphoma develop SVCS. Although Hodgkin's disease commonly involves the mediastinum, it is an uncommon cause of SVCS.

Breast cancer is the most common metastatic disease causing SVCS. Rarely, thymoma, germ cell tumors and Kaposi's sarcoma also may cause SVCS. Metastatic cancers are responsible for 5–10% of all cases of SVCS.

8. What are the nonmalignant causes of SVCS?

Traditionally, nonmalignant cases of SVCS have been caused by infectious agents. The first described case of SVCS was caused by a syphilitic aortic aneurysm, reported in 1757. Historically, tuberculosis mediastinitis was a common cause of SVCS, accounting for up to 45% of cases before the development of effective antiinfective agents. With the increasing incidence of AIDS and the corresponding increasing incidence of tuberculosis and syphilis, some clinicians warn that infectious causes must again be considered in the differential diagnosis.

Currently the most common nonmalignant cause of superior vena cava syndrome is thrombosis. This iatrogenic complication is seen most commonly in the presence of central venous catheters or pacemakers. Mediastinal fibrosis, a narrowing or stricture of the superior vena cava, may be caused by radiation therapy to the mediastinum or histoplasmosis. This cause is exceedingly rare. Other nonmalignant causes include goiters, idiopathic mediastinal fibrosis, and histoplasmosis.

9. How is the diagnosis of SVCS made?

Clinical signs and symptoms, along with imaging studies such as chest radiograph or chest computed tomography scan, are usually sufficient to make the diagnosis. Current practice demands a tissue diagnosis before instituting treatment unless the patient has a malignancy known to cause SVCS. The only exception to this dictum is when respiratory and neurologic status are so compromised that a delay in treatment would pose a threat to life; this situation is rare.

IMAGING STUDY	COMMENTS
Chest radiograph	Shows right superior mediastinal mass (widening) and mediastinal and paratracheal lymphadenopathy. May be normal despite obstruction.
Computed tomography (CT) of chest	Gives more detail about superior vena cava, its tributaries, and other critical structures (bronchi and spinal cord). Can identify intrinsic vs. extrinsic causes of obstruction. May guide attempts at biopsy.
Contrast venography	Controversial because of invasive nature and use of contrast. Carries risk of thrombosis. Can confirm clinical diagnosis, outline anatomy, and define pattern of collateral flow. Largely replaced radionuclide studies (SPECT scan or technetium-99 scan) but is useful if surgery is contemplated.*
Magnetic resonance imaging	Because of multiplane capabilities, better than CT to show relationship of nodes, vessels, and other mediastinal structures and to demonstrate vessel patency. Chest wall collaterals easier to see on CT scan.

SPECT = single-photon emission computed tomography.
* Concern that interrupting the integrity of a vessel wall in the presence of increased intracranial pressure may lead to excessive bleeding has been refuted by clinical experience.

10. What procedures are used to obtain tissue for diagnosis?

As a general rule, the least invasive method of obtaining tissue is used first. The likelihood of getting a diagnostic sample must be factored into this decision.

DIAGNOSTIC PROCEDURE	COMMENTS
Sputum cytology	For patients with suspected lung carcinoma; approximately 50% chance of diagnostic success.
Thoracentesis	Indicated if pleural effusion present.
Bone marrow biopsy	Rarely done; only if bone marrow involvement suspected.
Bronchoscopy	Useful if small cell lung cancer is suspected.
CT-guided needle biopsy	Effective and safe alternative to open biopsy or mediastinoscopy.
Mediastinoscopy	If all other procedures fail; carries some risk because of difficulty with hemostasis in presence of large, dilated veins.
Thoracotomy	If all other procedures fail, risk of hemorrhage because of dilated veins in operative field; parasternal approach is known as Chamberlain procedure

11. SVCS is listed among oncologic emergencies. Is there an urgency to begin treatment?

SVCS has long been considered a potentially life-threatening medical emergency. Only patients with airway compromise, cardiovascular collapse, or increased intracranial pressure are at high risk and require emergent treatment. Historically it was common to give emergent radiotherapy with initial high-dose fractions, sometimes even before histologic diagnosis was established. Invasive diagnostic procedures were avoided because they were considered to be dangerous because of the high intraluminal pressure and the presumed increased risk of hemorrhage. In fact, a study done by Ahmann revealed an approximate 1% complication rate with invasive procedures, none of them life-threatening. Biopsy does not carry an excessive risk in patients with SVCS. Concern about exposure to anesthesia in patients with SVCS was also allayed. Whenever possible, the standard of care demands that time be taken to establish a histologic diagnosis so that proper treatment may be initiated.

12. What is the goal of treatment?

The goal of treatment is to decrease the size of the tumor or obstruction, thereby relieving the pressure and restoring normal venous drainage. This strategy brings rapid resolution of symptoms. Secondarily and simultaneously, the goal is to attempt a cure of the primary malignant process. Small cell lung carcinoma, non-Hodgkin's lymphoma, and germ cell tumors constitute 85% of the malignant causes of SVCS and are potentially curable.

13. Once the diagnosis is made, how is SVCS treated?

Treatment of SVCS varies, depending on the underlying cause: lung cancer, non-Hodgkin's lymphoma, or thrombus.

14. Describe the treatment for SVCS due to lung cancer.

Small cell lung cancer is a chemosensitive tumor treated initially with combination chemotherapy alone. If there is no response or if disease progresses, radiation therapy is used. The mean time to resolution of symptoms for small cell carcinoma treated with combination chemotherapy is 7 days (range = 7–10 days). The presence of SVCS is not an adverse prognostic factor for small cell lung cancer. In this setting, onset of SVCS develops quickly because of the characteristic rapid doubling time of small cell lung cancers.

Non-small cell lung cancer is not considered chemosensitive. The initial treatment is radiation therapy. The likelihood of relieving symptoms is high, but overall prognosis is poor.

15. How is SVCS due to non-Hodgkin's lymphoma treated?

The most common subtypes of non-Hodgkin's lymphoma are diffuse large cell and lymphoblastic lymphoma. Both are high-grade lymphomas and are considered chemosensitive and curable in the earlier stages. Patients should undergo a complete staging work-up before treatment is initiated if time permits (as is usually the case). For patients with lymphoma, chemotherapy is the treatment of choice. It provides both local and systemic therapeutic activity. Local consolidation with radiotherapy may be beneficial in patients with bulky mediastinal disease (> 10 cm or > one-third the diameter of the chest on chest radiograph). In this setting, radiation is used to treat the obstruction of the superior vena cava; chemotherapy follows and is used to treat systemic disease. Chemotherapy alone is mandated if the patient has already undergone previous mediastinal radiation. Most patients achieve complete relief of symptoms within 2 weeks after beginning treatment.

16. Describe the treatment of thrombus-related SVCS.

If obstruction is caused by a thrombus, fibrinolytic therapy with streptokinase or recombinant tissue-type plasminogen activator (tPA, a highly selective fibrinolytic agent) is a common intervention. Another alternative is to remove the catheter that induced thrombus formation with simultaneous anticoagulant therapy to prevent embolization. Surgical removal of a thrombus (mechanical thrombectomy) is rare.

17. When and how is thrombolytic therapy used?

Thrombolytic therapy is limited to catheter-induced SVCS. Until recently, urokinase was the most commly used thrombolytic therapy. With the unavailibility of urokinase, other thrombolytic therapies are being explored. Recently tPA (Alteplase, Activase), administered as a continuous infusion, has been used with great success. It has selective action on a clot and can be used safely when thrombolytic therapy is administered systemically. The total dose (1.25 mg/kg) is administered over 3 hours; 60% is given in the first hour and the remaining 40% over 2 hours. Compared with urokinase, tPA is less likely to cause hemorrhagic complications, has a shorter time to clot lysis, and is more likely to dissolve a clot formed more than 5 days before the start of the infusion. These advantages must be balanced against the added cost of tPA. As always, thrombolytic therapy is contraindicated in patients with cerebral metastases or at risk for intracranial hemorrhage.

18. What monitoring is required for thrombolytic therapy?

Patients receiving tPA are monitored closely for bleeding complications. Vital signs are monitored every 15 minutes for the first hour, then every 30–60 minutes for the duration of the infusion, depending on the clinical situation. Monitoring for bleeding complications should continue beyond the discontinuation of thrombolytic therapy because the effects last for several hours. Any thrombolytic agent must be administered with an infusion pump. No other invasive monitoring is necessary.

19. What other drugs may be used to treat SVCS?

In addition to the thrombolytic agent, patients also receive a heparin infusion and are converted to an oral anticoagulant before discharge. The patient must be educated about discharge medications and periodic laboratory studies (protime measurement with an international normalized ratio). Compression of the superior vena cava by tumor or adenopathy can be complicated by a secondary thrombosis. Venous stasis distal to the obstruction may allow a clot to form. For this reason, heparin or oral anticoagulants may be used to reduce the extent of thrombus formation and prevent progression.

20. What is the role of surgery in the treatment of SVCS?

Surgery is rarely needed for malignant SVCS. It is considered when the obstructive process progresses rapidly. In general, surgery is reserved for patients with chronic or recurrent SVCS who have a good prognosis and in whom all other treatment options have been exhausted. There are two types of surgical procedures:

1. Superior vena cava bypass graft creates a new vessel that circumvents the obstruction.
2. Placement of a stent into the superior vena cava to dilate and expand the narrowed lumen of the vessel provides immediate relief of symptoms for both malignant and benign causes. Complications include stent migration, misplacement, and occlusion.

21. Discuss the morbidity and mortality associated with surgery for SVCS.

Surgical intervention has been shown to be an effective technique for the handful of patients reported in the literature. All patients had immediate relief of symptoms. At long-term follow-up, 80% of bypass grafts remained patent up to 15 years, and most patients were symptom-free. There were no reports of operative mortality. It must be remembered that surgery is a rare intervention done only in highly selective situations.

22. What are the alternatives to surgery in select situations?

The most effective alternative is transluminal angioplasty using a balloon technique similar to that used for cardiac vessel disease, with insertion of expandable wire stents through the angioplasty device. If a thrombus is causing the obstruction, thrombolytic therapy may be administered directly to the clot via the angioplasty device.

23. What are the major differences in presentation and behavior between superior vena cava caused by benign and malignant causes?

Patients who present with a benign obstruction of the superior vena cava often have symptoms long before seeking medical advice. Short duration of symptoms (3–4 weeks) usually indicates malignancy. It often takes more time to establish the diagnosis of benign SVCS, but survival is markedly longer for a nonmalignant etiology.

24. Do steroids have a role in the treatment of SVCS?

The role of steroids is controversial, although some studies show that corticosteroids may help in reducing symptoms associated with tumor necrosis and inflammation. An inflammatory reaction is usually not associated with SVCS. Steroids are probably indicated when respiratory distress is present.

25. What is the role of radiation therapy?

Radiation therapy is the initial treatment of choice when the histologic diagnosis cannot be established and the patient's clinical status is deteriorating. This situation, however, is exceedingly rare. In a true emergency, the bronchus is likely to be obstructed. Other critical structures, including the esophagus, trachea, vocal cords, and pericardium, may be involved. The total dose of radiation ranges from 3,000–5,000 cGy, depending on the underlying malignancy. Initially, 2–4 large daily fractions (300–400 cGy) are followed by conventional fractionation (180–200 cG/day). The radiation field includes gross tumor with appropriate margins plus mediastinal, hilar, and supraclavicular lymph nodes. Usually improvement is seen within 24–72 hours. More rapid responses are seen with non-Hodgkin's lymphoma than with small cell carcinoma. Clinical improvement may be due to development of collateral circulation in addition to decreased obstruction of the superior vena cava by a smaller tumor mass.

26. What important nursing interventions are involved in the care of patients with SVCS?

1. **Maintain airway patency.** Bedrest with the head of the bed elevated (Fowler's position) plus use of supplemental oxygen may temporarily relieve dyspnea and other symptoms caused by decreased cardiac output and increased venous pressure. Assistance with activities of daily living is also recommended to decrease energy expenditure.

2. **Monitor fluid and electrolyte balance.** Overhydration may exacerbate symptoms of SVCS. Although diuretic therapy and reduced salt diets have been used to decrease edema, their efficacy has not been demonstrated. Conversely, dehydration and the associated increased risk of thrombosis should not be ignored.

3. **Monitor vital signs and level of consciousness.** The patient should be observed for respiratory stridor and changes in mental status. Respiratory and neurologic changes may signal onset of a true emergency (from extension of thromboses to cerebral veins).

4. **Avoid accessing veins of the involved extremity** (usually the right arm) because of the risk of poor circulation, venous stasis, phlebitis, thrombosis, and hemorrhage. Postprocedural bleeding as a result of venous engorgement is a major concern. If chemotherapy is administered, decreased circulation may result in local accumulation of drug with poor absorption into the systemic circulation. This tendency is of particular concern when vesicant or irritant drugs are used. The safety of administering chemotherapy into the peripheral veins of lower extremities is controversial. Therefore, surgical cannulation of the femoral vein with a Broviac or Hickman-type catheter is recommended.

5. **Avoid invasive or constrictive procedures of the involved extremity.** Rings and restrictive clothing should be removed. Blood pressure measurement can be done on the thigh. Venipunctures can be done on the lower extremities.

6. **Reduce anxiety.** A calm, restful environment with visible support is helpful. Analgesics and tranquilizers may be administered for discomfort and anxiety. Interventions to avoid the Valsalva maneuver (e.g., stool softeners, cough suppressants, antiemetics) may be indicated to keep intrathoracic pressure as low as possible.

7. **Assist with medical intervention.** Coagulation profiles should be monitored if anticoagulants are used. Emergent treatment must be instituted for symptoms of cerebral edema, decreased cardiac output, or airway obstruction.

8. **Assess teaching needs.** For some patients, malignancy is diagnosed after the onset and diagnosis of SVCS. Such patients must deal with the emergency of SVCS as well as the

unexpected diagnosis of malignancy and need teaching related to the disease process, treatment of SVCS, treatment of the malignancy, and body image changes. The nurse should stress that changes in physical appearance are temporary; body image changes secondary to facial edema and plethora subside with successful treatment.

9. **Treat side effects related to therapy.** For most patients with SVCS, chemotherapy or radiation therapy is used to treat the underlying malignancy. Radiation side effects may include skin reactions, dysphagia, esophagitis, dry cough, nausea, vomiting, and fatigue. Chemotherapy has its own set of side effects and toxicities, depending on the specific agents used.

27. What is the prognosis of SVCS?

Prognosis strongly correlates with prognosis of underlying disease. Important prognostic variables include underlying malignancy (histology), extent of the primary tumor (stage), responsiveness of the tumor to radiation therapy or chemotherapy, patient's performance status at the time of diagnosis, treatment history, and availability of remaining treatment options. The prognosis for lymphoma is better than that for lung cancer. For untreated malignant SVCS, survival is often less than 6 weeks.

28. What is the risk of recurrence after successful treatment of SVCS?

Recurrence is rare in patients with non-Hodgkin's lymphoma; unfortunately, it is more common with small cell carcinoma of the lung. Patients with SVCS related to malignancy have an approximately 10–19% chance of recurring SVCS.

REFERENCES

1. Abner A: Approach to the patient who presents with superior vena cava obstruction. Chest 103:394S–397S, 1993.
2. Ahmann FR: A reassessment of the clinical implications of the superior vena cava syndrome. J Clin Oncol 2:961–969, 1984.
3. Baker GL, Barnes HJ: Superior vena cava syndrome: Etiology, diagnosis, and treatment. Am J Crit Care 1:54–64, 1992.
4. Escalante CP: Causes and management of superior vena cava syndrome. Oncology 7(6):61–68; discussion, 71–72, 75–77, 1993.
5. Gray BH, Olin JW, Graor RA, et al: Safety and efficacy of thrombolytic therapy for superior vena cava syndrome. Chest 99:54–59, 1991.
6. Greenberg S, Kosinski R, Daniels J: Treatment of superior vena cava thrombosis with recombinant tissue type plasminogen activator. Chest 99:1298–1301, 1991.
7. Holland JF, Bast RC, Morton DL, et al: Oncologic Emergencies: Cancer Medicine, 4th ed. Baltimore, Williams & Wilkins, 1999.
8. Rantis PC, Littooy FN: Successful treatment of prolonged superior vena cava syndrome with thrombolytic therapy: A case report. J Vasc Surg 20:108–113, 1994.
9. Sitton E: Superior vena cava syndrome. In Yarbro CH, Frogge MH, Goodman M, Groenwald SL (eds): Cancer Nursing Principles and Practice, 5th ed. Boston, Jones & Bartlett, 2000, pp 900–912.
10. Tighe DA: Superior vena caval syndrome: Color flow Doppler detection of collateral venous channels. J Am Soc Echocardiogr 13:780–784, 2000.
11. Yahalom J: Oncologic emergencies: Superior vena cava syndrome. In DeVita V, Hellman S, Rosenberg SA (eds): Cancer: Principles and Practice of Oncology, 6th ed. Philadelphia, Lippincott Williams & Wilkins, 2001, pp 2609–2619.

56. SYNDROME OF INAPPROPRIATE ANTIDIURETIC HORMONE

Leigh K. Kaszyk, RN, MS, and Debra Adornetto, RN, MS

1. What is the syndrome of inappropriate antidiuretic hormone (SIADH)?

SIADH is a syndrome of hyponatremia due to abnormal secretion or production of antidiuretic hormone (ADH). ADH levels are inappropriate for the osmotic or volume stimuli that normally cause the release of ADH. Despite a normal intravascular volume, the urine osmolality is inappropriately high (concentrated) compared with plasma osmolality. ADH causes water retention, which leads to decreased sodium and inability to excrete dilute urine. Cancers, particularly small-cell lung cancer, are the most common causes of SIADH.

2. What physiologic mechanisms maintain normal plasma osmolality and plasma sodium concentrations?

1. ADH, also known as vasopressin, helps to conserve water. It is secreted by the posterior pituitary in response to hypotension, decreased fluid intake, and blood loss. Water is conserved when ADH is released; hence the word "antidiuretic" in its name. ADH acts on the distal renal tubules to increase permeability, resulting in increased reabsorption of water from the kidney.

2. Thirst mechanism is activated by osmoreceptors located in the hypothalamus in response to dry mouth, hyperosmolality, and plasma volume depletion. A water loss of 2% of body weight or increase in osmolality activates the thirst mechanism.

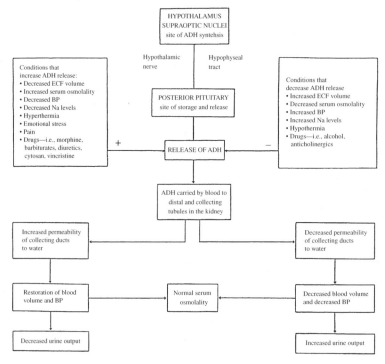

Mechanisms of ADH release. (From Poe CM, Taylor LM: Syndrome of inappropriate antidiuretic hormone: Assessment and nursing implications. Oncol Nurs Forum 16:373–381, 1989, with permission.)

3. How does ADH affect the body?

When blood levels of ADH increase, the epithelium of the cortical collecting ducts of the kidneys becomes water-permeable. Water enters the extracellular fluid through osmosis, less water is excreted, and urine osmolality increases. The results are excessive water retention and dilutional hyponatremia.

4. What causes SIADH?

Any patient presenting with symptoms of SIADH without a known cause should have a complete malignancy work-up; 60% of patients with SIADH are diagnosed with cancer. Only 1–2% of patients with cancer, however, develop SIADH. The most common malignancy causing SIADH is lung cancer. Up to 15% of patients with small cell lung cancer (SCLC) have SIADH at presentation, and ADH levels are increased in 50% of the cases. SIADH is not a negative prognostic factor in SCLC; it is also not related to the patient's potential response to chemotherapy.

Causes of SIADH

Malignant tumors	Central nervous system disorders
Lung cancer	Trauma
Thymoma	Stroke
Mesothelioma	Infection
Prostate cancer	**General surgery**
Lymphomas	
Hodgkin's disease	**Pharmaceutical agents**
Gastrointestinal cancer	Cytotoxic agents
	Vinca alkaloids
Pulmonary disease	Cisplatin
Acute respiratory failure	Cyclophosphamide
Tuberculosis	Tricyclic antidepressants
Positive pressure ventilation	Morphine

5. Why do people with cancer develop SIADH?

SIADH most often results from ectopic production or release of ADH by the tumor. There is evidence that the production or release of atrial natriuretic peptide (ANP) by itself or in conjunction with ADH is a factor in SIADH. People with cancer often receive drugs, such as cytotoxic agents, morphine, and tricyclic antidepressants, which release or potentiate the action of ADH. In addition, certain lung conditions that patients with cancer often develop (e.g., pneumonia, empyema) may result in SIADH.

6. What other pathophysiologic mechanisms are responsible for SIADH?

One pathologic mechanism is inappropriate secretion of ADH from the supraoptic hypophyseal system. This mechanism is seen in postoperative patients and patients with central nervous system disorders, shock, positive pressure ventilation, and other conditions that increase intrathoracic pressure or decrease venous return (e.g., intrathoracic tumors).

7. What is the cause of SIADH in patients infected with the human immunodeficiency virus (HIV)?

Most HIV-infected patients with SIADH have *Pneumocystis carinii,* or bacterial pneumonia. Other diagnoses include central nervous system infections or malignant disorders.

8. What other factors contribute to the development of SIADH in patients with cancer?

- Chemotherapy with or without hydration due to water-retaining properties of agents (e.g, cisplatin) in combination with vigorous hydration
- Nausea (common side effect of chemotherapy) stimulates ADH release.
- Tricyclic antidepressants may potentiate the action of ADH.
- Narcotics for pain relief may enhance ADH secretion or its effect on the distal nephron.

- Presence of pulmonary infections (abcesses, pneumonia)
- History of infections or lesions of the central nervous system
- Concurrent cardiac, renal, or hepatic diseases

9. How is SIADH diagnosed?

First the patient must be assessed clinically (history and physical exam) to determine whether intravascular volume is normal, low, or expanded. Low volume status must be corrected. Then blood and urine specimens are obtained for assessment of sodium and osmolality. The patient has SIADH if the intravascular volume is normal or increased; urine osmolality is high compared with plasma osmolality; and renal, thyroid, and adrenal function are normal. Observe for fluid overload: weigh patient, maintain strict input and output values, and test urine for specific gravity. To make a diagnosis of SIADH, adrenal insufficiency and hypothyroidism must be ruled out, because both may increase ADH secretion.

10. Which laboratory values should the nurse observe in patients with SIADH?

SIADH levels	Normal levels
Low serum sodium (< 130 mEq/L)	135–145 mEq/L
Low serum osmolality (< 280 mOsm/kg)	280–300 mOsm/kg
High urine sodium level (> 20 mEq/L)	40–220 mmol/L
High urine osmolality (> 1400 mOsm/kg)	200–800 mOsm/kg
Low blood urea nitrogen (BUN)	6–23 mg/dl
Low creatinine	0.6–1.1 mg/dl
Low uric acid	Male, 3.4–7.0 g/dl; female, 2.4–5.7 g/dl
Low albumin	3.4–5.0 g/dl

11. What are the clinical symptoms of SIADH?

Signs and symptoms are a reflection of water intoxication.

Mild hyponatremia (sodium level = 115–130 mEq/L)
Constitutional: fatigue, weakness
Gastrointestional: nausea, vomiting, anorexia, thirst, diarrhea
Neurologic: headaches, lethargy, confusion, irritability
Renal: decreased urine output, weight gain
Muscular: myalgias, muscle cramping (edema is rarely seen)
Severe hyponatremia (sodium level = 100–110 mEq/L)
Altered mental status
Confusion, personality changes
Psychosis
Seizure activity
Progressive lethargy, coma

12. What are the goals of treatment of SIADH?

The primary goal in patients with cancer and SIADH is treatment of the underlying tumor with systemic chemotherapy. Initial interventions are aimed at correcting the sodium–water imbalance. Discontinue agents that contribute to SIADH, such as diuretics, morphine, and antidepressants.

13. How are symptomatic patients treated until the tumor is affected by chemotherapy?

Symptomatic treatment consists of restriction of fluids to 500–1,000 ml/day for mild-to-moderate SIADH (sodium level > 125 mg). In the presence of life-threatening hyponatremia, an intravenous solution (200–300 ml) of 3% hypertonic saline is infused over 2–3 hours, and furosemide is administered concurrently to increase fluid excretion. Fluid is restricted to 500 ml/day. Care must be taken not to increase the serum sodium level too quickly, or neuronal damage may result, causing cerebral edema and seizures.

14. **What fluids with a high sodium concentration may be offered to patients with SIADH?**
Tomato juice, V-8 juice, beef or chicken broth, and Gatorade have high sodium concentrations.

15. **What nursing interventions may decrease the severity of symptoms (e.g., thirst and neurologic changes) associated with SIADH?**
Divide the amount of fluids the patient consumes among day, evening, and night hours. Rinse the patient's mouth every 2 hours, and offer sugar-free candy/gum to stimulate salivation. Orient the patient to person, time, and place using cues such as calendars and clocks. Implement seizure precautions as necessary.

16. **What is done for patients with chronic or recurrent SIADH despite chemotherapy?**
Chronic or recurrent SIADH is treated with drugs that inhibit the renal effects of ADH, such as demeclocycline, furosemide, and lithium carbonate. Demeclocycline is the treatment of choice. It may take 5–7 days after initiation of treatment for symptoms to decrease. Demeclocycline, an antibiotic, is given orally in a dose of 900–1200 mg/day. This tetracycline derivative interferes with ADH action by decreasing the renal response to ADH, causing isotonic or hypotonic urine and an increase in serum sodium. Absorption may be impaired if the drug is taken with milk or milk products. Side effects include photosensitivity, hematologic changes, azotemia, superinfection, and mild nephrotoxicity.

17. **Does recurrent SIADH mean that the cancer is returning?**
Not always. SIADH usually resolves once the cancer is treated. However, it may return during stable disease while the patient is receiving maintenance chemotherapy. Nurses need to be aware of the patient population at risk for developing SIADH. Involving patients in the management of SIADH is critical in reversing symptoms. The ability to manage this syndrome and enhance the patient's quality of life depends on how the patient is taught about SIADH and how well the patient understands and accepts the treatment.

REFERENCES

1. Block JB: Paraneoplastic syndromes. In Haskell CM, Berek JS (eds): Cancer Treatment. Philadelphia, W.B. Saunders, 1995, pp 245–264.
2. Ezzone SA: SIADH. Can J Oncol Nurs 3:187–188, 1999.
3. Haapoja IS: Syndrome of inappropriate antidiuretic hormone. In Yarbro CH, Frogge MH, Goodman M, Groewald SL (eds): Cancer Nursing: Principles and Practice, 5th ed. Boston, Jones & Bartlett, 2000, pp 913–919.
4. Itano JK, Taoka RN: Core Curriculum for Oncology Nursing, 3rd ed. Philadelphia, W. B. Saunders, 1998.
5. John WJ, Foon KA, Patchell RA: Paraneoplastic syndromes. In DeVita VT, Hellman S, Rosenberg SA (eds): Cancer: Principles and Practices of Oncology, 5th ed. Philadelphia, Lippincott-Raven, 1997, pp 2397–2422.
6. Keenan AM: Syndrome of inappropriate secretion of antidiuretic hormone in malignancy. Semin Oncol Nurs 15:160–167, 1999.
7. Kovacs L, Robertson GL: Syndrome of inappropriate antidiuresis. Endocrinol Metab Clin North Am 21:859–875, 1992.
8. Moore JM: Syndrome of inappropriate antidiuretic hormone secretion. In Johnson BL, Gross J: Handbook of Oncology Nursing, 3rd ed. Boston, Jones & Bartlett, 1998.
9. Moses AM, Streeter DHP: Disorders of the neurophysis. In Fauci AS, Breunwold E, Isselbacker KJ, et al (eds): Harrison's Principles of Internal Medicine, vol. 2, 14th ed. New York, McGraw-Hill, 1997.
10. Poe CM, Taylor LM: Syndrome of inappropriate antidiuretic hormone: Assessment and nursing implications. Oncol Nurs Forum 16:373–381, 1989.
11. Sorensen JD, Andersen MK, Hansen HH: Syndrome of inappropriate secretion of antidiuretic hormone (SIADH) in malignant disease. J Intern Med 238: 97–110, 1995.
12. Tank WW, Kaptien EM, Feinstein EI, Massry SG: Hyponatremia in hospitalized patients with the acquired immunodeficiency syndrome (AIDS) and the AIDS-related complex. Am J Med 94:169–174, 1993.

57. TUMOR LYSIS SYNDROME

Anne Zobec, MS, RN, CS, ANP, AOCN

1. Define tumor lysis syndrome.

Tumor lysis syndrome (TLS) is an oncologic emergency that may lead to life-threatening complications such as cardiac arrhythmias and renal failure. TLS is a complication of cancer therapy that occurs when a large number of tumor cells are destroyed. It is most common during aggressive treatment of large, rapidly dividing tumors.

2. Describe what happens in TLS.

Chemotherapy given to fast-growing tumors causes massive necrosis of cancer cells. As tumor cells die, they release cellular contents into the bloodstream. When the cell membrane is ruptured, nucleic acids that form DNA and RNA are released along with potassium and phosphorus. The nucleic acids are converted by the liver into uric acid. Abnormally high levels of uric acid, potassium, and phosphorus cause a host of metabolic alterations.

3. What are the harmful effects of TLS?

The high levels of intracellular contents that are liberated from the tumor cells overwhelm the kidneys. High levels of uric acid may crystallize in the distal tubules and collecting ducts, leading to obstructions and eventually acute renal failure. Increased levels of potassium and phosphorus may cause cardiac, neurologic, and gastrointestinal toxicities.

Clinical Manifestations of Tumor Lysis Syndrome

Renal problems	Neuromuscular irritability	
Decreased urine output	Tetany	
Elevated blood urea nitrogen and serum creatinine	Carpopedal spasm	
	Muscle cramps	
Elevated serum uric acid	Confusion, delirium, or hallucination	
Uric acid crystallization in renal tubules	Seizures	
Acute renal failure	Digital and perioral paresthesias	
Cardiac arrhythmias	**Gastrointestinal effects**	
Atrioventricular blocks	Nausea and	Anorexia
Ventricular tachycardia	vomiting	Intestinal colic
Cardiac arrest	Diarrhea	Hyperphosphatemia

4. In which kinds of cancers is TLS more common?

TLS is seen most often in patients with high-grade lymphoma or acute lymphoblastic leukemia. It also occurs in patients with acute myelogenous leukemia, chronic myelogenous leukemia in blastic transformation, Burkitt's lymphoma, and non-Hodgkin's lymphoma. These kinds of cancers have a high growth fraction; that is, they multiply and grow very quickly. Tumors with rapid growth rates are highly sensitive to the effects of chemotherapy drugs. When treatment begins, the tumor cells are rapidly destroyed.

5. Does TLS present in patients with solid tumors?

TLS is rare in patients with solid tumors because they respond more slowly to chemotherapy. Large, bulky tumors (> 8–10 cm in size) increase the risk. TLS can occur in lung cancer, metastatic breast cancer, melanoma, and metastatic medulloblastoma. Newer chemotherapeutic agents that have greater efficacy against tumors may contribute to more cases of TLS.

6. Can TLS occur in patients who are not treated with chemotherapy?

TLS occasionally occurs with radiation therapy. In untreated patients with cancer, TLS may develop if a rapidly growing, large tumor mass undergoes profound cell destruction. This syndrome also has been reported in patients receiving corticosteroids, hormonal therapy, and biologic response modifiers. Surgical procedures in which the tumor mass is manipulated also may cause spontaneous TLS.

7. What are the identifying laboratory features of patients at risk for TLS?

Patients with elevated levels of blood urea nitrogen (BUN), creatinine, uric acid, and electrolytes before treatment are at a greater risk of developing TLS. These abnormal laboratory studies indicate that the patient may have problems with renal function or dehydration. Patients with increased levels of lactate dehydrogenase (LDH) are also at a greater risk for TLS. LDH levels are correlated with large tumor masses. Other risk factors include splenomegaly, lymphadenopathy, high white blood cell count, and presence of a catabolic state.

8. What are the most common metabolic abnormalities in TLS?

The four hallmark signs of TLS are hyperuricemia, hyperphosphatemia, hyperkalemia, and hypocalcemia. These abnormalities result when the kidneys are unable to process and excrete the huge amount of intracellular products and metabolites that are released when the tumor cells are destroyed.

9. What contributes to a decrease in uric acid excretion?

Uric acid is not excreted well in the following situations: low urinary flow rate in the 24 hours before treatment, history of hyperuricemia or renal failure, renal insufficiency, dehydration, and acidic urine. Uric acid is poorly soluble in acid urine (pH < 5.5).

10. What are the signs and symptoms of hyperuricemia?

The patient usually complains of gastrointestinal symptoms first, before signs of renal failure. Initial signs and symptoms of hyperuricemia include nausea, vomiting, and diarrhea. Flank pain, anuria, oliguria, and cloudy sedimented urine indicate serious problems.

11. When does TLS occur?

TLS develops within hours to a few days after treatment. It most often occurs within the first 24–72 hours after chemotherapy is initiated. TLS may persist for 5–7 days after therapy; this is the period when the most significant tumor cell destruction occurs. TLS also may develop later, with signs and symptoms appearing 4 days after treatment.

12. What are the goals of treatment of TLS?

The primary goal is prevention of renal failure and severe electrolyte imbalances. This goal is accomplished by increasing urine production, decreasing uric acid concentrations, and increasing the solubility of uric acid in urine.

13. How can TLS be prevented?

When patients are identified as being at high risk for developing TLS, special treatments can be initiated to prevent its development. Preventive measures should be started before chemotherapy is initiated and continued for at least 7 days after chemotherapy. Being alert for early symptoms and close monitoring of laboratory values can reduce the risk of TLS.

14. Describe the important treatment strategies.

Prevention is the best strategy. The medical management of TLS includes aggressive hydration, forced diuresis, alkalinization of urine, administration of allopurinol, and prompt correction of metabolic alterations. Dialysis may be necessary in severe cases.

15. What is the role of allopurinol in TLS?

Most patients at risk for TLS are treated with allopurinol before and during initial chemotherapy. Allopurinol decreases uric acid concentration and inhibits the enzyme xanthine oxidase, which, in turn, blocks the conversion of uric acid precursors into uric acid and prevents uric acid nephropathy. Allopurinol reduces both serum and urine levels of uric acid. Intravenous allopurinol has been found to be safe and effective in patients who are unable to take the oral medication.

16. What side effects are associated with allopurinol?

Some patients may experience a hypersensitivity reaction with side effects of fever, eosinophilia, rash, or dermatitis. Allopurinol should be stopped when it is no longer needed because it can sometimes cause drug fever.

17. Why is alkalinization of the urine important?

Uric acid is only slightly soluble in acid urine, but it is much more soluble (> 10 times) in alkaline urine. When the urine is acidic, high levels of uric acid form crystals in the tubules of the kidneys. To prevent crystallization, intravenous fluids are given to hydrate the patient and to increase the amount of fluids flowing through the kidneys. Sodium bicarbonate is frequently added to the intravenous fluids to create alkaline urine (50–100 mEq sodium bicarbonate to each liter of intravenous fluid). Urine pH values are obtained and should be kept at a level above 6 or 7.

18. Can other drugs be used to alkalinize the urine?

Acetazolamide, a diuretic, may be given in addition to or in place of sodium bicarbonate. It inhibits the reabsorption of bicarbonate, preventing its excretion in the urine. Urate oxidase is an investigational medication that promotes the excretion of uric acid.

19. What problems may be associated with alkalinizing the urine?

Caution should be used in alkalinizing the urine because calcium phosphate precipitation may occur. Some physicians choose not to alkalinize the urine to minimize further problems.

20. Describe the most important nursing interventions.

Nursing care should focus on prevention and management of symptoms caused by metabolic disturbances. Serum electrolytes may be ordered as often as every 4–6 hours in the initial crisis period. Nursing assessment should center on the symptoms of hyperkalemia, hypocalcemia, and hyperphosphatemia. Hyperkalemia results in cardiovascular change that may lead to atrioventricular block, ventricular tachycardia, ventricular fibrillation, or asystole. Neuromuscular effects of hyperkalemia include muscle cramps, weakness, and paresthesia. Gastrointestinal effects are nausea, diarrhea, and intestinal colic. Symptoms of hypocalcemia include ventricular arrhythmias, 2:1 heart block, and cardiac arrest. Neurologic symptoms include muscle cramping and twitching, carpopedal spasms, tetany, laryngospasm, paresthesia, confusion, delirium, and convulsions. Hyperphosphatemia primarily causes renal problems: anuria, oliguria, and azotemia.

21. What simple assessment tests can detect a low calcium level?

Low levels of serum calcium cause neuromuscular irritability. A low calcium level can be detected by Chvostek's and Trousseau's signs. Chvostek's sign is tested by lightly tapping the facial nerve area below the zygomatic process in front of the ear. A positive response (low calcium level) is indicated if the facial muscles and upper lip contract or twitch. Trousseau's sign is tested by inflating a blood pressure cuff to a level slightly above the patient's systolic blood pressure for 1–3 minutes. The sign is considered positive if contractions of the hand result.

22. How is hyperkalemia treated?

Hyperkalemia can be treated with oral Kayexalate, 15–30 gm, and 50 ml of 20% sorbitol given 2–4 times/day. Kayexalate also can be given rectally in enema form, if the patient cannot take oral medications. Fifty grams of Kayexalate in 200 ml of 20% sorbitol is given as a retention enema and held for 30–60 minutes. Diuretics, calcium gluconate, sodium bicarbonate, hypertonic dextrose, and regular insulin also may be used to treat hyperkalemia. These medications promote a shift of potassium into the cells or excretion of potassium.

23. What is significant about the patient's fluid level?

Maintaining optimal fluid balance is crucial to the patient's recovery. Intravenous fluids are frequently given at rates of 150–300 ml/hr to ensure that the patient is well hydrated. Hourly assessments of urine output are essential in evaluating kidney function. The urine output goal should be 100 ml/hour or more, with or without the use of diuretics. Nurses should be aware that fluid volume overload may occur. Monitoring blood pressure and pulse at least every 4 hours, auscultating lung sounds, watching for signs of edema and cough, and checking the patient's weight every 12–24 hours can demonstrate early signs of fluid overload.

24. Describe the treatment for elevated phosphate levels.

Phosphate-binding antacids, such as Amphojel or Basaljel given orally in doses of 30–60 ml every 4–6 hours, reduce the serum phosphate level. These antacids may cause constipation, however; stool softeners may be advised.

25. Which medicines should be avoided in patients at risk of TLS?

Aspirin, radiographic contrast, probenecid, and thiazide diuretics should be avoided because they block tubular reabsorption of uric acid. Phosphate and potassium-containing medications also should be avoided.

26. When should hemodialysis be considered?

Patients may require hemodialysis if the above strategies are not successful in removing uric acid and correcting electrolyte abnormalities. Dialysis is usually indicated in patients with serum potassium ≥ 6 mEq/L, serum uric acid ≥ 10 mg/dl, serum phosphorus ≥ 10 mg/dl, symptomatic hypocalcemia, and signs of volume overload.

27. List important patient education topics.

Patients and their families should be taught about treatments and chemotherapy drugs. Signs and symptoms of side effects and problems to report should be explained in detail. Patients should understand the importance of drinking plenty of fluids and also should watch to make sure they have an adequate output of light-colored urine.

REFERENCES

1. Castro M, VanAuken J, Spencer-Cisek P, et al: Acute tumor lysis syndrome associated with concurrent biochemotherapy of metastatic melanoma. Cancer 85:1055–1059, 1999.
2. Ezzone S: Tumor lysis syndrome. Semin Oncol Nurs 15:202–208, 1999.
3. Flombaum C: Metabolic emergencies in the cancer patient. Semin Oncol 27:322–334, 2000.
4. Hogan D, Rosenthal L: Oncologic emergencies in the patient with lymphoma. Semin Oncol Nurs 14:312–320, 1998.
5. Persons DA, Garst J, Vollmer R, Crawford J: Tumor lysis syndrome and acute renal failure after treatment of non-small-cell lung carcinoma with combination irinotecan and cisplatin. Am J Clin Oncol Aug 21:426–429, 1998.
6. Smalley R, Guaspari A, Haase-Statz S, et al: Allopurinol: Intravenous use for prevention and treatment of hyperuricemia. J Clin Oncol 18:1758–1763, 2000.

VII. Caring for the Person with Cancer

58. COMMUNICATION IN CANCER CARE: MAKING EVERY WORD COUNT

Constance Engelking, RN, MS, OCN

1. What is communication?

Communication is everything that occurs between two minds. It is a means for one person to relay a message to another and, in doing so, to stimulate a response. Behavior is communication, and all communication produces behavior. As such, communication is a process that involves both sending and receiving information (i.e., attitudes, feelings, and facts) by verbal and nonverbal means. The "message" from the sender produces feedback or "response" from the receiver, which, in turn, produces reaction or acknowledgement from the sender. Thus, the process of sharing information is:
- A continuous, dynamic, and circular process that relies on feedback mechanisms
- Composed of three key elements, including sender and receiver, message to be conveyed, and medium by which the message is conveyed (verbal and nonverbal)
- Executed according to a common set of rules that are both linguistic and behavioral

2. Explain the meaning of communication in health care.

In health care, the communication process is narrower in scope, addressing specifically how people seek to achieve or maintain health and how they handle issues of health and illness. According to the Northouse model, health care communications involve specific participants, including the health care professional, patients, family members, and significant others. Participants engage in transactions that have both content and relationship dimensions.

The goal of health care transactions is to exchange information about the health and well-being of patients and family members. These transactions take place within certain health care settings, such as a busy clinic or acute care hospital room, and with various participants (e.g., groups on clinical rounds vs. one-on-one interactions). Each of these variables in the process sets the stage for the character of the interaction. Health care providers must be alert to and build their interactive approach in accordance with these dimensions in order to achieve the most effective or therapeutic interaction.

3. What are the essential functions of communication in cancer care?

Communication skills are essential to the practice of oncology nursing because our interactions with patients, family members, and significant others are the vehicle through which we achieve positive clinical outcomes. Chief among the functions of communication in cancer care are:
- Minimizing fears associated with images of pain, suffering, and death that compose the stigma of cancer.
- Facilitating informed decision-making about options for treatment and care, including participation in clinical trials, by assisting patients to formulate and present relevant questions and concerns.
- Interpreting complex medical information about disease and treatment to permit patients and family members to understand the concepts as applied to their clinical situation.
- Providing instruction about self-monitoring, complication identification, and symptom management to empower patients and their family members.
- Navigating patients and their families through the health care system and acting as a liaison among clinical services and settings to ensure continuity.

- Counseling, coaching, and guiding patients and families over the enormous physical and emotional hurdles imposed by cancer.
- Promoting family functioning and mobilizing supportive resources within the patient's network and the community.

4. What are the barriers to effective communication in cancer care?

Internal factors have to do with our personal beliefs, values, and attitudes and are primarily associated with the myths and fallacies surrounding malignant illnesses. Examples include the perceptions that: (1) a diagnosis of cancer equates to pain, suffering, and death; (2) cancer is a contagious illness easily spread to those in close contact; (3) getting cancer is in some way a consequence of or punishment for bad deeds; and (4) people with depressive personality traits are prone to develop cancer. Belief in these myths can produce in nurses feelings of uneasiness and reluctance to initiate relationships with patients and family members. Myths may be further embedded in the nurse's mindset if he or she has personal fears or a previous negative experience with cancer.

External factors relate to the milieu in which cancer care is delivered. Often the setting deters engagement in the interactive dimensions of cancer patient care. In an era of downsizing and resource reallocation, pulling up a chair next to an anxious patient to spend time listening to his or her concerns may not be as highly valued as performing a reimbursable procedure, such as chemotherapy administration.

Internal and External Factors that Hamper Communication Skill Development in Cancer Care

INTERNAL FACTORS	EXTERNAL FACTORS
Focus: Loss of professional credibility. *Worry:* Behaving unprofessionally or losing composure by becoming tearful or visibly distressed during patient/family interaction.	• Abstract nature and difficulty measuring both performance and outcome of clinician/patient/family interactions; subsequent perception that interactive skills are of lower priority for resource allocation than physical care skills.
Focus: Fatalistic attitudes about cancer. *Worry:* "Leaking" the truth about poor prognosis or personal biases/beliefs about cancer and its outcome (e.g., futility of medical intervention, resource waste).	• Limited resources and time constraints associated with restructured health care system; heightened complexity of care produced by technologic advancements.
Focus: Uncertainty about rules for information-sharing (who, what, and how) about cancer. *Worry:* Having to face the consequences of overstepping professional boundaries with patients, family, physicians, and institutions.	• Relational conflicts, strained interpersonal relationships and disagreement among cancer care team about: • type, amount, and timing of information to be shared with patient and family • team member designated as primary patient/family contact
Focus: Concern about emotional attachments. *Worry:* Enduring the sadness of loss and being drawn into patient/family grieving experiences that are emotionally exhausting.	• Lack of peer support for time expenditure to engage in the communicative aspects of cancer care. (Clinicians who expend time talking with patients and families often are viewed by fellow staff members on a busy unit or in high-volume clinic settings as "not carrying their load.")
Focus: Perceived communication skill deficit. *Worry:* Responses to patients and family will be emotionally harmful to them.	• Limited formal educational preparation and lack of role models in the system to provide opportunities for observation of effective interactions.

Adapted from Engelking C: Overcoming barriers to effective communication in cancer care. In Lindley C, Wickham R (eds): Issues in Managing the Oncology Patient. New York, Philips Healthcare Communications, 1999, pp 58–74.

5. Describe the connection between the interactive aspects of oncology nursing and the job-related stress experienced by oncology nurses.

Underdeveloped communication skills are a major source of stress for clinicians who treat patients with cancer. In studies examining stress responses associated with patient/family care in critical care and oncology nursing during the past three decades, interpersonal relationships, which rely heavily on communication, are consistently cited as a primary source of stress. The "diagnostic," "treatment decision-making," and "terminal care" dimensions of cancer often are especially stressful for nurses because the most intimate and emotionally charged interactions with patients and family members take place during these times. Stress is compounded for nurses who are pulled into tumultuous interactions with not one patient or family member at a time but rather simultaneously with a variety of different people in the patient/family networks. Furthermore, nurses often are not able to bring patient/family relationships to closure because the patient is discharged, dies, or is reassigned to a coworker when the nurse is not on duty, thus producing cumulative unresolved grief and raising the level of stress.

6. What are the potential sources of personal stress associated with cancer care communications?

Actual and anticipated encounters with patients, family members, and other members of the health team about sensitive topics such as prognosis, treatment challenges, and end-of-life issues can create feelings of discomfort and significant distress in the nurse who feels unprepared or inadequate in the interactive aspects of clinical practice. Personal discomfort can arise from (1) the content of a discussion; (2) the context in which the exchange takes place; (3) projected patient, family, or physician responses and their consequences; or (4) a combination of factors. For example, nurses can feel overwhelmed when patients and families express strong emotions or misplace/direct outpourings of anger and rage provoked by cancer at nurses because they are a convenient target.

7. How can the nurse deal with such stressors?

Acknowledging feelings of discomfort is an important first step in minimizing associated stress and, ultimately, in cultivating effective communication skills. The following questions can help you get in touch with your own personal reactions:

1. How often do you equate symptoms that you experience with cancer? What is your response to such thoughts?

2. Have you ever borne the brunt of patient/family reactions to the diagnosis and its consequences? How did it make you feel?

3. Have you been asked difficult existential questions, such as "Why did I get cancer?" and "How long do I have to live?" At the time, what was your reaction to the questions?

4. Have you encountered situations in which you worry that you will "reveal the truth" to a patient or family member and thus cause harmful emotional effects? What did you do and why?

5. Have you ever held back tears or avoided a patient's room because you were worried that the patient and family members would read your fatalistic attitudes?

6. Have you ever been in a position of disagreement with patient decisions, family opinions, or physician recommendations? What was your response?

8. What types of patient/family statements can trigger distress in nurses?

A structured self-assessment tool helps to pinpoint specifically what types of patient/family statements trigger distress. The inventory lists anxiety-provoking questions or statements commonly posed by patients, family members, or significant others in the patient's support network. Each question or statement is rated on a simple 5-point Likert scale, ranging from least to most discomfort. The most critical aspect of this introspective exercise is to determine personal reasons for the discomfort ratings that you assign. Space is provided in the far right column to jot down brief narrative notes describing associated personal "fears" or "fantasies" that engender distress in each instance.

Communication Discomfort Self-Inventory

Instructions: The following are questions that might be raised during interactions with patients or their family members. Frequently these questions trigger discomfort in the nurse. Read each trigger statement. Estimate your discomfort level by circling a representative number on the scale provided. Jot down your immediate reactions or concerns about what might happen if/when you respond to the question.

TRIGGER STATEMENT	DISCOMFORT LEVEL					FEARS/CONCERNS
	LEAST				MOST	

The adult patient asks:

1. What's wrong with me? My doctor hasn't said anything.	1	2	3	4	5	
2. My doctor said I have a tumor. Does that mean cancer?	1	2	3	4	5	
3. Have you known other people getting the same treatment as I am? How did they do?	1	2	3	4	5	
4. Do you think I'm going to die?	1	2	3	4	5	
5. How will I look after this radical neck?	1	2	3	4	5	
6. Do you think I'm doing the right thing to take this treatment?	1	2	3	4	5	
7. Why do I have this terrible smell? Do you think the cancer is getting worse?	1	2	3	4	5	
8. How much pain do you think I am going to have?	1	2	3	4	5	
9. How much longer can I go on like this?	1	2	3	4	5	
10. I've taken good care of myself. I don't understand why this had to happen to me.	1	2	3	4	5	
11. I don't want to see anyone. They all feel sorry for me.	1	2	3	4	5	

The young adult patient asks:

12. What will I tell my children?	1	2	3	4	5	
13. Will I see my children grow up?	1	2	3	4	5	
14. How will my wife ever manage?	1	2	3	4	5	
15. Does this mean the end of my sex life?	1	2	3	4	5	
16. If feel I can't go on like this. Is there any point in prolonging the inevitable?	1	2	3	4	5	
17. I can't continue these treatments. They, not the cancer, are what's making me sick.	1	2	3	4	5	

The parent or family member asks:

18. How can I tell my child he won't get better?	1	2	3	4	5	
19. Can't we stop this treatment? We know our mother wouldn't want this despite what our father says.	1	2	3	4	5	
20. How much should we make our father do for himself even if he doesn't want to?	1	2	3	4	5	
21. Will my wife try to kill herself? She seems so depressed.	1	2	3	4	5	
22. This type of cancer runs in our family. Do you think I'll get it too?	1	2	3	4	5	
23. My mother wants to be home, but I don't think I can take care of her. What can I tell her?	1	2	3	4	5	
24. What will I do if my husband dies? I can't face life without him.	1	2	3	4	5	

© Constance Engelking

9. Are there specific guidelines for responding to patients and family members in difficult interactive situations?

There are no recipes or pat answers to give to patients and family members facing the crisis of cancer. However, incorporating some simple concepts into daily practice can help to keep your own feelings of uneasiness in check.

1. Keep in mind that responding to every patient/family question with "the right answer" is neither expected nor realistic. Often questions are merely a way for patients or family members to organize and express their thoughts and concerns. The nurse's silent presence or a simple comforting gesture communicates interest and provides reassurance that they will not be abandoned despite the difficult situation. It may not be as important to give answers as it is to listen, understand, and discover the patient's or family member's real issues and meaning.

2. To avoid confusion, preface any response with a quick assessment to gather data about the most recent information that has been shared with the patient or family member by a physician or other health team member. Sometimes patients or family members have already received answers to their questions and may be testing to determine your level of honesty, the accuracy of the information, or compatibility of your answer with messages from others.

3. It is perfectly acceptable to reveal personal reactions to a patient or family member's situation so long as they are appropriately handled. Examples include statements such as, "It concerns me that you seem so sad," "I'm sorry that you have received this difficult news," or "I too am disappointed that your disease has not responded to the treatment." Tears associated with a genuine spontaneous response are also permissible. Sharing feelings with the patient can help to create a level of empathy and develop the transpersonal relationship necessary for deep and meaningful therapeutic interactions. Self-disclosure is acceptable provided the disclosure is brief and relevant to the situation and patient rather than provider-focused.

4. Consider what patients' or family members' actual motivation might be for posing the question or statement; then realize that this reason is only your assumption and remain skeptical until it is validated with them. A patient found alone crying in his or her room is not necessarily upset. The tears may be an expression of relief or joy at receiving good news.

5. Do not assume family relationships based on age or gender. Often a spouse may be considerably younger or older, and today there are new family constructs. Always validate your assumptions before initiating dialogue. Acting on assumption alone can be embarrassing and, at worst, have negative outcomes for patients and their families or on your relationship.

6. Steer clear of labeling responses to patients and family members as "right" or "wrong." Instead, think of interactions as being "helpful" or unhelpful." This strategy makes the prospect of close encounters much less threatening to your sense of competency with the interactive aspects of cancer care.

10. What can I do if I find myself feeling uneasy with patient/family interactions?

To help determine the source of your discomfort, ask yourself the following questions:

1. What is it about this particular statement/question that really makes me feel uncomfortable?

2. What are all of the possible reasons that the patient/family member might have for making this statement/asking this question?

3. Is my assumption about the patient/family member's motivation valid? Why or why not?

4. Does the patient/family member expect me to respond to this statement/question, or is it rhetorical?

5. Would the most helpful response in this situation be verbal or nonverbal?

11. What are closed communication behaviors? How do they diminish the potential therapeutic benefit of patient/family/nurse interactions?

In addition to the internal and external factors that can hamper communication in cancer care, another significant barrier is closed communication. It is human nature to use both verbal and nonverbal behaviors (consciously and unconsciously) to protect ourselves from emotional discomforts triggered by the content or tone of a discussion and its potentially negative psychological impact.

Nurses, because of the intimate relationships they have with patients and family members, often engage in such behaviors. For example, content categorized as "breaking bad news" (e.g., a new diagnosis of cancer, discovery of metastatic disease, poor response to anticancer therapies, limited availability of curative options) or end-of-life decision-making discussions can evoke distressing images of pain, suffering, and death. Particularly when time is limited, nurses are often hesitant to initiate or participate in such discussions and may protect themselves unconsciously by physically "escaping" the encounter. Nurses also use closed verbal approaches that discourage discussion of intimate subject matters by keeping the level of the dialogue superficial and redirecting or completely closing off the discussion when sensitive topics are broached . Closed communication is also characterized by the use of position or status to maintain control over the interaction.

Closed Communication Patterns and Syndromes

PATTERN	PRESENTATION	
False reassurances Used to "lighten the emotional load" for patient/family but close the door to further exploration of uneasy feelings; minimize patient/family concerns but discourage problem-solving.	**Nurse promises something that may not or cannot happen.** *Clinical situation:* Patient is going to surgery for biopsy of suspicious lesion.	
	Unhelpful: "It's probably nothing. I know things will work out for the best."	*Helpful:* "You seem anxious. What worries you the most?" "Tell me what you're thinking about."
	Nurse says something that is not true. *Clinical situation:* Patient is scheduled for chemotherapy and at high risk for adverse effects.	
	Unhelpful: "Calm down. You have nothing to worry about." "I've seen sicker patients do just fine."	*Helpful:* "I think you have reason to hope for the best with this treatment." "What are you thinking will happen with this therapy?"
	Nurse provides statements that are incongruent with demonstrated behaviors. *Clinical situation:* Nurse, distracted during interaction, focuses on his or her own next actions, not patient.	
	Unhelpful: Says, "I feel for you" while nervously looking around the room to avoid eye contact.	*Helpful:* "I have some other things on my mind. Let me get collected for a moment."
Changing the subject Redirecting the discussion in response to the introduction of sensitive or uncomfortable topics into the discussion.	*Unhelpful:* "Let's talk about that later." "Before we talk about that, I wanted to tell you about…"	*Helpful:* "That sounds important. Tell me more." "I know this is painful to discuss, but try to tell me how you are feeling."
Moral imperatives/judgmental behavior Statements that reflect clinician judgment based on personal values and admonishment of patient/ family member. This approach directs patient/family to suppress true feelings, blames or belittles, and restrains the interaction.	*Unhelpful* "Don't get angry." "You shouldn't feel that way." "You must be strong at times like these." "You are overreacting. Things are not that bad." "We know what's best for you."	*Helpful* "You seem really angry. Can I help you?" "It must be difficult to bear up with the stresses you're facing." I can see that you are very upset. Tell me what's happening." "What do you think would be best for you?"

Table continued on following page

Closed Communication Patterns and Syndromes (Continued)

PATTERN	PRESENTATION	
Advice-giving Advice is nothing more than an individual's opinion. Giving advice centers the interaction on the clinician's needs and perspective rather than patient/family. It sets the clinician up to take an inappropriate level of responsibility for patient/family decisions.	*Unhelpful* "If I were in your situation, I would…" "If you want my opinion, I think you should/should not pursue the therapy." "You shouldn't be seeing that doctor. You need to be cared for by a specialist."	*Helpful* "What are the pros and cons of each choice for you?" "How are you thinking about handling the decisions about your care?" "How did you use to choose your doctor? Did you use any particular criteria?"
Generalizing Responding to patient/family expression of feeling with broad, sweeping or trite statements. Turns focus away from uniqueness of individual and his/her response to the situation.	*Unhelpful* "Everyone feels this way before starting chemotherapy (radiation)." "Keep your chin up."	*Helpful* "I can understand how frightening it must be to be starting therapy. What concerns you most?" "You're smiling. Does that mean you feel better?"
Overuse of "why" questions Clinician becomes the interrogator, putting patient/family on the defensive; clinician controls dialogue.	*Unhelpful* "Why didn't you report the fever earlier?" "Why do you feel so anxious?" "Why are you so depressed?" "Why didn't you tell the doctor?"	*Helpful* "You didn't call right away. What happened?" "Tell me more about your anxious feelings." "What's been going on with you?" "Tell me what held you back from talking about it with the doctor."

Poor listening styles

Stage hog: interested only in presenting own ideas.
Ambusher: focuses on collecting information for counterattack.
Selective: responds only to aspects of dialogue in which he/she is interested.
Insulated: ignores aspects of the dialogue perceived to be unpleasant or uncomfortable.
Defensive: all statements perceived to be a personal attack with defensive replies.
Insensitive: unable to look beyond the spoken word to cues to hidden meanings; takes the interaction at face value.

Adapted from Engelking C: Overcoming barriers to effective communication in cancer care. In Lindley C, Wickham R (eds): Issues in Managing the Oncology Patient, 2nd ed. New York, Philips Healthcare Communications, 1999, pp 58–74.

12. Give examples of how nurses escape patient interactions.

Nonverbal escape behaviors include physically avoiding patients by becoming absorbed in other "work," such as documentation, delivering care in a rushed manner in the patient's presence, and consistently referring the patient to other team members. Each of these behaviors sets up the invisible protective shield of distance. On inpatient hospital units, nurses may seek to place distance between themselves and patient/families by (1) assigning the patient to a room far from the nursing station or otherwise keeping the patient out of sight (e.g., with a pulled curtain or closed door); (2) rigidly limiting family visitation or participation in care; (3) using the intercom to address patient calls rather than going to the room for face-to-face interactions; and (4) depersonalizing the situation by referring to patients as their diagnoses or room numbers (e.g., "the leukemic in room 10"). Awareness of the potential negative impact of such behaviors helps nurses to avoid using them and ultimately enhances the connectivity among nurse, patient, and family members.

13. Do patients also engage in closed communication?

Yes. Patients with cancer and their family members also engage in specific closed communication syndromes. These behaviors systematically close the door to meaningful exchange, thus denying opportunities for therapeutic interaction between patients/family members and the cancer care team. Nurses who recognize early indicators of closed communication patterns and syndromes can more easily avoid them, thereby optimizing opportunities for therapeutic interaction.

Closed Communication Syndromes

SYNDROME	INDICATORS
Conspiracy of silence (Shields) Withholding information. Occurs when people in patient support network are guided by the belief that hope is the main ingredient of the patient's remaining happiness and that it cannot coexist with knowledge of the severity of his/her clinical situation.	*Between health team member and patient:* clinician elects not to inform patient of diagnosis or reveals diagnosis as an isolated point of information then fails to discuss patient's symptoms or health status within the context of cancer. *Between patient and family member:* family member chooses not to address the subject of cancer with patient, attributing all health problems to some other cause (e.g., pain is due to arthritis or flu). *Between patient and clinician/family:* clinician and family enter into collusion. Family insists that clinician withhold diagnosis and clinician agrees. In this situation, the clinician is freed of responsibility for the deception because family has made the decision and because they all agree that they are operating in the best interest of the patient.
Denial/protection syndrome (Rogers and Mengel) Responsibility for facilitating dialogue about the illness experience is dispersed diversely among health team and family members, leaving no one fully accountable and providing everyone with an avenue for avoiding the topic of cancer.	Patient/family complains that physician is not providing them with adequate information but have not arranged to meet him/her to discuss the situation. Patient/family does not address the issue of cancer directly, request clarification or pursue concerns on difficult topics such as prognosis during their interaction with clinicians. Family places blame for patient's depression on clinician, who openly shares the facts with the patient, because they believe the patient was not "ready to hear the news" or "couldn't handle it."
Disconfirming interaction cycle (Northouse and Northouse) Interaction patterns that deny the existence of patient/family and invalidate their worth and competence, creating defensive posturing as protection. Includes variety of disconfirming responses, often in combination.	*Impervious:* ignores or disregards the patient/family attempt to communicate. *Interruptive:* cuts patient/family off before they have completed or fully elaborated topic. *Irrelevant:* responds in unrelated way by shifting or introducing new topic. *Impersonal:* responds in third person in intellectualizing tone with cliches/euphemisms. *Incongruous:* acts in a way that differs from what is being said verbally. *Incoherent:* responds with long, rambling, difficult-to-follow sentences or monologues.

Adapted from Engelking C: Overcoming barriers to effective communication in cancer care. In Lindley C, Wickham R (eds): Issues in Managing the Oncology Patient, 2nd ed. New York, Philips Healthcare Communications, 1999, pp 58–74.

14. What is "therapeutic" communication?

Therapeutic communication refers to the deliberate use of interactional techniques specifically designed to achieve positive outcomes within the context of the patient's illness experience. Therapeutic communication is an intervention to improve or restore the patient's emotional health and well-being.

15. How can I become a better communicator with patients and family members?

Athough it is inevitable that on occasion nurses will not make the best choice of words and phrases or will "say the wrong thing," the important point is that we acknowledge such incidents and seek to discover alternative responses to make our interactions more effective. Unlike the way in which we regard physical care procedures, we do not typically consider our responses to patient/family questions and concerns as discrete techniques or a practice skill. Yet, as with physical care, recognizing the components of communication skills and knowing how best to select and combine these elements helps to maximize the therapeutic nature of patient/family interactions. Practicing interactive skills and techniques helps you to develop and refine your existing repertoire of communication skills.

Basic Therapeutic Communication Techniques and Sample Responses

TECHNIQUES	DESCRIPTION	SAMPLE RESPONSES
• **Attending behaviors**	Listening and communicating to the patient/family that you are listening through effective use of:	
	• Posture	Sits close to and faces patient; leans forward; may use touch.
	• Eye contact	Makes eye contact as appropriate.
	• Accurate verbal follow-through	Responses match content of patient statement or question.
• **Encouraging verbal interaction**	Interactive behaviors that open and expand the communication:	
	• Open questions	"How do you think you might react if you learn you have cancer?" "Can you tell me more?"
	• Minimal leads	"And then..." "Go on..." "I see..."
• **Paraphrasing**	Determine and restate the cognitive content of patient/family statement.	"You say your pain is caused by the cancer in your spine?"
• **Reflecting feeling**	Identify emotional content and validate with patient/family.	"You feel angry because your treatment has been delayed—is that right?"
• **Summarization**	Select and tie together priority concepts.	"So, you've said that you are confused and upset about this change in your chemotherapy regimen and you want the doctor to discuss it with you again when your wife is present?"
• **Self-disclosure**	• Sharing personal reaction to patient/ family interaction	"It makes me feel sad to see you so upset."
	• Revealing relevant personal experience and/or feeling	"I can understand what you mean. I often felt angry when my mother had cancer and needed so much of my time."
• **Confrontation**	Express observed discrepancies between patient/family statement and demonstrated behaviors.	"You have often said how much you miss seeing your children when you are in the hospital, but you have asked your husband not to bring them to visit."

From Engelking C: Overcoming barriers to effective communication in cancer care. In Lindley C, Wickham R (eds): Issues in Managing the Oncology Patient, 2nd ed. New York, Philips Healthcare Communications, 1999, pp 58–74, with permission.

16. Besides gathering data, what are some tips to "set the stage" for interactions with patients and family members?

Setting the stage involves ensuring that everyone is "on the same page" from the outset. This means recognizing and testing personal assumptions about patient/family knowledge base, feelings, attitudes, and motivations. It is also critical to provide a therapeutic milieu or framework within which the exchange can take place. Preparative questions, which help determine whether the environment is conducive to therapeutic interaction, include:

- Are the right participants present to carry on the discussion?
- Have the participants demonstrated or indicated readiness?
- Is there adequate privacy to ensure confidentiality?
- Has a supportive (rather than defensive) climate been established?
- Were arrangements made with coworkers to handle other responsibilities during the session to avoid interruption?

Establishing mutual goals for the exchange clarifies for all participants the desired outcomes of the session, thus promoting a meaningful discussion. What is the primary intent of the interaction? Is it to collect data, deliver information, or provide support and reassurance? Although these discretely different goals are intertwined, knowing patient/family priorities beforehand helps to match the character of the interaction with their specific needs at the time. Similarly, establishing rapport and trust permits the interaction to extend beyond the superficial, to the deeper level necessary to provide emotional support.

17. How do I communicate therapeutically on a busy, short-staffed inpatient oncology unit or ambulatory clinic setting?

Although most exchanges between the nurse and patient or family members take place during the delivery of physical care or "on the fly" in hallways or corridors rather than during organized sessions, it is still possible to apply the communication principles and techniques presented in this chapter. While you are bathing a patient, performing dressing changes, or other procedures (e.g., drug administration), you are afforded precious time to get information, deliver education, and offer support and reassurance. You will be amazed at how much can be accomplished during brief exchanges if you take a few moments at the beginning of the shift to set specific goals that you want to achieve through your interactions with each of your assigned patients that day. Maintaining awareness of your communication approach, remaining flexible and open, and using the described communication techniques and skills will enhance the quality of each interaction. Most patients and family members respond immediately to the genuine interest in them and their circumstance conveyed through your focused attention (i.e., attending behaviors) and direct open-ended statements (e.g., "I can only imagine how difficult/frightening this must be for you. How can I help?").

18. What are some general guidelines about "therapeutic" communication?

1. Stop, watch, and listen when you are involved in patient/family interactions.
2. Avoid excessive questioning, which can make patients feel as though they are being interrogated.
3. Avoid giving advice without taking time to hear the patient's concerns and opinions.
4. Let the patient or family member's demeanor and reactions guide the interaction.
5. Center attention on the patient while he or she is talking. Listen carefully instead of focusing on what you are planning to say next.
6. Make use of silence to absorb what the patient or family member has told you.
7. Always check to see whether the patient understood your explanations, then clarify and validate your statements.
8. Maintain awareness of and avoid being drawn into verbal and nonverbal closed communication patterns and syndromes.

19. What statements can nurses use to facilitate communication?

1. "Tell me about yourself. Go on...tell me more...um hmm...."
2. "Give me an example from your own experiences. Describe it further."
3. "What do you mean? Please explain. Help me to understand better."
4. "What do you see as the reason for/cause of that?"
5. "What was the importance of that event/person/interaction to you?"

6. "If I hear you correctly, you are saying that...."
7. "Let me restate what I think I heard you say."
8. "What would you do if a situation like this arises again?"
9. "It sounds as if you think you will/will not be okay on your own."

20. What assessment parameters are most useful in determining the type of communication techniques and approach selected for interactions with patients and family members?

Although each interaction is unique, an essential step in shaping the communication approach is to complete an accurate assessment of the patient or family member's readiness to interact, support network dynamics, and key issues or concerns. The nurse must know "where they are coming from" to plan the approach. Information about patient/family member experience, style, expectations, support system, and priorities is important data to establish the goal, tone, and content of the interaction. Observing for nonverbal messages conveyed by expression and body language is another equally important source of data. The patient/family profile is dynamic, changing in character as the patient progresses through the course of the illness. A person who appears calm and collected at the outset can become frazzled and demanding as the situation becomes more intense and the protective cloak of denial is more difficult to maintain. Interpersonal understanding is facilitated and interactions optimized when the nurse's response is compatible with the patient or family member's style, expectations, and specific needs.

Sizing Up Your Patient: An Interaction Preassessment Tool

Expression
- What are the patient/family member nonverbal cues?
- Does she/he look physically or emotionally uncomfortable?

Experience
- Is your patient newly diagnosed or experienced with cancer?
- Where in the illness continuum is the patient right now?
- Has the patient/family had negative past experiences with cancer, the health care team, or the health care system?
- How has the patient coped with past crises? Has it been effective?

Expectations
- What does the patient/family think will happen right now? Later?
- How does the patient/family think the you can help right now?

Style
- Does the patient swallow or disclose emotions and concerns?
- Does the patient have an internal or external locus of control?
- Is the patient open or closed to your intervention right now?

Network
- Does the patient have a support network available right now?
- Is it limited to family, or is it an expanded network?
- Who are the key supporters? How does the patient use them?
- What supportive resources, if any, has the patient used in the past?

Priority issue
- What is most bothersome for the patient/family right now?
- Is the issue physical or emotional or a combination?
- Is/are the issue(s) immediately manageable?

21. How significant is the nurse's role in enhancing communication with patients and family?

Of all the cancer care team members, nurses are in the most strategic position to assist patients and family members over the emotional hurdles imposed by cancer and its consequences.

Unlike other members of the team, who have episodic contacts with patients and family members, nurses have a more constant presence. Consequently, nurses are able to evaluate patient/family responses not only to physical care procedures but also to interactions with all members of the team. Nurses, therefore, can coordinate the sharing of information and serve as liaisons, preparing other members of the team to communicate therapeutically with patients and family members. It is likely that in the future, the nursing role will become increasingly focused on the interactional dimensions of care. Outcome indicators and studies reflecting improved patient compliance, shortened hospital stays, and enhanced patient/family satisfaction as a result of enhanced communications will help to build the value of these interventions and gain support for the development and integration of communication skills as part of the required therapeutic plan. Oncology nurses who develop and incorporate communication skills into their practice now will be ready for the future focus on this aspect of cancer nursing practice and at the same time experience greater satisfaction with the care that they deliver.

ACKNOWLEDGMENT

The author wishes to thank the hundreds of patients and family members who have helped her to develop insights and skills in communicating effectively with those facing the crisis of cancer.

REFERENCES

1. Bradley JC, Edinbergh MA: Communication in the Nursing Context. New York, Appleton Century Crofts, 1982.
2. Engelking C: Overcoming barriers to effective communication in cancer care. In Lindley C, Wickham R (eds): Issues in Managing in the Oncology Patient, 2nd ed. New York, Philips Healthcare Communications, 1999, pp. 58–74.
3. Engelking C, Steele N: Overcoming barriers to primary cancer nursing care. In Caliandro G, Judkins B (eds): Primary Nursing Practice. Boston, Scott, Foresman., 1988, pp 266–306.
4. Engelking C, Garis G, Steele N: Using therapeutic communication skills as a stress management strategy for oncology nurses. Oncol Nurs Forum 12:84, 1985.
5. Greisinger AH, Lorimor RJJ, Aday LA, et al: Terminally ill cancer patients: Their most important concerns. Cancer Pract 5:759–763, 1997.
6. Heinrich AP, Bernheim KF: Responding to patients' concerns. Nurs Outlook July:428–433, 1981.
7. Herschbach P: Work-related stress specific to physicians and nurses working with cancer patients. J Psychosoc Oncol 10:79–99, 1992.
8. Northouse LL, Northouse PG: Health Communications Strategies for Health Professionals, 2nd ed. Norwalk, CT, Appleton & Lange, 1992.
9. Ravert P, Williams M, Fosbinder DM: The interpersonal competence instrument for nurses. West J Nurs Res 19:781–791, 1997.
10. Rogers BJ, Mengel A: Communicating with families of terminal cancer patients. Top Clin Nurs 1:55–61, 1979.
11. Shields P: A supportive bridge between cancer patient, family and health care staff. Nurs Forum 21:31–36, 1984.
12. Thorne SE: Helpful and unhelpful communications in cancer care: The patient perspective. Oncol Nurs Forum 15:157–172, 1988.
13. Welch D: Promoting change in patterns of nurse communication. Nurs Administr Q 5:77–81, 1981.

59. CANCER AND PREGNANCY

Linda U. Krebs, RN, PhD, AOCN

1. How common is cancer associated with pregnancy?
Although generally considered to be a rare event, the incidence of cancer associated with pregnancy is increasing. Cancer is one of the most common diagnoses and the second leading cause of death during the reproductive years. Approximately 1 of every 118 pregnancies will be complicated by a cancer diagnosis.

2. Why is the incidence of cancer associated with pregnancy increasing?
As women delay childbearing until later in life (into their 30s and early 40s), the likelihood of having concomitant pregnancy and cancer has increased. In addition, the incidence of some of the more common types of cancer (e.g., breast cancer, cervical cancer) appears to be increasing in younger women. The combination of delayed childbearing and younger incidence of specific cancers has led to the increase.

3. What is the time frame for pregnancy associated with cancer?
Most authors include not only the 9 months of pregnancy but also the 6 months (some include up to 1 year) before becoming pregnant or after delivering as the time frame for a pregnancy-associated cancer.

4. What are the predominant types of cancer diagnosed during pregnancy?
In descending order, the cancers most commonly diagnosed during pregnancy are breast cancer, cervical cancer, ovarian cancer, colorectal cancer, lymphoma, and leukemia. Malignant melanoma, although rare, is often included in any discussion of cancer associated with pregnancy because its incidence is rising, and it is frequently found during the reproductive years. Breast cancer occurs in approximately 1 of every 3000 pregnancies. Cervical cancer occurs in approximately 1 of every 400 pregnancies; the majority of cases, however, are not invasive but rather carcinoma in situ. Ovarian masses are a common finding during pregnancy. Between 1 in 9,000 and 1 in 25,000 will be malignant. Pregnancies associated with colorectal cancer, Hodgkin's disease, non-Hodgkin's lymphoma, leukemia, and malignant melanoma are even less common.

5. Is cancer arising during pregnancy more aggressive than the same type of cancer in a nonpregnant woman?
Cancer arising during pregnancy was previously believed to be more aggressive because the stage of disease was more apt to be advanced (stage III or IV) at diagnosis. However, in depth review of the stage of disease at diagnosis, treatment regimens, and overall survival statistics has shown that women at equivalent stages and treatments have similar survival statistics regardless of pregnancy. What appears to be the most likely cause for advanced disease is delay in making the diagnosis. This delay is due, in part, to the difficulty of recognizing the signs and symptoms of cancer in pregnant women.

6. Is therapeutic abortion of benefit in the management of cancer associated with pregnancy?
Scientific studies have not shown therapeutic abortion to be of any benefit in controlling disease or prolonging survival. In general, the pregnancy does not affect the outcome of the cancer, and the cancer does not affect the pregnancy. Therapeutic abortion may be of benefit if the planned treatment would be detrimental to the fetus, and altering treatment to spare the fetus would have a negative impact on the mother's survival. The decision to have a therapeutic abortion should not be made until the risks of maintaining the pregnancy during delivery of optimal

cancer treatment have been thoroughly explained and discussed with the pregnant woman and her significant others.

7. Is it difficult to differentiate between body alterations found with routine pregnancy and signs and symptoms of cancer?

Making the diagnosis of cancer during a pregnancy may be difficult because of similarities among common symptoms associated with pregnancy and the signs and symptoms often associated with cancer. Nausea and vomiting, constipation, breast changes, changes in moles, fatigue, backache, and other constitutional symptoms are common to both cancer and pregnancy. A breast mass is often believed to be related to a plugged milk duct, whereas the changes in the size and pigmentation of a mole may be believed to be part of normal changes in the skin during pregnancy. Patient concerns must be fully evaluated. In addition, the patient's history and current risks for cancer must be taken into consideration.

8. Are there any specific contraindications to the use of radiographs, radioisotopes, or other diagnostic methods in pregnant patients?

Radiographs should be used sparingly, if at all, in pregnant patients. When they are necessary, adequate fetal shielding must be used. Chest radiographs deliver minuscule doses of radiation and, with appropriate shielding, appear to be safe during pregnancy.

Mammography may be safely undertaken if the abdomen is adequately shielded. Mammography is not considered to be highly reliable, however, because of increased breast density, decreased fatty tissue, and increased water content of the breasts during pregnancy.

Ultrasound and magnetic resonance imaging may be safely used. Computed tomography and isotope studies are not recommended.

Tumor markers (e.g., alpha-fetoprotein, beta-human chorionic gonadotropin, lactate dehydrogenase, CA-125) are of limited benefit because many markers are routinely elevated during pregnancy.

Fine-needle aspiration, Papanicolaou smear, and colposcopy are considered safe. Biopsy under local or general anesthesia is also safe if adequate fetal oxygenation and circulation are maintained. Although cone biopsy may be undertaken, complication rates may be as high as 30%; specific complications include infection, hemorrhage, and premature delivery. Most recently, the loop electrode excision procedure (LEEP) has been suggested as an alternative to the complications known to occur with cone excision. However, LEEP has been associated with an increased incidence of cervical hemorrhage and thus probably is of no true advantage.

9. How should cancer associated with pregnancy be treated?

As a general rule, a woman diagnosed with cancer during pregnancy should receive the same treatment options as a nonpregnant woman with the same malignancy. Some modifications may be necessary to minimize fetal exposure to chemotherapy or radiation. In some instances, definitive therapy may be delayed until after delivery with little or no risk to the patient. In other instances, therapeutic abortion may be undertaken to provide aggressive therapy that could be potentially lethal to the fetus. In all cases, therapeutic decisions should be individualized. Recommendations for specific cancer types include the following:

Breast cancer. Modified radical mastectomy with lymph node sampling is the standard treatment. Lumpectomy with lymph node sampling also may be undertaken. Radiation therapy is not generally recommended for pregnant patients and is usually delayed until after delivery. Adjuvant chemotherapy may be safely given after the first trimester or may be delayed until after delivery.

Cervical cancer. For carcinoma in situ, the pregnancy can be allowed to continue, with definitive therapy delayed until after delivery. Close follow-up with intermittent biopsy is imperative. For invasive disease, radical surgery or radiation therapy, without therapeutic abortion, is recommended. If the patient is near delivery, viability can be awaited, the infant delivered by cesarean section, and definitive therapy then completed.

Ovarian cancer. Early-stage disease may be safely managed by unilateral oophorectomy and biopsy of the contralateral ovary. The pregnancy can be continued. For advanced disease, treatment consists of a radical hysterectomy, omentectomy, node biopsies, and peritoneal washings. The uterus is removed without prior evacuation of the fetus.

Colorectal cancer. Definitive therapy with a colectomy or abdominoperineal resection can generally be undertaken in the first 20 weeks of gestation without hazard to the fetus. For more advanced disease, involving the uterus or impeding access to the rectum, radical hysterectomy may need to be included. For the second half of gestation, viability is awaited, if possible, with definitive therapy after delivery. If an obstruction is present, a colostomy may be performed in the interim.

Lymphoma. Combination chemotherapy is generally the treatment of choice. In the first 20 weeks of gestation, a therapeutic abortion is recommended. In the second half, chemotherapy may be given or, if the fetus is near viability, treatment may be delayed until after delivery.

Leukemia. Treatment with chemotherapy should be instituted without delay. If the fetus is viable, delivery should occur as soon as possible. Therapeutic abortion is suggested for patients in the first trimester.

Malignant melanoma. Primary treatment consists of wide local excision with skin graft, if necessary. Lymph node dissection remains controversial. The benefits of adjuvant therapy are unclear.

10. Is the survival rate of pregnant patients diagnosed with cancer different from that of nonpregnant patients?

A stage-for-stage comparison reveals no difference in survivorship between pregnant and nonpregnant patients diagnosed with cancer, regardless of the type of cancer.

11. What are the effects of cancer treatment on the fetus?

Surgery. Maternal surgery involves minimal risk to the fetus if hypotension is prevented and adequate oxygenation is ensured. General anesthesia is well tolerated after the first trimester. Pelvic surgery is more easily achieved during the second trimester.

Radiation therapy. Fetal damage is unlikely at doses < 50 cGy. Radiation doses > 250 cGy have been associated with fetal damage, including spontaneous abortion, mental retardation, microcephaly, sterility, cataracts, and skin changes. Radiation exposure during the first trimester is of greatest concern. Even with adequate shielding, radiation scatter may be sufficient to cause harm or fetal demise. Radiation therapy should be avoided if possible.

Chemotherapy. Chemotherapy during the first trimester has been associated with low birth weight, fetal malformations, and fetal demise. The incidence may be minimized or avoided by careful selection of agents or combinations of agents and/or delaying chemotherapy until after the first trimester. Unexpected or more severe toxicities may occur in the fetus because of alterations in individual drug pharmacokinetics due to the normal physiologic changes associated with pregnancy. This is of particular importance if chemotherapy is administered close to delivery. The neonate's metabolism and excretion of chemotherapeutic agents may not be sufficient when its primary mechanism of drug excretion, the placenta, is no longer present; thus, increased exposure to drugs and enhanced toxicities may result.

12. What is the incidence of malformation in fetuses exposed to chemotherapy during gestation?

Fetal malformation is estimated to be < 10%. Examples of malformation include skeletal malformations, hydrocephalus, atrial/septal defects, cranial dysostosis, various limb deformities, and cerebral anomalies. Methotrexate and aminopterin (a folic acid antagonist developed before methotrexate) have been most commonly implicated. The incidence is higher when combination therapy is given. The incidence is highest when chemotherapy is given in the first trimester and lowest when chemotherapy is given in the second or third trimester. The incidence of major congenital malformations in all births is approximately 3%, whereas it may reach 9% for minor malformations.

Fetal Abnormalities Associated with Exposure To Chemotherapy/Biologics

AGENT	ABNORMALITY/MALFORMATION
Aminopterin	Spontaneous abortion Aminopterin syndrome: cranial dysostosis, hypertelorism, wide nasal bridge, micrognathia, external ear anomalies Skeletal malformations Cerebral anomalies
Methotrexate	Spontaneous abortion Skeletal malformations Intrauterine growth retardation
5-Fluorouracil	Spontaneous abortion Intrauterine growth retardation
Cyclophosphamide	Spontaneous abortion Intrauterine growth retardation
Busulfan	Spontaneous abortion Skeletal malformations
Procarbazine	Atrial/septal defects
Thalidomide*	Skeletal malformations/deformities Fetal death
Epirubicin	Spontaneous abortion
Interferons	Spontaneous abortion

* Pregnancy contraindicated when taking this drug

13. Does the mother's cancer ever spread to the fetus?

Maternal-to-fetal spread is extremely rare, although scientific reports have included malignant melanoma, non-Hodgkin's lymphoma, leukemia, breast cancer, lung cancer, and gastrointestinal malignancies. A variety of single case reports also can be found in the literature. In all instances, the mothers had widely disseminated disease. In most reported series, malignant melanoma is the most common form of cancer associated with fetal spread. In some instances only the placenta is involved; in other instances, the cancer spreads to the fetus. Some infants have died of the disease.

14. What are the specific recommendations about delivery?

The type of delivery, vaginal versus cesarean section, is controversial for women with cervical cancer. Some health care professionals are concerned that, in the presence of active disease, vaginal delivery will spread the cancer or cause infection or hemorrhage; thus cesarean section is recommended. Others report that vaginal delivery does not increase risk of disease dissemination, hemorrhage, or infection, and, in fact, may be associated with increased maternal survival. Four cases of recurrence of disease in the vaginal episiotomy have been reported. The definitive answer for cervical cancer remains unclear. Careful follow-up for recurrence is mandatory in all women who have vaginal deliveries. Cesarean section is the method of choice if the woman is to undergo radical hysterectomy after delivery.

For all other cancer types, the type of delivery depends on disease status, fetal gestation, immediacy of delivery, and whether definitive treatment, requiring an abdominal incision, is to be done after delivery. For ovarian cancer, treatment is often undertaken at delivery; thus, a cesarean section is performed, followed by radical hysterectomy.

If possible, delivery should be timed so that patients receiving chemotherapy will have recovered from bone marrow suppression and other therapy-related toxicities. A complete blood count and other appropriate laboratory parameters should be evaluated before delivery, and extra precautions to minimize bleeding and infection should be taken as necessary.

15. What types of neonatal monitoring should occur at delivery?

The fetus exposed to chemotherapy may be premature and also may weigh less than expected for gestational age. Because of the potential for increased toxicities, particularly if treatment is given close to delivery, laboratory evaluation should include a complete blood count. The neonate should be evaluated carefully for chemotherapy-induced malformations, including skeletal and internal organ abnormalities. The placenta and neonate also should be evaluated for signs of metastatic involvement, particularly if the mother has disseminated disease.

16. Is it possible to breastfeed an infant during or after treatment for cancer?

Breastfeeding is contraindicated when the mother is receiving chemotherapy or undergoing tests that use radioactive materials; these agents or their metabolites can be found in breast milk and may be detrimental to the infant. Breastfeeding can be safely recommended for all other patients. Women with breast cancer who have received breast radiation may have diminished or absent lactation on the radiated side. They are generally discouraged from attempting to breastfeed on the radiated side because of an increased risk of developing mastitis.

17. Are future pregnancies possible or recommended after a diagnosis of cancer?

The ability to become pregnant after a diagnosis of cancer depends on the primary site, stage of disease, type and extent of therapy, and age of the woman. For women who wish to conceive and remain physically capable of doing so, there are no known contraindications. Most clinicians recommend a waiting period of 1–5 years after completion of therapy, depending on stage of disease. This recommendation minimizes the possibility of recurrence during the future pregnancy and allows the woman to regain physical and emotional health before undergoing the rigors of pregnancy.

18. What are the specific recommendations for prevention and early detection of cancer while a woman is pregnant?

All initial prenatal visits should include a Papanicolaou smear and a thorough breast examination. Women should be instructed to do breast self-examinations (BSE) monthly throughout pregnancy. In addition, women should be taught self-examination techniques for skin cancer and encouraged to complete them on a monthly basis. A thorough history for cancer risks should be obtained, and special precautions and evaluations should be included in prenatal care as appropriate. Pregnant women should be encouraged to discuss all abnormal findings or concerns with health care providers. All concerns should be evaluated thoroughly.

19. What is known about the long-term survival and future cancer risk of children exposed to cancer treatment in utero?

There appear to be no alterations in long-term survival and no increased risk of cancer, beyond that which is related to heredity, in children exposed to cancer treatment in utero. Rare abnormalities with no obvious pattern have been shown in long-term studies of children exposed to chemotherapy. Long-term effects of low-dose radiation are currently unknown. Follow-up of children exposed to higher doses of radiation is limited. Concerns for such children remain, and follow-up over many generations will be necessary to determine the exact effects.

20. Is nursing management of pregnant women with cancer any different from management of a woman who has cancer or a woman who is pregnant?

Nursing management for pregnant women with cancer is much more complex. Primary nursing roles include assessment, physical care, emotional support, and provision of information and education. The team approach, involving oncology, obstetrics, neonatology, and various support services, is essential. In addition to routine medical and nursing management strategies, educational, psychosocial, and ethical interventions need to be incorporated into the plan of care. Because of disease, treatment, fears for the fetus, concerns about survival, and numerous other anxieties, normal activities of pregnancy may be deferred or prevented. Ethical dilemmas may occur as treatment needs are weighed against fetal survival. Emotional support is essential and can take its toll on the health care provider as well as on the patient and family.

21. What are the risks to the health care professional who mixes, administers, or handles chemotherapeutic agents while pregnant, breastfeeding, or attempting to conceive?

Risks vary, depending on whether one is mixing or administering chemotherapy or handling chemotherapy-contaminated excreta. The highest risk occurs when admixing drugs, the lowest when handling excreta. The Occupational Safety and Health Administration notes a lack of in-depth information available to quantify exact risks. Previous studies showing increased risk to women handling chemotherapeutic agents were conducted when adequate guidelines were not available or recommendations for protection had not been followed. Possible risks include spontaneous abortion and an increased incidence of ectopic pregnancy. Adequate protection should minimize, if not eliminate, potential risks.

22. Do special precautions in the mixing, administration, and handling of chemotherapeutic agents apply only to women who are trying to conceive?

Both women and men who are attempting pregnancy should minimize exposure to chemotherapeutic agents through the use of appropriate protective equipment.

REFERENCES

1. Boulay R, Podczaski E: Ovarian cancer complicating pregnancy. Obstet Gynecol Clin North Am 25:385–399, 1998.
2. Connor JP: Noninvasive cervical cancer complicating pregnancy. Obstet Gynecol Clin North Am 25:331–342, 1998.
3. Dow KH (ed): Pocket Guide to Breast Cancer. Sudbury, MA, Jones & Bartlett, 1999, pp 183–190.
4. Ferreira CM, Maceira JM, Coelho JM: Melanoma and pregnancy with placental metastases. Report of a case. Am J Dermatol 20:403–407, 1998.
5. Krebs LU: Sexual and reproductive dysfunction. In Yarbro CH, Frogge MH, Goodman M, Groenwald SL (eds): Cancer Nursing: Principles and Practice, 5th ed. Boston, Jones & Bartlett, 2000, pp 831–854.
6. Krebs LU: Sexuality and reproduction. In Yasko J (ed): Nursing Management of Symptoms Associated with Chemotherapy, 5th ed. Philadelphia, Meniscus (in press).
7. Peleg D, Ben-Ami M: Lymphoma and leukemia complicating pregnancy. Obstet Gynecol Clin North Am 25:365–383, 1998.
8. Pelsang RE: Diagnostic imaging modalities during pregnancy. Obstet Gynecol Clin North Am 25:287–300, 1998.
9. Samuels TH, Liu FF, Yaffe M, et al: Gestational breast cancer. Can Assoc Radiol J 49:172–180, 1998.
10. Shivvers SA, Miller DS: Preinvasive and invasive breast and cervical cancer prior to or during pregnancy. Clin Perinatol 24:369–389, 1997.
11. Sood AK, Sorosky JI: Invasive cervical cancer complicating pregnancy. Obstet Gynecol Clin North Am 25:343–352, 1998.
12. Sorosky JI, Scott-Connor CEH: Breast disease complicating pregnancy. Obstet Gynecol Clin North Am 25:253–263, 1998.
13. Surbone A, Petrek JA: Childbearing issues in breast carcinoma survivors. Cancer 79:1271–1278, 1997.
14. Teplitzky S, Sabates B, Yu K, et al: Melanoma during pregnancy: A case report and review of the literature. J LA State Med Soc 150:539–543, 1998.

60. CANCER IN THE ELDERLY

Deborah A. Boyle, RN, MSN, AOCN, FAAN

1. Why is cancer in the elderly a critical issue in cancer care?

The geriatric oncology imperative is a concern for two critical reasons. First, cancer is primarily a disease of aging. More than one-half of all cancers occur in people over age 65, despite the fact that the elderly represent only 12% of the U.S. population. Thus, most cancers occur disproportionately in relatively few Americans.[16] Second, despite the prevalence of cancer with advancing age, there has been little investigation of cancer in the elderly. Research is necessary to explain a host of questions: Why is there a heightened risk of cancer in the elderly? How do the elderly respond to treatment? What is the incidence and severity of treatment-related toxicities in this age group? What are the psychosocial responses and challenges unique to this subset of cancer patients? Cancer in the elderly also has significant implications for the future. With the aging of the "baby boomers" (currently the largest developmental subset of Americans), we can expect increasing numbers of cancers due to a higher volume of vulnerable adults in the coming decades.

2. How can we explain the lack of research in this population?

Ageism, or societal prejudice toward the elderly, promotes negative social and medical views about growing old.[13] This phenomenon has fostered a historical lack of interest in addressing the special needs of the elderly who face cancer. For example, there is no dedicated subspecialty of geriatric oncology parallel to pediatric oncology. Yet children represent less than 10% of all Americans who develop cancer. The social worth phenomenon emphasizes the value of children in our culture. We perceive the actual or potential loss of a child to be significant not only to the immediate family but also to society as a whole. Therefore, health professionals and the public alike can justify the occurrence of a life-threatening illness in an elder but struggle to do so in the case of a child.

3. How has the lack of attentiveness to the elderly affected what we know and do not know about cancer?

Historically, we have not treated cancer in the elderly aggressively, based on the assumption that they could not withstand the rigors of aggressive therapy. We have presumed that physiologic and chronologic age are equivalent. Rather than determine the appropriateness of therapy based on individual physiologic parameters, many elderly people have been judged unfit for potentially curative therapies.

Until recently, the elderly have been excluded from participation in clinical trials on the basis of chronologic age, with age 65 as the cutoff point. This exclusion has resulted in two important phenomena. First, by not allowing the elderly to participate in clinical trials, we have minimal quantitative data to substantiate how the elderly fare in a variety of cancer treatment regimens. This lack of information perpetuates the practice of treating the elderly based on assumption and speculation rather than on the results of vigorous research. Second, the lack of research facilitates the delivery of substandard treatment regimens when, in fact, the elderly may benefit from a more aggressive intervention. An important article by European oncologists published in *Lancet* a decade ago states the following:

> There is widespread misconception that the elderly are always poorly tolerant of chemotherapy or radiotherapy with the inevitable result that many elderly patients with cancer are undertreated. In current practice the elderly, disenfranchised as they are from entry to clinical trials, receive either untested treatments, inadequate treatment or even none at all, at the whim of their clinician. Any novel therapy, if only used for those aged less than 70 years, will have a reduced effect on population mortality statistics because only half of those with that disease will receive adequate treatment.[11]

4. How should the elderly be treated for cancer?

The elderly individual's physiologic age should be the major determinant of appropriate cancer therapy recommendations (rather than chronologic age). The patient's baseline function—in particular, the presence or absence of comorbid disease—is an important consideration. Comorbid diseases influencing cardiovascular, pulmonary, and renal function as well as diabetic conditions often preclude the administration of regimens with potential related organ impairment. Functional status must also be considered and measured as outcomes of therapy are quantified.

5. Why is cancer so prevalent in the elderly?

There are nine major theories of cancer's etiology in the elderly. These theories are, in most respects, complementary, multifocal, and highly interrelated. Additionally, the process of carcinogenesis in the older host is most likely characterized by a paradigm of latency. Major theories include:

- Longer duration of carcinogen exposure
- Accumulation of somatic mutations with longevity
- Decreased ability to repair DNA
- Oncogene activation or amplification
- Tumor suppressor gene loss
- Decreased immune surveillance
- Increased cell-mediated immune senescence
- Increased sensitivity to oncogenic viruses
- Increased tendency toward hormone imbalance

6. What are the major cancers in the elderly?

The major cancers in the elderly are primarily solid tumors that are postulated to evolve over decades. The metastatic potential of these tumors is significant, resulting in the prominence of cases that are diagnosed at late stages. The major tumors in the elderly include the following:

Male: prostate, lung, colorectal, and bladder.

Female: breast, lung, colorectal, and uterine.

7. Are other cancers prominent in the elderly?

Yes. Other malignancies, although not significant in number, are important because they occur almost exclusively during old age. Examples include gastric malignancies, cancers of the vulva and gallbladder, multiple myelomas, and chronic leukemias. Approximately two-thirds of these malignancies occur in the elderly population. Additionally, the incidence of acute nonlymphocytic leukemias (variants of acute myelogenous leukemia) and lymphomas are rising in the above-60-years-old population.[4]

8. How does this heightened incidence rate correspond to mortality rates in the elderly subset of cancer patients?

Until recently, it was generally thought that the elderly demonstrated poor treatment outcomes due to their advanced age. However, close scrutiny of major clinical trials reveals that the stage of disease at initial diagnosis is an important determinant of cancer outcome. Many more elderly people are initially diagnosed with advanced stages of cancer than their younger counterparts. Greater tumor burden, then, may be more responsible for poorer outcomes from treatment than chronologic age alone.

9. Who is responsible for the lack of early detection: health professionals or the patient?

Both parties share this responsibility. Treatment aversion and cancer fatalism among the elderly often negate prompt solicitation of medical advice for suspicious symptoms. The patient, as well as physicians and nurses, may attribute potentially suspicious symptoms of cancer to factors related to advancing age or other comorbid diseases. Cohen described this phenomenon as cancer symptom confusion in the elderly. Some examples are listed below.

SYMPTOM OR SIGN	POSSIBLE MALIGNANCY	AGING EXPLANATION
Increase in skin pigment	Melanoma, squamous cell	Age spots
Rectal bleeding	Colon or rectal cancer	Hemorrhoids
Constipation	Rectal cancer	Old age
Dyspnea	Lung cancer	Old age, out of shape
Decrease in urinary stream	Prostate cancer	Dribbling—benign prostatic hypertrophy
Breast contour change	Breast cancer	Normal atrophy or fibrosis
Fatigue	Metastatic or other	Loss of energy due to aging
Bone pain	Metastatic or other	Arthritis: aches and pains of aging

10. What is the best approach to educate the elderly about early cancer detection?

Despite the fact that cancer is primarily a disease of the elderly, few public education programs target this population. Public education programs should consider barriers to community education specific to the elderly. Examples include problems with transportation (can they get to the programs and screenings?), neurosensory impairment (can the person read, see, and hear the information?), misperceptions (does the individual understand the varieties of cancer and the factors that influence outcomes?), and acknowledgment of the benefit of early detection in terms of treatment outcomes (does the individual have a fatalistic attitude, assuming that all cancer is a death sentence and thus viewing screening and early detection as useless?). Interventions that address both human and system barriers must be considered to enhance cancer screening opportunities for the elderly (see figure below).

The two most problematic cancers are breast and prostate cancers. The majority (> 50%) of these malignancies occur in the elderly; hence, the elderly should be the focus of major efforts in public awareness and screening. Lack of risk knowledge based on advanced age and embarrassment

Human Factors

Interventions to Motivate Patients to Obtain Screening
• Social marketing campaign
• Culturally sensitive, tailored messages and media
• Information about new affordable screening options

Interventions to Make it Easire for Providers to Screen
• Increased emphasis on screening in medical school training
• Continuing education programs on screening guidelines and techniques; patientcommunication skills; office reorganization systems; legal issues and referral databases
• Policies mandating insurance coverage for patient education
• Physician incentives for mammography referrals

System Factors

Interventions to Help Providers Integrate Screening into Office Practice
• Reminder systems
• Increased use of support staff for patient education referral

Strategies to Increase Accessibility to Screening
• Mobile vans, flexible clinichours
• Policies requiring free screening by mammography facilities and acceptance of walk-ins and self-referrals

• Providers encounter less patient resistance.
• Providers have more time to screen.
• Providers become more aware of screening resources.

• Providers feel more confident about screening.
• Providers more likely to "seize the opportunity" to screen underserved groups of older women.

Increased utlization of screening among unerserved groups of older women

Potential interventions to help providers seize the opportunity to screen for breast and cervical cancer. (From Gulitz E, Bustillo-Hernandez M, Kent EB: Missed cancer screening opportunities among older women: A review. Cancer Pract 6:289–295, 1998. Reprinted by permission of Blackwell Science, Inc.)

due to the nature of the examinations may preclude willingness to participate in early intervention programs and educational offerings. Monthly breast self-examinations and yearly mammograms are recommended for women over age 50. Annual digital rectal examinations and prostate-specific antigen (PSA) evaluations are recommended for men over age 50.

11. Is surgery usually problematic for older cancer patients because of advanced age?

Normative changes in physiologic function occur with advancing age. The major changes, which have implications for invasive interventions, include reductions in the following parameters:
- Cardiac index
- Standard glomerular filtration rate
- Vital capacity
- Standard renal plasma flow
- Maximal breathing capacity

These changes, however, are highly variable based on genetic, nutritional, and self-care practices. The presence of comorbid conditions, rather than advanced age, is the major predictor of operative complications.

12. What are the most important comorbid conditions affecting outcomes of treatment for elderly patients?

Comorbid conditions (sometimes referred to as intercurrent illnesses) that are most problematic include cardiovascular conditions (i.e., cardiac and cerebrovascular disease, hypertension, thromboembolism), pulmonary compromise, diabetes, renal problems, and malnutrition. These problems rather than chronologic age alone also contribute to the incidence and severity of toxicities associated with cancer therapy. They also may place the older patient at heightened risk for poorer outcome from treatment because of the inability to deliver optimum doses and full courses of therapy.

13. In general, do the elderly have more problems with medication tolerance than their younger counterparts?

Important pharmacologic parameters of medication tolerance in the elderly include consideration of pharmacokinetics (i.e., how the elderly person activates, metabolizes, distributes, and excretes drugs) and pharmacodynamics (how the drugs affect the elderly person's target organs and toxicity prevalence). Despite acknowledged changes in both processes with advanced age, there is little information to help with dose titration guidelines compared with what is available for pediatric dosing recommendations. The exception is information about renal toxicity and dose modification in the elderly when a renally toxic drug is prescribed. In general, however, drugs with bone marrow toxicity are most problematic in the elderly. Limited bone marrow reserve may preclude the older cancer patient's ability to recover from bone marrow compromise caused by chemotherapeutic agents. This is of particular concern when the older patient has a hematologic malignancy in which bone marrow dysfunction predates administration of antineoplastic therapy.

14. What other problems may be medication-related in the elderly?

An important issue in the elderly is polypharmacy. When multiple drugs are prescribed to treat a variety of ills, several phenomena influence adherence.

First, the elderly may not take the drug(s) as prescribed because of confusion, forgetfulness, or the fact that taking pills becomes burdensome. On the average, two drugs are prescribed per chronic illness, and many elderly people are dealing with multiple chronic conditions. Evidence suggests that when the elderly are asked to take more than three drugs on a routine basis at least one of the drugs will be mishandled. Hence, cancer clinicians should anticipate that the medications taken routinely for pain, emesis, bowel alterations, infection, hormonal therapy, and those consumed for other chronic illness(es) will be at risk for misuse. Polypharmacy in the elderly is a critical consideration in the assessment of untoward effects during cancer treatment, yet it remains a predominantly unstudied area of practice.

Second, it is unclear how the many drugs consumed by the elderly interact with one another to cause adverse events. This is particularly true when over-the-counter medications are taken with prescription drugs. Hence, in acknowlegment of the physical functional decline with age and the presence of comorbid conditions that influence drug synthesis, in conjunction with the consumption of a variety of drugs to treat the malignancy and other chronic conditions, the pharmacologic paradigm within geriatric oncology becomes a critically important one.

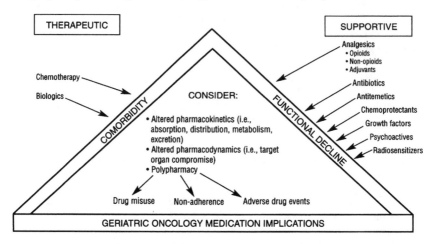

The paradigm of pharmacological management in geriatric oncology. (Adapted from Boyle DM: The geriatric imperative in cancer nursing practice. Oncol Nurs Today 2:12–15, 1997.)

15. Is confusion often related to problems with drug therapy?

Confusion in elderly cancer patients is often acute, reversible, and related to medications and metabolic compromise. Infection, hypoxia, hypercalcemia, and hyponatremia are just a few of the common physiologic etiologies. Additionally, the use of drugs for central nervous system activity, particularly those with central anticholinergic effects (drugs with atropine), are troublesome to the elderly. Administration of these drugs increases the likelihood of acute confusion. When assessing the nature of confusion in an elderly patient, it is critical to ask family members, "Is the confusion new, or is it a gradual worsening of an insidious problem?" If the confusion is new, an acute confusional state must be considered and a metabolic or drug-related etiology should be considered. Once the source of the confusion is determined and treated, the confusion should resolve. A history of ongoing and progressive mental status changes reported by the family, however, may indicate the presence of an organic dementia rather than an acute confusional state. Symptoms associated with acute confusion versus dementia are listed below.

Characteristics and Distinctions of Acute Confusion and Dementia

CHARACTERISTIC	ACUTE CONFUSION	DEMENTIA
Onset	Acute	Insidious
Duration	Hours to weeks	Months to years
Course	Short, diurnal fluctuations with lucid intervals	Enduring effects without diurnal component; progressive yet stable over time
Alertness	Fluctuates	Normal
Orientation	Variably impaired, usually for time	Variably impaired
Memory	Recent and immediate impaired	Recent and remote impaired
Perception	Distorted, often visual	Normal

Table continued on following page

Characteristics and Distinctions of Acute Confusion and Dementia (Continued)

CHARACTERISTIC	ACUTE CONFUSION	DEMENTIA
Psychomotor behavior	Variable with hypo-, hyper-, or mixed variants	Normal
Sleep/wake cycle	Disrupted with cycle reversal	Fragmented
Associated conditions	Physical illness commonly present	Absent
Treatment	Protect the patient while treating the cause; reversible	Protect the patient while treating the behaviors; permanent

Adapted from Foreman MD: The cognitive and behavioral nature of acute confusional states. Schol Inq Nurs Pract Intl J 5(1):3–16, 1990; Lipowski ZJ: Transient cognitive disorders in the elderly. Am J Psychiatry 140:1432, 1983; and Ignatavicius D: Resolving the delirium dilemma. Nursing99 29(10):41–46, 1999.

16. Why are bowel problems a concern in elderly patients?

Like acute confusion, there are multiple causes of bowel alterations in the elderly. With constipation, alterations in mobility, changes in eating patterns, decreased fluid and insufficient fiber intake, and use of drugs that induce peripheral neurotoxicity are factors to consider. In particular, opioids and vinca alkaloid chemotherapeutic agents (vincristine, vinblastine, etoposide) are major offenders in the elderly. When these drugs are prescribed, a prophylactic bowel regimen should be started immediately to counter the likelihood of constipation. Lower pelvic irradiation is a frequent cause of diarrhea and should be aggressively managed to minimize fluid and electrolyte disturbances. Other causes include the administration of parenteral nutrition, surgical manipulation of the bowel, and laxative misuse. Just as multiple factors may contribute to the problem, so must multiple factors be considered in treatment. Medications should be administered along with dietary modifications.

17. What about depression in the elderly?

Many nurses and other health professionals expect depression to be a major corollary to cancer in the elderly. The older adult may have numerous losses to adapt to such as depletion of work or financial independence, change in living arrangements, and loss of health, spouse, significant others, or physical stamina. Hence, the elderly person must adapt to these losses, which result in normal sadness. The most important predictor of a major depressive response in elderly cancer patients, however, is not old age alone, but rather a premorbid history of depression. A careful precancer history is paramount for the early recognition and treatment of a major depression.

18. What other important psychosocial issues should I be aware of?

For the elderly patient facing cancer, prominent themes include the anticipation of death and undertaking a critical life review. These two processes prepare the older adult for the reality of dying. Also, the older patient has had significant encounters in dealing with crises; this emotional rehearsal offers them strategies for dealing with a life-threatening illness. A prominent dilemma for the family is caregiver burden. Providing care for aged parents in conjunction with meeting the competing demands of one's own family often exacerbates stress and family system disequilibrium. With daughters and daughters-in-law commonly assuming most of the responsibility of caregiving, this social support dilemma has evolved into a major women's health concern.

19. What are the prominent areas I can learn more about to provide better care for older patients with cancer?

We would all be well served to learn more about general principles of gerontologic nursing and then to apply them to what we know about cancer nursing. The "graying of America" demands not only greater understanding of the biobehavioral science of aging, but creative use of that knowledge base clinically.[15] For example, conditions linked with aging have numerous implications for nursing care of elderly cancer patients, including falls, acute confusion, altered nutrition, bowel and bladder dysfunction, skin integrity, and sleep disturbances. Application of gerontologic nursing expertise to the clinical, educational, and research domains of oncology nursing will improve the quality of nursing care for elderly cancer patients and their families.

20. What are the major initiatives for the future of geriatric oncology?
Many issues related to the care of the elderly with cancer are becoming the focus of research and clinical innovation. Ten major themes address the following quandaries:

- Investigation of how the age of the host influences carcinogenesis and patterns of metastasis
- Study of the impact of prevention initiatives begun in old age
- Examination of subsets of elderly (i.e., young-old vs. old-old) and their responses to treatment
- Determination of screening guidelines for cancers unique to the elderly
- Development of model programs to facilitate optimum early detection behaviors
- Creation of cancer clinical trials specific to elderly patients
- Elucidation of toxicity profiles in the elderly receiving antineoplastic therapies
- Evaluation of drug therapy regimens to treat symptom distress in the elderly
- Provision and impact of novel social support interventions
- Management of psychosocial correlates of coping with cancer during advanced age

REFERENCES

1. Balducci L, Parker M, Sexton W, Tantranond P: Pharmacology of antineoplastic agents in the elderly patient. Semin Oncol 16:76–84, 1989.
2. Benowitz S: Wanted: Senior citizens for cancer treatment trials. J Natl Canc Inst 92:446–447, 2000.
3. Blair KA: Cancer screening of older women. Canc Pract 6:217–222, 1998.
4. Boyle DM: The geriatric imperative in cancer nursing practice. Oncol Nurs Today 2:12–15, 1997.
5. Boyle DM: Realities to guide novel and necessary nursing care in geriatric oncology. Canc Nurs 17:125–136, 1994.
6. Boyle DM, Angert V: Lymphoma at the extremes of age. Semin Oncol Nurs 14:302–311, 1998.
7. Boyle DM, Engelking C, Blesch KS, et al: Oncology Nursing Society position paper on cancer and aging: The mandate for oncology nursing. Oncol Nurs Forum 19:913–933, 1992.
8. Bruner DW, Pickett M, Joseph A, Burggraf V: Prostate cancer elder alert: Epidemiology, screening and early detection. J Gerontol Nurs 26:6–15, 2000.
9. Cohen HJ: Oncology and aging: General principles of cancer in the elderly. In Hazzard WR, Bierman EL, Blass JP, et al (eds): Principles of Geriatric Medicine, 3rd ed. New York, McGraw-Hill, 1994.
10. Extermann M, Overcash J, Lyman GH, et al: Comorbidity and functional status are independent in older cancer patients. J Clin Oncol 16:1582–1587, 1998.
11. Fentiman IS, Tirelli U, Monfardini S, et al: Cancer in the elderly: Why so badly treated? Lancet 335:1020–1022, 1990.
12. Gulitz E, Bustillo-Hernandez M, Kent EB: Missed cancer screening opportunities among older women: A review. Canc Pract 6:289–295, 1998.
13. Knight JA: Ethics of care in caring for the elderly. South Med J 87:909–917, 1994.
14. Kurtz ME, Kurtz JC, Stommel M, et al: Symptomatology and loss of physical functioning among geriatric patients with lung cancer. J Pain Sympt Manage 19:249–256, 2000.
15. McBride AB: Nursing and gerontology. J Gerontol Nurs 26:18–27, 2000.
16. Monfardini S, Yancik R: Cancer in the elderly: Meeting the challenge of an aging population. J Natl Canc Inst 85:532–538, 1993.
17. Raveis VH, Karus D, Pretter S: Correlates of anxiety among adult daughter caregivers to a parent with cancer. J Psychosoc Oncol 17:1–26, 1999.

61. CULTURE AND CANCER

Patricia W. Nishimoto, RN, MPH, DNS, COL, AN, USAR,
and Joanne Itano, RN, PhD, OCN

1. Define culture and ethnicity.

Culture defines reality for members of a social group, including the individual's purpose in life and proper, sanctioned behavior within the group. **Ethnicity** refers to an ethnic quality or affiliation with a particular ethnic group (large groups of people classed according to common traits and customs). The world view of a culture affects the values, beliefs, and practices held by group members about health promotion and illness prevention; the causation, detection, and treatment of illness; the care of ill and well people; whom to ask for assistance; and the social roles, relationships, and expectations that guide encounters between members and health care providers.

2. How does the culture of the nurse affect nurse–patient interactions?

In addition to the nurse's own ethnic culture, she or he is also part of the westernized culture of medicine with its own set of values and beliefs. Health care beliefs and practices of many cultural groups may not be congruent with those of mainstream, westernized medicine. Conflicts and nonadherence may result because of a natural tendency to be ethnocentric—to view people unconsciously by using one's group and one's own customs as the standard for all judgments. For example, being on time and keeping appointments is a value of the westernized health culture. Some cultures have a present-time orientation and value living in the present. A patient who is consistently late for appointments may be viewed negatively by health care providers who are using their own belief system as the basis to judge a patient's behavior. It is extremely important to *avoid stereotyping*. It is also important to acknowledge differences across and within cultural groups.

3. What is the cultural distribution in the U.S.?

Until recently, the cultural diversity of the United States was limited largely to White immigrants from Europe. In the 1950s nine out of every 10 Americans were of European descent. In the 1990s one out of every four adults and one out of every three children were of African, Latin American, or Asian origin. The U.S. Census Bureau projects that by 2050 the population distribution will be as follows: White, 52.5%; Hispanic/Latino, 22.5%; Black, 14.4%; Asian Pacific Islander, 9.7%; and Native American, 0.9%. Thus, nurses will care for patients from diverse cultures.

4. What aspects of a cancer diagnosis may be affected by culture and ethnicity?

Cultural norms and expectations affect many aspects of the cancer diagnosis, including responses to treatments, their side effects, and pain; concepts of body image and sexuality; expectations about suffering; public and private behavior; interactions with authority figures; determination of who constitutes the family; dynamics within the family unit in response to a life-threatening illness; how health care decisions are made and by whom; and how dying and death are conceptualized, approached, and commemorated.

5. How are ethnic and cultural groups categorized?

A person's ethnic group should be described as he or she identifies it. Black Americans include immigrants from such countries as Africa, the West Indies, Dominican Republic, Haiti, and Jamaica. Asian Pacific Islanders, the fastest growing cultural minority group in the U.S., include people from 28 countries and 25 identified Pacific Island cultures. They are a highly diverse group consisting of recent immigrants as well as groups that have been in the U.S. for several generations. Native Americans include American Indians and Alaskan Eskimos. *Note:* Categories used to describe race (more specific to distinct, inheritable physical traits) may differ from ethnic or cultural categories.

6. Summarize the differences in cancer incidence and mortality among cultural groups.

Overall cancer incidence and mortality rates vary among cultural and ethnic groups. Blacks are more likely to develop cancer than persons of any other ethnic group. They are 60% more likely to develop cancer than Asian Pacific Islanders, and Hispanics/Latinos are more than twice as likely to develop cancer as American Indians.[5] Blacks are also about 33% more likely to die of cancer than Whites and are two times more likely to die of cancer than Asian Pacific Islanders, Native Americans, and Hispanics/Latinos. Generally, Hispanics/Latinos rank in the middle for cancer incidence and mortality. As a group, Asian Pacific Islanders have the second highest incidence and lowest mortality rates compared with Blacks, Hispanics/Latinos, and Native Americans. Native Americans have the lowest cancer incidence and mortality among the four major ethnic groups. Based on data collected by the National Cancer Institute's Surveillance, Epidemiology, and End Results (SEER) program and the American Cancer Society, the following table displays the most common cancers in various ethnic groups.

CANCER TYPES	PREDOMINANT ETHNIC GROUPS
Lung	Higher incidence in Blacks than Whites; mortality rates in Blacks are twice those in Whites.
Prostate	Incidence higher by 50% in Blacks compared with Whites; mortality rates also are higher in Blacks than in Whites.
Breast	White women are more likely to develop breast cancer; Black women have higher mortality rates.
Colorectal	Blacks have the highest incidence and mortality rates.
Pancreas	Blacks have higher incidence than Whites (60%); Black mortality rate is also higher.
Hepatocellular	Prevalent in Asian Pacific Islanders. Vietnamese men have the highest incidence; Chinese women have the highest mortality rate.
Cervical	Vietnamese women have the highest incidence rates, followed by Hispanic/Latino women. Black women have the highest mortality rates, followed by Hispanic/Latino women.
Ovarian	Increased incidence and mortality rates in White women.
Bladder	Hispanic/Latino men have the second highest incidence after Whites. Whites have the highest mortality rates, followed by Blacks.
Esophageal	Blacks have highest incidence and mortality rates.
Nasopharyngeal	Asian Pacific Islanders (Chinese men) have the highest incidence and mortality rates.
Gastric	More prevalent in Asian Pacific Islanders. Highest incidence in Korean men and Vietnamese women; highest mortality rate in Japanese men and Hawaiian women.
Non-Hodgkin's lymphoma	Highest incidence in Whites followed by Vietnamese men; highest mortality rates in Hawaiian men, followed by Whites.

7. Describe the major types of health beliefs as affected by culture.

Magicoreligious view: belief that health and illness are controlled by supernatural forces. Illness is seen as punishment for misbehavior or opposing God's will.

Scientific or biomedical view: life and life processes as controlled by physical or biochemical processes that can be manipulated by humans.

Holistic view: the forces of nature must be maintained in balance or harmony to maintain health.

8. What is folk medicine?

Folk medicine is a type of healing practice in which beliefs and practices related to illness and health are derived from cultural traditions rather than from a scientific base. Because cancer may be viewed as an unnatural illness caused by supernatural or sinful behavior, some cultures may have a fatalistic view that cancer cannot be treated effectively by Western medicine and prefer to use folk medicine. Folk healing is regarded as more comfortable and less frightening than traditional Western medicine. It is thought to be more humanistic and holistic because healing is a restoration of a person to a state of harmony between body, mind, and spirit. People may consult a folk healer first because he or she understands the problem within a cultural context, speaks the same language, and shares a similar world view as the patient. The consultation and treatment take place in the community of the patient, usually in the home of the healer. The folk healer is often a woman in the community knowledgeable about home remedies or a spiritualist who combines rituals, spiritual beliefs, and herbal medicines. The healer typically prepares the treatment and frequently either the healer or the patient performs some type of ritual practice.

9. Summarize common differences in healing practices among cultural groups.

The holistic view of health is held by many **Asian Pacific Islanders**, whose healing practices include the use of herbs, traditional healers, and healing ceremonies. Balance and harmony in body, mind, and spirit with nature and the universe are necessary for good health. The balance between hot and cold elements is also significant. Cancer is viewed as a cold illness and treated with foods, herbs, and healing ceremonies that possess "hot" properties. A widespread belief among some Asian Pacific Islander groups that suffering is part of life may lead to delay in seeking treatment.

A common **Hispanic/Latino belief** is that health is the result of good luck or a reward from God for good behavior. Fatalism and the concept of illness resulting from an imbalance of hot and cold is also seen in Hispanic/Latino groups. Their first line of treatment often includes home remedies and visits to the family folk healer.

Native Americans commonly link health beliefs and religion and view health as living in harmony with nature. Some tribes believe that illness is caused by witchcraft. The traditional healer in the Native American culture is the medicine person who is "chosen" and wise in the ways of the land and nature. The goal of treatment is to enhance total healing; healers take time to determine first the cause of illness and the proper treatment. Treatment typically includes special or healing ceremonies, herbs, prayers, or songs.

10. How is screening affected by ethnicity and fatalism?

Ethnic background, health beliefs, and fears as well as level of education, acculturation, age, and insurance coverage can affect and prevent screening practices. For example, Hispanic/Latino women who believe that caressing the breast, injury to the breast, or multiple sexual partners increase the risk of breast cancer as a punishment of God may not go for screening because they do not want to know. If they are diagnosed with breast cancer, their concern is how to tell their family that God is punishing them. Women who are not sexually active may believe screening is not necessary until a partner begins to touch their breasts. Screening is not a customary event for West Indians, Hmongs, male Puerto Ricans, and American Indians who follow traditional healing practices.

Fear that all cancer is fatal promotes the belief that there is "no use" in screening. The incidence of fatalism is higher in women, Blacks, and people with low income and low educational levels. Fatalism also may be expressed by some Asian Pacific Islander groups. The sense of fatalism can be decreased in people who have a strong spiritual core through the interventions of ministers, prayers, and prayer groups.

Fatalistic beliefs about screening can delay diagnosis, resulting in advanced stage of disease at presentation. This scenario reinforces the impression of the community that cancer is an automatic death sentence: "My auntie was feeling poorly and three weeks after she saw her doctor, she was lying in her coffin."

People who are fatalistic may interpret self-breast examinations as a monthly stressor. To engage in screening is to "name the disease" and can cause "bachi" (bad luck that makes the thing feared actually happen). A fear that you are "destined" to die after a diagnosis of breast cancer can be reinforced when a friend dies of breast cancer. Studies reporting that the behavior of breast cancer at the molecular level is affected by ethnicity can reinforce the belief that ethnicity alone predicts survival. It is the role of the nurse to answer patients' questions honestly while helping them to interpret the statistics that they may have read.

11. What can be done to increase screening in different ethnic groups?

The overall consensus is that patients need to understand the rationale for the screening test and to feel the concern and respect of the health care provider who asks them to participate in screening. This is particularly true for Arab Americans, Cambodians, Central Americans, Cubans, Filipinos, Gypsies, Iranians, Haitians, Japanese-Americans, Koreans, Vietnamese, and Samoans.

When West Indians are agreeable to screening, be extremely cognizant of their high level of modesty and need for privacy. This also holds true for Samoans, female Puerto Ricans, Mexican Americans, Koreans, Filipinos, Ethiopians/Eritreans, Chinese Americans, and Cambodians. Matching the provider's gender to the patient's may help. A strategy to help increase screening among Puerto Rican males is to get their wives to encourage them to go for screening.

Screening in many Brazilians, Russians, and Hmongs can be accomplished when they come for an office visit for an illness or other symptoms. It is uncommon for them to come for screening while they are feeling well. Native Americans may comment that they do not believe in "silent disease," and Brazilians may avoid screening to prevent hearing "bad news."

Blacks may think that there is no need for screening or treatment because God's will determines whether you live or die; everything is left in God's hands. They also may believe that cancer is caused by not following God's will. Using knowledge about these beliefs and the help of Black leaders, the American Cancer Society developed a video, "Telling the Story—To Live is God's Will," to urge people to go for cancer screening. The video uses gospel music while Blacks speak about their personal experiences with cancer screening.

12. How can the use of groups facilitate screening?

The American Indian Women's Talking Circle focuses on wellness to increase cervical cancer screening. The Western approach of screening to prevent death may seem strange because "all people die." The women meet weekly for 16 sessions where time is flexible and open to allow conversation, sharing, and prayer. Each session begins with a traditional story, and culturally sensitive strategies are used to encourage discussion. This is similar to the Native Hawaiian kokua groups, in which lay leaders or navigators increase cervical and breast cancer screening. (*Kokua* means to give help voluntarily without the request for assistance. The term *navigator* connotes the ancient Polynesians who navigated canoes to Hawaii.)

Peer educators are used in Arizona with Companeros en la Salud (Partners in Health). Women meet after church to discuss screening and are given low-cost vouchers for screening tests. In the Witness Project in Arkansas, Black survivors of breast cancer meet with women after church services to discuss the importance of early screening and treatment. The group's name incorporates the spiritual importance in the lives of the women, who can witness the importance of screening, just as they witness the blessings of the Lord at church.

13. How does culture affect the family and its decision making?

Cultural behaviors (how one acts in certain situations) are acquired through the family, the basic unit of society and major social network for most people. Cultures vary in their definition of family and beliefs about the role of the family in health and illness. For example, the Samoan and Hispanic/Latino cultures expect a large gathering of family members in the patient's room and in the waiting room when a person is hospitalized.

To meet the patient's needs, it is important to know who makes the health care decisions. Depending on the culture, however, the patient may not be the person who makes the health care decisions. For example, the wife or mother in a Black family generally is charged with the responsibility of protecting the health of the family. Family members may enter the health care system at the advice of the matriarch of the family. In contrast, in the Hispanic/Latino culture men typically assume a dominant role and may need to be involved in decision-making.

14. How does ethnicity affect the process of informed consent?

Informed consent is based on the value of patient autonomy, truth telling, and the belief that people should be in control of their lives. Although this is a European-American approach, it may not be acceptable to people from Micronesia. When families believe that the patient should not know the diagnosis of cancer, informed consent for treatment and especially for clinical trials is impossible. If they believe being truthful and forthright is disrespectful and rude, the sharing of detailed information about possible side effects may conflict with the goal of providing culturally sensitive care.

Asian Americans who believe that being told a diagnosis of malignancy makes a person "give up and die" may view informed consent as a threat to the patient's well-being. Memorizing which ethnic groups believe that cancer is a death sentence is neither practical nor reliable because each person individualizes cultural beliefs based on personal life experiences. It is important to remember, however, that informed consent is not an "automatic given" to include with all patients. Instead of assumptions, in the initial meeting with the patient remember that people deal with disease in many ways. Inform patients that you want them to tell you how they want to be given information about their diagnosis and tests results. This begins a conversation that encourages them to teach you about how they view life and how they want to be treated as your patient.

Informed consents tend to be written in English, are often lengthy, and continue to be written in language that is technical and difficult to understand even by people for whom English is a first language. If they have been translated into other languages, careful attention is needed to check who translated them and if back translation was done to ensure correctness.

15. Does ethnicity affect participation in clinical trials?

Multiple efforts have been made to include diverse populations in clinical trials. Yet the majority of people who participate in clinical trials are Whites who are well educated with a higher socioeconomic status. People participate because of great trust in physicians, a sense of hope, a belief that there is a chance of cure even when the prognosis is fatal, and the opportunity to feel "in charge" of the disease. When fatalistic beliefs are strong, people may feel no need to participate in a treatment that may have increased side effects. When people believe that outcome is based on God's will alone, there may be hesitation to participate because it may seem to be a lack of faith not to trust the Lord. Cultural beliefs about whether a person should even know the diagnosis also affect participation.

16. How does culture affect support group attendance?

Age, gender, ethnicity, and levels of acculturation, education, and socioeconomic status can affect support group attendance. The distance to travel to a meeting does not seem to affect support group attendance. Young adults who continue to work full-time during treatment may not attend traditional support groups but find it helpful to participate in on-line chat groups via the computer. Young teens often find it more comfortable to talk openly in a group if they are "not looking at each other." When running a support group for teens, it is helpful to plan a physical activity during the session to allow them to look at their hands.

Japanese American women who value cultural norms of reciprocity, social obligation, harmony, and respect may avoid groups. This is further influenced by the concept of *giri* (social obligation), according to which it is necessary to repay favors with an equivalent gesture; the high level of nonverbal communication that considers it rude to discuss or ask about feelings; and the expectation that if a person cares about you, they will *know* how you feel without asking. The need for harmony and not appearing different from others is not dissimilar in the Hong Kong Chinese. This need can cause people to hesitate to join a group, but once they attend and meet others in a similar situation, they form connections and are able to voice common concerns. Communal values of some Hispanic/Latino, Black, and/or Native American cultures may positively influence participation in a group with others of similar background. Many Samoans may have a strong family support network and view it as disrespectful if the patient attends a support group of nonfamily members.

Men may be more likely to participate if an educational component is identified as the reason for the group and if the group is made up of men. Some men may be more interested if recreational activities are offered as part of the meeting.

17. How do culture and ethnicity affect pain expression?

Ethnic and cultural backgrounds contribute to variations in pain perception, meaning of pain, and responses to pain. Multiple studies have documented inadequate assessment and treatment of pain in people of ethnic diversity. This finding may be due to difficulty in reducing the complexity of pain to a number. Perhaps a cultural background of stoicism results in underrated pain, or cultural expressiveness may lead to overtreatment of pain. Many patients want to be seen as "good patients" who do not complain. For example, some Asian Americans may value harmony so highly that they do not want to cause disharmony with a provider or make the provider "lose face" if they are unable to relieve the pain. Some ethnicities are known for their stoicism but caution must be applied because not all Russians, Filipinos, Irish, Japanese Americans, Samoans, Cambodians, Chinese Americans, and Mexican Americans are stoic. Some American Indians may use only general terms to tell staff about pain level and, if pain is not relieved, will not ask again. They may not tell staff directly but use a family member or friend to tell about pain.

Ethnic groups known to express pain openly include gypsies, Puerto Ricans, Iranians, Central Americans, Brazilians, Arab Americans, Haitians, Koreans, and Cubans. Furthermore, verbal expressions of pain may be accelerated when the family is present. For example, Korean Americans may moan loudly "chagetta" ("I could die") when visited by their families.

18. What factors contribute to ethnic differences in the metabolism of pain medications or other drugs.

Studies have reported that ethnicity can affect how people respond to drugs. Factors contributing to the various reactions to drugs among ethnic groups include environment (e.g., diet, smoking, use of alcohol), culture (values and beliefs), and genetics. A person's race can influence drug responses because metabolism of drugs is genetically determined (genetic polymorphism).

19. Give examples of genetic polymorphism.

Three types of genetic polymorphism have been identified with many drugs metabolized via these pathways: acetylation polymorphism, debrisoquine polymorphism, and mephenytoin polymorphism. Japanese and Inuit populations have more rapid acetylators than slow acetylators. Poor metabolizers of debrisoquine (an antihypertensive compound) are found in approximately 3–9% of Whites in the U.S., Canada, Britain, Denmark, Sweden, and Switzerland; the lowest percentage (0–2%) of poor metabolizers are from China, Japan, Malaysia, and Thailand. Some opioids, antihypertensives, antipsychotics, and antidepressants are metabolized similarly to debrisoquine. For example, codeine is more likely to be effective in Chinese or Japanese patients than in patients from Sweden. There is a higher percentage (about 20%) of poor metabolizers of mephenytoin (anticonvulsant agent) in China and Japan than in other countries. Drugs metabolized via the mephenytoin pathway include various barbiturates and diazepam. The examples of genetic polymorphism highlight the need to consider ethnicity as well as age, gender, and weight in the type and dosages of drugs that are prescribed.

20. What factors should be considered in addressing advance directives with different cultural groups?

Health care providers may see advance directives as a means of empowerment and a sign of respect, but they also can be seen as disrespectful, insulting, or immoral. For many Chinese and Japanese, it is considered bad luck even to talk about death. Those who place value on family and harmony also may find the concept of power of attorney as burdensome and incongruent with the value of deciding as a family. Advance directives imply knowledge of prognosis, which may not be desired by Korean, Chinese, or Mexican Americans.

Many Japanese Americans may ask their family to make end-of-life decisions for them. Chinese Americans value respect for elders. A do-not-resuscitate (DNR) order may imply disrespect or giving up if the family is asked to make the decision. Samoans believe that if you dishonor a dying patient's wishes, he or she will haunt and harm the youngest child in the family. Navajos may believe that saying something aloud shapes reality and causes it to occur.

Recent immigrants or former refugees may not have trust in giving a physician power over a life-and-death decision. Requiring advance directives to be written implies that the physician does not trust or honor the word of an Arab American. Trust issues also may affect DNR decisions for Hispanics/Latinos or Blacks, who may worry that their care will be substandard if they choose a DNR status.

21. How are cultural or religious rituals related to the dying process?

The nurse needs to take time to learn the unique ways that each person and family want to approach the dying process. For example, the Hindu faith may forbid non-Hindu staff from touching the body. The Muslim religion has prescribed behaviors for the dying patient that may take precedence over their ethnic beliefs about the dying process. If able to do so, the patient recites the Declaration of Faith: "There is no God but God and Mohammed is his Messenger." After death, a family member washes the body. Autopsy is not permitted because of the need for the body to be buried intact. Countries that share a Muslim world view include Senegal, Somalia, Saudi Arabia, Qatar, Pakistan, Nigeria, Morocco, Maldives, Malaysia, Libya, Lebanon, Kuwait, Jordan, Iraq, Iran, Indonesia, Guinea, Ethiopia, Egypt, and Bangladesh.

For religious reasons, it is extremely important not to remove items placed in the dead person's body. For example, Buddhists may place jewelry, money, or rice into the dead person's mouth to help him or her travel into the next life. Strings placed around the neck or wrist by a Hindu priest should not be removed because they are blessings for the dead person. (For more information about religion and spirituality, see Chapter 62).

22. How does one communicate effectively with patients from different cultures?

When communicating with patients from a different culture, nurses should ask the patient what name they would like to called and whether note-taking is permissible. They should speak in an unhurried manner, validate information rather than interpret silence or head nodding as agreement, and listen carefully, allowing time for responses and giving full attention to the patient.

Nonverbal communication includes touch, facial expressions, body movement, or posture. In some cultures, direct eye-to-eye contact is considered disrespectful, impolite, and an invasion of privacy. For example, some Native American tribes consider eye-to-eye contact as looking into one's soul, which may result in its loss. Touch may be important because it conveys approval, empathy, caring, or trust. However, in some groups, touch between the nurse and patient may be viewed negatively. For example, in some Asian Pacific Islander groups, the head is sacred, and touching or patting the head may be perceived as a rude gesture. Some Native Americans consider a firm handshake as a sign of aggression. Navajos extend their hand and lightly touch the hand of the person whom they are greeting.

The amount of physical space that is considered appropriate between people also varies among cultures. Nurses must be sensitive to patients' reactions to movement toward them. A patient may physically withdraw or back away if the nurse is perceived as being too close. Cultural groups also differ in their use of body language. Some are often more dramatic in their body language, whereas others are characterized as stoical or nonexpressive of emotion.

23. What if you need an interpreter?

A professional interpreter with a health care background is preferred rather than a family member, employee, or visitor. Patients may be uncomfortable discussing intimate issues with a family member or visitor as an interpreter. In addition, the interpreter may be uncomfortable asking the patient personal questions. When seeking an interpreter, be sure to clarify whether the patient is speaking a specific dialect of the language. For example, Filipinos may speak Tagalog, Visayan, Ilocano, or Cebuano. Matching the gender of the interpreter to the patient is preferable. Age also may be a concern. An older, more mature interpreter is preferred over someone younger than the patient. It may be important to consider socioeconomic differences between the patient and interpreter and to avoid an interpreter from a rival tribe, state, or nation.

24. What culturally sensitive resources are available to oncology nurses?

The **American Cancer Society** has developed multiple programs to reach out to different ethnic groups. Examples include the Witness Program, a breast cancer screening program for Black women, and the video, "Telling the Story—To Live is God's Will."

Professionals often recommend the **National Cancer Institute website** to patients who want to learn more about their diagnosis. It is available only in Spanish and English (at a twelfth-grade reading level). Overall, the United States population has a lower reading level, and if English is a second language, the site may be less useful. Many of the nutritional suggestions are helpful for people with a European background but not for those who may use kim chi, tortillas, or sushi in their diet.

The following addresses and web addresses are a slight sampling of useful resources.

- Office of Minority Health Resource Center
  P.O. Box 37337
  Washington, DC 20013-7337
  (800) 444-6472
  www.omhrc.gov
- National Black Leadership Initiative on Cancer
  (800)-4-CANCER
- Celebrating Life Foundation
  P.O. Box 224076
  Dallas, TX 75222-4076
  (800) 207-0992
  www.celebratinglife.org
  (Promotes awareness of breast cancer among women of color)
- Chinese-American Cancer Foundation (affiliated with American Cancer Society)
  Orange County office:
  9092 Talbert Ave, # 1
  Fountain Valley, CA 92708
  (714) 378-6067
  National organization:
  8232 E. Garvey Avenue, # 201
  Rosemead, CA 91770
  (818) 280-0610

The American Cancer Society (ACS) has three units that focus on Chinese Americans:
- ACS, Queens Division, Chinese Unit
  41-25 Kissena Blvd, Room 103
  Flushing, NY 11355
  (718) 886-8890
  CACA-ACS@worldnet.att.net
- ACS, Northern California, Chinese Unit
  39277 Liberty St, #D14
  Fremont, CA 94538
  (888) 566-6222
- ACS, New Jersey Division, Chinese-American Affiliate
  669 Littleton Road
  Parsippany, NJ 07054
  (210) 334-2249

Two units of the ACS have Korean-speaking staff members: ACS Queens Division (718-263-2224) and ACS Los Angeles Unit (213-386-7660). Many ACS divisions have Native American materials specific to cancer screening, including the Oklahoma Division, Minneapolis, MN, and South Dakota Division.

• National Asian Women's Health Organization (NAWHO)
Suite 1500, 250 Montgomery St.
San Francisco, CA 94104
(415) 989-9747
www.nawho.org (information available in English, Catonese, Laotian, Vietnamese, and Korean)
• American Indian Health Care Association
St. Paul, MN
• National Hispanic Leadership Initiative on Cancer
En Accion Texas Center
University of Texas Health Sciences Center at San Antonio
7703 Floyd Curl Drive
San Antonio, TX 78284-7791
(210) 567-7826

REFERENCES

1. Douglas M: Pain as the fifth vital sign: Will cultural variations be considered? J Transcul Nurs 10:285, 1999.
2. Ersek M, Kagawa-Singer M, Barnes D, et al: Multicultural considerations in the use of advance directives. Onc Nurs Forum 25:1683–1690, 1998.
3. Geissler EM: Cultural Assessment, 2nd ed. St. Louis, Mosby, 1998.
4. Gotay CC, Wilson ME: Social support and cancer screening in African American, Hispanic, and Native American women. Cancer Pract 6:31–37, 1998.
5. Greenlee RT, Hill-Harmon MB, Murray T, Thun M: Cancer Statistics 2001. CA Cancer J Clin 51:15–36, 2001.
6. Itano J, Brandt J, Ishida D, et al: Multicultural Outcomes: Guidelines for Cultural Competence. Pittsburgh, Oncology Nursing Society, 1999.
7. Itano J: Cultural issues. In Itano J, Taoka K (eds): Core Curriculum for Oncology Nursing, 3rd ed. Philadelphia,W.B. Saunders, 1998, pp 60–76.
8. Jang M, Lee E, Woo K: Income, language and citizenship status: Factors affecting the health care access and utilization of Chinese Americans. Health Soc Work 23:136–142, 1998.
9. Joslyn SA, West MM: Racial differences in breast carcinoma survival. Cancer 88:114–123, 2000.
10. Kagawa-Singer M, Chung R: A paradigm for culturally based care in ethnic minority populations. J Commun Psychol 22:192–208, 1994.
11. Krizek C, Robers C, Regan R, et al: Gender and cancer support group participation. Cancer Pract 7:86–92, 1999.
12. Kudzma EC: Culturally competent drug administration. Am J Nurs 99:46–51, 1999.
13. Lipson JG, Dibble SL, Minarik PA: Culture and Nursing Care: A Pocket Guide. San Francisco, UCSF Nursing Press, 1996.
14. Makabe R, Hull MH: Components of social support among Japanese women with breast cancer. Onc Nurs Forum 27:1381–1390, 2000.
15. Meisenhelder JB, Chandler EN: Faith, prayer, and health outcomes in elderly Native Americans. Clin Nurs Res 9:191–203, 2000.
16. Mok E, Martinson I: Enpowerment of Chinese patients with cancer through self-help groups in Hong Kong. Cancer Nursing 23:206–213, 2000.
17. Phillips JM, Cohen MZ, Moses G: Breast cancer screening and African American women: Fear, fatalism, and silence. Onc Nurs Forum 26:561–571, 1999.
18. Powe BD, Weinrich S: An intervention to decrease cancer fatalism among rural elders. Onc Nurs Forum 26:583–588, 1999.
19. Purnell L, Paulanka B: Transcultural health care: A culturally competent approach. Philadelphia, F.A. Davis, 1998.
20. Strickland CJ, Squeoch MD, Chrisman NJ: Health promotion in cervical cancer prevention among the Yakama Indian women of the wa'shat longhouse. J Trancult Nurs 10:190–196, 1999.
21. Taoka K, Itano J: Cultural diversity among individuals with cancer. In Yarbro C, Frogge M, Goodman M, Groenwald S (eds): Cancer Nursing: Principles and Practice, 5th ed. Boston, Jones & Bartlett, 2000, pp 100–134.
22. Vaughn G, Kiyasu E, McCormick WC: Advance directive preferences among subpopulations of Asian nursing home residents in the Pacific Northwest. J Am Geriatr Soc 48:554–557, 2000.
23. Wilson FL, Baker LM, Brown-Syed C, et al: An analysis of the readability and cultural sensitivity of information on the National Cancer Institute's web site: Cancer Net (TM). Onc Nurs Forum 27:1403–1409, 2000.

62. RELIGION AND SPIRITUALITY

Julie R. Swaney, MDiv

1. What is the difference between religion and spirituality?

Spirituality is not necessarily religion. Many more people are spiritual than religious. Religion is a type of spirituality that refers to a disciplined, dogmatic set of beliefs usually set forth in writings (Koran, Bible, Creeds, and Confessions) and institutions (synagogues, churches). Spirituality refers to patterns or habits that human beings practice "for the purpose of grounding their ordinary lives in a life of the spirit which has meaning for them and to which they commit and re-commit themselves."[8] Spirituality has to do with meaning-making.

Some people find meaning in religion; others find or make meaning in their own spirituality. Spirituality asks and helps to answer crucial questions: How does this illness make sense in my life? How does my life make sense with this illness? What meaning does this cancer have for me? What meaning do I have with this cancer? What meaning do I have to my family? To God? To myself? What is spiritual has to do with what is essential; that is, what is of essence. We often think of spirituality as an external relationship with God—"out there"—rather than the more accurate notion of God within us.

2. What is the importance of religion and spirituality in illness?

Religion and spirituality provide the interpretive lens or framework within which persons make sense of living and dying. Being left to the whim of fate is universally terrifying. Patients with cancer and their caregivers often believe in something that helps to maintain hope. Patients may believe in chemotherapy, radiation, doctors, vitamins, macrobiotic diets, God's faithfulness to them, superstitious ritual, or their immune system. What they believe in provides a way of making sense of themselves and their experiences. As one patient stated, "believing in my immune system is everything. . . . It's the peg to hang my hat on." When people are coping with cancer, what they believe about themselves—what they hold in their spirits—profoundly affects their experience. Many studies indicate a positive correlation between spirituality and illness as well as spirituality and healing. Spiritual care is an important component of today's healthcare milieu. Spiritual care criteria has been articulated by the Joint Commission on Accreditation of Healthcare Organizations (JCAHO) providing a framework to help guide nurses' spiritual caregiving.

3. How do religious beliefs help people to cope with terminal illness?

People with healthy faith are better able to face reality, maintain hope, tolerate uncertainties, and retain their self-esteem and dignity. Religious beliefs that promote the constancy of God's presence help patients to realize their significance and permanence and to accept the ambiguity of God's ways. Prayer and meditation can reduce anxiety and strengthen coping skills. Certain beliefs answer the question "why?," whereas other beliefs provide comfort in the midst of the question itself.

The crisis of cancer prompts questions about meaning and existence: How much do I want to live? How much time do I have? Why did this happen to me? What did I do or not do? Why does God allow this? Why do I have to suffer? Am I a good person? Is God punishing me? Where is God? If I promise to go to church, will God heal me? Many people understand their existence in relation to God, whereas others do not. These existential questions of the human spirit are significant because they affect coping skills. "Being religious" does not guarantee survival, but it does guarantee a qualitative difference in the experience of cancer.

4. Can beliefs impede the healing process?

What people believe to be true may be what they will experience. Belief systems centered on punishment and guilt or even satanic forces may impede the healing process. Such beliefs lead people to think that they "deserve" the cancer and cannot be well again, whereas beliefs centered on forgiveness and hope facilitate healing and wholeness. Unhealthy faith provides an escape from reality and hinders adaptation to the experience.

5. How does hospitalization affect religion and spirituality?

Impressive human changes may occur during illness and hospitalization. During hospitalization, patients journey along a path with hope and healing on one side and terror and tragedy on the other. In a study of changes in hospitalized patients, 90% of the patients claimed to use their hospitalization to review and reorder their central values.[4] Over 50% of patients reported major shifts in their perception of the importance and quality of their relationships. Other changes reported in the study included the following: 71% reported that illness had changed their understanding of the purpose of their lives; 85% reported being more aware of the passing of time; 81% reported a decreased sense of being in control of their lives; 58% reported that illness had deprived them, to some extent, of the sense of being like other people; and 70% reported changes in their religious faith and practice.

6. What are the common religious beliefs and rituals related to illness and death?

Because a religion's stated positions may influence individual medical decisions, it is important to be familiar with some of the beliefs of particular religions, as outlined below. The nurse may ask patients about their beliefs and make use of religious authorities to assist them.

Buddhism (Tibetan)

Illness rituals	Prayer and meditation
Meaning of illness	Natural part of life
Faith healing	Possible through prayer and meditation
Sacraments	Respect intermediate state; preparation for death very important. Death signals entry into intermediate state of great intensity. Do not interrupt period of great concentration as deceased travels through intermediate state. Environment to be peaceful, focused, and intimate for terminally ill or deceased. Do not move body for 72 hours after death. Spiritual goal: extinction.
Autopsy	Permissible
Burial	Cremation
Meaning of death	Enlightenment

Roman Catholicism

Illness rituals	Baptism, reconciliation, Sacrament of the Sick, Eucharist, Prayer
Meaning of illness	Natural part of life; preserve dignity of patient; some suffering considered meaningful.
Faith healing	Possible through prayer, Sacrament of the Sick (anointing)
Sacraments	Sacrament of the Sick
Autopsy	Permissible
Burial	Burial or cremation
Meaning of death	Release to God

Christian Science

Illness rituals	Prayer
Meaning of illness	Mental concept that can be destroyed by altering thoughts and discovering "spiritual truth." Use Christian Science practitioners.
Faith healing	Primary means of healing; emphasize spiritual healing.
Sacraments	None
Autopsy	Unlikely, but permissible
Burial	Burial or cremation
Meaning of death	Return to God

Mormon (Church of Jesus Christ of Latter-day Saints)

Illness rituals	Prayer
Meaning of illness	Natural part of life; revelation of meaning through individual visions
Faith healing	Laying on of hands for divine healing
Sacraments	Adult baptism essential, even after death; preach gospel. Wash body; dress body in white robe.
Autopsy	Permissible
Burial	Burial; no cremation
Meaning of death	Death a blessing; return to God

Hindu

Illness rituals	Prayer
Meaning of illness	Punishment
Faith healing	Possible through prayer and meditation
Sacraments	Tie thread of blessing. Pour water in mouth. Washing of body. Particular about who touches body.
Autopsy	Permissible
Burial	Cremation (Ganges)
Meaning of death	Death an endless passage through cycles of life; natural part of life. Hope for better existence in next life. Death is liberation.

Jehovah's Witness

Illness rituals	Prayer
Meaning of illness	Natural part of life; strong sanctity of life
Faith healing	Possible through prayer
Sacraments	None
Autopsy	Acceptable; body intact
Burial	Burial or cremation
Meaning of death	Natural part of life

Judaism (Orthodox)

Illness rituals	Prayer
Meaning of illness	Natural part of life; strong sanctity-of-life ethic requiring all possible medical care to preserve life.
Faith healing	Demand medical attention; possible through prayer
Sacraments	Goses, Shiva, Yetziat Neshamah, Kevod Hamet
Autopsy	Rarely permissible; consult rabbi.
Burial	No cremation, quick burial
Meaning of death	Natural part of life; no afterlife

Presbyterian (Protestant)

Illness rituals	Baptism, communion, anointing, prayer
Meaning of illness	Natural part of life; quality of life valued over quantity of life
Faith healing	Prayer, communion
Sacraments	Prayer
Autopsy	Acceptable
Burial	Burial or cremation
Meaning of death	Resurrection into afterlife

7. How do religious beliefs affect ethical decision-making?

At times of uncertainty, people often turn to their moral or religious community for guidance in ethical decision-making. What appears to others to be non-beneficial or "futile" treatment may, in fact, be perceived by a patient to be beneficial as defined by the religious community or doctrine to which he or she belongs. A Muslim patient may demand "futile" treatment because the tenets of Islam dictate that life must be prolonged regardless of its quality. A Jehovah's Witness patient may refuse blood, even if the outcome is death, because of religious tenets. Suicide is not condoned by religious groups and denominations;

however, religious authorities should be consulted if suicidal ideation or suicide becomes an issue with any patient. Other common religious beliefs that affect ethical issues are outlined below.

Buddhism

Drugs, blood, artificial life support	Acceptable
Organ donation	Allowed if enhanced possibility of enlightenment
Termination of treatment	Allowed
Withholding/withdrawing life support	Allowed. Death is natural, to be accepted. Avoid unnatural intrusion of dying process
Active euthanasia	Prohibited

Roman Catholicism

Drugs, blood, artificial life support	Acceptable
Organ donation	Justified
Termination of treatment	Allowed except in cases of pregnancy
Withholding/withdrawing life support	Allowed. "Ordinary but not extraordinary" duty to prolong life. Importance of dignity. Exception: pregnancy.
Active euthanasia	Prohibited

Christian Science

Drugs, blood, artificial life support	Unacceptable
Organ donation	Unlikely
Termination of treatment	Allowed. Rely on faith healing.
Withholding/withdrawing life support	Allowed. Unlikely to accept in first place; unlikely to prolong dying process.
Active euthanasia	Prohibited

Mormon (Church of Jesus Christ of Latter-day Saints)

Drugs, blood, artificial life support	Acceptable
Organ donation	Individual decision
Termination of treatment	Allowed
Withholding/withdrawing life support	Allowed. Inevitable death viewed as a blessing.
Active euthanasia	Prohibited

Hindu

Drugs, blood, artificial life support	Acceptable
Organ donation	Permissible
Termination of treatment	Allowed
Withholding/withdrawing life support	Allowed. Death is liberation.
Active euthanasia	Prohibited

Jehovah's Witness

Drugs, blood, artificial life support	Some drugs; no blood or blood products; life support acceptable
Organ donation	Forbidden
Termination of treatment	Allowed
Withholding/withdrawing life support	Allowed. Rely on individual conscience in this decision. Duty not to accept blood or blood products.
Active euthanasia	Prohibited

Judaism (Orthodox)

Drugs, blood, artificial life support	Acceptable
Organ donation	Consult rabbi.
Termination of treatment	Not allowed. Consult rabbi.
Withholding/withdrawing life support	Not allowed. Consult rabbi.
Active euthanasia	Prohibited

Presbyterian (Protestant)

Drugs, blood, artificial life support	Acceptable
Organ donation	Acceptable
Termination of treatment	Allowed
Withholding/withdrawing life support	Allowed. Quality of life valued over quantity of life. Importance of dignity.
Active euthanasia	Prohibited

8. How do I understand a belief system different from my own?

Listen intently. *Ask* with sincerity. *Respect* what you hear. Some people have specific religious views to fashion their understanding, whereas others have their own theology, which may not fit any particular religious tradition. Even if you do not agree with all of a patient's beliefs, you can still help the patient by allowing him or her to articulate personal beliefs. It is not appropriate to try to convert patients to your belief system during vulnerable times. It is important to remember that beliefs exist for a reason.

9. How does one make a spiritual assessment?

The first step is to assess one's own view of the role and importance of spirituality and religion in health and illness. Person-centered nursing requires tending to the human spirit. The second step is to assess one's personal comfort level with addressing spiritual issues. The nurse who is uncomfortable with such issues should refer the patient to someone else. The third step is to offer one's self in a genuine, honest, empathic way. Empathy and respect for the patient's questions and views are more important than providing answers. One may help the patient simply by listening. The final step is to do a spiritual assessment. While there are many ways to do a spiritual assessment, one recommended approach is the FICA spiritual assessment tool.[10] This tool simply asks:

F (FAITH):	Do you consider yourself to be spiritual or religious? What things do you believe in that give meaning to your life?
I (IMPORTANCE):	Is faith important to you? How have your beliefs influenced your behavior during this illness?
C (COMMUNITY):	Are you part of a spiritual or religious community? Is there a person or a group of people who are really important to you?
A (ASSESSMENT):	How would you like me, your healthcare provider, to address these issues in your health care?

Answers to these questions will help you to understand your patient's spiritual state, including recent changes, and need for any special religious resources.

10. What are key nursing interventions to promote the spiritual well-being of patients?

Perhaps the most important nursing intervention is to offer genuine concern and empathy in eliciting the patient's spiritual strengths, beliefs, doubts, and confidences. Nurses should not impose their beliefs on patients; instead, they should assist patients in discovering and utilizing their own beliefs. A nursing care plan should include assisting patients to meet their spiritual goals, facilitating patients' spiritual practices or rituals, and providing privacy to do so.

A study asked Protestant, Catholic, and Jewish respondents if they thought that nurses could be helpful to them in establishing or maintaining a relationship with God.[9] Only 5 (20%) of Jewish subjects said "yes," whereas 42 (91%) of Protestant respondents and 26 (72%) of Catholic respondents said "yes." The table below summarizes Protestant and Catholic views of specific nursing activities thought to be most helpful.

NURSING ACTIVITY	CATHOLICS RESPONDING YES	PROTESTANTS RESPONDING YES
Read to me Bible passages I have chosen	15/20 (75%)	36/41 (88%)
Read or recite Bible passages of nurse's choice	12/22 (55%)	31/40 (78%)
Listen to me talk through my problem	22/24 (95%)	32/40 (80%)
Pray with me at my bedside	20/24 (83%)	37/40 (93%)
Tell me that the nurse is praying for me (when not with me)	23/24 (96%)	36/39 (92%)

11. What is spiritual distress?

Spiritual distress is a condition in which a person experiences or is at risk of experiencing a disturbance in a belief or value system that provides strength, hope, and meaning to life. Spiritual distress or faith crisis, as a nursing diagnosis, refers to "a disruption in the life principle that pervades a person's entire being and that integrates and transcends one's biological and psychosocial nature."[12] Spiritual distress occurs when religious ideology or accepted beliefs suddenly hold no integrity for an individual. Such a faith crisis is generally accompanied, if not precipitated, by anger and distress. Ways of interpreting life ("I always thought God would protect me"), of making sense, of finding meaning, fall apart. Sources of spiritual distress may be the crises of illness, suffering, or death itself; the inability to practice spiritual rituals; or conflict between beliefs and treatment regimen.

12. List common signs of spiritual distress.

Signs of spiritual distress range from obvious expression to subtle clues:
• Statement of spiritual distress or crisis
• Withdrawal, depression
• Anger
• Crying
• Loneliness, loss of self-esteem
• Hopelessness, helplessness
• Changes in reading or not reading religious literature
• Expression of feeling abandoned by persons and God
• Inability to cope with illness or treatment
• Refusal of or demand for treatment
• Praying for a miracle
• Tenacious grip on a rigid set of beliefs

13. What are nursing interventions for spiritual distress?

If spiritual distress is related to the inability to practice spiritual rituals, the nurse may help by addressing the disruptive factors and enabling the patient to engage in important (health-aiding) rituals. When spiritual distress is related to the crisis of illness, suffering, or dying, the nurse can help the patient verbalize a sense of meaning, sense of forgiveness, and sense of belonging and love. Such distress may be expressed in such questions as "Why is this happening to me?" (meaning), "What did I do to deserve this?" (forgiveness), or "Why do I feel so alone?" (love/relatedness). The nurse can help patients use their own inner resources to address such questions and may also enlist the help of external resources (clergy, family, friends, literature, health care professionals). Spiritual distress related to conflict between religious or spiritual beliefs and the prescribed health regimen can be relieved by providing thorough and accurate information for informed consent or informed refusal. The health care team should support the patient in his or her stated wishes and goals.

14. Why do people with faith tend to suffer less than those without it?

"Being religious" offers a qualitative difference in one's experience of cancer. People with healthy faith are generally more able to remain centered, to come to terms with their suffering, if not their death, because they seek to know themselves as God knows them. Their sense of significance, permanence, and self-esteem is determined in this larger context.

People suffer less when they are able to maintain a sense of personal worth, dignity, significance, even permanence in the wake of death. "Being religious" does not guarantee positive self-regard but does reduce sources of suffering. Religious individuals may suffer less from fear of dying because of their belief in spiritual permanence. Discovering themselves as God knows them makes people aware that they belong to a greater order in which they matter and in which attachment to God is fundamental. Patients with healthy faith believe that "in life and death, we belong to God"; thus, they are more able to accept the ambiguity of God's ways and to maintain hope in the midst of uncertainty.

15. What is the difference between suffering and pain?

Bodies do not suffer; people do. Pain refers to a physical sensation, whereas suffering refers to the quest for meaning, purpose, and fulfillment. Although pain is often a source of suffering, suffering may occur in the absence of pain. For example, a nuclear physicist with malignant melanoma metastatic to his brain is paralyzed on the left side of his body and dying. He describes suffering over the perceived lack of meaning in his life and death with cancer: "My life has meant nothing. It ends here." He is suffering because he has lost his centeredness and feels himself to be fragmenting and disintegrating in terms of personal significance. Suffering may occur when a person perceives death as meaningless or as a form of personal disintegration. People who have not made the most of their lives have a hard time facing death.

Other sources of suffering are the effects of disease and treatment, such as change in identity, loss of control, isolation, not feeling understood, perception of a foreshortened future (i.e., "nothingness," death), and threats of losing relationships, mobility, independence, finances, control, and self-worth. Theologically and existentially, suffering occurs when we are threatened by something not in our control. In this sense, some suffering is inevitable, because we are always facing things we cannot control. Suffering is more bearable when we remain centered, when we can plumb the depths of our suffering to discover life's ultimate meaning for us.[3]

16. What difference does faith make in the experience of pain and suffering?

How people view their pain and suffering affects their healing or dying process. The early Greeks and Romans emphasized the practice of euthanasia as an honorable way to manage pain. *Euthanatos* translates as "a good death." For the ancients, it was important to die a good death with self-control. Plato, Socrates, and many Greek and Roman physicians who administered poisons claimed that when a person became "useless to society," dying decently was a measure of the final value of life. Pain and suffering were meaningless.

The Judeo-Christian tradition transformed pain and suffering into meaningful experiences. After the second century A.D., this influential tradition in western thought and culture emphasized the importance of enduring suffering. Pain and suffering were believed to be the sign of God's presence in one's life. Suffering meant that one belonged to God and had to endure the life that one was given. The goal, then, was not to alleviate suffering but to endure it.

Many people still believe that pain and suffering are meaningful signs of God's presence and must be endured. Others are outraged by the pain and suffering that they endure and demand alleviation. Both positions may be more than simple attitudes; they may be deep religious convictions. The nurse may verify patient's beliefs and give the patient permission to verbalize personal points of view. When in doubt, the nurse should err on the side of alleviating pain and suffering.

17. How does spiritual care contribute to healing?

The most powerful healing emotion is expectant faith. Healing is the product of a human bond between caregiver and patient. Faith, hope, respect, compassion, trust, and empathy are essential elements of that bond that contribute to healing. The heart of nursing or caring is a healing relationship, and the heart of healing relationships is trust, acceptance, and empathy.

To cure (Latin: *curare*) means to take care of, to take charge of. It implies successful medical treatment. To heal (Anglo-Saxon: *haelen*) means to make or become whole, to recover from sickness, to get well. Helping someone to become whole is accomplished through a healing relationship as well as technical competence. Both are important. Healing is a process and comes from the same root word as holy. Both refer to wholeness. To facilitate healing is to facilitate greater wholeness. Through relationships and skills, the nurse can facilitate healing, wholeness, and even that which is holy in patients. It is hoped that nurses can experience the same processes in themselves.

18. What is the connection between prayer and healing?

"The science of prayer" has generated much debate and controversy. Prayer seems to be effective, but how and why? Why does prayer "work" for some people and not for others? To answer this question, as well as to define the relationship between prayer and healing, we must remain open to the mystery and ambiguity of healing, and perhaps of God.

Both theologians and physicians are enlarging their frameworks for understanding the connection between faith and healing. Historically, all physicians were priests, nurses were nuns, and religious orders ran hospitals. Spiritual and physical healing were recognized as intimately connected. Early 19th century rationalism, with its mechanical view of the body, increasingly separated the body from the mind and spirit. Religion left medicine, and medicine left the church. Yet there remained a holistic notion of persons that emphasized the integration of body, mind, and spirit.

Prayer is one way of attending to the spirit. Prayer grounds people in what gives them meaning and in their relationship with God. Prayer puts important words to their experiences. Prayer also evokes important feelings for healing—safety, hope, love, seeing oneself as one is seen by God, personal worth and self-esteem, and feeling cared about and "not alone." Prayer helps people to face reality; to tolerate ambiguity and uncertainty; and to confront the unknown, which is so constant in illness. At the very least, prayer helps to reduce anxiety, to remain centered, to remember that one is part of God's greater order; it helps patients to relax. And at the very most, prayer is an expression of a profound and empowering relationship with God.

Positive effects of prayer have been reported in patients with high blood pressure, wounds, heart attacks, headaches, and anxiety. One study showed that intercessory prayer (prayer for others) was a contributing factor to the healing of cardiac patients. The positive effects of prayer have also been indicated on nonhuman subjects such as water, enzymes, bacteria, plants, yeast, mice, and red blood cells.

19. Is prayer magic?

Prayer is not magic, religion is not magic, and God is not a magician. Many people use prayer and religion as a way of invoking "divine magic"; they are likely to be disappointed. One cannot manipulate God through piety or ritual. The adage, "there are no atheists in foxholes," is especially true when the foxhole is cancer. It is not wrong to pray when one is frightened, regardless of one's relationship with God. But it is wrong to try to manipulate God. The power to affect the outcome of prayer is in God, not in the person praying.

Miracles are not magic. Many people say that they are "praying for a miracle." A miracle is a purposeful intervention from God that is often a process and not an instant. "Praying for a miracle" does not relieve one of continuing personal responsibility, such as pursuing treatment or making difficult decisions. Miracles happen as part of God's order, not our magical wishes for situations to change. It is fine for people to pray for miracles as long as they also face the reality before them.

20. When should a chaplain be called?

Chaplains are frequently called for deaths, although religion and faith are not just about death. The goal of pastoral care is healing of the spirit, whether a person is living or dying. As nurses become acquainted with the hospital chaplain, they come to know how he or she approaches the nuances of a patient's concerns. Very often this is accomplished through an empathic relationship that encourages and allows patients to use their own inner resources to affect healing and strength.

Chaplains generally represent all denominations and faith traditions—Protestant, Catholic, Jewish, Hindu, Islam. Staff chaplains can assist the nurse in finding a representative from a particular faith. Chaplains are available for sacramental purposes such as baptism, communion, anointing, weddings, funerals, and confession. They are also available for pastoral purposes such as counseling, prayer, support, and assistance in decision-making. Although there are many times and reasons to call a chaplain, some of the most common are when the patient:

- uses religion as a source of support
- is withdrawn, depressed, restless, complaining, or irritable
- is anxious (notably preoperatively)
- worsens, becomes terminally ill, or dies
- expresses interest or curiosity about religious questions or issues
- reads scripture and other religious literature
- is struggling with loss or grieving
- exhibits spiritual distress
- has ethical dilemmas, decisions to make
- asks to see a chaplain, asks about worship services, desires a Bible
- has no visitors, cards, or flowers in room
- expresses a desire for sacraments

21. What does a chaplain do during a visit?

Chaplains respond to the presenting need (e.g., fear of dying, anxiety about procedures, grief over a diagnosis, hopelessness of ongoing treatment, need for prayer and reassurance, anger at God). One of the most valuable pastoral interventions is to offer an empathic relationship. This means entering into the world of the patient and listening to his or her experience, conflict, dilemma, or fear. Chaplains should not try to convert people unless requested to do so by the patient. Chaplains encourage a person's inner strengths. They assist persons in finding hope when they feel hopeless and help persons to recover or discover for the first time who they are in relationship with God. Because of the intimacy of the process of illness, dying, and death, many chaplains perform funerals and memorial services for patients who have died. Chaplains also assist in discussions about code status, requests for organ donation, and mortuary arrangements.

22. Are chaplains available to staff?

Most chaplains are available to staff members as well as patients and families. Oncologic nurses must take care of themselves, allow themselves to suffer with their patients, acknowledge their own pain and losses, and utilize supportive people around them. Chaplains are also available for support, clarification, encouragement, and hope. Chaplains may offer periodic memorial services for the staff to gain closure in regard to patient deaths.

23. What is a parish nurse?

A parish nurse is a registered nurse licensed to practice within the state whose practice setting is the congregation. The parish nurse is available to congregation members as a personal health counselor, health educator, resource referral agent, volunteer facilitator, and integrator of faith and health.

24. How can parish nurses and oncology nurses work together?

Parish nurses and oncology nurses can be resources to one another when they share the care of an oncology patient. The parish nurse can facilitate the use of community resources and support, including spiritual support, for oncology patients and their families. Oncology nurses can educate parish nurses on how to prepare patients, families, and congregational staff with what to expect in the oncology disease process. Oncology and parish nurses can work together as partners in providing health care to oncology patients along the continuum of care from the health-care institution to the community.

ACKNOWLEDGMENT

The author thanks Mary Jo Bay, RN, MSN, Pastoral Nurse/Health Ministry Consultant, Spiritual Care Department, Centura Health/Penrose–St. Francis Health Services, Colorado Springs, Colorado, for her contributions on parish nursing.

REFERENCES

1. Baumann A, Johnston N, Antai-Otong D: Decision Making in Psychiatric and Psychosocial Nursing. Philadelphia, B.C. Decker, 1990.
2. Bay MJ: Healing partners: The oncology nurse and the parish nurse. Semin Oncol Nurs 13:275–278, 1997.
3. Cassell E: The nature of suffering and the goals of medicine. N Engl J Med 306:639–645, 1982.
4. Gibbons J, Miller S: An image of contemporary hospital chaplaincy. J Pastor Care 43:355–361, 1989.
5. Highfield MEF, Taylor EJ, Amenta MD: Preparation to care: The spiritual care education of oncology and hospice nurses. J Hosp Palliat Nurs 2:53–63, 2000.
6. Joint Commission on the Accreditation of Healthcare Organizations: Automated Comprehensive Accreditation Manual for Hospitals: The Official Handbook. Oakbrook Terrace, IL, 1999.
7. Marty M, Vaux K (eds): Health/Medicine and the Faith Traditions: An Inquiry into Religion and Medicine. Philadelphia, Fortress Press, 1982.
8. Mitchell K: Spirituality and pastoral care. J Pastor Care 43:93–95, 1989.
9. Murray R, Zentner J: Spiritual and Religious Influence on the Person. Nursing Assessment and Health Promotion Strategies Through the Life Span. New Jersey, Prentice-Hall, 1989.
10. Puchalski CM: Taking a spiritual history: FICA. Spirituality and Medicine Connection 3:1, 1999.
11. Sheldon JE: Spirituality as a part of nursing. J Hosp Palliat Nurs 2:101–108, 2000.
12. Taylor EJ, Amenta M, Highfield M: Spiritual care practices of oncology nurses. Oncol Nurs Forum 22:31–39, 1995.

63. FAMILY AND CAREGIVER ISSUES

Karen J. Stanley, RN, MSN, AOCN

A diagnosis of cancer is analogous to the ripples of a stone thrown into still waters. The person diagnosed with cancer is certainly affected, but so, too, are those in the patient's constellation of family, friends, and significant others. In fact, this constellation becomes the focus of professional caregiving. An ability to promote healthy interaction among family, friends, and significant others serves the patient well.

1. Describe the typical family response to a diagnosis of cancer.

There is no typical response from patients and families. Shock, anger, fear, denial, disbelief, generalized anxiety, and feelings of helplessness and vulnerability are common initial responses to what is perceived as a life-threatening diagnosis. Communication among the patient and significant others, healthcare team, and well-meaning friends who relate similar personal or second-hand experiences contribute to the initial and ongoing intellectual and emotional responses. Some people become frozen and withdrawn in response to tremendous fear and anxiety, whereas others respond by seeking as much information as possible from the healthcare team and external sources. It is also quite common for both patients and families to search for some kind of existential meaning to the experience in an attempt to explain in an orderly way why the cancer has occurred.

2. How do you deal with a patient or family who denies or refuses to discuss the diagnosis and its implications?

Professional ethical standards demand both truth-telling and nonmaleficence (the concept of doing no harm). These two ethical constructs may seem to be mutually exclusive in attempting to move the patient and family beyond initial reactions of denial and/or withdrawal. Denial can be healthy for a certain period because it provides a "buffer zone" or respite for the patient and significant others to absorb the reality of the diagnosis and its implications. Confronting the patient, family, and friends with the raw truth when they are not prepared to integrate that information can be harmful in many ways. Mistrust and anger can result, and the chance for an ongoing therapeutic relationship may be permanently destroyed. The professional must use prior experience, intuitiveness, kindness, and a focused approach on the ultimate goal, which is to allow the patient and significant others to hear appropriate information as they are able to tolerate its implications.

3. How can you facilitate communication about the diagnosis and its implications between the patient and family/significant others?

It may not always be possible to facilitate healthy communication between the patient and other people, but responsible health care professionals should encourage an atmosphere of open and honest communication when culturally appropriate. It may be helpful to remind family and friends that refusing to discuss the illness and its implications can isolate the patient and increase anxiety, fear, and sadness. When patients tell professional caregivers that their families will not allow discussion of the issues despite repeated requests, the healthcare team must make every effort to ease the way for family and friends to participate in what the patient views as an essential dialogue. A frank but private discussion with family and friends about the patient's need to take care of unfinished business may be helpful. It is also appropriate to encourage family members and friends to "practice" difficult discussions with each other and with healthcare professionals. Family and friends may be encouraged by reminders that their personal grieving and bereavement may be positively enhanced by the knowledge that they were able to have meaningful conversations with the patient over the illness continuum. Families require encouragement, support, suggestions, and permission to try and fail without fear of censure.

4. What other communication techniques are possible when conversation is difficult?

Family and friends may find that they are unable to consistently participate in what may be viewed as highly intimate and frightening conversations. They can be encouraged to communicate by touch, by providing gifts of comfort (e.g., a particularly loved book or video, a comforting story, a photo album or scrapbook), or just by remaining present when the patient is frightened or lonely.

5. How can a healthcare professional balance appropriate and effective communication with a patient's need for and right to control the flow of information?

Multiple issues are involved in the patient's right to control how, when, and to whom information is conveyed. Privacy may be a priority for the patient who requests that others not be told of the diagnosis, prognosis, or treatment plan without permission. In such instances, healthcare providers must refer family and friends to the patient when questions are asked. Of equal importance are circumstances in which family members request that patients not be told of their diagnosis for fear that they will become depressed or lose hope. It is *not* appropriate for a healthcare professional to promise a family member or friend that the patient will not be told the circumstances of the illness. The health care provider has an ongoing responsibility to confirm repeatedly with the patient the amount of information that the patient requires. Patients may delegate a family member or friend to receive the information and make decisions for them. When patients ask for information, it is always appropriate to explore exactly what they would like to know and respond accordingly.

6. Do families cope with the stressors of the illness in similar ways?

A family's ability to deal with the unexpected stressors of a cancer diagnosis is predicated on various factors: educational background, cultural expectations and norms, communication techniques, established coping mechanisms, family dynamics (including dysfunctional behaviors), prior history and/or experience with life-threatening illness, and confidence in the ability to be an effective caregiver. Each family employs a set of behavioral norms that may not be verbalized or readily apparent but are nevertheless operative. The health care provider must learn the family's behavioral norms to communicate and intervene effectively. Healthy families may use humor, good communication techniques, and willingness to be flexible to deal with unexpected happenings, but the healthcare provider may need to coach families who do not have such skills. It may be necessary to diffuse tension, to assist the patient and family in conversational techniques, and, above all, to ensure that the patient's needs in the greater family circle are prioritized and met.

7. What are the warning signs that families may require assistance in coping with the stressors of the patient's illness?

Many families are not emotionally prepared to respond in a supportive way. Although it may seem reasonable that the patient with cancer should be the primary focus of the healthcare team, it is impossible to separate the constellation of family and significant others involved in the patient's life and care. They become integrated into the concept of "patient" because they have many of the same fears, anxieties, and difficulties in coping with the stressors of the illness, and their concerns, if not attended to, can negatively affect the primary patient. Some warning signs:

- Persistent anger, hostility, resentment, or denial
- Conflict between the patient and caregiver(s)
- Missed healthcare appointments when the patient is dependent on others
- Caregiver illness or health problems
- Decreased patient self-care abilities accompanied by increasing caregiver responsibilities
- Signs of caregiver burden (e.g., weariness, depression, physical complaints)
- Inadequate or inappropriate caregiving: increasing inability to manage the caregiving regimen, inability to use necessary equipment (e.g., ambulatory infusion pumps, patient-controlled analgesia devices, oxygen tanks and tubing, special air mattresses), inappropriate administration of medications, forgetfulness, poor patient hygiene, signs of physical abuse or neglect
- Inadequate number of caregivers in relationship to the care required
- Detachment or withdrawal at diagnosis, during illness progression, or at the terminal phase of illness

8. Identify issues and stressors that can emerge in significant relationships after a diagnosis of cancer.
- Weeks and/or months of disruption and emotional upheaval throughout the treatment process
- Restructuring of family roles and responsibilities
- Exacerbation of preexistent dysfunctional relationships
- Overprotectiveness of parents, spouses, or children
- Overidentification and intensification of feelings by siblings
- Distancing of significant family members and friends by others in the constellation
- Resentment of new responsibilities or anger that the burden may not be equally shared by family members and friends

9. How may families be helped to adapt to the rigors of the diagnosis and caregiving?
- Practice of family-centered care
- Emotional support: acknowledgement of the difficulties engendered by the cancer diagnosis accompanied by offers to listen, to assist with problems, and to be available
- Acknowledgment of actual and potential losses
- Communication of realistic hopes and goals
- Informed and honest discussions about treatment options and expected side effects, the right to solicit a second opinion, effective ways to communicate with other members of the healthcare team, consistent feedback on the patient's response to treatment and pending diagnostic assays, clarification of misinformation or misunderstanding of previous discussions about the patient's health, and/or a review of options in unexpected circumstances (e.g. recurrence of disease)
- Detailed instruction (both written and verbal) about medical appointments, management of side effects of the illness and treatment regimen, medication administration, use of infusion devices or other equipment
- Informed description of what to expect both physiologically and psychologically
- Encouragement of the patient to articulate healthcare choices and prepare an advance healthcare directive, if needed
- Assistance in redefining roles and organization of additional responsibilities
- Referral to outside resources when necessary and/or possible
- Consistent attention to family members who otherwise may be neglected as the patient's needs become the center of attention
- Keeping other friends and family members informed
- Offer to hold family conferences when necessary (e.g., conflict arises, patient and family require support to discuss a difficult issue, a new family member arrives on the scene)
- Review of financial and legal issues that may require outside assistance

10. What basic, essential tenets should caregivers know?
The National Family Caregivers Association recommends "four messages to live by":
1. Choose to take charge of your life. Do *not* let your loved one's illness or disability always take center stage.
2. Honor, value, and love yourself. Self-care is not a luxury; it is a necessity and your right as a human being.
3. Seek, accept, and at times demand help.
4. Stand up and be counted. Stand up for your rights as a caregiver and a citizen.

11. How can families be assisted to extend their informal support network?
It is easier to solidify relationships with and ask help from people whom one already knows. Emotional energy, often a scarce resource at this time, is required to make new friends. Most old friends genuinely want to offer assistance but may not know how to do so. Requests for help are usually welcome and well-received. Families often need significant encouragement to ask for

help. It is useful to assist family members to draw up lists of tasks that can be delegated to others. It may be helpful to ask a close family friend to coordinate requests for help and relieve the family of both the emotional and physical burdens of acknowledging need. Community agencies may be able to offer assistance such as Meals on Wheels or varied programs sponsored by the American Cancer Society or other cancer support organizations. Faith communities can be welcome sources of much needed help.

12. What formal resources are available for caregivers?

1. The **National Family Caregivers Association** (NFCA) is a membership organization promoting self-advocacy and self-care for people caring for a family member. They can be contacted at 10400 Connecticut Avenue #500, Kensington, MD 20895 (800-896-3650). Their website at www.nfcacares.org has an extensive section on caregiving tips.

2. The **Cancer Survival Toolbox**, jointly developed by the National Coalition for Cancer Survivorship, the Oncology Nursing Society, and the Association of Oncology Social Work, contains a free set of audiotapes that focus on issues such as communication, decision-making, finding ways to pay for care, and topics for older people. The tapes may be ordered by calling 877-TOOLS-4-U or visiting the Oncology Nursing Society website at www.ons.org

3. **Strength for Caring**, developed at the University of Pennsylvania, Philadelphia, focuses on caregiver confidence and competence and validates the importance of the role of the caregiver. The four main sections are (1) What is Cancer?; (2) Cancer and the Family; (3) The Role of the Caregiver; and (4) The Caregiver's Role in Symptom Management. Ortho-Biotech recently began to fund this project. The Oncology Nursing Society Education Department may be contacted for local resources (412-921-7373).

4. The website **www.caregivers.com** is spiritually focused. Its intent is to provide spiritual and emotional support for all caregivers. The site offers a free newsletter that touches on many of the emotional issues that caregivers experience.

5. The **Rosalynn Carter Institute** at Georgia Southwestern State University recently launched the Caregivers Corner website (www.rci.gsw.edu/corner/). The site hosts an active online support group on Mondays at 9 P.M. EST.

13. How may nurses ease the transition for patients and families from active treatment to palliative care?

If the healthcare provider and patient/family constellation have consistently discussed the illness, response to treatment, and disease progression, the transition from active care to comfort care may be easier. One should not minimize this transition in any way, and communication should focus on the changing goals of care, not an abandonment of care. This transition may require several conversations as hopes are readjusted and expectations clarified. Decisions that have life and death implications for patients and families should not be made in isolation. The nurse may need to provide assistance by outlining options and explaining the consequences of various choices. Patients and families need to hear repeatedly that they will not be abandoned, that attention to symptom management will be meticulous and professional, that the healthcare team is committed to maximizing the patient's quality of life, and that all involved in care are privileged to participate. Most importantly, the healthcare provider must listen and learn.

14. What have patients identified as important contributors to quality end-of-life care?

Patients have singled out the following issues: adequate pain and symptom management, no inappropriate prolongation of dying, promoting a sense of control, relieving the burden on families and caregivers, and strengthening relationships with loved ones.

15. How do these concerns affect family and friends?

These important concerns, if known to family and friends, may be addressed along the continuum of illness. Patients and families should be empowered to ask for and receive adequate pain and symptom management when the need arises. Families should be encouraged to have frank discussions with the patient about desired healthcare interventions over the illness contin-uum, most particularly at the end of life. These discussions should clarify how much control the patient chooses to have over personal circumstances and whether the patient chooses to relinquish control to another family member or friend at any point during the illness. Families should be en-couraged to explore at length and on repeated occasions the patient's perception of burden to the caregivers. This particular concern may be monumental to the patient, and planned interventions to provide respite or relief to family and friends may provide as much, if not more, comfort to pa-tients than to caregivers. Many people are distinctly uncomfortable at the prospect of being depen-dent on others; they deserve the opportunity to discuss and remedy the problem, inasmuch as it is possible. Lastly, strengthening relationships with loved ones is important at all times. Many pa-tients, when faced with a diagnosis of cancer, regard the time remaining to them as a gift, a time in which to make amends, to enjoy precious time with family and friends, to do what is most mean-ingful to them, and to live every day to the fullest. If the people nearest the patient share and/or un-derstand this outlook, the potential for the richest life possible can be realized.

16. What can be done to help the family of a terminally ill patient?
- Encourage difficult questions and/or seek out unasked questions.
- Validate the amount of information desired.
- Respect individual expressions of grief as distinct and worthwhile.
- Encourage active storytelling from patients and family members as a way of dealing with loss and honoring the life that has been lived.
- Explore previous family member's experiences with terminal illness and their remem-brances of the circumstances.
- Provide open and ongoing communication about how pain and other symptoms will be managed, reassuring the family that everything possible will be done to avoid suffering.
- Assist other members of the healthcare team in speaking honestly with each other and with the patient and family.
- Encourage communication with the patient's religious or spiritual community, if appropriate
- Assist in the translation of what is heard, seen, and experienced.
- Encourage family members and friends to discuss what the future will be like after the pa-tient has died; allow fears, resentments, and unspoken feelings to emerge.
- Consistently reinforce nonabandonment and the privilege of participating in the process.

REFERENCES

1. Beckwith S: Creating a team approach to care: Professionals and caregivers. Last Acts Fall:6–9, 2000.
2. Gorman LM: The psychosocial impact of cancer on the individual, family and society. In Carrol-Johnson RM, Gorman LM, Bush NJ: Psychosocial Nursing Care Along the Cancer Continuum. Pittsburgh, Oncology Nursing Press, 1998, pp 3–25.
3. Gomez E: Family caregivers can find resources, support on the internet. ONS News 15(11):7, 2000.
4. Goselin TK: Family caregivers need nurse support. ONS News 15(11):1, 4–5, 2000.
5. Ingebrigtsen P, Wallio Smith M: Family issues. In Gates RA, Fink RM: Oncology Nursing Secrets. Philadelphia, Hanley & Belfus, 1997, pp 459–462.
6. Singer PA, Martin DJ, Kelner M: Quality end-of-life care: Patients' perspectives. JAMA 281:163–168, 1999.
7. Stanley KJ: Silence is not golden: Conversations with the dying. Clin J Oncol Nurs 4:34–40, 2000.

64. SURVIVORSHIP

Susan A. Leigh, BSN, RN, *and* Debra Thaler-DeMers, BSN, RN, OCN, PHN

> From the time of its discovery and for the balance of life, an individual diagnosed with
> cancer is a survivor. *F. Mullan*

1. Why should nurses who care for patients in a hospital or clinic be interested in cancer survivors?

Historically, a diagnosis of cancer has elicited feelings of fear, dread, terror, doom, mutilation—words that describe the underlying notion that the person surely will die of the disease. This myth about cancer can psychologically paralyze the person who receives the diagnosis; it can also evoke negative reactions from nurses and other caregivers. Negative reactions from nurses can decrease the sense of hopefulness and future orientation that is vitally necessary during the early stages of survival. The knowledge that people survive different types of cancer— many are actually cured, and others live for long periods with cancer as a chronic illness—helps nurses to introduce the potential for survival, to decrease the sense of helplessness, and to transform a passive acceptance of fate into a proactive sense of control. Thus quality of life is improved for both survivor and caregiver.

2. How long after diagnosis is a patient considered to be a survivor?

The traditional medical definition is 5 years after the diagnosis of cancer. The National Coalition for Cancer Survivorship (NCCS), which was founded in 1986, has crafted a definition that focuses on the qualitative aspects of survival: "From the time of its discovery, and for the balance of life, an individual diagnosed with cancer is a survivor."

3. What does cancer survivorship mean?

Cancer survivorship is a process rather than a fixed point in time. It is *how* we survive the experience of living with cancer, adapting to it as a part of the life process and incorporating it into the broader perspective of overall life experiences. Many survivors have provided valuable insight into the experience of living with cancer by writing about the impact of cancer on their lives. Such books and stories indicate that the experience of living with cancer can have profound positive repercussions. Newly diagnosed cancer survivors, as well as nurses and physicians who care for them, must understand the importance of quality of life.

4. How many cancer survivors are there in the United States?

The most recent estimate is that approximately 8.4 million people in the United States have histories of cancer. About half are long-term survivors (5 or more years). Taking into consideration all types of cancer, the relative 5-year survival rate (the ratio of observed survival rate for survivors vs. the expected survival rate of the general population) has reached 51%, according to the latest American Cancer Society Facts and Figures. Although this percentage is much higher for some and much lower for others, depending on the specific type and stage of cancer, it means that approximately one-half the number of people diagnosed with cancer today will be long-term survivors.

To put these statistics in perspective, consider the fact that the number of cancer survivors in the United States has more than tripled over a 10-year period. With recent advances in the early detection of cancer , the development of supportive therapies, and genetic studies that have identified specific cancer-causing genes, the number of cancer survivors is expected to continue its rapid growth.

5. Do cancer survivors go through discernible stages?

Yes. The two obvious stages are B.C. (before cancer) and A.D. (after diagnosis). Each survivor has different issues to deal with, depending on life circumstances B.C. The stages of coping with death, as first described by Elisabeth Kubler-Ross, can be applied to almost any situation involving loss, including cancer survival. In addition, the continuum of cancer survivorship has been described by Mullan in terms of the seasons of survival: acute, extended, and permanent.

6. What are the stages described by Kubler-Ross?

Shock, anger, denial, bargaining, and acceptance. Nurses should keep in mind that no one progresses through these stages in the same way. A person may move back and forth between stages or may not experience one or more of the stages at all. As with any model, the stages act essentially as guidelines.

7. Summarize the acute stage of survival as described by Mullan.

Acute survival begins with the diagnosis of cancer. During this period the survivor's life is dominated by the illness. The focus is on medical treatment, whether it be surgery, radiation, chemotherapy, or biotherapy. Survivors may be feeling sick and considering their mortality. It is also a time when the survivor has more access to support services. Physicians, nurses, social workers, and many community resources are available through the hospital, clinic, physician's office. or local cancer agencies to assist the survivor and family members in dealing with the immediate needs surrounding the cancer diagnosis and treatment.

8. Summarize the extended stage.

During the season of extended survival, the survivor enters remission or discontinues routine treatment, making a transition from life as a patient to reintegration into everyday activities. The focus shifts from the medical environment to the community. Survivors may return to work, school, or the responsibility of managing a household. Support is crucial during this transition time. Nurses are encouraged to be available as a source of information, reassurance, and support. Survivors may benefit from referral to community support groups or resource centers, legal services, or professional counseling services. An increasing number of national organizations offer a wide variety of services specific to different types of cancer, such as breast, ovarian, prostate, brain, or lung cancers as well as leukemia, lymphoma, and myeloma.

9. Summarize the permanent stage.

The season of permanent survival is equated with the word "cure"; cancer is no longer a major focus of the survivor's life. During this extended remission, the cancer experience is integrated into the broader experience of the survivor's entire life. Cancer survivors must remain in contact with the medical community. Long-term follow-up of survivors, with at least annual examination, is important for screening for long-term and late effects of cancer treatment. Legal, economic, and insurance issues may arise or continue to be a problem. Referral to appropriate resources may be helpful, but fewer programs or agencies focus on long-term survivors. The NCCS has advocated for continued attention to this population since 1986. The National Cancer Institute (NCI) created the Office of Cancer Survivorship to help address survivorship-related issues.

10. What issues are of primary importance in the acute stage of survival?

During the acute stage of survival, patients focus on issues pertaining to treatment options, such as gathering information about the disease process, methods of treatment (surgery, radiation, chemotherapy, brachytherapy, bone marrow transplant, stem cell procedures, biotherapy), and survival statistics related to their particular type of cancer. Nurses must assist survivors in communicating their needs to the health care team. Survivors are entering the environment of the medical community where a foreign language is spoken — "medicalese." It is a language filled with abbreviations (CBC, CT, MRI, ABVD, HCT) and words that may be unfamiliar to the survivor. The problem becomes more difficult if the survivor's primary language is not English. A survivor may not know what questions to ask, particularly during the initial consultation with the oncologist. Excellent resources are available through national advocacy organizations and the NCI to assist survivors during the acute stage. In addition, support groups benefit many survivors by introducing those who are newly diagnosed to those who are cancer "veterans."

11. What can nurses do to help survivors make informed decisions about treatment during the acute stage of survival?

A newly diagnosed survivor is faced with gathering information quickly to make critical life-altering decisions and receives a great deal of information during a time when the ability to concentrate may be impaired. During this confusion, nurses can help survivors make informed decisions about treatment. Because people learn in various ways — through visual or auditory input or through a written format—nurses can use various teaching methods to convey information. Videotapes, written information, audiotapes, pictures, and verbal communication can be used to share important information with survivors and significant others.

12. List helpful hints for communicating information to cancer survivors.

1. Repeat information numerous times; less than 50% of what is conveyed is usually retained by the survivor.

2. Use a variety of settings and contexts, both to reinforce the information and to elicit questions from the survivor.

3. Encourage survivors to bring a family member or friend to consultations and conferences to take notes and help recall information.

4. Assess the survivor's ability to read and understand the language of printed material.

5. Encourage survivors to keep a journal or log of their experiences, questions, and concerns. The journal can be kept at the bedside so that if questions or concerns arise during the night, the survivor can write them down and deal with them at a later time.

6. Suggest using a tape recorder. Teaching sessions, consultations, and conferences with survivors and/or caregivers can be recorded. If questions arise later when the survivor returns home, the recorded information can be used as a reference. The question may have been answered during the conference, and listening to the tape saves additional phone calls to the physician's office. In addition, family members who may not have been able to attend the conference can hear the information. The tape becomes a resource for both survivors and families.

13. What is Cancer Survival Toolbox ©?

An excellent new resource that can be offered to the entire family is *Cancer Survival Toolbox ©: Building Skills That Work for You*. This free set of audio programs was developed jointly by the Oncology Nursing Society, the Association of Oncology Social Work, and the NCCS. It was funded by Genentech BioOncology and is available free of charge by calling 877-NCCS-YES or ordering through the NCCS website at www.cansearch.org.

14. Who else is available to help the multidisciplinary health care team deliver support, information, resources, and treatment?

It is helpful to have the survivor's insurance company assign a case manager. The case manager's name and office number should be available to both the treatment team and the survivor. Ideally, the insurance company also should provide a way to reach the case manager outside normal business hours. Family, friends, and community support groups can provide support and help the survivor to gather and process information.

15. What problems or barriers may cause survivors to discontinue treatment?

Treatment for cancer is difficult and takes its toll in many different ways. Any number of problems—physical, psychological, social, financial, cultural—can prompt survivors to interrupt or stop therapy.

Problems Prompting Discontinuation of Therapy

Physical
Uncontrollable or unacceptable acute effects (e.g., nausea and vomiting, fatigue, pain)
Chronic or long-term effects of treatment (e.g., peripheral neuropathy)
Inability to concentrate or think clearly
Increasing disability or dependence

Table continued on following page

Problems Prompting Discontinuation of Therapy (Continued)

Psychological
    Fear of disfigurement (e.g., scarring, hair loss)
    Fear of permanent disability, including impotence
    Fear of late effects (e.g., infertility, second malignancies)
    Decreased quality of life
Social
    Lack of transportation
    Fear of losing job
    Inadequate or unaffordable child care
    Insufficient support with family responsibilities
    Decreased social interactions (e.g., dating, marriage)
Financial
    Unable to miss work or survive on reduced paycheck
    Un- or underinsured
    Unaffordable out-of-pocket expenses
    Ineligible for government assistance (e.g., Medicaid, Medicare, Social Security Disability)
Cultural
    Language barriers
    Lack of understanding
    Erroneous information or belief in myths
    Conflicting attitudes, beliefs, and values

16. What resources are available to assist survivors and families with problems and barriers?
    After specific problems or barriers are identified, nurses must find the appropriate resources to help deal with them. Consultations with other professionals within the hospital or community may involve specially trained nurses, attending physicians, social workers and social services, translators, psychologists, chaplains, legal assistance, and financial and government consultants. Other resources include written publications, cancer-related videos, educational programs, on-line services (Internet), and support groups. Local cancer organizations also may be accessed, (e.g., Leukemia and Lymphoma Society, American Cancer Society, Wellness Communities). The important point is to be aware of available resources.

Selected National Resources for Cancer Survivors

National Cancer Institute (NCI)
    Cancer Information Service (CIS)   800-4-CANCER
    Physician Data Query (PDQ)   800-4-CANCER
    CANCERFAX   301-402-5874
    Website   www.cancer.gov
National Coalition for Cancer Survivorship (NCCS)
    General Information   877-NCCS-YES
    Website: www.cansearch.org
Candlelighters Childhood Cancer Foundation
    General Information   800-366-2223
    Local (Washington, DC)   301-657-8401
    Website   www.candlelighters.org
American Cancer Society (ACS)
    General Information   800-ACS-2345
    Website   www.cancer.org
Leukemia and Lymphoma Society of America
    Educational Materials   800-955-4LSA
    General Information   212-573-8484
    Website   www.leukemia.org

Table continued on following page

Selected National Resources for Cancer Survivors (Continued)

Cancer Care, Inc.	
General Information	800-813-HOPE
Local (New York)	212-302-2400
Website	www.cancercare.org
Y-ME National Breast Cancer Organization	
General Information	800-221-2141
24-hour Hotline	312-986-8228
Website	www.y-me.org
US TOO International, Inc (prostate cancer)	
General Information	800-808-7866
Local (Hinsdale, IL)	708-323-1002
Website	www.ustoo.com
National Brain Tumor Foundation	
General Information	800-934-CURE
Local	415-284-0208
Website	www.braintumor.org
National Alliance of Breast Cancer Organizations (NABCO)	
General Information	800-719-9154
Website	www.nabco.org
National Ovarian Cancer Coalition (NOCC)	
General Information	888-OVARIAN
Website	www.ovarian.org

Note: Many websites link to additional resources.

17. What issues are specific to adolescent survivors and young adults?

Issues important to younger cancer survivors include fertility, cognitive deficiencies, and growth problems. Chemotherapy protocols that may preserve fertility should be used whenever possible, and young men should be encouraged to bank sperm before treatment.

Therapy involving the brain or central nervous system of a child should minimize cognitive problems after treatment. Such children may need long-term follow-up, which includes assessment for learning disabilities, memory deficit, distractability, and decreased verbal ability and IQ scores. If children are treated before puberty, they should receive long-term follow-up with specialists who can address potential growth problems.

18. Are treatment options less toxic to the reproductive system available for younger survivors?

In some types of cancer, such as Hodgkin's disease, it is possible to shield the reproductive tissue from direct radiation. Oophoropexy, a procedure in which the ovaries are surgically placed midline in front of or behind the uterus, reduces ovarian exposure in women receiving pelvic irradiation. Testicular shields can reduce testicular exposure to < 10% of the prescribed dose. When a male patient undergoes retroperitoneal lymph node dissection, nerve-sparing techniques should be used to preserve fertility. When nerve damage occurs, techniques such as electroejaculation and sperm banking can be used to preserve fertility options for the future. Furthermore, in female patients with Hodgkin's disease, ovarian suppression during therapy, cyclic estrogen replacement, and alternative chemotherapy protocols have been used to preserve fertility. Infertility in a significant number of long-term survivors has been caused by the MOPP (Mustargen [nitrogen mustard], Oncovin {vincristine], procarbazine, prednisone) protocol. Use of the ABVD (Adriamycin [doxorubicin], bleomycin, vinblastine, dacarbazine) protocol has proved to be less toxic to ovarian function and equally effective in inducing long-term remissions. Long-term follow-up of young survivors is important to identify late physiologic effects or psychosocial problems. Continued research to develop effective and less toxic treatment protocols is an essential component of cancer treatment.

19. As the initial phase of treatment is completed, the extended stage of survival begins. Does life automatically return to normal?

Anticipating the end of treatment provokes an array of mixed emotions. Ambiguity defines this stage as survivors experience a mixture of joy and fear, relief and anxiety, security and uncertainty. Although no longer a patient, the survivor is not entirely healthy and tries to balance both physical and emotional recovery. This stage encompasses learning to live with the fear of recurrence, uncertainty about the future, and loss of treatment-based support systems. The survivor also must learn to assess and trust his or her body again and to resume prior family and social roles and relationships. Often this period is characterized by a feeling of being in limbo. The sense of "normal" has changed; it will never be the same as before the cancer. A "new normal" specific to the suvivor must be created gradually. This process takes time; it will not happen overnight. For many survivors, the "new normal" is actually better than the original.

20. How can nurses prepare survivors for potential problems once therapy is completed?

Knowledge helps to decrease fear of the unknown. As survivors complete treatment, an individualized exit interview assists with the transition into life after therapy. Components of the interview may include information about medical follow-up appointments with specific diagnostic tests; possible late effects from therapy; symptoms that require attention or symptoms that may be expected; cancer prevention, health promotion, and wellness education; referrals for physical, psychological, and social rehabilitation; support networks, educational programs, and survivor publications; and continued access to specific members of the health care team.

21. When does permanent or long-term survival begin?

The long-term stage of survival begins at different times for different people. Much depends on the type and extent of the original disease and the risk for recurrence. Although no specific time frame or event defines this stage, freedom from disease for 2 or more years begins to yield a certain level of trust, and a sense of comfort gradually returns. This stage may be labeled sustained remission or possibly cure, although the definition of cure is controversial (see question 23). Some survivors can breathe a little easier after 2 years, such as those who are diagnosed with testicular cancer or Hodgkin's disease. Others who have non-Hodgkin's lymphoma or ovarian cancer may need 5 or more years to feel out of the woods. Survivors of breast cancer are watched closely for recurrence for 10 years or more. All of these numbers are arbitrary and act only as guidelines for increased vigilance; they are not meant to hinder survivors from living life to the fullest.

22. What problems are associated with long-term survival?

A lack of guidelines to optimize disease-free survival continues to be a major problem for long-term survivors. Although many survivors have no physical evidence of disease and appear fully recovered, the life-threatening experience of having had cancer takes its toll in many ways. Physically, the survivor is at risk for other malignancies and organ system failures; psychologically, the survivor must live with the constant fear of recurrence; socially, the survivor frequently encounters employment and insurance discrimination; and spiritually, survivors struggle with the meaning of life and the identification of new goals and priorities. Although survivors are often praised for overcoming adversity, identification of real problems can be hampered as they are reminded how lucky they are to be alive. In this age of managed care and cost-containment, long-term survivors need continued access to appropriate specialists and guidelines for systematic follow-up.

23. Is there any guarantee of "cure" for survivors who remain disease-free for 5 years?

The concept of cure implies successful treatment of disease or restoration to health. Surely cure is the ultimate hope for anyone treated for cancer. Yet no one can say for sure that a disease as ruthless and secretive as cancer will never return; thus, guarantees are not realistic. Probabilities for cure can be estimated and are available in the American Cancer Society's annual publication, *Cancer Facts and Figures*. The 1960s and 1970s brought a new sense of hopefulness to researchers and clinicians who treated people with cancer. With the development of potentially curative therapies, specialists carefully followed their patients for signs of disease recurrence.

Many believed that patients who are disease-free for 5 years have a greatly increased chance of cure and a normal lifespan. Many patients "walked on egg shells" or "held their breath," anxiously waiting to reach the magic 5-year landmark. They were not considered survivors until they reached this point. Unfortunately, many survivors have recurrent disease even after 5 years, or they are diagnosed with other cancers. Because there are multiple types of cancers with different stages of disease, a wide variety of treatment options, and circumstances unique to each survivor, it is literally impossible to guarantee cure.

24. Do survivors face employment discrimination due to their history of cancer?

Approximately 25% of people with histories of cancer experience some type of employment discrimination. Examples include not being hired for a particular job, being selected for a company lay-off, being demoted or having duties cut back, or being denied a promotion or increase in salary. Some employers believe that cancer survivors are less productive and use more sick days than other employees. Studies have not supported this belief. In fact, studies have shown that survivors use fewer sick days and tend to be more productive than other workers, often because they are fearful of losing their job if they appear to be sick.

25. What problems do survivors face in terms of health insurance?

Cancer survivors also experience "job lock"; that is, they feel unable to apply for a change in employment because of fear of losing health insurance benefits attached to their current employment. Survivors also may feel that they cannot accept employment from a company that does not provide adequate health insurance benefits. For this reason, they may accept employment in a position where they are overqualified to obtain needed health insurance. Recently enacted federal legislation allows cancer survivors to obtain health insurance when they change jobs without having to endure a long waiting period, but there are no restrictions on the cost of such coverage.

Insurance companies also tend to give survivors a higher rating designation in setting insurance premiums. The higher rate applies to both health and life insurance. Some life insurance carriers will not insure cancer survivors until they have been disease-free for 5 years or more. Others charge very high premiums. Cancer survivors should be encouraged to check with a number of insurance providers before agreeing to a premium amount. A financial planner may be able to present options other than life insurance that will serve the same purpose for survivors and their families.

Another situation finds survivors dependent upon their spouse for health insurance benefits. In most states, the survivor is no longer able to obtain insurance benefits from their former partner once a divorce takes place. Survivors may feel themselves locked into a marriage because of the need for insurance coverage. Along with an insurance consultant, an attorney specializing in family law may provide the survivor with options for obtaining individual or group insurance. Organizations such as university alumni associations, American Association of Retired People, professional associations, fraternal organizations, and other special interest groups may provide insurance to members at group rates.

26. How long should cancer survivors be followed by an oncologist after termination of treatment?

The "how long" question is of major concern in the changing health care delivery system. Before managed care and cost containment, long-term follow-up was left to the discretion of the oncologist and survivor. Many oncologists wanted an ongoing relationship with people whom they had treated, even if it was once a year. Furthermore, many survivors felt bonded to the specialists who had helped them overcome a life-threatening disease. The establishment of trust over the years made the yearly follow-up exam easier to bear, and many oncologists still believe that they know best how to assess survivors for potential treatment-related problems.

The current system of managed care and cost containment has changed this once sacred, ongoing relationship by decreasing both utilization of services and referrals to specialists. Oncologists now are more inclined to see the survivor for a limited number of years after therapy, as prescribed by the individual plan. They then refer the survivor to the primary care provider—a family practitioner or internist—for long-term follow-up.

Because little systematic long-term follow-up has been done in adult cancer survivors, there are no guidelines for continued care. Researchers and clinicians in oncology must develop standards of care that can be shared with the generalist physicians who see and assess survivors. Survivors are best served through cooperation among oncologists, primary care providers, and other specialists; education of primary care providers about the special needs of this expanding population; and timely referrals to the appropriate specialist when complicated or unusual problems arise.

27. What are the physical aftereffects of cancer therapy?

Even as we celebrate successful therapy, we must be cognizant of long-term and late effects of treatment or disease. Surgery, radiation therapy, chemotherapy, biotherapy, or combinations of therapy may cause chronic or delayed problems that impede full recovery from the original diagnosis. These problems or effects fall into three categories: system-specific, cancer-related, and general related problems:

System-specific problems

Organ damage or failure	Reproductive problems, cardiomyopathy, thyroid dysfunction, pulmonary fibrosis
Premature aging	Cataracts, muscle atrophy
Compromised immune system	Increased infections

Cancer-related problems

Increased risk of recurrence	Primary malignancy
Increased risk of other malignancy	Related to primary cancer (e.g., breast cancer after ovarian cancer)
	Related to therapy (e.g., breast cancer after Hodgkin's disease)

General related problems

Functional changes	Lymphedema, pain syndromes, fatigue
Cosmetic changes	Amputations, ostomies, scars
Chronic illness	Osteoporosis, arthritis

Although physical aftereffects do not preclude the necessity of the original therapy, they validate the need for research into long-term and late effects, improvements in therapy, continued medical surveillance, and survivor education.

28. How can survivors optimize their healthcare follow-up?

The era of personal responsibility has arrived. Consumers of health care can no longer stand by passively and allow others to make unilateral decisions about cancer care and follow-up. Cancer survivors must learn to make informed choices, to understand treatment options, and to request changes or alternatives when their needs are not met. To ensure optimal long-term follow-up care, survivors are encouraged to do the following:

1. Keep all medical records, including types and doses of chemotherapy, sites, and amounts of radiation.

2. Develop a personalized health maintenance plan with oncology caregivers that covers time frames of check-ups, specific diagnostic tests, rehabilitation practices, and healthy behavioral modifications.

3. Carefully study and select, if possible, health insurance plans that offer flexibility and choice.

4. If warranted, negotiate a price for an annual follow-up visit outside the insurance plan, and pay out of pocket if the rate is affordable. Survivors must decide for themselves whether this added expense is worth the peace of mind that it may bring.

5. Learn to identify and communicate needs, and obtain assertiveness training if necessary.

6. Know individual rights as a health care consumer and how to take appropriate legal action if warranted.

7. Advocate insurance reform and standardized guidelines.

REFERENCES

1. Cancer Facts and Figures. Atlanta, GA, American Cancer Society, 2000.
2. Clark EJ, Stovall EL, Leigh S, et al: Imperatives for Quality Cancer Care: Access, Advocacy, Action, and Accountability. Silver Spring, MD, National Coalition for Cancer Survivorship, 1996.
3. Clark EJ: You Have the Right to be Hopeful. Silver Spring, MD, National Coalition for Cancer Survivorship, 1996.
4. Hoffman B: Working It Out: Your Employment Rights As a Cancer Survivor. Silver Spring, MD, National Coalition for Cancer Survivorship, 1999.
5. Keene N, Hobbie WL, Ruccione KS: Childhood Cancer Survivors: A Practical Guide to Your Future. Sebastopool, CA, O'Reilly, 2000.
6. Leigh S: Defining our destiny. In Hoffman B (ed): Cancer Survivors Almanac: Charting Your Journey. Minneapolis, Chronimed Publishing, 1996, pp 261–267.
7. Mullan F. Seasons of survival: Reflections of a physician with cancer. N Engl J Med 313:270–273, 1985.
8. National Coalition for Cancer Survivorship, Oncology Nursing Society, Association for Oncology Social Work: Cancer Survival Toolbox©: Building Skills That Work for You. Genentech BioOncology, 2000. Unrestricted grant through Genentech BioOncology, Inc.
9. Surveillance, Epidemiology, and End Results Program: Annual Cancer Statistics Review. Bethesda, MD, National Cancer Institute, 1997.

65. HOSPICE CARE

Janelle McCallum Orozco, RN, BSN, MSM

1. Define hospice.
Hospice is an interdisciplinary program of care focused on the relief of symptoms and suffering of the dying and support for their families. In the United States the Medicare Hospice Benefit has become the major source of funding for palliative care.

2. When is hospice care appropriate?
A person is ready for hospice care whenever he or she chooses palliative, noncurative holistic care instead of aggressive, curative medical care for a life-limiting illness. Typically hospice care has been available for people with a prognosis of 6 months or less. More recently patients have been referred close to the week of death. The average length of stay for hospice patients in the U.S. is 48 days. The median length of stay is 29 days (National Hospice and Palliative Care Organization, 1999.) Unfortunately, such late referral may preclude much of the benefit offered by the interdisciplinary team. To meet the needs of people and physicians who are reluctant to accept hospice care earlier in the course of illness, many hospices offer pre-hospice services. Pre-hospice services are for patients who are clearly terminal but who choose aggressive palliative care such as second- or third-line chemotherapy.

Historically, the majority of hospice patients have had cancer. Now patients with non-cancer diagnoses are using hospice services. Hospice-appropriate diagnoses include:
- Organ cancers (e.g., pancreas, liver)
- Cancers with metastatic processes
- Life-threatening congenital defects
- Massive cerebrovascular accidents (CVAs)
- Endstage chronic diseases, such as chronic obstructive pulmonary disease (COPD), multiple sclerosis (MS), amyotrophic lateral sclerosis (ALS), and acquired immunodeficiency syndrome (AIDS)
- Failure to thrive or significant weight loss secondary to debility
- Discontinuation of treatment or medications that prolong life (e.g., dialysis, antirejection medications, ventilators)
- Bone marrow transplant failure
- Patients with a do-not-resuscitate (DNR) order
- Patients with complex pain symptoms who need expert management
- Patients with repeat hospitalizations
- Patients with social, psychological, or spiritual challenges dealing with terminal illness and disease process
- Patients in whom aggressive treatment does not have a favorable outcome
- Patients with frequent changes in treatment plan due to slow but declining status
- Patients who decline treatment or diagnostic interventions for life-threatening illness

3. Where can a patient receive hospice care?
Hospice care can be provided in almost any setting: home, apartment, assisted living facility, nursing home, hospital, specialized inpatient hospice unit, or prison.

A 1992 Gallup poll revealed that 9 of 10 Americans surveyed would choose the services offered by hospices if faced with a terminal illness. Most people prefer to remain in their homes as they die. A Medicare expenditure report for 1982–1986 showed that 80–84% of Medicare hospice beneficiaries remained in their homes to die.[3]

Some people, however, need or choose an inpatient setting, including (1) patients who have no family or caregivers, (2) patients and families who desire an inpatient setting for personal reasons, and (3) patients with extreme medical or social conditions that make it necessary to transfer to an inpatient setting.

4. Who should bring up the subject of hospice care?

This can be a tricky area in which intuition and diplomacy are warranted. As the patient's nurse, you can do the following:

1. Begin your discussion and assessment with the patient's physician.
2. Offer to be present for the physician's discussion with the patient and family.
3. Offer to present the hospice option yourself. (In many hospitals discharge planners may be given the role of discussing hospice care.)

Often a hospice referral comes abruptly in the eyes of the patient and family. They believe that an aggressive curative course is under way, and the next day everything changes. The patient "suddenly" needs hospice care and, if hospitalized, must leave the hospital that same day. Proactive public education about palliative care and hospice philosophy is the key to diminishing the frequency of this scenario.

5. What if hospice care is clearly appropriate, but the physician refuses to discuss it with the patient or family?

First, discuss your concerns with the patient's physician. Try to follow Covey's axiom, "Seek first to understand, then to be understood." Perhaps more information or a more complex dynamic is involved than is readily apparent. The physician may be more open to "palliative or supportive care." In any case, consider the following questions as guides when introducing hospice or palliative care to the patient or family:

1. How are things going with your body?
2. What do you think is going on with your medical condition?
3. What do you think the future holds for you?

Depending on the patient's answer, follow the appropriate path. Let the patient know that you are open to hearing and discussing the unthinkable—dying.

6. What do I say when patients ask me if they are dying?

Be truthful. Chances are good that the patient has already been told that he or she is dying but may need to hear it again as conditions change. Approaches to answering this question include:

- What does it seem like to you? Then confirm the answer, if appropriate.
- What has your doctor told you? Then build or expand on what the patient already knows.

Reassure the patient that symptoms will be controlled. One hospice nurse emphasizes that someone given a "terminal diagnosis" often has time to do and say almost anything they want to before they die. Many people do not have this gift of time and die without saying and doing what they may have wanted. The bottom line is to follow the patient's lead. Ask, "Do you think you are dying?" Then take the conversation from there. This question helps to discover what the person really wants to know.

7. What promises should I never make to a dying person?

The premise is simple: Don't make promises you can't keep. Remember that the dying person has less time in which to have the promises fulfilled. Examples of key promises not to make include:

- I promise I'll be with you when you die.
- I promise I'll see you before you go.
- I promise I'll help you die.
- I promise I won't be depressed after you die.

It is also important to encourage family members *not* to make promises that they cannot keep.

8. What if I'm not sad when every patient dies?

One hospice nurse recalls that when she first started taking care of hospice patients, she expected that she should be sad when every patient died. Then she realized that she was connected to some patients and families and not so connected to others. Another hospice nurse says, "It's okay not to be sad. We don't like everyone we meet in life, so we won't like everyone we meet in death." Death is the natural conclusion of life. Hospice nurses strive to make the final hours or days a period of quality time for patient and family. Hopefully when they look back on that time, the actual death will be only a small part of a greater event.

9. How can I show respect for life after the patient has died?

Handle the patient in death as you did in life—with respect and care; make no distinction. Specific interventions include:

- Allow families private time with the body, and respect families' wishes, traditions, and customs.
- Be gentle and caring when removing lines and tubes and washing the body.
- Close the patient's eyes. Cover the patient to the neck; there is no need to cover the face.
- Brush the hair off the forehead and touch the face of the deceased in a gentle, loving manner.
- Reminisce with the family about the patient.
- From a chaplain's perspective: touch the body by laying on hands in blessing and talk as if their spirit is still present in the room. Sit in silence and reverence with the body.

10. What matters to families immediately after the death of the patient?

Ask the family what matters to them. Each family is different, and we must give them space to tell us what would be helpful. For example, some families want to spend lots of time with the dead body, whereas other families want the body removed as soon as possible. For some, the patient's appearance is of great concern (e.g., hair, make-up, clothing, position). However, families seem to have some fairly universal needs:

1. Show them that someone cares about them and the patient.

2. Let them know that you will take care of necessary details (e.g., with the physician, coroner, mortuary, equipment company, medications).

3. Provide a time and a place to make phone calls.

4. For deaths that occur in a private residence, it may be important to have the medical equipment (e.g., bed, wheelchair, oxygen) removed as soon as possible.

5. Explain bereavement services and leave written materials about grief for later reading.

Be sure to ask about rituals and spiritual needs. Be sensitive to cultures unlike your own. Most families want reassurance that their loved one will be treated with respect even in death.

11. What is anticipatory grief?

In the context of hospice care, anticipatory grief refers to emotions of loss and grief and even relief *before* the person's death. Many people expect profound anguish, but they feel guilt as they find themselves planning for the future—before the person actually dies. Hospice workers encourage anticipatory grief and help to normalize such emotions. Planning for the future is a healthy sign of anticipating life after the death of a loved one. It does not mean the survivors do not love the dying person or wish that the person would die sooner. It is what healthy people do when facing such life-changing circumstances as losing a loved one to terminal illness.

12. What can I do to help during the grieving process?

Simply stated, listen to the person's fears, ask about strategies to deal with the fears, and assist as appropriate. Ask about future plans. If the person has none, encourage thinking about the future. Reassure the person that future planning is normal and may cause some feelings of guilt. If a severely depressed survivor speaks of having no plans or future, this may be a red flag. Refer the person immediately to a social worker or chaplain.

Not all people who die are "loved ones." Be open to relief in family members or friends, who may make such statements as "He was so abusive," "We had a terrible marriage," or "I hated her." We tend to expect everyone to be sad about the patient's death, but this is not always the case.

Know that even though a person may be relieved that the patient died, the associated guilt must be resolved eventually.

13. Is it professional to go to the patient's funeral and maintain contact with the family?

In an inpatient setting, if scheduling allows and you feel a need to attend the funeral for your own closure, it is appropriate to do so. Continued contact with the family is generally *not* appropriate. Refer the family to a local hospice for bereavement assistance.

In a hospice setting, staff are encouraged to attend the patient's funeral and to make bereavement follow-up. Generally the staff who knew the patient attend the funeral, and a grief counselor does the follow-up bereavement work. The goal of follow-up is to assist the grieving person to heal in a healthy way.

Continued contact by direct care staff is discouraged because it continues a relationship that was begun during a time of crisis and death. The nurse's job is to assist the patient and family along the journey to death. The journey after death is equally important and may be assisted by another caregiver (e.g., bereavement counselor). There are always exceptions to this advice, however. Be careful to consider whose needs are primary—yours or the family's. Your goal in caring for the family after death is the same as when the patient was alive: *Do what is best for the patient and family first; meet your own emotional and social needs secondarily.*

Furthermore, it is known that morbidity and mortality increase significantly after a spouse's death. A recent study by Connor and McMaster evaluated the impact of psychosocial intervention on the use of inpatient and outpatient health care services by bereaved spouses. The results showed that spouses treated with hospice services used hospitals and clinics significantly less than spouses in the nonintervention and limited intervention groups. This study helps to describe the positive health and economic benefits provided by hospice bereavement services.

14. What is the role of the hospice in discontinuation of life-sustaining treatments?

Unfortunately, hospice staff are not consulted enough in such situations. The interdisciplinary hospice staff can be of great assistance in discussing options and supporting choices from many perspectives. They can help in determining the patient's decision-making capacity and ensuring that all parties are informed and advised. Whereas the medical model typically addresses only the physical domain, hospice staff consider the physical, emotional, social, and spiritual domains as the patient and family struggle with the decisions to end life-sustaining treatment.

For example, Emily was a patient whose family had made the decision to remove her from the ventilator. But they wanted her to die at home. They wanted to dress her in her prettiest nightgown, play her favorite country music, and have the smell of apple pie coming from the kitchen. After much negotiation, the hospice was able to assist the family to bring Emily home in the ambulance with an ambu bag. When she arrived home, the whole family was there. Her husband, who needed a wheelchair, was able to sit next to her on the couch and hold her hands as the ambu bag was discontinued. The sounds of country music mixed in with the clatter of kitchen noises. Emily died smelling apple pie and the other familiar scents of her own home. The family was touched and felt that they had influenced her death as well as her life. They were proud of themselves.

15. How can the hospice staff help to assess a patient's decision-making capacity with regard to discontinuation of life-sustaining treatments?

Ultimately the physician determines patient capacity, but staff can assist by asking the following questions:
- Is the patient able to communicate feelings and desires clearly to others?
- Is the patient clearly stating (via his or her method of communication) the desire for discontinuation of technical support?
- Is the patient able to articulate (via his or her method of communication) various options and consequences of actions?
- Is the patient depressed? Have antidepressant therapy and counseling been attempted?
- What are the patient's and family's spiritual concerns or understanding about discontinuation of treatment?

- Has the patient talked with others outside the health care team about this decision? If not, would this be helpful?
- Does the patient require more time for a thoughtful decision?
- Does the patient have an advance directive consistent with this decision?

16. What areas of agreement or disagreement should be addressed before discontinuing life-sustaining treatments?
- Does the patient have capacity? If not, who can make decisions for the patient?
- Are family and friends in agreement?
- Are current health care providers in agreement?
- Is there a physician's order for discontinuation?
- Which physician will preside at removal of the ventilator?
- Does the decision seem reasonable to staff who have assessed patient and family?

17. Is it true that it does not matter whether a terminally ill person is addicted to narcotics?
No. The point is that less than 1% of people who need narcotics for terminal pain actually display symptoms of true addiction. To alleviate the patient's and family's fears, it is helpful to understand and be able to teach the three components of the addiction scenario (tolerance, physical dependence, and psychological dependence.) As Foley points out, "The truth is that addiction is not the issue for cancer patients, and informing health care professionals and patients about the distinctions between tolerance, physical dependence, and psychological dependence is crucial."

Challenge the statement, "Who cares if he is addicted in the last months of his life anyway?" It is important to explain the following points:

1. In almost all cases the patient is not addicted.

2. Thinking that the family member was addicted to narcotics may be a stumbling block in the bereaved person's road to recovery.

3. The myth of addiction serves only to continue the public's misunderstanding of narcotics and appropriate pain management.

18. How can I remain compassionate yet not go crazy caring for dying patients and their families?
Here is how several hospice workers answer this question:

Ed: Take care of yourself. If you don't, you can't care for others. Cherish your life and all who are in it. Nurture your spiritual being to sustain you in times of need. Be aware of how this vocation can affect you. Talk about your feelings with your co-workers, and don't be afraid to seek outside help.

Jean: I get energy from the courage and love of so many of the families. I get two hugs for every one I give.

Micki: I maintain the philosophy that everyone dies, and if I can in any way facilitate meeting the patient's needs and wishes surrounding this one-time event, it is rewarding. Educating, reassuring, and guiding families is great.

Phyllis: When I close the door of the hospice inpatient unit, I am symbolically closing that part of my life until the next day. Recipe for success: do fun things, let the inner child out.

Janelle: If you're going to work with people who die, you had better learn how to live, decide what's important to you, and say what needs to be said. Every now and then, someone will wrap their soul around your heart, and it hurts when they suffer or die. This then is the essence of life.

Kay: When I feel valued and supported by the people I work for, it helps me remain focused. Use the support of other team members. Talk about what is going on.

Sandi: For me the key has been finding a clear theology for this work. Theology really helped me with "What's it all about, Alfie?" This work has given me a non-anxious paradigm about death.

Sally: Working part-time helps. I take care of myself physically (exercise and rest) and especially spiritually (meditation). I nurture friendships outside of hospice, and I spend as much time as possible with people who make me laugh.

Suzette: Have a life. Do for yourself. Forget all work issues on the weekend. Get away from your normal environment. Don't be a caregiver for all the people in your life. Have a person who listens to your problems—even a therapist. Maintain inner balance. Exercise, shop, have parties.

Paula: Don't overidentify with patients and families. Know your limits. Use the support of others.

Michelle: Set limits. Take care of yourself. Have outside interests and activities. Accept the laughter and the tears. Take opportunities for closure.

19. What if the patient wants to stay at home alone, but this option really is not safe?

Our job as nurses is to assess the safety and competency of the patient in whatever setting the patient resides. At times it is hard to be objective. We often think of a preferred arrangement because it would put our minds at ease. In the case of a live-alone patient, we need to identify true safety hazards and look at our own personal tolerance for marginal situations. The following checklist may be used:

Functional, Physical, and Environmental Concerns

1. Patient residence is ( ) multiple-family dwelling ( ) single-family dwelling
2. Personal emergency response system in use: ( ) Yes   ( ) No

	Y	N	
3.	( )	( )	Bedbound
4.	( )	( )	History of falls
5.	( )	( )	Fire hazards
6.	( )	( )	Hearing and/or vision
7.	( )	( )	Home alone
8.	( )	( )	Lives alone
9.	( )	( )	Medication compliance
10.	( )	( )	Decision maker
11.	( )	( )	Transportation assistance
12.	( )	( )	Oxygen: as needed _____ continuous _____
13.	( )	( )	Smoker
14.	( )	( )	Basic utilities
15.	( )	( )	Telephone

Psychosocial concerns

	Y	N	
16.	( )	( )	Financial Management
17.	( )	( )	Psychiatric Problems: Current _____ Hx _____
18.	( )	( )	Alcohol/Drug Problems: Current _____ Hx _____
19.	( )	( )	Suicidal Ideation: Current _____ Hx _____
20.	( )	( )	Violence or Potential: Current _____ Hx _____

Y = observed and/or reported; N = not observed, not reported, or denied; Hx = history.
Adapted from Hospice of Metro Denver, Denver, Colorado.

Equally important as the safety assessment is whether the patient has the capacity to make decisions. It is important to note that capacity is situational. Generally, the patient needs only to understand the consequences of a decision to have capacity. A person may have capacity and make poor decisions. In the case of poor decision making that puts the patient or others at risk, a call to Adult Protective Services is probably the best course of action.

Unfortunately, safety assessment is not an exact science. We must try to assess objectively the social, emotional, and physical strengths, weaknesses, needs, and desires of the patient and family, then make a decision to the best of our ability. Advice: maybe a plan to stay at home can work for a while; then regroup and make a new plan.

Example: Molly is a 78-year-old woman whose primary caregiver is her daughter. The daughter works full-time and is afraid to ask for time off despite the Family Medical Leave Act. Molly is alert but bedridden. The daughter plans to leave Molly alone while she works. Certified nursing assistants will visit Molly every day for personal care and to fix lunch. The daughter leaves water and snacks. Molly has an indwelling Foley catheter and can move herself in bed somewhat. Telephone, television remote control, water, and snacks are within Molly's reach. The daughter will call to check on Molly every 2–3 hours. Molly agrees to the plan, which works for 2 months. Then Molly tells the nursing assistant that she is afraid to be alone. A family conference is held to put a new plan in place. The daughter cannot hear her mother's fears. The hospice has to advocate for the patient. Finally Molly and her daughter agree to inpatient placement.

Molly's case was not an easy one. The hospice had to define its limits and advocate for the patient and her daughter. Unfortunately, conflict around caregiving needs is not uncommon. Helping families find a tolerable middle ground is a reasonable outcome.

20. What if a hospice patient talks about suicide or tries to commit suicide?

Many people who have been told that they have a terminal illness think about suicide at some point. Most work it through and decide that suicide is not really what they want to do. However, some continue to have a strong desire to kill themselves. In talking about suicide it is important to let the patient know three points:

1. It is okay to talk about such thoughts. (In fact, it is imperative that staff ask for more details to assess the seriousness of the threat.)
2. Suicidal ideation cannot be kept a secret; other team members need to know.
3. Support and assistance will be provided to the patient to work through fears and to continue living until the illness runs its course. The patient will not be abandoned.

When a patient talks about suicide, keep the following points in mind:

1. Do not be afraid to use the "s" word. For example: "Are you considering suicide?" "Have you thought about hurting yourself?" "Do you want to do something that would end things sooner?" By speaking the words aloud, you allow the person the option of responding either yes or no. If the patient says yes, ask whether the patient has a plan and get all the details. If the patient says no, ask what keeps the patient from doing it. This information may be helpful at another time.
2. Find out what specifically is intolerable for the patient. Is it pain, fear of pain, anxiety, lack of support, worry about being a burden, worry about losing dignity, or some other concern? Often we can eliminate the issue that makes the patient want to leave life early.
3. Explain that the discussion of suicide cannot be a secret. You will have to tell the physician and social worker, who will ask further questions and assist as possible.

21. When are invasive measures appropriate for a hospice patient?

Generally, invasive measures are not appropriate for hospice patients. However, there are exceptions. The goals of therapy are patient and family choice and optimal quality of life. Examples of invasive treatments that may be used include:

- Intravenous fluids (when used judiciously and discontinued as fluid begins to accumulate)
- Intravenous or intraspinal pain medication
- Gastric feedings
- Rectal tubes
- Paracentesis and thoracentesis (for a limited time)
- Surgery to repair fractures (often Buck's traction and pain management are used instead)
- Certain chemotherapies (to achieve palliation of symptoms)
- Total parenteral nutrition (for a limited time)

22. What do I do when the patient insists on experiencing pain, even though I know that medications and other treatments would help?

1. Listen to the patient; hear the request to decline pain medications.
2. Ask why medications and treatments are not acceptable.

3. Ask for permission to explain pain relief measures. Describe the medications, expected actions, and side effects. Remember to explain the concept of addiction and the surrounding myths.

4. If the patient still declines, accept the answer. But check again to make sure no intervention is wanted. (Suggest starting out with a very low dose to decrease fear and build trust.)

5. Comfort the family and friends of the patient. They, too, find it difficult to watch their loved one suffer. In your conversation with the family use the term *declined*, as explained below.

6. Assess reasons why the patient declines pain relief. Often there is a spiritual component to why people choose to suffer (e.g., "I want to suffer the way Christ did").

7. In your charting and discussion about the patient, consider using the words *declined medication* instead of "refused." The simple change of wording often evokes a change in the nurse. The word *refused* conjures up the image of a noncompliant patient. By the using the word *declined* we imagine a person with dignity making an informed decision. Be sure to document the teaching you have done if the patient continues to decline the offer of pain medication.

23. What about the young patient whose body just will not die?

Younger, actively dying patients tend to linger longer than older, actively dying patients. Even though the body is full of cancer, the younger person's heart can last longer. The stage called "actively dying" is the time just before a person dies when the kidneys begin to shut down, blood pressure decreases, oral intake stops, alertness diminishes (although not always), and mottling of the extremities may occur. An older patient may be in the "actively dying" stage for 1–3 days, whereas a younger person may be "actively dying" for days to weeks. Although longer death vigils are grueling for all involved, they seem to serve an important purpose for the patient as well as the family.

24. Who makes the decision about what constitutes palliative treatment and when it is appropriate to discontinue blood transfusions, palliative radiation, total parenteral nutrition, or enteral feedings?

Generally the patient's primary physician, in conjunction with the hospice medical director, makes the decision as to what constitutes palliative treatment. Of great importance is how we talk to the patient and family about these issues. It is helpful to describe the physiologic reasons why the treatments are not effective and are probably more uncomfortable to continue. Be sure to speak with the physician about discontinuation before discussing it with the family. Here are general rules of thumb for discontinuing treatment within a hospice context:
- When the physician believes that the treatment is no longer effective.
- When the patient can no longer make the trip to the hospital or clinic (e.g., taking the patient by ambulance to receive a blood transfusion does not usually make sense. However, it is often the patient or family member who says, "You know, I'm just too tired to make the trip—even with an ambulance").
- When the patient no longer tolerates the treatment.
- When the treatment causes more pain than comfort.

25. What does normal grief look like?

Grief takes time. It often takes a year or more to regain balance in life after a loss. The following are all natural and normal grief responses, listed in "A Few Words about Grief and Loss" (published by Hospice of Metro Denver, 1996).
- Tightness in the throat or heaviness in the chest
- Hollow feeling in the stomach and loss of appetite
- Need to tell and retell the story of the events leading up to the death and its aftermath
- Restlessness and need to fill time with activity, but often with difficulty in concentrating and getting organized
- Feeling as though the loss is not real, that it did not really happen
- Sensing the deceased person's presence; perhaps expecting him or her to walk in the door at the usual time, hearing the voice, or seeing the face on a stranger in a crowd
- Aimless wandering, forgetfulness, trouble with finishing projects at work or home, or absent-mindedness

- Intense preoccupation with the life of the deceased
- Crying at unexpected times
- Feeling guilty or angry over things that happened or did not happen in the relationship with the deceased
- Intense anger at the deceased for leaving
- Taking on mannerisms or traits of the deceased
- Sense of relief, sometimes followed by pangs of guilt or regret
- Unpredictable, rapid, and sharp mood swings
- Avoidance of talking about feelings of loss around others
- Weakness or lack of energy

If any of the above symptoms persists for more than 2 years or is exaggerated to the point of bodily injury, refer the person to a mental health counselor.

26. What can be done to help the grieving person?

1. Normalize the person's grief experience. "Because grief often feels so painful and overwhelming, it can be frightening. Many people worry that they are not grieving in the 'right' way or wonder if the feelings they have are normal."[4]

2. Encourage grieving people to tell their story. Telling the story is a major part of the healing process because the death event is so important. To embed every detail in one's memory, one must tell the story—over and over.

3. Encourage grieving people to take care of their own health and nutrition.

4. Advise them to make as few major changes in their life as possible.

5. Encourage them to ask for what they need from a few friends on whom they can rely.

27. How do I respond when a patient's family member rushes from the room and says, "I think he just died!"?

Give the person your immediate attention. You may say, "Okay, let's go." It is important to attend to the situation immediately. As you enter the room, all of the family may be at the bedside, waiting. At times it is hard to be sure that the patient has really died. Take the necessary time to be sure that the heart has stopped and there are no respirations. Telling the assembled family members that their loved one has died can be difficult. Do your best to "read" their expectations in terms of the language you may use. Possible phrases for telling the news include "He's gone" or "He's passed on." Often the family will ask, "Is he dead?" or "Is she gone?" Then you can affirm the question, using the words they have chosen.

In my experience, using the "d" word (dead) has not been perceived as "sensitive" by the family. It seems that at the time of death, the word "dead" rings hollow and cold. The death of the loved one is obvious, and perhaps euphemisms are appropriate comfort at this time.

28. What do I say to a patient's wife who is upset because her husband will not eat the food she fixes?

First, realize that loss of appetite can be traumatic for the patient's family. Eating and drinking are not only physiologic acts but also important social activities. Adjusting to an ill person's lack of interest in food and fluids can make the family feel helpless. In the above example, acknowledge the wife's frustration and fear. Explain that the food she fixed probably did sound good to her husband, but the disease prevents him from enjoying the meal she prepared. Explain the following:

- Loss of appetite is normal in a terminally ill person. The body needs less food when a person has cancer and is inactive; eating less does not shorten a person's life in serious disease, and in this case, low food intake does not cause hunger.
- Eating may become a difficult activity for a very ill person. Food may be offered, but the person should eat only if he wants. In some cases, the person may eat more than he desires because he believes that it is expected and then feels sick afterward.
- The person who is ill may develop new food preferences because some foods may taste different or have no taste at all.

29. What do I do when a patient insists on believing in a cure or miracle?

First, listen to the patient's belief. Do not try to talk the patient out of it. However, it may be possible to reframe what a "miracle" looks like. Hope is always appropriate. People must be allowed to hope for a miracle that can save their life. It is *not* necessary that they go through all stages of death and dying and reach acceptance. Some people are in denial until the end.

It is our task to be present to patients wherever they are. In our love and support they may find that the miracle for which they had been hoping is the nurse who is an excellent pain manager and who is present in their time of suffering and need.

30. What does it mean when a patient is discharged from hospice?

Patients that stabilize or improve as a result of team-oriented hospice care may be discharged if they no longer fit the definition of a "hospice patient" under the Medicare Hospice Benefit. The patient may be readmitted at a later date when his or her condition has deteriorated. There is no limit to the Medicare Hospice Benefit as long as the patient meets diagnostic and functional criteria. Hospices are trying to find other ways of providing palliative care without relying solely on the Medicare Hospice Benefit. However, changes in public policy and community awareness will be required to keep the Medicare Hospice Benefit from shrinking further. Other funding options for palliative care are needed.

From a patient and family perspective, discharge from hospice can be difficult. The patient and family have come to expect death and often have difficulty readjusting to "chronic illness" and the lack of interdisciplinary support to which they have become accustomed. In many ways, discharge from hospice is a "good news, bad news" scenario. The good news: you have graduated from hospice care. The bad news: you no longer have hospice services and need to get on with life without the support and quality of life that hospice helped to provide.

31. List important resources.

National Hospice and Palliative Care Organization: (703) 837-1500; website: nhpco.org

Hospice and Palliative Nurses Association: (412) 361-2470; website: hpna. org

Canadian Palliative Care Association: (613) 241-36663 or 1-800-668-2785; website: cpca.net

Hospice Information Service (United Kingdom): + (44) (0)20-8778-9252; website: www.hospiceinformation.co.uk

ACKNOWLEDGMENTS

The author thanks the staff of the Hospice of Metro Denver, who contributed to many of these questions. Specifically, they are Phyllis Walker, Caitlin Trussell, Michelle Taylor, Bob Severin, Sally Pyle, Micki Potter, Edward Orozco, Kay Johnson, Carolyn Jaffe, Jean Fredlund, Paula Dybinski, Vicki Dodson, Sandra Daniel, Mary Curtin, and Suzette Baca. The author also thanks the patients, families, volunteers, and other staff members who provided many life lessons as they shared the journey toward death.

REFERENCES

1. Conner SR, McMaster JK: Hospice, bereavement intervention and use of health care services by surviving spouses. HMO Pract 3:20–23, 1996.
2. Covey S: Seven Habits of Highly Effective People. New York, NY, Fireside, Simon & Schuster, 1989.
3. Foley KM: The cancer pain patient. J Pain Sympt Manage 3:S18, 1988.
4. Horne BK: Hospice care for the terminally ill: A logical, compassionate, and cost effective choice for case managers. NHO Newsline, November 15, 1995, pp 2–4.
5. Hospice of Metro Denver: Policy and Procedure Manual: 2000. Denver, Colorado, Hospice of Metro Denver, 2000. Specific entries include discontinuation of life-prolonging treatments, safety assessment, home alone/live alone protocol flow chart, when eating or drinking becomes a problem, and a few words about grief and loss.
6. Jaffe C, Ehrlich C: All Kinds of Love: Experiencing Hospice. Amityville, NY, Baywood Publishing, 1997.
7. Martinez JM, Wagner S: Hospice and palliative care. In Yarbro CH, Frogge MH, Goodman M, Greenwald SL (eds): Cancer Nursing: Principles and Practice, 5th ed. Boston, Jones & Bartlett, 2000, pp 1681–1698.
8. Purdue Frederick Company: Up-to-date answers to questions about pain medication. Norwalk, CT, 1986, p 7.

66. ADVANCE DIRECTIVES AND END-OF-LIFE DECISIONS

Jane Saucedo Braaten, RN, MS, CCRN,
and Paula Nelson-Marten, RN, PhD, AOCN

1. What are advance directives?

Advance directives include any kind of directions, either written or oral, by which the person makes his or her wishes for medical treatment known and/or appoints a surrogate to make decisions should he or she become unable to do so. Advance directives were created to help facilitate communication and to make end-of-life care a more positive experience. They are grounded in the principle of autonomy, or the patient's right to choose or refuse treatment.

2. What is the Patient Self-Determination Act (PSDA)?

The PSDA is federal legislation that requires all health care institutions receiving Medicare or Medicaid funds to give patients information about advance directives. It also specifies that patient preferences be queried and documented in the medical record. The PSDA specifies that a patient has the right to refuse therapy, including potential life-saving therapy.

3. What kind of information should be provided?

Although the PSDA requires that advance directive information be given to patients, the quality of information is not specified. Frequently, advance directive brochures are given to the patient without being fully discussed. Many patients do not understand options at the end of life. Thus, it is important not only to give the information, but also to answer questions and promote discussion.

4. What is the difference between a living will and a medical durable power of attorney?

A **living will** is a document signed by the patient stating that he or she does not want artificial life support in the event of terminal illness. The will takes effect when two physicians agree in writing that the patient has a terminal condition. A living will can be used to stop tube feeding and intravenous fluids only if this condition is stated specifically. Two witnesses need to sign the living will. Persons who cannot witness or sign include patients in or employees of the facility in which the patient receives care; any doctor or employee of the patient's doctor; the patient's creditors; or anyone who may inherit the patient's property.

A **medical power of attorney** is a document signed by the patient naming someone to make medical decisions in the patient's behalf. Anyone can act as a medical durable power of attorney as long as that person is at least 18 years of age, mentally competent, and willing to serve as the patient's agent. Examples include spouses, significant others, siblings, or parents. This type of advance directive covers more decisions than a living will and is not limited to terminal illness. A medical durable power of attorney can be effective immediately or when the patient becomes unable to make decisions. It is crucial to stress the importance of a thorough discussion of health care wishes between the patient and the person whom the patient has chosen.

5. Why do patients with living wills receive cardiopulmonary resuscitation (CPR)?

A living will is not an automatic do-not-resuscitate (DNR) order. Living wills do not cover acute conditions such as infection or bleeding. The living will goes into effect only when the condition is deemed irreversible.

6. What is surrogate decision-making or substituted judgment?

In the event that a patient becomes unable to make decisions and is critically ill, health care providers often ask the family or friends of the patient to inform them of what decision the patient would have made under such circumstances. This practice is based on a standard of substituted judgment and is accepted by many legal and medical authorities. The family and/or friends are the surrogate or substitute decision makers.

7. Has surrogate decision-making proven to be accurate?

Studies have shown that when given hypothetical end-of-life situations, surrogates did not accurately choose what the patient would prefer. A factor that greatly increased accuracy was a prior discussion of end-of-life preferences between patient and surrogate. This finding illustrates two clear needs: (1) the patient is the only one who can predict what kind of care he/she would want at the end of life, and (2) these wishes need to be clearly communicated to those who may act as surrogates.

8. What is a CPR directive?

A CPR directive is a document that refuses CPR if the patient goes into respiratory or cardiac arrest. It does not refuse other medical care. On admission to the hospital, it acts as a valid physician's order. It is available to patients from their physician, hospice, hospital, or nursing home. It must be signed by the patient or proxy and a physician. Many states now offer an outpatient CPR directive.

9. Why don't more patients come into the hospital with an advance directive?

Studies have shown that fewer than 5% of patients in various settings had written advance directives. One reason is that written advance directives require a bit of formal paperwork, which sometimes deters people from completing them. Another reason is fear that with an advance directive even basic care will be denied. In addition, the public and health care providers lack a clear understanding and hold misconceptions about advance directives.

10. What is the role of the oncology nurse in advance directives?

As the patient's advocate, it is the nurse's role to help the patient make an informed decision and to ensure that the patient's wishes are followed. The nurse should provide educational material and programs, schedule time for discussion, and communicate patient wishes to all members of the health care team. Educating patients during home and office visits and through community presentations is also important, because the best time to discuss advance directives is before an acute hospitalization. Most people are more likely to discuss a sensitive topic when they are in a comfortable, nonthreatening environment.

11. How should the nurse bring up the subject of advance directives?

Studies have shown that most patients welcome a discussion of advance directives but are uncertain of how to bring up the subject and prefer that health care providers initiate the discussion. The subject of advance directives may be introduced with a brochure or pamphlet with an explanation that this reading is part of the standard admission process. The nurse should emphasize that he or she (or another health care provider, such as a clinical nurse specialist, physician, chaplain, social worker, or patient representative) is available to answer questions after the patient has read the brochure. A time should be scheduled to discuss this issue with the primary care provider. The nurse should explain that advance directives include preferences about CPR and DNR orders as well as other levels of care, such as hydration, further chemotherapy, antibiotics, blood products, and analgesics. For the patient with cancer whose wishes have not yet been discussed but whose condition may be terminal, the subject of advance directives also may be brought up with a brochure or a statement that it is standard practice to query patients about their code status and other levels of care. If possible, health care providers who best know the patient should discuss the patient's wishes well in advance of a critical situation.

12. Give general guidelines for initiating discussion with cancer patients about code status:

1. The nurse may begin by saying, "Nobody can tell you for certain how much time you have left to live, but based on past experiences and knowledge about your particular condition,

we believe you have a short time left to live. In order to honor your wishes, we need to ask you some questions about your care." The nurse should ask patients what they understand about their condition, prognosis, and goals of therapy; give the patient sufficient time to ventilate feelings and questions; and continue the dialogue if the patient can acknowledge the condition and wants further discussion.

2. The nurse may begin by saying, "Knowing that your condition cannot be cured or that you may have only a short time left to live, do you want us to attempt CPR or try to bring you back when your heart stops or you stop breathing?" The nurse should be prepared to explain and clarify terms such as CPR, resuscitation, and mechanical ventilation and to discuss chances of success as well as possible complications. The nurse also should explain to the patient that CPR is most likely to be successful in generally healthy patients with sudden and reversible conditions and that patients with serious underlying medical conditions, such as advanced cancer, have a poor chance of successful CPR and a higher chance of serious complications (see question 19). The DNR order should be clarified, and the patient should be reassured that all other levels of care, including comfort care and other therapies, will continue as the patient requests.

13. What problems related to advance directives may occur in the hospital?

Many problems related to advance directives are specific to the hospital environment:

1. Paperwork may be lost during transfer to the hospital or misplaced within the hospital.

2. Patients may not be asked about their treatment preferences because of the fast-paced, cure-oriented environment or reluctance of the healthcare provider.

3. Misinterpretation may result from ambiguous language used in the advance directive.

4. The patient may have no advance directive and no surrogate decision-maker.

5. Advanced directives may be ignored or misunderstood by the hospital staff.

14. What is an ambiguous advance directive?

Sometimes an advance directive is ambiguous because of the lack of detail needed to understand completely the person's wishes. An example is a verbal or written statement such as "I do not want to be kept alive on life support," with no further instructions or guidance for the health care provider. This statement is difficult to interpret because it fails to specify in what situations the person wants it to apply and which interventions the patient considers life support. When encountering such an advance directive, the oncology nurse needs to act as patient advocate, using ethical principles to clarify the advance directive with the patient and/or family. Using other available tools to clarify what the patient values and what he/she would want in specific situations further strengthens an advance directive.

15. Are oral advance directives valid?

Oral advance directives are valid and are the most common type of advance directive in the hospital. Courts have consistently upheld decisions to withhold therapy on the basis of clear and convincing oral advance directives. However, oral directives often are vague, made long before the situation at hand, and highly subjective, especially when being recalled by another person. Family disagreement about the meaning of a patient's prior statement can also complicate the decision-making.

16. Is legal assistance required to make out an advance directive?

A patient does not need a lawyer to make out a living will, appoint a medical durable power of attorney, or write a CPR directive.

17. Can advance directives be changed?

Advance directives can be changed at any time. The patient needs to destroy the previous advance directive and inform anyone who may have a copy that it has been changed. It is wise to revoke the advance directive in writing and to give copies of the revocation to all who may have received the original document.

18. What can be done if a member of the healthcare team acts contrary to the patient's wishes?

As patient advocate, the nurse has the obligation to help make the patient's wishes known and followed by the healthcare team. If a member of the team is not following these wishes, the member simply may not have understood the advance directive. A meeting among nurse, healthcare team member, and patient or family may clear this misunderstanding. If not, the nurse may request that the nursing supervisor or medical director access the hospital ethics committee.

19. What advice can the nurse give to patients who want to ensure that their wishes will be followed?

1. Encourage patients to talk to their relatives or other potential surrogates about their wishes before illness or hospitalization.

2. Encourage use of a combination of living will and medical durable power of attorney. This combination ensures that wishes are followed if the living will is unclear in a specific situation.

3. Use clear language and specific examples, such as "I do not wish to be placed on a ventilator if it is deemed that my disease process is terminal and it is unlikely that I would be able to survive without ventilator support." Do not use terms such as "artificial" or "extraordinary"; these terms have different meanings to different people.

4. Be sure that the primary care physician knows and agrees to carry out the patient's wishes.

5. Encourage patients to give copies of paperwork to relatives and primary care physician and also to bring a copy to the hospital.

20. What factors do nurses see as obstacles to their ability to provide adequate end-of-life care?

In a recent study, nurses stated that obstacles to providing good end-of-life care include (1) family behavior that removed the nurse from the bedside; (2) family requests for more aggressive therapy than the patient wanted; (3) family's failure to understand care or prognosis; (4) family disagreement about options; and (5) physician behaviors, such as disregarding patient wishes, avoiding the family, giving false hope, disagreement with the healthcare team about treatment, and failure to provide nurses with orders for adequate pain relief.

21. What factors do nurses see as aids to their ability to provide adequate end-of-life care?

Examples of practices that help end-of-life care include (1) agreement among physicians about the plan of care; (2) communication among all of the healthcare team so that the plan of care is well understood; (3) environmental factors, such as allowing the family to adjust the room to offer a peaceful, comforting bedside scene and flexible visitation; (4) staffing adjustments that allow the nurse to spend enough time with the patient and family; and (5) nursing education and support for end-of-life care.

22. Do patients with a DNR order receive different nursing care from other patients?

The DNR order is defined simply as no CPR. Nonetheless, a DNR order is often thought to imply that other life-sustaining interventions, such as mechanical ventilation, blood products, and dialysis are not desired. In a study by Henneman and colleagues, nurses reported that they would be less likely to perform various interventions for a patient with a DNR order, whereas they would be more likely to provide more psychosocial interventions and comfort care. Some people believe that the amount of time spent in caring for the patient with a DNR order will be decreased. A recent study of cancer patients in the ICU showed the same amount of nursing care expended and comfort care given on behalf of the patients with or without DNR orders.

Realistically, nursing care of patients with DNR orders depends on the specific wishes of the patient and has little to do with the order itself. For example, the patient or family may request comfort care or want aggressive therapy only to a certain point. Generally, such wishes are not conveyed in a DNR order and need to be explored and documented through other more specific advance directives.

23. How successful is CPR in patients with advanced illness?
CPR was originally intended for use after acute situations in otherwise healthy people. It is now widely used in hospitals despite its limited effectiveness (0–28% survival rate to hospital discharge). Patients most likely to benefit from CPR are those with sudden circulatory or respiratory collapse in the setting of acute cardiovascular illness. Those least likely to survive are patients with multisystem organ failure, metastatic disease, age > 70, and severe chronic or acute conditions. These facts should be discussed with patients with advanced illness.

24. Is a "slow code" ethical or legal?
A so-called "slow code" is not an ethical or a legal order. An unofficial slow code order is usually an indication that the subject of advance directives has not been adequately discussed with the patient or family. Orders to resuscitate or not to resuscitate should be made clear and understandable to all hospital staff.

25. "They can't sue me for saving their lives." Is this statement true?
Legal action can be brought against a healthcare provider who ignores an advance directive. Intentionally administering a treatment against a patient's wishes, such as performing CPR on a patient with a CPR directive, may be regarded as assault and battery.

26. Is there a difference between withdrawing and withholding care?
Most ethicists agree that legally and ethically there is no difference. In either case, the decision achieves the same outcome—inevitable death. However, many healthcare professionals feel that there is a difference between withdrawing treatment and not starting it in the first place. It may be that withdrawing treatment is seen as taking a more active role in the death of the patient.

27. Can treatment be withheld if the patient is not terminally ill or unconscious?
Courts have allowed treatments to be withheld in various situations, including bleeding from trauma, gangrene, respiratory failure, renal failure, cancer, and quadriplegia. The patient also may refuse any and all treatment.

28. Can fluids and nutrition be withheld?
Courts have consistently declared that fluids and nutrition are to be handled as other medical interventions and may be withdrawn or withheld in appropriate circumstances. Patients can refuse these interventions through clear and convincing oral advance directives or through a durable power of attorney. A living will may specify a time frame chosen by the patient in which to administer and then withdraw tube feedings or fluids.

29. What is the difference between active and passive euthanasia?
Active euthanasia is administering an intervention with the intent to kill the patient. This practice is not legal in the United States, although Oregon has passed a law that allows physicians to prescribe, but not administer, drugs to be used for euthanasia. Passive euthanasia allows a disease to continue its natural course. Withholding and withdrawal of care fit into this category.

30. If I give pain medication that knocks out the respiratory drive, am I performing active euthanasia?
No. The intent in giving pain medication is to relieve pain and suffering, not to knock out the respiratory drive. Some clinicians undermedicate patients because of this fear. According to the American Nursing Association's Code for Nurses with Interpretive Statements, "The nurse may provide interventions to relieve symptoms in the dying client even when the interventions entail substantial risks of hastening death."

31. Why is the subject of end-of-life decision-making so difficult to discuss?
The subject of death is never an easy topic for the patient, family, or healthcare provider to discuss because of the overwhelming societal view that death is something to be avoided at all

costs. Healthcare providers may not want to accept the limits to their interventions. Furthermore, discussion about death and dying has not been a routine part of medical or nursing school curricula. In a recent study, oncology nurses rated their basic preparation for end of life care as inadequate. In addition, the patient may not want to accept the fact that death is inevitable and that his or her disease process may result in death. Whatever the reasons for avoidance, death must be seen as an inevitable part of life. Planning and discussion can help to make death and dying more acceptable. This planning, while often uncomfortable, helps to facilitate transition to terminal illness and resolution for both patient and family.

32. How has end-of-life care improved?

SUPPORT (Study to Understand Prognosis and Preferences for Outcomes and Risks of Treatment), a large, 4-year, multicenter study funded by grants from the Robert Wood Johnson Foundation, examined end-of-life care in hospitals and concluded that for many patients it was less than optimal. Fifty percent of patients suffered moderate or severe pain in their last days of life; 38% of patients who died spent 10 or more days in the intensive care unit; and physicians did not accurately understand or ignored the patient's preferences for advance directives. Of the patients (79%) who had a written DNR order, the DNR was written within 2 days of death.

Since this study, many groups have focused on improving end-of-life care. One group from the Institute of Medicine published guidelines and recommendations focusing on palliative care, elimination of legal obstacles, improved education for healthcare providers, and research focused on the end-of-life experience.

33. How can education about end-of-life care be improved for healthcare providers?

Improving end-of-life care requires educating current healthcare professionals and faculty in schools of medicine and nursing. They, in turn, will educate their colleagues and students. National courses have been designed for physicians and nursing faculty. The course for physicians is Education for Physicians on End-of-Life Care (EPEC). The core curriculum educates physicians about essential clinical competencies required to provide high-quality end-of-life care. The course for nursing faculty is End-of-Life Nursing Education Consortium (ELNEC), a comprehensive education program designed to develop a core of expert nursing educators and to coordinate national nursing efforts in end-of-life care.

CONTROVERSIES

34. Who determines "futility" when the family or patient wants more intervention than the health care providers think is appropriate?

Some patients and/or family members may request care that is excessive or inappropriate. A determination of medical futility can limit such requests. The problem is that medicine is not an exact science and no prognostic indicators are completely accurate. As a result, futility, more often than not, is a value judgment. Who makes this judgment—health care providers or patient and family—is a highly controversial topic.

Proponents of determination by clinicians or hospitals argue that futility can be judged ethically and that excessive use of scarce resources can be limited. They believe that hospitals are within their rights to create guidelines or policies for futile care that include referring the patient to a different facility or clinician for the treatment that is deemed futile. Opponents argue that determination by clinicians or hospitals is an example of paternalism (deciding for the patient) and conflicts with the principle of autonomy. Some believe that shared decision-making between clinician and patient or surrogate is the ideal solution.

35. Will assisted suicide soon be legal?

This issue has received attention because of the common belief that patients have little control over end-of-life care. Approximately a dozen states have drafted legislation to legalize physician-assisted suicide. Oregon voters passed the Death with Dignity Act in 1994. Since then, there have been 43 cases of physician-assisted suicide. Recently, euthanasia was legalized in the Netherlands.

For: Right-to-die advocates (e.g., the Hemlock Society) state that society has an obligation to relieve pain and suffering if the patient wishes. They argue that competent patients should be allowed to control the time and manner of their death. They base their position on the principles of beneficence (obligation to do good) and autonomy.

Against: Opponents state that if assisted suicide is legalized, less attention will be focused on pain management and groups such as the elderly, mentally compromised, and poor patients may be coerced into this decision. In an era of managed care and emphasis on cost control, they argue that giving physicians the right "to kill" may be abused. They base their position on the principle of nonmaleficence (obligation to inflict no harm).

WEBSITES OF INTEREST

Last Acts: www.lastacts.org/
Before I Die: www.wnet.org/bid/
Partnership for Caring Inc.: www.partnershipfor caring.org
Education sites:
    End-of-Life Nursing Education Consortium (ELNEC): www.aacn.nche.edu/elnec
    Education for Physicians on End-of-Life Care (EPEC): www.epec.net

REFERENCES

1. Aiken TB, Catalano JT: Legal, Ethical, and Political Issues in Nursing. Philadelphia, F.A. Davis, 1994.
2. American Nurses Association: Code for Nurses with Interpretive Statements. Kansas City, MO, American Nurses Association, 1985.
3. Beland DK, Froman RD: Preliminary validation of a measure of life support preferences. Image 27:307–310,1995.
4. Cugliari A, Miller T, Sobal J: Factors promoting completion of advance directives in the hospital. Arch Intern Med 155:1893–1898, 1995.
5. Dautzenberg P, Brockman T, Hooyer C, et al: Review: Patient related predictors of cardiopulmonary resuscitation of hospitalized patients. Age Aging 22:464–475, 1993.
6. Ferrell B, Virani R, Grant M,. et al: Beyond the Supreme Court decision: Nursing perspectives on end-of life care. Oncol Nurs Forum 27:3:445–454, 2000.
7. Field M, Cassel C: Approaching Death. Washington, DC, Institute of Medicine, 1997.
8. Hall J: Nursing, Ethics and Law. Philadelphia, W.B. Saunders, 1996.
9. Henneman E, Baird B, Bellamy P, et al: Effect of do-not-resuscitate order on the nursing care of critically ill patients. Am J Crit Care 3: 467–472, 1994.
10. Hoffman M: Use of advance directives: A social work perspective on the myth versus the reality. Death Stud 18:229–241.1994.
11. Kaplow R: Use of nursing resource and comfort of cancer patients with and without a DNR in the ICU. Am J Crit Care 9:87–95, 2000.
12. Kirchhoff K, Beckstrand R: Critical care nurses' perceptions of obstacles and helpful behaviors in providing end-of-life care to dying patients. Am J Crit Care 9:96–105, 2000.
13. Laffey J: Bioethical principles and care-based ethics in medical futility. Cancer Pract 4:41–46, 1996.
14. Larson D: Resuscitation discussion experiences of patients hospitalized in a coronary care unit. Heart Lung 23:53–58, 1994.
15. Lo B: Resolving Ethical Dilemmas: A Guide for Clinicians. Baltimore, Williams & Wilkins, 1995.
16. Meisel A, Snyder L, Quill T: Seven legal barriers to end of life care. JAMA 284:2495–2501, 2000.
17. O'Keefe S, Redahan C, Daly K: Age and other determinants of survival after in-hospital cardiopulmonary resuscitation. Q J Med 81:1005–1010, 1991.
18. Suhl J, Simons P, Reedy T, Garrick T: Myth of substituted judgment: Surrogate decision making regarding life support is unreliable. Arch Intern Med 154:90–96, 1994.
19. SUPPORT Principle Investigators: A controlled trial to improve care for seriously ill hospitalized patients: The Study to Understand Prognoses and Preferences for Outcomes and Risks of Treatment (SUPPORT). JAMA 274:1591–1598, 1995.

67. COMMON ETHICAL DILEMMAS

Paula Nelson-Marten, RN, PhD, AOCN, and
Jane Saucedo Braaten, RN, MS, CCRN

Since ethics is fundamentally a practical discipline, it is concerned with what we should do and how we should live.
Churchill, 1989

1. Why is it important for nurses to understand ethics?

An understanding of ethics and ethical decision-making should be applied in daily nursing practice. Ethical dilemmas occur often and in every aspect of nursing practice. Without a basic knowledge of ethics, the nurse will miss opportunities to advocate for patients and families and to enhance care. In a survey of 900 nurses from various settings, conducted by the American Nurses' Association (ANA) Center for Ethics and Human Rights, 43% reported that they deal with ethical issues in their nursing practice on a daily basis and 36% on a weekly basis.

2. How can the nurse use ethics in everyday nursing practice?

The nurse uses ethics in everyday nursing practice when he or she is alert to moral conflicts, identifies ethical issues, uses the ANA Code of Ethics as a basis for practice, advocates for patients, shares decision-making with patients, and helps to implement moral decisions.

3. How does the nurse distinguish an everyday dilemma from an ethical dilemma?

A dilemma occurs whenever a situation requires a choice between two equally desirable or undesirable alternatives. All people are confronted by daily dilemmas that involve choice. A dilemma acquires moral qualities when the person can justify alternative courses of action through use of fundamental moral rules or principles. An ethical dilemma arises when moral claims conflict with one another.

4. What is the difference between morals and ethics?

Morals and ethics are often used interchangeably. Each word, however, has a distinct derivation and meaning. The word *morals* is derived from the Latin word *mores*, which means custom or habit and refers to a set of values or rules that are peculiar to each individual. These values and rules are based on conscience and cultural or religious beliefs; they serve as a guide in personal decision-making regarding right and wrong. The word *ethics* is derived from the Greek word *ethos*, which means customs, conduct, and character. Ethics is the study of how one determines right from wrong. The use of ethics involves a process based on the use of principles and decision-making frameworks.

5. What ethical codes provide guidance for nursing practice?

The ANA Code of Ethics and the International Council of Nurses (ICN) Code make explicit the ethical values of the nursing profession. The professional nurse makes a moral commitment to practice within the expectations set by ethical codes. The ANA Code, which was first adopted in 1950 and has undergone subsequent revisions, includes 11 statements that define ethical responsibilities of nurses in terms of the following topics: respect for human dignity, safeguarding the client's right to privacy, client safety, responsibility for nursing judgment, competence, informed judgment, development of nursing knowledge, standards of practice, conditions of employment, protection of a client from misrepresentation, and collaboration to meet health needs of the public. The ICN Code, which was adopted in 1973, contains statements relating to ethical practices of the nurse in five areas—with people, in practice, in society, with coworkers, and for the profession. For complete texts of ANA and ICN Codes for Nurses, see reference 3.

6. Describe four goals that provide an ethical basis for planning and providing health care.

An international project, conducted by the Hastings Center in the mid-1990s, determined where medicine has been and defined future priorities. Representatives from the World Health Organization and 14 countries were included. The project defined the following four goals of medicine that provide an ethical basis from which to plan and provide care:
1. Prevention of disease and injury and promotion and maintenance of health
2. Relief of pain and suffering caused by maladies
3. Care and cure of those with a malady and care of those who cannot be cured
4. Avoidance of premature death and pursuit of a peaceful death

7. Explain the two major traditions in Western ethics.

The general perspective of **biomedical ethics** is based on justice and/or equity in distribution of resources. This tradition is commonly used in medicine. The **ethic of care** involves a perspective on relationship. Care for the individual patient becomes highly important. This ethical tradition is closely aligned with nursing. Neither tradition is gender- or discipline-based. Physicians and nurses may operate out of either tradition.[6]

8. What are the major ethical decision-making processes in biomedical ethics?

The two major schools of thought in Western biomedical ethics, defined by philosophers in the eighteenth and nineteenth centuries, have resulted in two major ethical decision-making frameworks. **Deontology or formalism** (from the work of Kant) indicates that the moral agent should consider the inherent nature of an act or rule rather than the consequences. This framework is principle-based and focuses on duties and obligations. The basic ethical principles are autonomy, justice, beneficence, and nonmaleficence. **Utilitarianism or teleology** (from the works of Mill and Bentham) indicates that the moral agent should consider consequences of rules and acts and seek the greatest possible balance of happiness over unhappiness for the greatest number. The two basic ethical principles are beneficence and nonmaleficence.

9. What are the major ethical principles in biomedical ethics?

1. **Autonomy.** This principle refers to self-rule, a person's right to self-determination, freedom of action, and noninterference to a degree consistent with respect for others. When an individual exercises autonomy, he or she determines what actions to take (self-determination). Freedom to act refers to a voluntary situation in which the individual is free of coercion and manipulation. The right of noninterference means that the individual's choices are respected whether or not they are in the individual's best interest. Use of this principle for major decision-making requires consideration of the individual's wishes, values, and goals. It opposes the use of paternalism (see question 11), by which the health care team and/or family determine what is best for the patient.

2. **Respect for persons.** This principle is broader than the principle of autonomy. It includes respect for individual autonomy and self-determination and at the same time acknowledges the interconnectedness of individuals, i.e., that we are all members of communities.

3. **Justice.** This principle refers to fairness. In health care ethics, its meaning narrows to distributive justice, which determines equal distribution of goods and services and addresses equality of treatment in conditions of scarcity. In using this principle, the moral agent attempts to find a balance between benefits and burdens. Current health care policies and reform represent a national effort to provide distributive justice.

4. **Beneficence.** This principle asks the individual to do good and has been defined by Frankena as the four "oughts": (1) one ought not to inflict evil or harm; (2) one ought to prevent evil or harm; (3) one ought to remove evil; and (4) one ought to do or promote good.

5. **Nonmaleficence.** This principle asks the individual to do no harm and relates to one of Frankena's four oughts—one ought not to inflict evil or harm.

10. Define rights vs. duties.

In ethical thought, for every right or privilege there is a corresponding duty or obligation. For example, if one considers health care to be a right, the corresponding duty on the part of the patient is to assume some personal responsibility for health and well-being. Often, one may become trapped into thinking that only patients have rights. However, everyone in the health care arena has rights and duties, including patients, family members, nurses, and all members of the health care team.

11. Define paternalism.

Paternalism, parentalism, and maternalism tend to be used interchangeably. All three terms refer to actions that override an individual's wishes or actions to benefit or avoid harm to the individual. Generally, paternalism occurs when two principles—beneficence and autonomy—are in conflict and the health care practitioner believes that he or she is making the best decision in relation to the patient's care. All members of the health care team are capable of paternalistic behavior, which often occurs daily in the oncology setting.

12. How should the nurse deal with paternalism?

The nurse needs to be alert so that he or she can recognize paternalism, continue to advocate for the patient, and foster self-determination and independence. Paternalism is not always negative, but when it occurs, it needs to be acknowledged. For example, if a patient's laboratory work and computed tomographic scan show evidence of recurrent disease, a physician may tell the patient that the cancer appears to be back but that the patient should not worry because a new course of chemotherapy will bring the recurrence under control. Nurses also need to be aware of their own actions in relation to paternalism. For example, the nurse may want to encourage the use of a pain medication that the patient rejects because of concern over the possible side effects of constipation and sedation. The nurse starts the pain medication and tells the patient, "It's important for you to get your pain under control!"

13. Why is confidentiality important?

Confidentiality, or the keeping of promises (principle of fidelity), is necessary both ethically and legally to care for the patient and to develop a relationship of trust. The ANA Code of Ethics states that the nurse should safeguard the client's right to privacy in a judicious manner that does not endanger the patient's welfare. For example, confidentiality may be violated whenever patient cases are discussed in public places or within hearing distance of others not involved in the case. The principle of fidelity needs to be considered in sharing and withholding information.

14. Explain the principle of veracity.

The principle of veracity (truth-telling) requires the nurse to consider whether communication is honest. At times "being truthful" may be difficult for the nurse, inconvenient for the health care team, and distressing for the patient and family. The nurse should consider four questions:
 1. Does the patient have the right to know?
 2. Does the patient have the right to refuse information?
 3. Does the family have the right to ask the health care team not to share all of the known information with the patient?
 4. Does the family have a right to know?

15. How is the principle of veracity applied in the nursing care of newly diagnosed patients and patients with recurrent disease?

In general, it is assumed that the patient has the right to full and accurate information about his or her situation. Withholding information may not be beneficial and may cause the patient to distrust the health care team. In cases of cognitive impairment or mental incompetence, the patient's level of comprehension should be considered so that the information is presented in a way that can be understood. Often patients who are not informed envision situations that are far worse than reality. Newly diagnosed patients and patients experiencing recurrence can assume no control over what is happening if they have not been told the truth. The facts may need to be restated several times in a way that promotes the truth, leads to open communication, and encourages questions. The nurse needs to be the patient's advocate. The right to information may be waived if the patient has good reason for requesting that information be withheld. The patient also may request that the family not be told. When the family requests nondisclosure, the nurse and health care team need to remember that the patient's right to confidentiality is primary.

16. What ethical issues are involved in informed consent?

Informed consent involves the principles of autonomy and nonmaleficence. The health care team needs to ensure that the patient has access to information and that the information is understood. The term *informed* assumes that the health care team will provide as much information as possible to the patient so that the decision is based on full knowledge. The information shared with the patient needs to be truthful. Informed consent is important in many areas of oncology—for any treatment (surgery, chemotherapy, radiation, clinical trials) and for participation in research. Patients must understand that they can withdraw from the treatment or research at any point and that withdrawal will not affect the level of medical or nursing care. Patients may refuse to give consent, and their refusal must be respected. It is a good idea to ensure that the patient gives informed refusal as well as informed consent.

17. When resources are scarce (principle of justice), who decides which patient receives priority treatment?

When oncologic resources are scarce (e.g., expensive chemotherapy, new protocols, new medications), some patients may not have access. One example is bone marrow transplant (BMT). Insurance companies have variable policies regarding BMT, and not all patients are covered. Another example is the use of antiemetic drugs. Ondansetron is fairly expensive, whereas droperidol is inexpensive. The physician may prefer the use of ondansetron for a specific patient, but the patient may not be able to afford the more expensive drug because of insurance coverage and limited ability for self-payment. The principle of distributive justice may assist the health care team in deciding which patient should get the scarce item. The team needs to consider the patient's illness, how the scarce item will or will not affect outcome, cost of the item, whether the patient can enter a clinical trial, and who will benefit most. The health care team must balance benefits and burdens. Sometimes there are no easy answers, but assessing all of the known facts and balancing outcomes, benefit, and burdens help the health care team to make the fairest decision possible.

18. Why is the ethic of care tradition more closely aligned with nursing?

The ethic of care is aligned with nursing because the nurse works closely with patients and families. Part of the nurses' role is to be an advocate for the patient/family. Advocacy is one of the moral concepts important in a care-based ethic.

19. Describe the main concepts of caring ethics.

Four major moral concepts are important for an ethic of care orientation: cooperation, advocacy, accountability, and caring. As Fry points out, these concepts have "enjoyed a special place of honor among nursing standards and statements over the years." The concept of cooperation encourages the nurse to participate actively with others, to collaborate, and to reciprocate. The concept of advocacy is closely aligned with the ANA Code of Ethics and is based on the principle that the freedom of self-determination is the most fundamental and valuable human right. Accountability is a concept which has two major attributes: answerability and responsibility. Caring is considered fundamental to the nursing role. Watson defines caring as the moral imperative of nursing. In other words, the nurse is called to be caring.

20. Describe a nursing model for ethical decision-making in the caring ethics tradition.

The Shared Decision Making Model of Bandman and Bandman encourages the nurse to be a patient advocate. The model has five basic steps, each of which has several components:

Step 1: Definition of the problem
- Assess the situation: does a problem exist?
- Assess the patient's perception of the situation.

• Clarify the problem in relation to the patient's lifestyle, value system, resources, family, and other personal factors.
• Decide whether further information is needed.
• Identify with the patient alternatives that are appropriate to goals.

Step 2: Analysis of factors to facilitate shared decision-making
• Is the patient competent to make a decision?
• Is the patient's decision fully informed and freely given?
• Are the ethical components of the decision clear?
• Does the patient/family have relevant information?
• Can the patient reverse the decision whenever he or she wishes?

Step 3: Identification of the ethical issue
• Discuss ethical choices with the patient.
• Identify sources of conflict among moral principles.
• Which moral principles can be justified for use in this situation?

Step 4: Decision regarding ethical choices
• The patient freely makes an informed decision consistent with his or her values, moral principles, lifestyle, and goals.
• The nurse and health care team are supportive of the patient's ethical choice.
• Family members and/or significant others are supportive of the patient's choice.

Step 5: Implementation of the moral decision. As the patient's advocate, the nurse supports the patient's decision.

21. Define sanctity of life.

Sanctity of life, also known as sacredness of life, is similar to the principle of avoiding killing. This principle is often relevant to end-of-life decisions. According to this viewpoint, life is sacred; therefore, you ought not to do anything that may hasten death, such as removing a feeding tube or discontinuing treatment. Before putting this principle into practice, you are obligated to consider the wishes of the patient and the risks/benefits of the intervention.

22. Who determines quality of life?

In the past it was common for the physician to determine the patient's quality of life (paternalism), especially in relation to the amount of remaining physical function and the likely outcome of continued interventions. From an ethical point of view, the patient should determine his or her quality of life (principles of autonomy and respect for personhood) unless the patient is not competent to assist in this determination. The family and health care team may become involved. The nurse must advocate for the patient and family and their goals for health care.

23. Explain the principle of double effect.

The principle of double effect refers to a situation in which an act intended to produce a good effect also produces a bad or unintended effect. In oncology, for example, titration of medicine to the level needed to relieve pain (a good intention) may hasten the patient's death (an unintended effect). This principle states that bad consequences of an action (i.e., giving pain medicine) are morally permissible if four conditions are met:

1. The action is good or neutral.
2. The nurse intends only the good effect (i.e., pain relief).
3. The bad effect (i.e., death) must not be a means to bring about the good effect (pain relief).
4. There must be a balance between the good and bad effects.

According to the ANA's Position Statement on the Promotion of Comfort and Relief of Pain in Dying Patients, "nurses should not hesitate to use full and effective doses of pain medication for the proper management of pain in the dying patient. The increasing titration of medication to achieve adequate symptom control, even at the expense of life, thus hastening death secondarily, is ethically justified." (See Appendix).

24. How does one determine ordinary vs. extraordinary means of preserving life?

Generally, the terms are used in conjunction with prolonging or preserving life. The best definition of the terms was given by Kelly in 1951: "Ordinary means are all medicines, treatments, and operations which offer a reasonable hope of benefit and which can be obtained and used without excessive expense, pain, or other inconvenience. Extraordinary means are all medicines, treatments, and operations, which cannot be obtained or used without excessive expense, pain, or other inconvenience, or which, if used, would not offer a reasonable hope or benefit."[2]

25. When are ethics committees needed? What is their role?

Institutional ethics committees provide a forum for review and discussion of ethical issues and dilemmas and share information as a guide for decision-making. In general, ethics committees provide advice and consultation and do not make the final decision. Any individual involved in an ethical dilemma (health care team member, patient, family member) can request a meeting of the ethics committee.

26. What is a nursing ethics round table? How are they useful for the practicing nurse?

A nursing ethics round table provides an opportunity for nurses to discuss ethical issues that are of concern in the care of a certain patient and family and/or more general patient situations that have ethical overtones. Usually an ethics roundtable is held monthly and facilitated by an ethicist or a person knowledgeable in ethics. The meeting gives nurses a chance to share experiences and to seek counsel and advice in planning care. Ethics round table meetings can help nurses to learn more about ethical issues, identify ethical dilemmas, and explore ways to resolve them.

27. To whom does the oncology nurse owe primary responsibility?

Oncology nurses, like all nurses, have many responsibilities, duties, or obligations of an ethical nature. Differing responsibilities may be of primary importance at any one time. There are responsibilities to patients, patient's families, employers, colleagues, one's own family, and self. In general, oncology nurses regard the patient as their primary responsibility. The ANA Code of Ethics outlines the nurse's responsibility to the patient.

28. What does the oncology nurse owe to the patient's family and significant other?

To care for the patient, the oncology nurse also may need to care for the patient's family and/or significant other. (In interest of space, the term *family* is used alone, but it is meant to refer to significant others that may be integral to or beyond the family unit). Often, family members are the patient's major source of social support; they need to be informed, along with the patient, about current disease and treatment status.

29. What ethical issues are involved with clinical trials?

Several ethical issues inherent in clinical trials are similar to those inherent in allocation of scarce resources. All patients cannot enter the clinical trial that they may wish, and sometimes the patient dies before the trial begins. Once the patient is in the trial, another ethical issue may arise in deciding when to remove the patient from the trial. If it is obvious that the trial is not benefiting the patient, the principles of beneficence and nonmaleficence may assist the health care team in decision-making.

30. How does the oncology nurse advocate for the patient when the nurse does not agree with the patient's decision?

Often the nurse faces an ethical dilemma if the patient decides either that he or she does not want further treatment or that he or she wants extraordinary treatment. In such situations, the nurse should follow the principles of respect for persons and autonomy. The nurse's role is to care for the patient, including advocating for the patient. The nurse or health care team must ensure that the patient is making an informed decision and that the patient and family understand the consequences of the decision. Once the patient or family has made a decision, the nurse's role is to care for the patient in a supportive manner, regardless of outcome. Three critical factors are maintenance of open communication, respect for the decision, and the patient-family's need not to feel abandoned by the health care team. In such situations, the healthcare team should discuss how each member feels about the patient-family's decision and support one another in delivering care.

31. How does the oncology nurse deal with ethnic and cultural differences from an ethical perspective?

To care adequately for a patient and family from another culture, the nurse needs to be mindful of the principle of respect for persons. To avoid offending the patient or family, the nurse should recognize and respect the ethnic and cultural traditions that influence the required care. Standards and protocols of care that incorporate cultural beliefs, rituals, and religious preferences need to be developed. An example is the development of protocols for the care of Hasidic Jewish women receiving bone marrow transplants for breast cancer.

32. How does the oncology nurse care for self from an ethical standpoint? Why is self-care important?

The oncology nurse needs to work at developing an ethical sense and becoming astute at recognizing ethical dilemmas with patients, team members, and self. Although the nurse must respond to many rights, he or she also has the duty to care for self. If one does not care for self, one cannot care effectively for others. At times, the nurse has an obligation to remind others that he or she needs to care for self. Often oncology nurses attempt to be all things to all people. Living a more balanced life affects positively all that the nurse does.

33. When is it ethical to let a terminal patient die without violating the principle of avoiding killing?

When it becomes obvious that treatment is of no further benefit, the nurse and health care team need to consider whether active treatment should be discontinued. Palliative or hospice care may be more appropriate. The patient and family may need guidance in making this decision. The patient may not wish to quit active treatment; for example, a patient who has responded to therapy for acute myelogenous leukemia in the past but whose clinical condition and laboratory values show no improvement with current therapy. In such a case, the doctor may be reluctant to continue aggressive treatment. The physician and nurse must be open and honest with the patient and family, explaining that the situation is now terminal and that supportive care (i.e., palliative and hospice care) is more appropriate. Supportive care should be given regardless of the patient's decision. The nurse can advocate for the patient, put shared decision-making into practice, and follow the principle of respect for persons. The decision to forego active treatment can be quite difficult for both patient and family, and a supportive atmosphere is of critical importance.

34. When should the determination be made that a patient is dying?

Because the topic of death is difficult to discuss, even among health care providers, the patient and family may not be told that death is a possibility until it is imminent. Telling the patient or family close to the time of death does not allow preparation for death and does not respect autonomy. A study investigated the care currently provided to terminally ill patients in a university hospital setting.[13] All disciplines (physicians, nurses, social workers, and chaplains) in various clinical specialties recognized that identifying patients as dying, at an appropriate point in their illness, is a major problem. One-third of the respondents (n = 346) believed that appropriate identification frequently or always occurred, while two-thirds believed that it did not occur. Fifty-four percent of respondents thought that transitioning patients from curative to palliative care occurred too late. The determination of when a patient is dying and who makes the determination are critical questions for health care professionals to consider in their care of seriously ill and dying patients and their families. If, how, and when patients and families are told about impending death are areas that engender the development of ethical issues and dilemmas.

35. Does the nurse have ethical responsibilities when caring for patients at the end of life?

Yes. Nurses face barriers and ethical dilemmas in providing quality end-of-life care. The nurse has the responsibility to be alert to ethical dilemmas, to call attention to them as they arise, and to advocate for patients and families so that their goals for end-of-life care can be obtained and implemented insofar as possible.

APPENDIX
American Nurses Association Position Statement on Promotion of Comfort and Relief of Pain in Dying Patients

Summary: Nurses should not hesitate to use full and effective doses of pain medication for the proper management of pain in the dying patient. The increasing titration of medication to achieve adequate symptom control, even at the expense of life, thus hastening death secondarily, is ethically justified.

Nursing has been defined as the diagnosis and treatment of human responses to actual or potential health problems (American Nurses Association, 1980). When the patient is in the terminal stage of life when cure or prolongation of life in individuals with serious health problems is no longer possible, the focus of nursing is on the individual's response to dying. Diagnosis and treatment then focus on the promotion of comfort, which becomes the primary goal of nursing care.

One of the major concerns of dying patients and their families is the fear of intractable pain during the dying process. Indeed, overwhelming pain can cause sleeplessness, loss of morale, fatigue, irritability, restlessness, withdrawal, and other serious problems for the dying patient (Spross, 1985, Amenta, 1988, Eland, 1989, Melzack, 1990). Nurses play an extremely important role in the assessment of symptoms and the control of pain in dying patients because they often have the most frequent and continuous patient contact. In planning nursing care of dying patients, "the patient has a right to have pain recognized as a problem, and pain relief perceived by the health care team as a need" (Spross, McGuire, Schmitt, 1990).

The assessment and management of pain should be based on a thorough understanding of the individual patient's personality, culture and ethnicity, coping style and emotional, physical and spiritual needs, and on an understanding of the pathophysiology of the disease state (Dalton & Fenerstein, 1998). The main goal of nursing intervention for dying patients should be maximizing comfort through adequate management of pain and discomfort as this is consistent with the expressed desires of the patient. Toward that end, the patient should have whatever medication, in whatever dosage, and by whatever route is needed to control the level of pain as perceived by the patient (Wanzer et al., 1989).

Careful titration of pain medication is essential to promote comfort in dying patients. The proper dose is "the dose that is sufficient to reduce pain and suffering" (Wanzer et al., 1989). Tolerance to pain medications often develops in patients after repeated and prolonged use. Thus, both adults and children may require very high doses of medication to maintain adequate pain control. These doses may exceed the usual recommended dosages of the particular drug for patients of similar age and weight (Eland, 1989, Foley 1989, Inturrisi, 1989, Schmitt, 1990).

While it is well known that pain medications often have sedative or respiratory depressant side effects, this should not be an overriding consideration in their use for dying patients as long as such use is consistent with the patient's wishes. The increasing titration of medication to achieve adequate symptom control, even at the expense of maintaining life or hastening death secondarily, is ethically justified. The nurse assumes responsibility and accountability for individual nursing judgments and actions (American Nurses Association, 1985). Nurses should not hesitate to use full and effective doses of pain medication for the proper management of pain in the dying patient.

From American Nurses Association: Position Statement on Promotion of Comfort and Relief of Pain in Dying Patients. Kansas City, MO, American Nursing Association, 1991, with permission.

REFERENCES

1. Bandman B, Bandman EL: Nursing Ethics through the Life Span, 2nd ed. Norwalk, CT, Appleton & Lange, 1990.
2. Beauchamp TL, Childress JF: Principles of Biomedical Ethics, 4th ed. New York, Oxford University Press, 1994.

3. Benjamin M, Curtis J: Ethics in Nursing, 3rd ed. New York, Oxford University Press, 1992, pp 216–220.
4. Benoliel JQ: The moral context of oncology nursing. Oncol Nurs Forum 20 (Suppl):5–12, 1993.
5. Callahan D:The Goals of Medicine: Setting New Priorities. Hastings Center Report, Special Supplement, S1–16, 1996.
6. Carse A: The "voice of care": Implications for bioethical education. J Med Philos 16:5–28, 1991.
7. Davis AJ, Aroskar MA: Ethical Dilemmas and Nursing Practice, 3rd ed. Norwalk, CT, Appleton & Lange, 1991.
8. Ethical Dilemmas in End of Life Care. Glaxo, 1995 [video].
9. Ersek M, Scanlon C, Glass E, et al: Priority ethical issues in oncology nursing: Current approaches and future directions. Oncol Nurs Forum 22:803–807, 1995.
10. Ferrell B, Virani R, Grant M, et al: Beyond the Supreme Court decision: Nursing perspectives on end-of-life care. Oncol Nurs Forum 27:445–455, 2000.
11. Frankena WK: Ethics, 2nd ed. Englewood Clifts, NJ, Prentice-Hall, 1973.
12. Fry S: Ethical dimensions of nursing and health care. In Creasia JL, Parker B (eds): Conceptual Foundations of Professional Nursing Practice, 2nd ed. St. Louis: Mosby, 1996, pp 260–284.
13. Kutner J, Vu K, Fink R, et al: The role of baseline data collection in implementing institutional initiatives to improve end-of-life care. Unpublished data.
14. Hall JK: Nursing: Ethics and Law. Philadelphia, W.B. Saunders, 1996.
15. Parker RS: Nurses' stories: The search for a relational ethic of care. Adv Nurs Sci 13:31–40, 1990.
16. Veatch RM, Fry ST: Case Studies in Nursing Ethics. Philadelphia, J.B. Lippincott, 1987.
17. Watson J: Nursing: Human Science and Human Care: A Theory of Nursing. Norwalk, CT, Appleton-Century- Crofts, 1985.

68. HUMOR

Lynn Erdman, RN, MN, OCN

1. What are the benefits of laughter for nurses and patients?

Benefits may be physiologic or psychologic. **Physiologically** laughter increases heart rate, quickens breathing, increases oxygen intake, improves circulation, and works the muscles in the face and stomach. William Fry, M.D., of Stanford University, has studied the effects of laughter for more than 30 years. He says that laughing 100 times/day is the cardiovascular equivalent of 10 minutes on a rowing machine. Laugher also releases enkephalins and endorphins, which are pain killers, and thus it is a natural way to reduce pain ranging from headaches to bone pain. Laughter also aids digestion by massaging the intestines. The last physiologic effect is probably the best: the body enters a relaxed state in which vital signs drop and tension eases. Unlike chemical tranquilizers and antidepressants, laughter is natural. It is also free.

Psychologically laughter reduces tensions, provides an outlet for release of negative feelings, softens personal interactions, helps to put matters into perspective, and lifts the spirit. As one patient put it, "I found that when I caught myself laughing, I realized I was beginning to enjoy life again." Laughter often helps to defuse anger or ease tensions so that difficult issues can be discussed. Laughter is a bonding emotion. It has been said that laughter is the shortest distance between two people. Think how good it feels to be around someone who makes you laugh. Patients and their families feel the same way, and the use of humor can make the health care environment much more friendly. As one nurse put it, "Laughing is a mini-vacation, an escape from reality, even if it lasts only 30 seconds. When I return to reality, I am able to look at things from a different perspective."

2. What are the benefits of using humor in the health care setting?

Humor has the following benefits:

- Feels good physically
- Offers emotional release
- Provides defense mechanism
- Releases stress and anxiety
- Relieves boredom
- Breaks down barriers between staff and patient
- Builds group cohesion
- Heightens productivity
- Improves decision-making and negotiating abilities
- Increases energy levels

3. How do you know if the time is right to use humor?

If the patient initiates humor, you know it is safe. Otherwise, assess three factors before initiating humor: timing, content, and receptivity. Is the time appropriate? (i.e., Did the patient just receive bad news?) Is the context of the humor appropriate? Is the patient receptive to humor? The nurse can determine the answers by asking a few questions:

1. Do you laugh?
2. Before you became ill, did you laugh?
3. What makes you laugh?
4. Do you feel better after you laugh?
5. Would you like to select a humorous video to watch while receiving your treatment today?

If you decide that humor is an appropriate intervention, jump in and remember something that most nurses have learned over the years: if it comes from the heart, you cannot go wrong.

4. Is humor appropriate in dealing with dying patients?

Yes. Dying is not death—it does not mean that life has ceased, and it certainly does not mean that emotions have stopped. The use of humor that produces laughter can be beneficial by releasing the tension and diffusing the anger that surrounds death. It can break the sadness even if just momentarily. I remember two daughters who were sitting patiently by their mother's bed, waiting for her to die. The mother had uttered no words during the past 24 hours and slept most of the time. Finally, one daughter turned to the other and asked in a loud whisper, "How much longer is this going to take?" At that moment the mother opened her eyes, looked at her daughters, and said in a clear voice, "A watched pot never boils." Everyone in the room began to laugh, and the whole tone of the room changed. Often humor occurs spontaneously and when we least expect it—so go with it! Most people agree that a good belly laugh makes them feel better. Now evidence shows that the benefits of humor may be even more powerful and longer-lasting.

5. Is there an inappropriate type of humor?

Yes. "Put-down" humor or humor with sexual overtones is inappropriate. Humor that can hurt someone's feelings should never be used. Much health care humor is appropriate only for other health care workers and should be kept behind closed doors so that patients and visitors do not hear.

6. How can you add humor to your work setting?

Try some of the following tips in the outpatient chemotherapy setting, radiation treatment room, inpatient unit, home care bag, or break room for staff:

1. Make a bulletin board or file of funny cartoons.
2. Create a basket of humorous items that the patient can borrow: bubbles, Play Doh, coloring books and crayons, finger paint, funny hats or wigs, water guns, humorous gadgets (e.g., big glasses, large noses, reflex hammer that squeaks when you tap it, mirror that laughs), and humorous books, audiotapes, and videotapes.
3. Make a laughter first-aid kit for your personal use or for patient use. (Develop your own—whatever makes you or the patient laugh.)
4. Show home movies.
5. Make funny pictures and display them.
6. Have dress-up day or theme day when staff and/or patients dress in funny outfits.
7. Create funny songs.

7. How can you add humor to your own life?

• Look for humor—try to see the amusing side of situations, and learn to laugh at yourself first!
• Keep a humor first-aid kit. Stock it with items that you think are funny, and pull it out when you need to laugh.
• Brighten your surroundings—use posters, cartoons, bumper stickers, pictures, or anything to make the workplace appear brighter and thus happier.
• Make time for fun—schedule some humor time each day (10 minutes).
• Be playful—spend time with a child or bring some of that childlike behavior into your life.
• Encourage laughter—laughter is contagious.

8. Give a few examples of humorous stories from oncology nursing.

• One day a young woman in her early thirties named Diane was admitted to our medical oncology unit with acute leukemia. She was a newlywed, and her husband, Joe, stayed by her side as she underwent induction chemotherapy. After several complications, the days turned into weeks, and she entered her seventh week with us. During her stay, when she and her husband wanted private time to share intimate moments together, they would place a "Do Not Disturb" sign on her door. This was continually ignored by the health care workers, who would simply knock and enter anyway. One night Diane and Joe decided to make sure they had privacy. Joe placed a sign on the door that read "SEX IN PROGRESS." That sign was not ignored; no one bothered them at all. The staff laughed until their sides hurt. Diane and Joe laughed too.

- Elsie was going to her plastic surgeon for a follow-up visit after having undergone a bilateral mastectomy and reconstruction 8 weeks earlier. When she arrived she was wearing a T-shirt that read, "Boobs by Dr. Smith, phone #333-8201." This message was painted on both sides of her shirt. When Dr. Smith saw Elsie, his first statement was, "I hope you haven't been sitting in the waiting room very long." Elsie responded, "Oh no, but I went to the mall to shop for an hour or two before I came here!" Dr. Smith's face turned bright red, and then he and Elsie burst into laughter.
- I was riding through a cemetery one day and saw a sign that read, "Pick flowers only from your own grave!" It made me laugh. I wondered whether anyone obeyed.
- Sophie was a patient in our inpatient hospice unit. She told her nurse Sally she was dying. She asked Sally to call her minister and the rest of her family to come quickly. Everyone arrived, and Sophie wanted to have a prayer service. She asked that candles be lighted in her room. On her table beside the candles, she had two pictures: one of her family and one of Jesus and his disciples. The candles were lit, and everyone bowed their heads as the minister began to pray. After a few seconds there was a burning smell that caused the group's eyes to open. To everyone's surprise, the picture of Jesus and his disciples had gone up in flames. Sophie's eyes got big, and she said, "Oh no, what am I going to do? The first thing Jesus is going to ask me is why I burned his picture?" Then Sophie began to laugh. The tension in the room eased as everyone joined in the laughter. Sophie died peacefully a few minutes later.

Remember, humor helps to balance our lives. It can occur in the most unexpected places and at the most unexpected times. Welcome it!

9. What humor resources are available to nurses and patients?
American Association for Therapeutic Humor
Networking source for practical applications of humor in all therapeutic modalities. Excellent newsletter and annual conference. Send $50 per year to: A.A.T.H., 222 S. Meramec, Ste. 303, St. Louis, MO 63105. Phone: 314-863-6232; fax: 863-6457; Web site: http://www.callamer.com/itc/aath

Hair by Chemo
T-shirts and hats with this logo and "Not by Choice" on backside. Box 216, Wauzeka, WI 53826 or call to order 800-729-9713

Humor and Health Journal
Bimonthly newsletter featuring interviews with humor experts, review of latest research and books published on humor and laughter. Send $22/yr to: Humor and Health Journal, PO Box 16814, Jackson, MS 39236. 601-957-0075.

Humor Project
Publishes *Laughing Matters*, an excellent quarterly journal, large catalog of humor books, annual humor conference. 110 Spring St., Saratoga Springs, NY 12866. 515-587-8770.

Journal of Nursing Jocularity
A hilarious quarterly publication about the funny side of nursing. For annual subscription, send $14.95 to J.N.J., 5615 W. Cermak Rd., Cicero, IL 60650-2290. For catalog and conference information, telephone 602-835-6165. Fax: 602-835-6922. E-mail: laffinm@neta.com Web site: http//www.jocularity. com

Too Live Nurse
Tape of funny songs about nursing, cardiac arrhythmias, and drugs. Send $17 each to PO Box 201, Cannan, NY 12029. Telephone 518-781-4943.

Whole Mirth Catalog
Access to many humorous items, toys, gags, books. 1034 Page Street, San Francisco, CA 94117.

A Little Book of Nurses' Rules
This book presents over 400 tips, helpful observations, and useful do's and don't's for nurses, offering insight into interactions with physicians, patients, and other nurses. It is a

128-page paperback book. Send $9.95 to Hanley & Belfus, 210 S. 13th Street, Philadelphia, PA 19107. Phone: 215-546-7293; fax 215-790-9330; Web site: http://www.hanleyandbelfus.com

The Best of Nursing Humor: A Collection of Articles, Essays, and Poetry Published in the Nursing Literature

This hardcover $8\frac{1}{2} \times 11$ book presents the best pieces of creative, humorous writing to appear in the nursing and related literature over the last 20 years. Addresses the funny side of interrelationships and communication between nurses and their colleagues, physicians, patients, and patients' families. Send $27.00 to Hanley & Belfus, 210 S. 13th Street, Philadelphia, PA 19107. Phone: 215-546-7293; fax 215-790-9330; Web site: http://www.hanleyandbelfus.com

Web sites

1. Humor for your health™
   Offers inspiring writings such as the "Gift of Laughter" and "Humor Tips at Work and School." Both by Dan Gascon, 1999.
2. "Put Laughter and Humor in Your Life", NF 98-389 by Herbert Lingren
   Describes benefits of laughter and helping the humor-impaired.

10. What are some funny books that may appeal to patients and health care professionals?

Barry D: Stay Fit and Healthy Until You're Dead. Emmaus, PA, Rodale Press, 1985.

Bonhom TD: The Treasury of Clean Jokes. Nashville, TN, Broadman, 1988.

Brillian A: I Want to Reach Your Mind—Where Is It Currently Located? Santa Barbara, CA, Woodbridge Press, 1994.

Klein A: Quotations to Cheer You Up When the World Is Getting You Down. New York, Sterling, 1991.

Metcalf CW: Lighten Up: Survival Signs for People Under Pressure. Reading, MA, Addison Wesley, 1992.

Mickie S, Hillman R: Death Is—A Lighter Look at a Grave Situation. Saratoga, CA, R & E Publishers, 1993.

Saltzman D: The Jester Has Lost His Jingle. Jester Company, 1995.

Wooten P: Heart, Healing and Humor. Salt Lake City, Commune A Key Publishing, 1994.

REFERENCES

1. Buxman K (ed): Nursing Perspective on Humor. Staten Island, NY, Power Publishers, 1995.
2. Cousins N: Anatomy of an Illness. New York, W.W. Norton, 1979.
3. Erdman L: Laughter therapy for patients with cancer. J Psychosoc Oncol 11(4):55–67, 1993.
4. Klein A: Healing Power of Humor. Los Angeles, Tarcher, 1989.

69. SELF-CARE STRATEGIES FOR NURSES: PREVENTION OF COMPASSION FATIGUE AND BURNOUT

Pamela J. Haylock, RN, MA

1. What is the result of negative job-related stress in the health care professions?

Inherent in the caregiving professions are stressors that are occupational hazards. High, unremitting, and unrelieved job-related stress in caregiving professions is linked to "burnout," also referred to as "compassion fatigue." Continual and consistent provision of compassionate care—the most basic tenet of the nursing profession—requires energy. Loss and grief, relationships with colleagues and physicians, constant exposure to pain and suffering, the need to make critical judgments about interventions and treatments, and balancing work and family commitments generate stress in nurses. But only a few nurses successfully use self-care skills to avoid reaching the end-stages of job-related stress that are recognized as burnout. Staff must assume the responsibility for self-care by finding ways not only to nurture the self but also ways to contribute to the caring support of colleagues in the work environment.

2. Why is job-related stress important for managers to consider?

More than a few healthcare organizations consider the concept of staff support as extraneous fluff. They are wrong. Supporting staff who work in any stressful environment is an essential component of wise business practices. Job-related stress has huge human costs, including turnover, absenteeism, and worker's compensation claims. Nurses finding satisfaction in their work convey a more pleasant and productive patient care setting and ultimately increase patient satisfaction. In the current market-driven healthcare environment, patient satisfaction is a critically important and cost-effective business goal.

3. Why is job-related stress in oncology nursing particularly complex?

Stress in the oncology care setting is complex. Nurses experience burnout because they are often idealistic, dedicated, and committed to their work but have minimal workplace support. Oncology nursing is recognized as a particularly stressful nursing specialty. The top three "stress clusters" in oncology nursing include those related to physicians, organizational factors, and frequent observation of suffering. The intense and turbulent healthcare environment is accompanied by workplace uncertainties due to downsizing, mergers, conflicts with management and/or co-workers, heavy workloads with limited autonomy, and minimal staff support. All of these factors can negatively affect and deplete nurses' coping reserves.

4. What are the warning signs of compassion fatigue and burnout?

Responses to job-related stress can be both physical and psychological as well as short-term or long-term. They are recognized as burnout warning signs.

Physical signs

• Physical fatigue	• Dry mouth	• Upper back pain
• Clammy hands	• Eating disorders	• Heart palpitations
• Diarrhea	• Halitosis	• Stiff neck or shoulders

Emotional signs

• Anxiety	• Frustration	• Poor self-image
• Depression	• Grief	• Sense of powerlessness
• Fear	• Isolation	• Sense of worthlessness

Characteristic behaviors

- Blaming others
- Crying, irritability
- Shortened attention span
- Overactivity
- Negative attitude
- Short temper
- Taking risks

5. How can compassion fatigue and burnout be prevented?

Once they reach the limits of their coping reserves, individual nurses, their coworkers, and the work environment suffer. Instead of dealing with nurses who are experiencing burnout, it is much more important and ultimately easier and more cost-effective to prevent this distressing problem in the first place. The following are common-sense self-care strategies for coping successfully with the stress inherent in oncology nursing:

1. **Practice responsible selfishness.** Engage in activities, pastimes, and pursuits that have no purpose other than to recharge and renew personal energies.

2. **Separate work from home.** Home/work conflicts can be a primary source of stress in oncology nurses. Apply creative transitional strategies that help you leave work at work. Some nurses find that physical exercise, mental imagery, and/or the distraction of favorite music, alone or collectively, helps to create a barrier between professional and personal stressors.

3. **Develop a positive support group.** Just as oncology nurses recommend peer self-help groups to patients and families, similar kinds of support offer nurses a way to mediate the negative effects of stress. Nurses can establish formal and/or informal groups in which participants listen, empathize, and solve problems with peers who share an understanding of common stressors.

4. **Be active in the larger professional arena.** Becoming an active member of a professional nursing organization helps nurses to see the bigger picture of the healthcare environment and to network with colleagues who face similar issues.

5. **Refuse to be a victim.** Despite perceived loss of control and autonomy in the current healthcare environment, we can make choices that focus on positive behavioral, cognitive, and affective responses to stress.

6. **Remember to laugh.** Humor and laughter are known palliative agents against negative effects of stress. Laughter can be intentionally provoked by writers, actors, and comedians, and it can erupt spontaneously as we see humor in events and situations around us.

7. **Redefine success.** Most nurses chose their profession out of a desire to help people. Whether or not nurses achieve this simple goal depends on how they ultimately define the word "help." Because nurses are highly committed and dedicated to their patients and work, a sense of personal failure and frustration can result when goals are not achieved. The work of oncology nurses offers limitless opportunities for personal success. Defining success in terms of the realities of oncology nursing takes us back to that simple goal of helping others and to greater satisfaction and joy in work.

6. What is the role of nurse managers and leaders in preventing and/or dealing with compassion fatigue and burnout?

Nurse managers and leaders must care for the psychological needs of their staff. Sources of job-related stress that contribute to compassion fatigue include:

- Role ambiguity
- Role conflict
- Role incongruity
- Role overload
- Role underload
- Role over- or underqualification

Astute managers, along with staff members, can investigate the extent to which any or all of these stressors contribute to job-related stress and implement strategies to mitigate negative elements in the work setting. Development of a comprehensive organizational stress management plan is invaluable in preventing compassion fatigue and burnout and thereby contributes to an organizational milieu conducive to job and patient satisfaction. Underrecognized and underutilized organizational and/or community-based resources may be tapped to resolve problems and assist in crafting long-range stress management strategies. Suggested interventions include addressing overall stress and coping via educational programming and implementation of strategies and structures that facilitate improvement in staff attitudes, self-esteem, and self-mastery—key elements to staff empowerment.

7. How can a nurse contribute to efforts to prevent compassion fatigue and burnout?

Changing an unhealthy work environment is too important to be left totally to managers and administrators. Every nurse can help to create and foster a supportive, healthy work environment. Individual staff members can be catalysts to positive change. A first step is to learn and use appropriate self-care skills, followed by a second step of sharing successful skills with colleagues. Learning, establishing, and maintaining good communication among all members of the healthcare team is a goal to which every nurse can aspire. Facilitation of staff support and provision of educational programming consistent with staff-empowerment efforts are roles that nurses are often particularly suited to fulfill. If a nurse faces irreconcilable differences in the work setting, walking away from the situation to gain perspective is often the best approach. In the interest of self-preservation, the nurse can consider the possibility of a job change. Moving to a more professionally fulfilling and satisfying role and work setting may make a huge difference. The oncology nursing specialty is rich with opportunities for nurses to change direction—to a different work setting (acute, ambulatory, office, home care), different foci of care (prevention, early detection, community education, hospice, rehabilitation), different patient populations (pediatric, young adult, adult, geriatric). All of these choices provide new opportunities to learn and grow while taking advantage of a nurse's wisdom, skills, and experience.

8. In what ways can involvement in a professional organization help an individual or group of nurses address the issues of compassion fatigue and burnout?

Active involvement in the larger professional arena nullifies the notion of isolation by providing nurses with a broader perspective and expanded network of like-minded colleagues. Through organizational involvement, nurses network with colleagues, some of whom may be dealing with similar challenges, while others have succeeded in creating positive change. A collective voice is more effective than a single voice and can be key to addressing issues and concerns that extend beyond one institution. Aside from the American Nurses Association, which addresses shared interests of all of America's 2.5 million nurses, several oncology specialty nursing organizations and others with subspecialty oncology-related interests have evolved over the past 25 years:

- Association of Pediatric Oncology Nurses (APON)
- Oncology Nursing Society (ONS)
- Society of Gynecologic Nurse Oncologists (SGNO)
- Association of Women's Health, Obstetric, and Neonatal Nurses (AWHONN)
- Wound, Ostomy, and Continence Nurses Society (WOCN)
- Society of Otorhinolaryngology and Head-Neck Nurses (SOHN)
- American Academy of Ambulatory Care Nursing (AAACN)
- American Holistic Nurses Association
- American Society of Pain Management Nurses

Depending on personal interests, skills, and practice area, a nurse should be able to find an organization that complements his or her professional and personal pursuits.

REFERENCES

1. Huber D: Managing time and stress. In Huber D (ed): Leadership and Nursing Care Management, 2nd ed. Philadelphia, W.B. Saunders, 2000, pp 123–140.
2. Lewis AE: Reducing burnout: Development of an oncology staff bereavement program. Oncol Nurs Forum 26:1065–1069, 1999.
3. Luban RJ: Is your fire going out? Maybe it's time you read the writing on the wall. Choicepoints.com, 1997–1999.
4. Santos SR, Cox K: Workplace adjustment and intergenerational differences between matures, boomers, and Xers. Nurs Econ 18:7–13, 2000.
5. Walsh DJ: Care for the caregiver: Strategies for avoiding "compassion fatigue." Clin J Oncol Nurs 3(4): 183–184, 1999.

70. ENDNOTES: COPING AND STORYTELLING

Rose A. Gates, RN, MSN, CNS/NP, and Regina M. Fink, RN, PhD, AOCN

> Every person is a volume: you just have to know how to read him.
> *Saying from a Chinese Fortune Cookie*

1. How do patients respond to the diagnosis of cancer?

Each person responds to the diagnosis of cancer in his or her unique way. The diagnosis may lead to a crisis or turning point in which past methods of coping do not work, or the diagnosis can be seen as an opportunity for discovery and growth.

Work-up. The work-up period is often described as the most difficult time because it is filled with uncertainty and a new world of medical jargon and procedures. It may take several weeks of anxious waiting before patients know their diagnosis. Some patients try to pretend that nothing is wrong and keep everything to themselves. Others get irritated easily and lash out at friends or family without realizing why. Patients may increase alcohol use or start taking antianxiety medications or sleeping pills. Often they tell you that "the not knowing is the worst."

Diagnosis. After they are given the diagnosis, patients may be emotionally overwhelmed and respond with fear, shock, disbelief, denial, anger, sorrow, bargaining, or "why me?" For some, the diagnosis is a confirmation of their worries, and they are relieved finally to have a diagnosis for their symptoms. Others nod their heads, ask pertinent questions, and then five minutes later seem to have forgotten the entire conversation. It may take several days for the reality of the diagnosis to become clear. Some respond with anger or believe that the "doctor made a mistake" or begin "doctor-shopping." Many express a feeling of vulnerability or helplessness, "feeling out of control," "being alone," and feeling that "no one understands." A few may feel hopeless and even contemplate "ending it all." Others may feel challenged and are motivated "to fight this battle" and want as much information as they can get.

Recurrence. Many patients respond as when they were initially diagnosed; however, news of an unexpected recurrence may result in more feelings of disappointment, despair, or sense of failure that they or others "did not fight hard enough." Other patients are glad for the extra time that they had and more accepting of their prognosis. Depending on the diagnosis and stage of disease, patients may be required to adjust from curative to palliative goals. Distress may be more evident as patients come to the realization that their time is limited or that death is close. They may start worrying about their last days and wonder if they will be a burden. Patients may become more spiritual or religious and seek resolution of conflicts and meaning in their living and/or dying.

As cancer progresses, goals change and patients hope for different things. Patients with cancer can remain hopeful despite limitations in activity or approaching death. Hope is an inner force that motivates and enriches a person's life. Initially the patient may hope for a cure, but if the cancer becomes terminal, he or she may hope for short-term goals such as relief of pain or seeing another sunrise.

2. How do patients cope with cancer?

Patients with cancer must cope with all kinds of stressors related to disease and treatment, health care providers, losses, body-image changes, and uncertainties. Coping refers to intentional problem-solving efforts to overcome or manage a stressor or threatening situation. Cancer patients usually use a combination of various coping strategies, as listed below:

Denial may be protective or detrimental. The nurse's role is to evaluate how long the denial lasts, how often it is used, and its intensity. From the beginning, it is important to establish what and how much information a patient wants and can handle at any one time. Denial can give the patient time to absorb and adapt to distressful or overwhelming information. Patients should not be forced out of denial if it helps them to cope. However, denial is detrimental if it prevents a patient from understanding consequences or if it potentially hurts others.

Search for meaning often begins with the question, "why me?," when patients attempt to make sense of their illness. Anxiety may be reduced by having an explanation or reason.

Spirituality identifies what is purposeful and valuable in life. Prayer and religion help many patients to find peace and meaning in their illnesses.

Downward comparison helps patients to feel better by comparing their condition to someone who is worse off or less fortunate. Patients may express relief that their condition is not as bad as another patient's.

Sense of mastery gives the patient a sense of control over the cancer or side effects related to therapy. Techniques that provide mastery include imagery, self-hypnosis, distraction, meditation, exercise, and dietary changes.

Reappraisal of life clarifies what is most important in a patient's life since the diagnosis of cancer. Patients often conclude that family and/or friends and health are more important than money and work.

Cognitive restructuring redefines or reframes the situation by finding positive aspects of the diagnosis, such as improvement in a patient's marriage since the diagnosis.

Emotional expression uses humor or talking with others to help with coping.

Wish-fulfilling fantasy wishes that the cancer would go away or that it was not as advanced.

Self-blame is feeling responsible or guilty for cancer. Patients may express regret for failing to get regular exams.

Information-seeking involves self-help and active engagement in learning about the disease and treatments.

Threat minimization is an attempt to focus on aspects of life other than cancer or to put cancer out of mind with distracting activities or simply talking about the cancer.

Benefit-reminding is when patients consciously remind themselves of a benefit that has come from their illness or situation.

3. What is storytelling? How does it relate to coping?

Stories are narratives that provide meaning in our lives. Since the beginning of time, storytelling has been used as a means of healing. Stories can have many different levels of meaning. They may deal with practical issues on the surface while exploring deeper life-meaning issues such as courage, love, grief, and hope underneath. Stories can order chaotic events in the lives of patients and caregivers. Because coping often depends on the meaning of cancer to the patient, storytelling or a narrative approach can be a valuable nursing intervention to help patients construct meaning and make sense of their experiences.

4. What is the value of storytelling for oncology nurses?

Storytelling helps us to learn about ourselves and others. By telling a story we give voice to our experiences and find meaning in who we are, who we have been, and where we are coming from. Stories can teach, heal, validate, offer reflection, and shape how we care for patients and others. Listening to the stories of patients and families helps nurses to understand the perceived meaning of the illness experience. Telling stories to others is a way to teach new things, to provide catharsis, to communicate more effectively while building trust, and to promote personal growth. They allow us to view experiences from different perspectives and provide a different lens through which a single event can be viewed.

5. How can nurses facilitate storytelling by their patients?

Most patients cherish the opportunity to tell their story from the beginning. Unfortunately, they are often not even asked to tell their story. Storytelling can be useful during difficult and changing times to present new perspectives and normalize concerns. Storytelling can be facilitated by the following guidelines:

• Be centered. Being centered is a key to storytelling. It means to be in the moment with another.

- Be present. Co-creation requires the physical and emotional presence of the nurse and the belief that the patient and nurse are mutually involved; both nurse and patient are changed.
- Be an active listener. An active listener nourishes, encourages, and enters into a caring relationship with the teller and helps find meaning in the story.
- Listen with empathy, and do not try to give moral advice or compare with other patients who are worse off.
- Be willing to share yourself. How can we get patients to tell their stories if we do not share part of our own? By telling our own stories we nurture a connection. Knowing what and how much to share is part of the art of nursing.
- Maximize privacy.
- Physically place yourself at the patient's level. If the patient is lying in bed, do not stand above the patient; sit down, lean forward to show interest, and face the patient.
  Encourage patients to keep a journal or notebook, and keep one yourself. Writing about experiences provides a technique to shed fears and concerns while renewing or replenishing inner resources. Photographs, mementos, videos, artwork, and music are other ways to start or shape stories.
- Be patient and wait for the time when patients are ready to tell their stories.

6. What do patients perceive as the most important nursing care behaviors?

Caring may not mean the same to patients as it does to nurses. For example, the nurse's willingness to listen may be ranked by patients as the most caring behavior or well below other behaviors. Although nurses place high value on psychosocial skills, Larson's study reported that cancer patients ranked competency of skills above the need to be listened to by the nurse. Listening and talking skills became more important only after the patient's "getting-better" needs were met. Other studies of nurse caring behaviors indicate that patients value "being accessible," "monitoring and following through," physical care, and professional knowledge. Nurses should not assume that what they define as caring or important has the same value to the patient.

QUOTES FROM ONCOLOGY NURSES

7. How do you respond to the question, "Isn't it depressing to work with cancer patients?"

- I take great pleasure in helping each patient live their life to the fullest, regardless of longevity.
- At times it is very sad, but I am clear that my job is to make the process the best it can be. I believe that we ultimately have little control over how things proceed. My job is one of support.
- I think of depression as a process, an evolving development. Working with cancer patients can be sad, yes. There are moments when you wish you weren't working that day, or moments when you wish you could change things somehow. But then there are those occasions when you have made a difference in someone's moment and that feels good. There are times when patients have done something that touched your moment.
- Working with persons who have cancer makes you realize that life is short, so don't sweat the small stuff.
- No, it's enlightening. It's a learning experience for me. Cancer patients have much to teach about life and living. I usually tell people, "I learn more about life and living working with these patients."
- After working with cancer patients for the past 20 years, I have felt sad at times but not depressed. I think this is because I have always been open to the energy of love and caring exchanged in each patient interaction. Yes, there have been a few difficult patients or families whom I felt were "psychic vampires," but I think I learned the most from those kinds of patients. Each patient encounter has been a lesson, challenge, or gift. From angry patients, I learned how difficult it was to let go of life. Lonely patients have taught me the value of letting the significant people in our lives know how much we care about them. Dying patients have taught me that the most important things in our lives are our families and our true friends:

"Nobody ever regretted spending too much time with their families; they did regret how much time was expended by working too many hours." I believe that if you truly love what you do or accept that you can't be everything to everybody, you may get tired but not depressed. If you dread going back to work, I think then it's time for a change or to take a break.

8. What advice may an experienced oncology nurse give to a new nurse?

- Trust your gut reactions. There's a reason you feel those vibes—act on them.
- Find balance. This type of work can be all-consuming. Understand that your gift is to guide, support, and encourage. Balance your life with the not-so-serious things. Take care of yourself so that you have good energy to share. A nurse can help a patient cope better if he or she is able to cope well. Balance the need to "be there" with your own needs.
- Remind yourself and your patients to take one day at a time.
- Stay centered in your own life so that when you are at home you are truly with yourself, your family, and significant others. At work you are centered on your patients at that particular moment.
- Listen and don't be afraid to feel; empathy is healing. Be aware of your feelings and talk about them
- Always leave room for hope and time for hugs.
- Be as competent in communication, as in you are in technical skills.
- Don't ignore your grief. Show your tears.
- Don't be afraid to confront the threat of death. "To maximize our professional passion for our work, we must embrace the pathos in our practice. With self-reflection and acceptance of our environment of sadness, we can create a culture of compassion that formally is heralded as oncology nursing's greatest asset."[3]

9. What are some secrets or quotes from patients?

The following excerpts are taken from actual patient stories:

- I wanted to give up, but you didn't give up on me. I never would have made it through my chemotherapy without you.
- Nurses and doctors tell you to call them when you have pain or another problem. But when you do, they come to check you and then go away. Sometimes they don't come back to tell you if it is or isn't time to have medication. If it isn't, they don't try to get another order to help. Be there. We need you.
- I want my caregivers to talk amongst themselves so they all know what is going on and coordinate my care. This would help me feel more secure about them. Knowing that they know me makes me feel better.
- Take time to know about individuals, their background, essence, and beliefs. This will help you know the person better. Everyone is unique and will act differently in different situations. This is perhaps the most important thing I want to tell you.
- Be sympathetic and helpful. I know you're busy. Be with us in the here and now. Don't rush.
- Caring goes a long way.
- A smile and a good attitude make a difference.
- When you're busy, don't lose sight of the person.
- Discover our uniqueness. Don't assume; don't stereotype. Put yourself in our shoes. That way you'll have a better understanding of what we need.
- Touching is a caring and reassuring gesture—continue to touch. Touching indicates a warmth and caring connection. It is a vital component of caring—maybe the most important aspect in my view.
- Talk with patients about their feelings.
- I want my caregiver to be someone with compassion.
- Physicians and nurses need to credit patients with the ability to take care of themselves and to think for themselves. We can be very self-reliant. Don't give me too much medication so

that I'm confused. I want to take responsibility for my care. To understand pain, you need to understand people, to listen to them. People heal from the inside out. Physicians try to heal from the outside in. There are times when I think no one is listening. My health care providers are opinionated and set in many ways. Healing can happen only when trust occurs.

• Who is going to listen to our stories? Doesn't anyone realize that there is more to healing than drugs?

10. What are some good books about patient's stories?

There are many good patient narratives, stories, or illness anthologies and books about patient experiences. Below are a few favorites:

Frank AW: At the Will of the Body: Reflections on Illness. Boston, Houghton Mifflin, 1991.

French M: A Season In Hell. New York, Ballantine Books, 1998.

Gullo S, Glass E (eds): Silver Linings: The Other Side of Cancer. Pittsburgh, PA, Oncology Nursing Society, 1997.

Jaffe C, Ehrlich CH: All Kinds of Love: Experiencing Hospice. Amityville, New York, Baywood Publishing, 1997.

Remen RN: Kitchen Table Wisdom: Stories That Heal. New York, Riverhead Books, 1994.

Rose G: Love's Work: A Reckoning with Life. New York, Schocken Books, 1995.

ACKNOWLEDGMENTS

The authors extend their thanks to the oncology nurses who shared their stories with us—Patricia Nishimoto, Becca Hawkins, Linda Krebs, Debi McCaffrey Boyle, Gari Jensen—and to our patients, who always have stories to share and just need to be asked.

REFERENCES

1. Affleck G, Tennen H: Construing benefits from adversity: Adaptational significance and dispositional underpinnings. J Personality 64:899–922, 1996.
2. Bolton G: Stories at work: Reflective writing for practitioners. Lancet 354:241–243, 1999.
3. Boyle DA: Pathos in practice: Exploring the affective domain of oncology nursing. Oncol Nurs Forum 27:915–919, 2000.
4. Byock I: Dying Well: The Prospect for Growth at the End of Life. New York, Riverhead Books, 1997.
5. Haber J, Krainovich-Miller B, McMahon AL, Price-Hoskins P: Comprehensive Psychiatric Nursing, 5th ed. St. Louis, Mosby, 1997.
6. Hagopian GA: Cognitive strategies used in adapting to a cancer diagnosis. Oncol Nurs Forum 20:759–763, 1993.
7. Heiney SP: The healing power of story. Oncol Nurs Forum 22:899–904, 1995.
8. Herth K: Fostering hope in terminally ill people. J Adv Nurs 15:1250-1259, 1990.
9. Larson PJ: Important nurse caring behaviors perceived by patients with cancer. Oncol Nurs Forum 11(6):46–50, 1984.
10. Nelson GL: Writing and Being. San Diego, Lura Media, 1994.
11. O'Berle K, Davies B: Support and caring: Exploring the concepts. Oncol Nurs Forum 19:763–767, 1992.
12. Post-White J, Ceronsky C, Kreitzer MJ, et al: Hope, spirituality, sense of coherence, and quality of life in patients with cancer. Oncol Nurs Forum 23:1571–1579, 1996.
13. Steeves RH: Loss, grief and the search for meaning. Oncol Nurs Forum 23:897–903, 1996.
14. ten Kroode HFJ: Active listening to cancer patients' stories. Netherlands J Med 53:47–52, 1998.
15. Watson J: Nursing: Human Science and Human Care. New York, National League for Nursing, 1988.
16. Williams J, Wood C, Cunningham-Warburton B: A narrative study of chemotherapy-induced alopecia. Oncol Nurs Forum 26 :1463-1468.
17. Witherell C, Noddings N (eds): Stories Lives Tell. New York, Teachers College Press, 1991.

INDEX

Page numbers in **boldface type** indicate complete chapters.